Wendy Iglesia

Aug '7?

1374 S. Pleasant Valley

Westminster Md. 21157

# Controversy in Surgery

EDITED BY

### RICHARD L. VARCO, M.D.
*Professor of Surgery,*
*University of Minnesota Medical School,*
*Minneapolis, Minnesota*

and

### JOHN P. DELANEY, M.D.
*Associate Professor of Surgery,*
*University of Minnesota Medical School,*
*Minneapolis, Minnesota*

W. B. SAUNDERS COMPANY • Philadelphia • London • Toronto

W. B. Saunders Company: West Washington Square
Philadelphia, PA 19105

1 St. Anne's Road
Eastbourne, East Sussex BN21 3UN, England

1 Goldthorne Avenue
Toronto, Ontario M8Z 5T9, Canada

**Library of Congress Cataloging in Publication Data**

Main entry under title:

Controversy in surgery.

1. Surgery.    I. Varco, Richard Lynn.    II. Delaney,
John Patrick. [DNLM: 1. Surgery. WO100 C764]

RD31.5.C63        617        75–12495

ISBN 0–7216–9016–5

Controversy in Surgery                                     ISBN   0-7216-9016-5

Last digit is the print number:    9    8    7    6    5    4    3

*To our wives,*
*with deep appreciation*
*for their essential role*
*in each of our lives,*
*and with full recognition*
*of how very fortunate*
*the editors are*

# CONTRIBUTORS

**W. GERALD AUSTEN, M.D.**

Edward D. Churchill Professor of Surgery, Harvard Medical School; Chief of the Surgical Services, Massachusetts General Hospital, Boston, Massachusetts.

**OLIVER H. BEAHRS, M.D.**

Professor of Surgery, Mayo Medical School; Consultant, Department of Surgery, Mayo Clinic and Mayo Foundation, Rochester, Minnesota.

**PHILIP E. BERNATZ, M.D.**

Professor of Surgery, Mayo Medical School; Consultant, Department of Surgery, Mayo Clinic and Mayo Foundation, Rochester, Minnesota.

**EUGENE F. BERNSTEIN, M.D., Ph.D.**

Professor of Surgery, University of California, San Diego, School of Medicine; Head, Vascular Surgery, University of California Medical Center, San Diego, and Veterans Administration Hospital, La Jolla, California.

**JOHN PETER BLANDY, M.A., D.M., M.Ch., F.R.C.S.**

Professor of Urology, University of London and The London Hospital Medical College; Consultant Urological Surgeon, St. Peter's Hospital, London, England.

**WILLIAM HENRY BOND, F.R.C.S., F.R.C.R., D.M.R.T.**

Senior Clinical Lecturer, University of Birmingham Medical School; Departmental Director and Consultant Radiotherapist, United Birmingham Hospitals, Birmingham, England.

**WALLY S. BUCH, M.D.**

Cardiovascular Surgeon, Stanford University Hospital, Palo Alto, California.

**HENRY BUCHWALD, M.D., Ph.D.**

Associate Professor of Surgery, University of Minnesota Medical School, Minneapolis, Minnesota.

**GEORGE E. BURCH, M.D.**

Emeritus Professor of Medicine, Tulane University School of Medicine; Consultant in Medicine, Charity Hospital of Louisiana, New Orleans, Louisiana.

**HAROLD BURGE**

Late Consultant Surgeon, Charing Cross Hospital, London, England.

**ROY E. CARLSON, M.D.**

Clinical Instructor in Surgery, University of California, San Francisco, School of Medicine, San Francisco, California.

CARL E. CASSIDY, M.D.

Clinical Professor of Medicine, Tufts University School of Medicine, Boston; Physician-in-Chief, Springfield Hospital Unit, Baystate Medical Center, Springfield, Massachusetts.

H. TAYLOR CASWELL, M.D.

Professor of Surgery, Temple University School of Medicine; Department of Surgery, Temple University Hospital, Philadelphia, Pennsylvania.

THOMAS CLARK CHALMERS, M.D.

Dean and Professor of Medicine, Mount Sinai School of Medicine of the City University of New York; Lecturer in Medicine, Harvard Medical School, Boston, Massachusetts; Attending Physician, The Mount Sinai Hospital, New York, New York.

EARLE M. CHAPMAN, M.D.

Associate Clinical Professor of Medicine, Emeritus, Harvard Medical School; Consulting Physician, Massachusetts General Hospital, Boston, Massachusetts.

ROBIN CHAPMAN, M.D.

Department of Urology, The London Hospital, London, England.

ORLO H. CLARK, M.D.

Assistant Professor, University of California, San Francisco, School of Medicine; Attending Surgeon, Veterans Administration Hospital and University of California Hospital; Consultant Staff, Letterman General Hospital, San Francisco, California.

SIDNEY COHEN, M.D.

Associate Professor of Medicine, The University of Pennsylvania School of Medicine; Chief, Gastrointestinal Section, Hospital of the University of Pennsylvania, Philadelphia, Pennsylvania.

RICHARD E. C. COLLINS, M.B., B.S., F.R.C.S.

Research Fellow, Beth Israel Hospital and Harvard Medical School, Boston, Massachusetts; Consultant Surgeon, Canterbury and Thanet Hospitals, Canterbury, Kent, England.

ROBERT E. CONDON, M.D.

Professor of Surgery, The Medical College of Wisconsin; Chief, Surgical Service, Wood Veterans Administration Hospital; Consultant and Attending Surgeon, Milwaukee County General Hospital and Columbia and Deaconess Hospitals, Milwaukee, Wisconsin.

DENTON A. COOLEY, M.D.

Clinical Professor of Surgery, The University of Texas Health Science Center at Houston Medical School; Surgeon-in-Chief, Texas Heart Institute; Consultant in Cardiovascular Surgery, St. Luke's Episcopal Hospital and Texas Children's Hospital, Houston, Texas.

T. P. CORRIGAN, M.D.

University College, Dublin, Ireland.

GEORGE CRILE, JR.

Emeritus Consultant, Department of General Surgery, Cleveland Clinic Foundation, Cleveland, Ohio.

CLYDE E. CULP, M.D.

Associate Professor, Mayo Medical School; Consultant, Proctologic Surgery, Mayo Clinic and Mayo Foundation; Proctologic Surgeon, St. Mary's Hospital and Rochester Methodist Hospital, Rochester, Minnesota.

W. ANDREW DALE, M.D.

Clinical Professor of Surgery, Vanderbilt University School of Medicine; Attending Surgeon, St. Thomas and Baptist Hospitals, Nashville, Tennessee.

W. CLAYTON DAVIS, M.D., F.A.C.S.

Chairman, Department of Surgery, York Hospital, York, Pennsylvania.

LAWRENCE DEN BESTEN, M.D.

Professor, The University of Iowa College of Medicine; Professor of Surgery and Vice Chairman, The University of Iowa Hospitals and Clinics; Chief, Surgical Service, Veterans Administration Hospital, Iowa City, Iowa.

M. MICHAEL EISENBERG, M.D.

Professor of Surgery, University of Minnesota Medical School; Attending Surgeon, University of Minnesota Health Sciences Center; Consultant, Veterans Administration Hospital and Abbott-Northwestern Medical Center, Minneapolis, Minnesota.

DONALD LESLIE ERICKSON, M.D.

Associate Professor, University of Minnesota School of Medicine, Minneapolis; Department of Surgery, University of Minnesota Hospital, Minneapolis; Chief of Neurosurgery, St. Paul-Ramsey Hospital, St. Paul, Minnesota.

JACK M. FARRIS, M.D.

Professor of Surgery, University of California, San Diego, School of Medicine, San Diego, California.

THOMAS J. FOGARTY, M.D.

Cardiovascular Surgeon, Stanford University Hospital, Palo Alto, California.

ELWIN E. FRALEY, M.D.

Professor and Chairman, Department of Urologic Surgery, University of Minnesota School of Medicine; Chief, Urologic Surgery Service, University of Minnesota Hospitals, Minneapolis, Minnesota.

EDGAR L. FRAZELL, M.D.

Clinical Professor of Surgery, The University of Texas Health Science Center at San Antonio Medical School, San Antonio, Texas; Consultant Surgeon and former Chief of the Head and Neck Service, The Memorial Hospital for Cancer and Allied Diseases, New York, New York.

THOMAS D. GILES, M.D.

Clinical Associate Professor of Medicine, Tulane University School of Medicine; Visiting Physician and Cardiologist, Hotel Dieu Hospital and Charity Hospital of Louisiana, New Orleans, Louisiana.

FRANK GLASSOW, M.A., M.B., B.Chir., L.R.C.P., F.R.C.S.

Senior Staff Surgeon, Shouldice Hospital, Toronto, Ontario, Canada.

**LEON GOLDMAN, M.D.**

Late Emeritus Professor of Surgery, University of California, San Francisco, School of Medicine, San Francisco, California.

**THEODOR B. GRAGE, M.D., Ph.D.**

Associate Professor of Surgery, University of Minnesota Medical School, Minneapolis, Minnesota.

**A. GERSON GREENBURG, M.D., Ph.D.**

Assistant Professor of Surgery, University of California, San Diego, School of Medicine; Chief, Surgical Intensive Care Unit, and Staff Physician, Veterans Administration Hospital; Attending Physician, University of California Medical Center, San Diego, California.

**DAVID V. HABIF, M.D.**

Morris and Rose Milstein Professor of Surgery, Columbia University College of Physicians and Surgeons; Attending Surgeon, Presbyterian Hospital, New York, New York.

**GEORGE A. HALLENBECK, M.D., Ph.D.**

Chairman, Department of Surgery, Scripps Clinic, La Jolla, California.

**SAMUEL HELLMAN, M.D.**

Alvan T. and Viola D. Fuller–American Cancer Society, Chairman, Department of Radiation Therapy, Harvard Medical School; Director, Joint Center for Radiation Therapy (Beth Israel Hospital, Boston Hospital for Women, New England Deaconess Hospital, Peter Bent Brigham Hospital, The Children's Hospital Medical Center), Boston, Massachusetts.

**FREDERIC P. HERTER, M.D.**

Auchincloss Professor of Surgery, Columbia University College of Physicians and Surgeons; Attending Surgeon, Presbyterian Hospital; Consulting Surgeon, Harlem and St. Luke's Hospitals, New York, New York.

**LUCIUS D. HILL, M.D.**

Clinical Professor of Surgery, University of Washington School of Medicine; Surgeon, Virginia Mason Medical Center, Seattle, Washington.

**EDWARD W. HUMPHREY, M.D., Ph.D.**

Professor of Surgery, University of Minnesota School of Medicine; Chief, Surgical Service, Veterans Administration Hospital, Minneapolis, Minnesota.

**ALFRED W. HUMPHRIES, M.D.**

Professor of Vascular Surgery, Cleveland Clinic Foundation, Cleveland, Ohio.

**RALPH E. JOHNSON, M.D.**

Chief of the Radiation Oncology Branch, National Cancer Institute, National Institutes of Health, Bethesda, Maryland.

**S. AUSTIN JONES, M.D.**

Professor of Surgery, University of California, Irvine, California College of Medicine; Department of Surgery, Veterans Administration Hospital, Long Beach, and Memorial Hospital of Glendale, Glendale, California.

VIJAY V. KAKKAR, F.R.C.S., F.R.C.S.E.

Senior Lecturer and Consultant Surgeon, Kings College Hospital Medical School, London, England.

KAILASH KEDIA, M.D.

Instructor, Department of Urologic Surgery, University of Minnesota School of Medicine; Staff Urologist, University of Minnesota Hospitals, Minneapolis, Minnesota.

THOMAS E. KERSTEN, M.D.

Medical Fellow in Surgery, University of Minnesota School of Medicine, Minneapolis, Minnesota.

DAVID P. KRAJCOVIC, M.D.

Instructor, Washington University School of Medicine; Department of Surgery, St. Louis County Hospital, St. Luke's East and St. Luke's West Hospitals, St. Louis, Missouri.

MORTIMER J. LACHER, M.D., F.A.C.P.

Clinical Assistant Professor of Medicine, Cornell University Medical College; Associate Attending Physician, Hematology-Lymphoma Service, Memorial Hospital for Cancer and Allied Diseases; Assistant Clinician, Sloan-Kettering Institute, New York, New York.

A. M. LAWRENCE, M.D., Ph.D.

Professor of Medicine and Biochemistry, Loyola University of Chicago Stritch School of Medicine, Maywood; Associate Chief of Staff for Education and Program Director, Endocrinology, Veterans Administration Hospital, Hines, Illinois.

WALTER LAWRENCE, JR., M.D.

American Cancer Society Professor of Clinical Oncology, Chairman, Division of Surgical Oncology, and Director, Cancer Center, Medical College of Virginia, Richmond, Virginia.

ROBERT I. LEVY, M.D.

Lecturer in Chronic Disease Epidemiology, Yale University School of Medicine, New Haven, Connecticut; Director, National Heart and Lung Institute, National Institutes of Health; Attending Physician, Lipid Metabolism (Molecular Disease Branch) Service, National Institutes of Health Clinical Center, Bethesda, Maryland.

JOHN L. MADDEN, M.D.

Clinical Professor of Surgery, New York Medical College; Attending Surgeon, St. Clare's Hospital and Health Center, New York, New York.

WILLIS P. MAIER, M.D., F.A.C.S.

Associate Professor of Surgery, Temple University School of Medicine, Philadelphia; Consultant in General and Thoracic Surgery, Veterans Administration Hospital, Wilkes-Barre, Germantown Dispensary and Hospital, St. Christopher's Hospital for Children, and Shriners Hospital for Crippled Children, Philadelphia, Pennsylvania.

COLIN MARKLAND, M.D.

Professor, Department of Urologic Surgery, University of Minnesota School of Medicine; Staff Urologist, University of Minnesota Hospitals, Minneapolis, Minnesota.

M. TERRY McENANY, M.D.

Assistant Professor of Surgery, Harvard Medical School, Boston; Chief of Thoracic and Cardiovascular Surgery, Mount Auburn Hospital, Cambridge; Junior Visiting Surgeon, Active Staff, Cambridge Hospital, Cambridge; Assistant Surgeon, Massachusetts General Hospital, Boston; Assistant in Surgery, Beth Israel Hospital, Boston, Massachusetts.

CHESTER B. McVAY, M.D., Ph.D.

Professor and Chairman, Department of Surgery, University of South Dakota School of Medicine, Vermillion; Chief of Surgery, Sacred Heart Hospital, Yankton, South Dakota.

KAZI MOBIN-UDDIN, M.B., B.S.

Director, Cardiovascular Surgery Section, Frederick C. Smith Clinic; Attending Cardiovascular Surgeon, Community-Med-Center Hospital, Marion, Ohio.

ELIZABETH A. MOLLAND, M.A., M.B., B.Chir., M.R.C.Path.

Lecturer, The London Hospital Medical College, London, England.

ELDRED D. MUNDTH, M.D.

Associate Professor of Surgery, Harvard Medical School; Co-Chief, Cardiac Surgery Division, Massachusetts General Hospital, Boston, Massachusetts.

ALTON OCHSNER, M.D.

Professor of Surgery, Emeritus, Tulane University School of Medicine; Consultant in Surgery, Ochsner Clinic and Ochsner Foundation Hospital; Consulting Surgeon, Charity Hospital of Louisiana; Honorary Staff, Division of General Surgery, Touro Infirmary, New Orleans, Louisiana.

CORNELIUS OLCOTT, IV, M.D.

Assistant Professor of Surgery, University of California, San Francisco, School of Medicine, San Francisco, California.

EDWARD PALOYAN, M.D.

Professor of Surgery, Loyola University of Chicago Stritch School of Medicine, Maywood; Associate Chief of Staff for Research and Chief of Endocrine Surgery, Veterans Administration Hospital, Hines, Illinois.

W. SPENCER PAYNE, M.D.

Professor of Surgery, Mayo Medical School, Rochester, Minnesota.

ERLE E. PEACOCK, JR., M.D.

Professor of Surgery and Chairman of the Surgical Faculty, University of Arizona College of Medicine; Department of Surgery, University of Arizona Medical Center, Veterans Administration Hospital, St. Mary's Hospital, and Tucson Medical Center, Tucson, Arizona.

DOROTHEE L. PERLOFF, M.D.

Clinical Professor of Medicine, University of California, San Francisco, School of Medicine, San Francisco, California.

HIRAM C. POLK, JR., M.D.

Professor and Chairman, Department of Surgery, University of Louisville School of

Medicine; Chief of Surgery, Louisville General Hospital; Consultant in Surgery, Veterans Administration Hospital; Attending Surgeon, Norton-Children's Hospitals, Louisville, Kentucky.

DAVID J. POLLOCK, B.S., M.B.Ch.B., M.R.C.Path.

Senior Lecturer and Consultant, The London Hospital Medical School; Consultant Pathologist, The London Hospital, London, England.

MARK M. RAVITCH, M.D.

Professor of Surgery, The University of Pittsburgh School of Medicine; Surgeon-in-Chief, Montefiori Hospital, Pittsburgh, Pennsylvania.

GEORGE J. REUL, JR., M.D.

Consultant Surgeon, St. Luke's Hospital, Texas Children's Hospital, and Texas Heart Institute, Houston, Texas.

BASIL M. RIFKIND, M.D., F.R.C.P.

Chief, Lipid Metabolism Branch, and Project Officer, Lipid Research Clinics Program, Division of Heart and Vascular Diseases, National Heart and Lung Institute, National Institutes of Health, Bethesda, Maryland.

GEORGE P. ROSEMOND, M.D., M.S., F.A.C.S.

Professor of Surgery, Temple University School of Medicine, Philadelphia; Surgeon, Temple University Hospital, Philadelphia; Consultant, Thoracic Surgery, Veterans Administration Hospital, Wilkes-Barre; Consultant, Department of Surgery, Paoli Memorial Hospital, Paoli; Consultant, Department of Surgery, Hanover General Hospital, Hanover, Pennsylvania.

EDWIN W. SALZMAN, M.D.

Professor of Surgery, Harvard Medical School; Associate Director of Surgery, Beth Israel Hospital, Boston, Massachusetts.

RICHARD D. SAUTTER, M.D.

Active Staff, St. Joseph's Hospital; Thoracic Surgeon, Marshfield Clinic, Marshfield, Wisconsin.

JOHN L. SAWYERS, M.D.

Professor of Surgery, Vanderbilt University School of Medicine; Surgeon-in-Chief, Nashville General Hospital, Nashville, Tennessee.

DAVID GEORGE SMITH, M.D.

Assistant Professor, University of Minnesota School of Medicine, Minneapolis, Minnesota.

JOHN B. STANBURY, M.D.

Professor of Experimental Medicine, Massachusetts Institute of Technology, Cambridge; Consulting Physician, Massachusetts General Hospital, Boston, Massachusetts.

MAUS W. STEARNS, JR., M.D.

Associate Professor of Surgery, Cornell University Medical College; Chief, Rectum and Colon Service, Memorial Sloan-Kettering Cancer Center, New York, New York.

H. HARLAN STONE, M.D.

Professor of Surgery and Director, Surgical Bacteriological Laboratory, Emory University School of Medicine; Director, Trauma, Pediatric, and Burn Surgical Services, Grady Memorial Hospital, Atlanta, Georgia.

RONALD J. STONEY, M.D.

Associate Professor of Surgery, University of California, San Francisco, School of Medicine, San Francisco, California.

S. TIMOTHY STRING, M.D.

Assistant Professor of Surgery, University of South Alabama College of Medicine; Chief, Vascular Surgical Service, University of South Alabama Medical Center, Mobile, Alabama.

ROBERT J. SWANSON, M.D.

Clinical Instructor in Surgery, University of California, San Francisco, School of Medicine, San Francisco, California.

W. GORDON WALKER, M.D.

Professor of Medicine, Johns Hopkins University School of Medicine, Baltimore, Maryland.

RALPH R. WEICHSELBAUM, M.D.

Instructor, Department of Radiation Therapy, Harvard Medical School; Assistant Radiation Therapist, Joint Center for Radiation Therapy (Beth Israel Hospital, Boston Hospital for Women, New England Deaconess Hospital, Peter Bent Brigham Hospital, The Children's Hospital Medical Center), Boston, Massachusetts.

VALLEE L. WILLMAN, M.D.

Chairman, Department of Surgery, St. Louis University School of Medicine; Department of Surgery, St. Louis University Hospitals (Firmin Desloge Hospital, Cardinal Glennon Memorial Hospital for Children, St. Mary's Health Center), St. Louis, Missouri.

LESLIE WISE, M.D., F.R.C.S., F.A.C.S.

Professor of Surgery, State University of New York at Stony Brook Health Sciences Center School of Medicine; Chairman, Department of Surgery, Long Island Jewish-Hillside Medical Center, New Hyde Park; Surgeon-in-Chief, Queens Hospital Medical Center, New York, New York.

EDWIN J. WYLIE, M.D.

Professor, University of California, San Francisco, School of Medicine; Chief, Vascular Surgery Service, University of California Hospital, San Francisco, California.

# PREFACE

The editors have sought to develop in this volume substantive analyses of specific, controversial issues which confront clinical surgeons. For each problem, a contributor examines and critically reviews the evidence supporting a particular approach to a specific problem. Proponents of *alternative* points of view are asked to bulwark, by as sound biologic information as is available, their respective positions. We believe the subjects selected to be of current clinical interest and to contain substantial elements of uncertainty. Indeed, the fact that a controversy exists implies that evidence leading to an unequivocally "correct" position is lacking.

The format, which is similar to that of the three very popular volumes of *Current Surgical Management* edited by Edwin H. Ellison, Stanley R. Friesen, and John H. Mulholland and published in 1957, 1960, and 1965 respectively, contrasts with that of textbooks, which customarily are devoted to reviewing accepted concepts and procedures in terms of historical, epidemiologic, pathologic, physiologic, and therapeutic considerations. Scientific articles in professional journals, too, tend to follow a standard sequence: introduction, materials and methods, results, discussion, and summary.

This book is not intended to be a substitute for textbooks or journals. Rather, the essayists and editors assume that the reader has a fundamental grasp of relevant anatomy, pathology, and pathophysiology or will fill in any such critical gaps from standard sources. A contributing author thus will make no attempt to outline an overall background but rather will devote himself to the sharp point of uncertainty or dispute. Although this book is not aimed at the beginning medical student, but rather at the practicing surgeon and the house officer, its analytical approach may stimulate critical thinking habits for the student.

We request that each author provide a critical evaluation of the evidence submitted. At times, in this real world, the champion of a particular point of view is not afflicted by serious doubts, even though there are weaknesses ranging from petty to gross in the evidence at hand. We urge, therefore, that the reader assess each presentation on the basis of the data presented rather than on the rhetorical skills of the writer. Too, where weaknesses in the argument presented are not readily apparent, we hope that the adversary, whose essay is in immediate juxtaposition, will hasten to point them out. We have advised the authors to be brief. The insistence on sound evidence, rather than anecdotal reporting, tends to promote brevity. As Oliver Wendell Holmes observed, "A few facts can ruin an otherwise good argument."

We suggest that the reader regard evidence as characterized by degrees of certainty. A double-blind study, for example, represents a rigorous clinical inquiry in search of those facts that determine logical decisions about therapy, but the situation in which neither patient nor physician is aware of the therapy employed is readily attained only in drug studies. Clearly, when surgical operations are under scrutiny, double-blind considerations are unlikely to prevail, for the surgeon will customarily know what procedure he is performing. With operative treatment protocols, even the single-blind situation may be quite difficult to achieve; it is rare for the patient to remain uninformed about the nature of the intervention.

The prospective randomized study is, at this time, the means most likely to provide definitive answers with respect to operative therapy. As a general consideration, credibility is enhanced if those individuals assessing the results of therapy are unaware of the details of the intervention, particularly when the assessment pivots upon subjective responses.

Of lesser reliability than randomization is the consecutive personal series in which each patient has been subjected to essentially comparable treatment and in which no conscious case selectivity has occurred. Under the most carefully pursued plan, however, some cryptic degree of patient selection invariably plays a role in determining the outcome. Hence subtle skew factors can deform seemingly obvious conclusions. We therefore have urged contributors submitting this type of evidence to identify, whenever possible, the bases for patient selection. In analyzing clinical series, careful writer and reader attention must be directed to recognition of significant differences in patient material, criteria of success, length of follow-up, method of follow-up, and other factors which could lead to variations in achievement quite unrelated to the particular mode of therapy espoused.

The clinical anecdote or "in my experience" type of surgical discussion has little stature in the hierarchy of evidence. The major weakness in a recalled episode is the nonreproducibility of the conditions that prevailed during the therapeutic event. However, the anecdote does have limited value as an observation which may justify attempts at duplication or which may provide clues to further understanding of the phenomena involved.

Each author has provided key references particularly relevant to the thesis supported to allow the reader access to all important information relating to the essayist's position.

The contributors were requested to identify not only the positive logical points for the position endorsed but also to acknowledge limitations created by unavailability of more solid evidence. Each was also asked to provide a brief analysis of basic deficiencies which he believes are inherent in alternative points of view.

Authors were invited to respond particularly to those specific issues which seemed to the editors to be unique to the topics under consideration. These issues are presented in a list of editorial questions at the beginning of each section; thus the reader can judge for himself just how effectively and with what degree of validation the author has dealt with those queries.

Ideally each author will: (1) state his position; (2) discuss the supporting evidence; (3) indicate gaps in his evidence; (4) point out flaws in opposing points of view; (5) provide references, with brief annotations for the key ones; and (6) answer the questions posed by the editors.

For most topics, the advocacy approach was employed; by this, we mean that two or more individuals take alternative and differing positions on a topic. However, some subjects, while controversial, do not lend themselves to this method. For these, we have asked one surgical scholar to review critically the evidence on various sides of a question. While this approach may provide a less sharply defined argument, it is no less useful in assessing available information.

The first article in the book, on controlled clinical trials, should be read carefully as an introduction to the concept of validating evidence.

If this book finds sufficient acceptance among those who labor with the problems and tools of surgery, further controversial topics may be dealt with in succeeding volumes.

RICHARD L. VARCO

JOHN P. DELANEY

# The tradition
# of respectful argument

JAMES P. SHANNON*

One mark of an educated man is his ability to differ without becoming angry, sarcastic or discourteous. Such a man recognizes that in contingent matters there will always be a place for legitimate difference of opinion.

He knows that he is not infallible, he respects the honesty and the intellectual integrity of other men and presumes that all men are men of integrity until they are proven to be otherwise.

He is prepared to listen to them when their superior wisdom has something of value to teach him. He is slow to anger and always confident that truth can defend itself and state its own case without specious arguments, emotional displays or personal pressures.

This is not to say that he abandons his position easily. If his be a disciplined mind, he does not lightly forsake the intellectual ground he has won at great cost. He yields only to evidence, proof or demonstration.

He expects his adversary to show conclusively the superior value of his opinions and he is not convinced by anything less than this. He is not intimidated by shouting. He is not impressed by verbosity. He is not overwhelmed by force or numbers.

His abiding respect for truth's invincibility enables him to maintain composure and balance in the face of impressive odds. And his respect for the person and the intellect of his opponent prevents him from using cheap tricks, caustic comments or personal attacks against his adversaries, no matter how brilliant or forceful, unjust or unfair, they may be.

Because of his large views of truth and of individual human respectability, he is prepared to suffer apparent defeat in the mind of the masses on occasions when he knows his position is right. He is not shattered by this apparent triumph of darkness, because he realizes that the mass-mind is fickle at best.

---

*Dr. Shannon, Executive Director of the Minneapolis Foundation, Minneapolis, Minnesota, is a regular contributor of a nationally syndicated newspaper column. We believe his essay is worthy of contemplative consideration by our readers, for its message speaks eloquently to certain concerns associated with controversy. — The Editors

He is neither angered nor shocked by new evidence of public vulgarity or blindness. He is rather prepared to see in these expected human weaknesses compelling reason for more compassion, better rhetoric, stronger evidence of his part. He seeks always to persuade and seldom to denounce.

The ability to defend one's own position with spirit and conviction; to evaluate accurately the conflicting opinions of others and to retain one's confidence in the ultimate power of truth to carry its own weight, are necessary talents in any society, but especially so in our democratic world.

In our day and in our land, there is some evidence that these virtues are in short supply. The venerable tradition of respectful argumentation, based on evidence, conducted with courtesy, and leading to the exposition of truth, is a precious part of our heritage in this land of freedom. It is the duty of educated men to understand, appreciate and perpetuate this tradition.

# CONTENTS

# 1

# *The Controlled Clinical Trial*

RANDOMIZED CLINICAL
TRIALS IN SURGERY
*by Thomas C. Chalmers*

# Randomized Clinical Trials in Surgery

THOMAS C. CHALMERS

*Mount Sinai Medical Center and Mount Sinai School of Medicine*

Gastroenterostomy and gastrectomy for the treatment of duodenal ulcer have been performed with varying popularity since the beginning of the 20th century. During the middle third of this century, partial gastrectomy was by far the most popular operation for patients with intractable ulcers. At one time, it was popular to remove more and more of the stomach in an effort to prevent recurrent marginal ulcers; however, now as little as possible is removed. Vagotomy was first introduced in 1943,[1] and more than 30 years later its modifications and efficacy are still being debated. As a replicate of the gastrectomy experience, many refinements of vagotomy have been devised in an effort to avoid annoying side effects without decreasing efficacy. At the present time, different combinations of vagotomy, gastroenterostomy, and various kinds of gastrectomy are being tried, most as consecutive series and only rarely in randomized clinical trials (RCT's). If one or more procedures do become established as superior, is it not a shame that it has taken so many years to reach a conclusion of such importance to the duodenal ulcer patient?

A distressingly high death rate from hemorrhage complicating peptic ulcer has led to advocacy of therapies ranging from prohibiting emergency intervention to operating on almost all patients. In 61 reports of 21,130 patients between 1930 and 1969,[2] the proportion of patients operated on as an emergency has risen in each decade—from 2 per cent in 1940 to 80 per cent in one series in 1964.[2] Yet the overall case fatality rate has stayed exactly the same. In three randomized clinical trials, emergency operation was no more effective than expectant therapy,[3-5] but these were not good examples of the RCT because too many patients in each study did not receive the therapy assigned at random. The age of patients with bleeding peptic ulcer has increased over the past three decades, and case fatality rates go up with age.[2] Does this mean that the operation has saved some lives? Or does the steady

3

case fatality rate, in spite of the increasing age of the patients, result from advances in the control of postoperative infection as well as of fluid and electrolyte problems?

Halsted introduced the radical operation for carcinoma of the breast in 1894.[6] It is still the operation of choice in the minds of the majority of surgeons, although probably not of the majority of completely informed patients. Simpler procedures have been and continue to be compared with the radical operation in RCT's,[7-10] and as yet, after several million have been performed, there is no conclusive evidence that the latter is the operation of choice for women with Stage I carcinoma.

Portacaval shunt surgery for the control of portal hypertension in patients with cirrhosis was introduced 30 to 40 years ago.[11] In this case, the value of the operation was not tested until thousands of patients had been treated surgically over a 20-year period, most clinicians having been fooled by dramatic differences in survival between patients operated on and historical or otherwise contrived controls. Now an accurate picture is emerging as a result of seven randomized trials.[12-17] Operation is apparently contraindicated in patients with esophageal varices who have not yet had a life-threatening hemorrhage; in patients who have bled, it prevents recurrence at the expense of an increased frequency of encephalopathy, and on the average life is prolonged a minimal amount. This logical conclusion from the seven controlled trials has had little influence on the opinions of the operation expressed in clinical reviews and textbooks, especially those written by surgeons (Table 1).

It has been estimated that over 25,000 coronary bypass operations are now being performed each year in the United States alone. As a result of dra-

**TABLE 1.   Opinions on Portacaval Shunt Surgery**

| Type of Shunt | Degree of Enthusiasm | | | Total |
|---|---|---|---|---|
| | *Marked* | *Moderate* | *None* | *Total* |
| *9 Textbooks and 5 Review Articles by Surgeons* | | | | |
| Therapeutic | 11 | 3 | – | 14 |
| Prophylactic | 1 | 1 | 4 | 6 |
| Emergency | 6 | 2 | 1 | 9 |
| For Ascites | – | 3 | 2 | 5 |
| *Total* | 18 | 9 | 7 | 34 |
| *11 Textbooks and 2 Review Articles by Internists and Gastroenterologists* | | | | |
| Therapeutic | 3 | 10 | 1 | 14 |
| Prophylactic | – | – | 7 | 7 |
| Emergency | 3 | 6 | – | 9 |
| For Ascites | – | 2 | 2 | 4 |
| *Total* | 6 | 18 | 10 | 34 |
| *Total of Opinions by Discipline* | | | | |
| Surgeons | 18 | 9 | 7 | 34 |
| Internists and Gastroenterologists | 6 | 18 | 10 | 34 |
| *Total*° | 24 | 27 | 17 | 68 |

°$\chi^2 = 9.53$, $p < .01$

matic relative efficacy in most patients with crippling angina, the indications have been expanded to include patients with early mild angina at one end of the scale, and patients dying of acute myocardial infarction at the other. Do patients at either extreme of the scale (in terms of expected operative mortality rate) have a better chance of survival in reasonable health than they would if they were treated expectantly? No studies are yet available to answer this critical question.[18]

Intestinal bypass operations for intractable obesity have now been performed for almost 20 years.[19] It is conceivable that the combination of operative mortality and serious long-term disability may bring about a reversion to conservative therapy. Yet individual surgeons continue to perform the procedure as if its safety and long-term efficacy have been established. How will they and their surviving patients feel if the operation is some day relegated to the status of colectomy for diseases of "auto-intoxication"? Will it prove to have been an experiment worth trying? Has it been an experiment at all?

It is probable that if proper and sufficient randomized clinical trials had been performed as soon as an operative treatment was devised, we would now know which patients would benefit from each kind of operation after medical therapy failed to cure peptic ulcer and who should be operated upon with bleeding, how simple a procedure is safe in early carcinoma of the breast, who should consent to a portacaval shunt, and which patients with intractable obesity or requiring coronary artery surgery should have short-circuiting procedures performed. If the answer were that easily obtainable, it is hard to understand why the latter two procedures have been so widely performed without controls, and why modifications of older operations are still being reported when it is impossible for the critical reader to properly evaluate them because inadequate controls are presented. There must have been serious obstacles to the conduct of proper RCT's. What were they, and how can they be overcome?

The author has previously discussed the reasons why more RCT's have not been performed.[20-24] From an ethical point of view, randomization has been hard to accept as a decision-making technique, and deciding when to stop studies has sometimes presented an insurmountable difficulty. The positive or negative pilot study has prevented many important RCT's from getting underway by prejudicing the investigator to the extent that he cannot bring himself to randomize patients into what he already believes to be the less effective therapy. RCT's are often considered impractical because large numbers of patients are necessary, often so large that cumbersome cooperative studies must be performed, or because they take so long that interest wanes after several years. Yet it has always amazed the author that clinicians have preferred to study consecutive series of patients instead of performing an RCT because the latter would take much longer, as if a useless answer obtained in a shorter time were not an even greater waste of time and effort, and sometimes of lives.

The deficiencies of the traditional custom of treating a consecutive series of carefully selected patients and reporting the results if favorable need some emphasis here. As innovative medicine and surgery have expanded, the "literature" has replaced personal experience as the principal source of data on which to base therapeutic decisions. Yet this tool has become more and more difficult to use effectively as the number of reported experiences has increased markedly and the complexities of patient selection and nuances of therapeutic modalities have become more apparent. In understanding the basis of patient selection, the details concerning the unsuitable and unselected patient may be critical to the surgeon who is trying to decide about a new procedure. Ideas so bad that even short uncontrolled series discouraged their originator are not likely to be reported. The "good" surgeons and clinics are more likely to report their results than the "bad" ones, and unusual results are more likely to be accepted for publication than those confirming preconceived notions.

There is only one condition under which the reporting of uncontrolled series of patients might be accepted as a poor substitute for widespread RCT's — when there is a network of reports of all patients treated by all kinds of surgeons using traditional as well as experimental procedures. The Veterans Administration has these data in its automated, system-wide patient treatment file. As analyses begin to appear in the literature, they will have to be interpreted with extreme caution, however, because therapeutic effects cannot be isolated from characteristics of patient referral and selection. Careful documentation of prognostic covariables[25] will be essential for proper interpretation. The decision on how to treat each patient is a probability decision based on how the patient fits into the data available in the literature. Without universal reporting of all cases treated, and even with it, multiple RCT's are the only reliable recourse for the surgeon who must predict what will happen to his patient.

In any clinical trial, controls must be concurrent because of the tremendous power of selection in determining outcome. Diseases are variable in the way in which they afflict people, and people are variable in their responses to operations; the combination is extremely variable. No study has ever admitted every conceivable patient in the population available for a given operation. There is bound to be some selection, and selection cannot take place without bias. If historical controls are selected, that choice will also be biased. If all patients in a given rubric are employed as historical controls, they cannot be comparable to a current group of selected patients. Informed consent, the taking of which always involves bias, is required of the experimental group but has seldom been obtained from the historical controls. Finally, subtle changes in therapy may take place in the period between the selection of the experimental patients and the compilation of the historical controls.[26]

In order to avoid the "RCT paralysis" that results from bias engendered by the uncontrolled pilot study, the very first patient to be subjected to a new procedure should be assigned at random to either the new or the standard operation. Admittedly there are strong scientific objections to this. Conclusions about relative efficacy could be influenced by an early "experience factor"; i.e., technical problems may result in an outcome distinctly worse than that from the standard therapy. So from the scientific standpoint alone, the technique should be fully developed before the randomized trial is begun. From the ethical standpoint, however, an early consecutive series would be wholly unacceptable unless the patient were told in the process of obtaining his informed consent that the technique was not yet fully developed and that he could not be expected to do as well as he would if he received the standard operation. Obviously, if properly informed, he would opt for the established operation. He might be expected to elect randomization, however, if convinced there was an equal chance that the new operation might be better than the old from the beginning. Randomization from the beginning, with truly informed consent, is the only *ethical* way to begin the exploration of new therapies.

Accepting the conclusion that an RCT must be designed and undertaken as soon as possible after the conception of a new surgical treatment, there are certain principles that must be followed if the results of the study are to be applied to future patients with the same disease. These are the aspects of design which the investigator must incorporate into the RCT, and they are the elements any reader should look for as evidence of a valid clinical trial. They will be presented from the latter point of view. This is not a "how-to-do-it" manual, but rather a "how-to-tell-whether-it-was-done-well" guide.

## The Biostatistician

There should be evidence that a competent biostatistician has had an integral part in the design, execution, and analyses of the study—this means that he should be a co-author. A note of thanks at the end of the report is not sufficient evidence that the biostatistician is willing to risk his reputation on the study. The reader can detect the magnitude of the biostatistician's contribution from the section on the estimates of numbers of patients required. Were the endpoints defined in the beginning, and the magnitude of a meaningful clinical difference defined? This is essential for the estimates of the numbers necessary to make it probable, at a selected $p$ value, that an observed difference was not due to chance and also to make reasonably sure that, according to accepted confidence limits, a clinically meaningful difference was not being missed by the study (power of the study). There are many other opportunities to detect the fine hand of the biostatistician in the other technical details of the good RCT, as described in the following sections.

## Selection of Patients

Ideally, all patients to whom the conclusions of a study will be applied should be included. This means that the exclusions must be as few as possible and must be confined to those who would be clearly harmed by one or the other of the treatments under consideration. Said in another way, the only exclusions should be those patients who would not be considered for the therapy eventually proved to be best by the study at hand, whichever therapy that might be. The reader should require a table summarizing the excluded patients who were seen by the investigator because they might be suitable and the reasons for their exclusion. To fulfill this need, the authors must have kept a log of such patients.

### Pre-randomization Data

The patients should be characterized as completely as possible before it is determined which therapy they will receive. Otherwise, bias can influence measurements which might later be used to interpret properly the differences encountered. Quantitative material should be accompanied by evidence that it was gathered in an objective manner and that reproducibility was measured.

### Randomization

The guiding principle of randomization is that chance and chance alone must determine which treatment is assigned to each patient. Since all available patients are never admitted to any study, the investigator must have no clues about which therapy is more likely to be next in the draw when he declares a patient eligible or obtains permission from the patient to be randomized. The latter is a critical issue because it is so easy for bias to influence the perseverance with which one seeks permission. This means that the chances of assignment to all treatments must be approximately equal at all times. This principle will be compromised whenever randomization is restricted in any of the ways described in the next three paragraphs. Efficient blinding reduces the magnitude of the problem, but blinding is obviously most difficult in the evaluation of surgical therapies.

STRATIFICATION. If it is known that certain pre-randomization factors are well-correlated with the outcome to be measured, and if they are qualitative factors for which effective adjustments cannot be made in the analyses, the authors may have wisely assigned the patients to pre-defined groups before randomization. If so, these should be described. However, some biostatisticians believe that it is seldom wise to stratify before randomization, because adjustments can be made in the analyses for non-treatment related differences in outcome.

RESTRICTION. If it is important that there be equal numbers in each treatment group, or if some sequential design is employed, or if differences in outcome are expected with time, the authors may have chosen to restrict the randomization to pairs or groups of four or eight. Beware of this in a study that is not successfully blinded with regard to both treatment and trends. The opportunity for distortion by bias is enormous if randomization is restricted and if the physician selecting a patient for a study and persuading him to volunteer knows what treatment the previous patient received and which way the overall results are trending.

PERMISSION OF THE PATIENT. There has been a gradual evolution in the attitude of both patients and investigating physicians toward the concept of randomization and the need for informing the patient in detail about the process when obtaining his consent. If the physician recognizes that it is ethically preferable to randomize his patient rather than to assign him arbitrarily to a treatment that may be inferior, then he should be willing and able to take the patient into his confidence, and there should be no difficulty in obtaining informed consent. If he thinks he knows the answer and needs to deceive his patient in order to obtain his permission, then he should not be undertaking the study.

### Post-randomization Removal of Patients from the Study

This is a most critical issue. All of the advantages of a valid randomization process are negated if an appreciable number of patients are removed from the study before the start or completion of treatment. Only when the investigator and the patient are totally blinded to both treatment and trends is removal not a hazardous procedure. Many randomized surgical trials, for instance those comparing emergency surgery with conservative therapy for gastrointestinal hemorrhage, are made less valid by the fact that patients opt out of the surgical group after they have been randomized. Obviously, if the surgeon has second thoughts about the suitability of his patient for surgery, he will be more likely to acquiesce to the patient's changing his mind; or if the patient is highly suitable, the physician may be more successful at persuading him to continue with the randomized treatment. Of course, this situation may also occur with the patient who was originally randomized to nonoperative treatment. A changing situation may require surgery for ethical reasons. Obviously, if either situation applies very often, the trial is no longer an RCT but is a comparison of two therapies applied to selected patients, and the outcome could result from the selections as well as from the therapies.

These are gross examples of a problem that is present in all RCT's that are designed so that patients can withdraw after randomization. Yet every study protocol must include a clause that patients are free to withdraw if they so desire. Bias is controlled only when the clinician dealing with the hesitant patient is blinded sufficiently to prevent undue influence on the outcome.

### How Can Surgical Procedures be Blinded?

Obviously, blinding is difficult. In the case of comparisons of no operation with operation, sham operations do not seem to be ethical because they have no place in medical care. When medical care is compared with an operation, a physician who was not involved in the initial randomization or therapy could follow the patient, but this is usually impractical. Possibly, the clinical endpoints could be judged once a year or so by someone who is not otherwise following the patient. When death is an endpoint, it is difficult for most people to determine how knowledge of the original treatment could bias the physician or surgeon following the patient. However, it may very well do so if other therapies employed should prove to be life-saving, since they could be more vigorously applied to the patient thought to be receiving the less effective therapy. Woe to the patient if the clinical investigator turns out to be wrong about the relative values of the original treatment and the additional life-saving measures.

In the comparison of two different surgical procedures, such as two different operations for peptic ulcer, it should be relatively easy to keep both the patient and the physician who will be following him from discovering the nature of the procedure performed. When this is done, the evaluations by both of efficacy and side effects can be valid. The reader should look for evidence of blinding in every RCT, and when there is none, should consider the possibility that this lack has invalidated the results.

### Measurements of Treatment Effects

Are they objective, and how might they be influenced by bias? Has observer variability been measured properly, and when influenced by bias, could it allow for more than one interpretation of the results of treatment?

### Analysis of the Data

Were the proper procedures employed? This is a problem requiring biostatistical expertise. Hopefully, all physicians and surgeons making decisions about new therapies described in the literature will have had some training in making these judgments. The reader should search in the data analyses for a section on validation of the randomization procedure. It is conceivable that the results could be influenced by the fact that the patients really were different on entry into the study.

### End of the Study and the Importance of a Policy Advisory Board

The reader should look for evidence that this most important aspect of any RCT has been adequately considered by the investigators. Here more than anywhere else, ethical considerations weigh heavily on those making the decisions. Toward the end of a study, a continuing awareness of trends by the clinical investigators makes it increasingly difficult to randomly assign patients to what could prove to be the inferior therapy. Because of this, the type of patient selected may change decidedly as the study nears its conclusion—patients less likely to respond to or be harmed by either therapy are admitted, thus postponing the appearance of a significant difference. These are the most important reasons for having a policy advisory board made up of experts from various fields who can be kept aware of the trends and can make the critical decisions in a less biased manner than the investigators. Their involvement should reassure patients volunteering for a study that their rights will be looked after by a respected group of clinicians and biostatisticians.

These are some of the factors to evaluate in deciding whether or not a trial is well designed and executed, but it is certainly not a complete list. Deficiencies of some features to varying degrees may explain why not all RCT's of new or old therapies produce the same conclusions. When faced with discrepancies, the reader should base his judgment on a careful examination of the strong and weak points of each study. All practicing surgeons should become experts in the RCT.

# References

1. Dragstedt, L. R., and Owens, F. M.: Supra-diaphragmatic section of the vagus nerves in treatment of duodenal ulcer. Proc. Soc. Exp. Biol. Med. 53:152–154, 1943.
2. Chalmers, T. C., Sebestyen, C. S., and Lee, S.: Emergency surgical treatment of bleeding peptic ulcer: an analysis of the published data on 21,130 patients. Trans. Am. Clin. Climatol. Assoc. 82:188–199, 1970.
3. Enquist, I. F., Karlson, K. E., Tanaka, A. M., et al.: Statistically controlled evaluation of three methods of management of upper gastrointestinal bleeding: a progress report. Gastroenterology 32:619–632, 1957.
4. Read, R. C., Huebl, H. C., and Thal, A. P.: Randomized study of massive bleeding from peptic ulceration. Ann. Surg. 162:561–577, 1965.
5. Spicer, F. W., Carbone, J. V., and Lyon, C. G.: Acute massive hemorrhage from gastroduodenal ulceration. Amer. J. Surg. 102:153–157, 1961.
6. Halsted, W. S.: Results of operations for the cure of cancer of the breast performed at Johns Hopkins Hospital from June, 1889 to January, 1894. Ann. Surg. 20:497, 1894.
7. Kaae, S., and Johansen, H.: Simple mastectomy plus postoperative irradiation by the method of McWhirter for mammary carcinoma. Prog. Clin. Cancer 1:453–461, 1965.
8. Brinkley, D., and Haybittle, J. L.: Treatment of stage II carcinoma of the female breast. Lancet 2:1086–1087, 1971.
9. Bruce, J.: Operable cancer of the breast: a controlled clinical trial. Cancer 28:1443–1452, 1971.
10. Atkins, H., Hayward, J. L., Klugman, D. J., et al.: Treatment of early breast cancer: a report after ten years of a clinical trial. Br. Med. J. 2:423–429, 1972.
11. Whipple, A. O.: The rationale of portacaval anastomosis. Bull. N.Y. Acad. Med. May, 1946, pp. 251–263.
12. Resnick, R. H., Chalmers, T. C., Ishihara, A. M., et al.: A controlled study of the prophylactic portacaval shunt. A final report. Ann. Intern. Med. 70:675–688, 1969.
13. Conn, H. O., Lindenmuth, W. W., May, C. J., et al.: Prophylactic portacaval anastomosis. A tale of two studies. Medicine 51:27–40, 1972.
14. Jackson, F. C., Perrin, E. B., Smith, A. G., et al.: A clinical investigation of the portacaval shunt. II. Survival analysis of the prophylactic operation. Am. J. Surg. 115:22–42, 1968.
15. Jackson, F. C., Perrin, E. D., Felix, R., et al.: A clinical investigation of the portacaval shunt. V. Survival analysis of the therapeutic operation. Ann. Surg. 174:672–701, 1971.
16. Resnick, R. H., Iber, F. L., Ishihara, A. M., et al.: A controlled study of the therapeutic portacaval shunt. Gastroenterology 67:843–857, 1974.
17. Reynolds, T.: Report of controlled trial of shunting for esophageal varices. Presented at the American Association for the Study of Liver Diseases, Chicago, Oct., 1973.
18. Chalmers, T. C.: Randomization and coronary artery surgery. (Editorial.) Ann. Thorac. Surg. 14:323–327, 1972.
19. Payne, J. H., DeWind, L. T., and Commons, R. R.: Metabolic observations in patients with jejunocolic shunts. Am. J. Surg. 106:273–289, 1963.
20. Chalmers, T. C.: The Boston inter-hospital liver group as an experiment in cooperative research. (Editorial.) Gastroenterology 57:339–341, 1969.
21. Chalmers, T. C.: A challenge to clinical investigators. Gastroenterology 57:631–635, 1969.
22. Shaw, L. W., and Chalmers, T. C.: Ethics in cooperative clinical trials. Ann. N.Y. Acad. Sci. 169:487–495, 1970.
23. Chalmers, T. C., Block, J. B., and Lee, S.: Controlled studies in clinical cancer research. N. Engl. J. Med. 287:75–78, 1972.
24. Chalmers, T. C.: Ethical aspects of clinical trials. Am. J. Ophthalmol. 79:753–758, 1975.
25. Feinstein, A. R.: Clinical biostatistics XIV. The purposes of prognostic stratification. Clin. Pharmacol. Ther. 13:285–297, 1972.
26. Chalmers, T. C.: Randomized versus historical controls. Submitted for publication.

# 2

# *Bowel Preparation for Resection of the Colon*

PREPARATION OF THE COLON
WITH NEOMYCIN-ERYTHROMYCIN
*by Robert E. Condon*

ROUTINE ANTIBIOTIC
PREPARATION IS UNWARRANTED
*by Frederic P. Herter*

## Statement of the Problem

*The issue relates to the merits and drawbacks of mechanical and antimicrobial measures to prepare the bowel for colon resection.*

*Describe in detail the routine you prefer to prepare for a left colon resection with a nonobstructing carcinoma of the sigmoid. Analyze data and include your own.*

*What mechanical measures should be used to clear the colon of stool? diet? laxative? enemas? Discuss antibiotic enemas.*

*Should nonabsorbable antibiotics be used? If so, what agents and for how long? Are systemic antibiotics useful in averting infection? Provide data on alterations in colonic bacterial population, qualitative and quantitative.*

*When the bowel is prepared with antibiotics, what is the frequency of clinically important bacterial overgrowth? of staphylococcal enterocolitis? chronic diarrhea? fungus overgrowth? wound infection? intra-abdominal abscess? anastomotic leak? tumor recurrence at the suture line?*

*Discuss colon preparation in the presence of a partially obstructing sigmoid lesion.*

# Preparation of the Colon with Neomycin-Erythromycin

ROBERT E. CONDON

*The Medical College of Wisconsin, Milwaukee, Wisconsin*

The major risk of serious morbidity in patients undergoing colon operation is wound infection caused by fecal organisms. Controversy over the use of antibiotics in preparation for colon operations has been continuous over the last 35 years.[16] Fortunately, recent studies have clarified this issue by providing evidence that antibiotics reduce both the numbers of bacteria in the colon and the risk of wound infection following colon operations.[1, 2, 5, 6, 18, 20, 21, 24]

## Microflora of the Colon

Some understanding of the numbers and kinds of bacteria found in the colon, their role in producing wound infections, and their sensitivity to antibiotics is essential if rational judgments are to be made about the use of antibiotics in preparation of the colon.[3, 4, 12, 23] The human colonic microflora is composed of two broad classes of organisms: aerobes and anaerobes. Aerobic organisms require oxygen for metabolism and reproduction. Anaerobic organisms, on the other hand, do not depend on oxygen and, indeed, many anaerobes are killed by exposure to low concentrations of oxygen.

Stool specimens (see Figs. 1 and 2) contain up to $10^9$ aerobes per gram, including $10^6$ to $10^8$ coliform organisms (*Escherichia coli*, Proteus, Pseudomonas, Klebsiella) as well as aerobic streptococci, lactobacilli, a few staphylococci, fungi, and a host of minor transient organisms. The major aerobe responsible for wound infections is *E. coli*, usually recovered either in pure culture or as a component of a mixed infection. Other varieties of coliforms, such as Proteus or Pseudomonas, rarely are found alone in infected wounds

15

but may occur together with *E. coli* and other fecal organisms in mixed infections. Although Proteus, Pseudomonas, and similar organisms are not primary solo wound pathogens, they may be selectively enhanced in a mixed infection as a result of antibiotic treatment and, in the later stages of some wound infections, become the predominant organisms.

Aerobic streptococci are found uncommonly in infected wounds and occur almost always in mixed infections with *E. coli*. Staphylococci and fungi are transients within the bowel; they are not the source of wound infections. When a staphylococcal wound infection occurs, the source is either the nares, skin, or perineum of the patient, or the organism has been acquired from the patient's environment.

*E. coli* are susceptible to a variety of antibiotics, including aminoglycosides (neomycin, kanamycin, gentamicin), ampicillin, cephalosporins, and tetracyclines. Most other coliforms show a narrower range of antibiotic susceptibility. Klebsiella, for example, are resistant to ampicillin; Pseudomonas are resistant to most antibiotics, with the exception of certain aminoglycosides and carbenicillin.

Stool specimens also contain up to $10^{11}$ anaerobes, including $10^7$ to $10^9$ *Bacteroides fragilis* per gram of wet feces. Compared with aerobes, the concentration of anaerobes in feces is $10^2$ to $10^3$ times larger. In other words, for each aerobe in a sample of feces, there will be 100 to 1000 anaerobes. In addition to the major anaerobe, *B. fragilis*, stool harbors other species of Bacteroides, Peptostreptococcus, Bifidobacterium and Clostridium. There also are a host of saprophytic and putrefactic organisms in feces. If sufficiently rigorous microbiologic technique is employed, an ordinary stool specimen may yield over 50 different species of anaerobes. Most, fortunately, are not pathogenic.

The anaerobe chiefly responsible for wound infections is *B. fragilis*. It is usually recovered mixed with aerobic coliforms and other varieties of anaerobes. Less often, but still accounting for about 15 per cent of wound infections, *B. fragilis* causes a totally anaerobic wound infection. Peptostreptococci are the other principal anaerobic pathogens; they usually occur in a mixed flora in a septic wound.

Clostridia, despite their virulent reputation among surgeons, are not especially virulent organisms, and most typically cause an indolent spreading cellulitis. The recovery of clostridia in mixed flora from an infected surgical wound should not be a cause for panic. While it is true that, if proper conditions are present, clostridia can produce extremely serious toxic infections, the fact is that the proper conditions—strict anaerobiosis and the presence of free hemoglobin or myoglobin—rarely are found in a well-managed primary surgical wound.

*B. fragilis* are resistant to penicillin, cephalosporins, and aminoglycosides, but regularly are susceptible to clindamycin and chloramphenicol. About 85 per cent of *B. fragilis* also are sensitive to erythromycin, and currently, about 65 per cent are susceptible to tetracycline; the incidence of tetracycline resistance seems to be increasing.[14] Most strains of other fecal anaerobes are sensitive to penicillin, particularly if high doses are administered.

## Rationale of Neomycin-Erythromycin Bowel Preparation

This method of bowel preparation was devised in collaboration with my colleagues, Ronald L. Nichols and Sherwood L. Gorbach. Each element in our method of preparing the colon for elective operation was deliberately chosen from among available alternatives.

### MECHANICAL PREPARATION: REMOVAL OF GROSS FECES

Each particle of feces contains billions of viable bacteria, in addition to undigested cellulose, dead bacteria, and other detritus. Removal of gross feces is the essential first step in colon preparation. Otherwise, the effect of any antibiotic is limited to bacteria on the surface of a fecal mass; organisms more deeply situated remain viable and constitute a reservoir from which the colon is promptly repopulated.

Removal of feces is accomplished by vigorous purgation and enemas. A low residue diet, which reduces the amount of undigestible cellulose fiber and thus decreases fecal bulk, is used during the early phases of mechanical colon cleansing. A liquid diet during the final phase of mechanical cleansing prevents re-entry of fiber into the evacuated colon and maintains a liquid bowel content to ease final evacuation.

Enemas soften feces and stimulate motility. Although right colon content is semifluid under normal circumstances, our experience is that in patients with noninflammatory colon disease, the right colon often is filled with solid, frequently scybalous, stool. In such patients, enemas alone may not remove all solid feces from the entire colon. In addition, use of enemas in the immediate preoperative period might remove antibiotic present within the colon lumen. Enemas also leave residual fluid within the colon.

Because of their limited effectiveness and the undesirability of using them immediately preoperatively, enemas in our method are used to aid evacuation of bulk feces only during the early phase of preparation. Enemas are specifically prohibited the evening before operation, so that residual fluid content will not be encountered intraoperatively and the residue of orally administered antibiotics will not be diluted or excreted.

Mechanical preparation is begun the evening of Day 1 (Table 1) with a 5 mg. tablet of bisacodyl, which facilitates emptying of fecal material stored in the rectum and distal colon. Purgation, using magnesium sulfate and following a vigorous schedule, is carried out on Days 2 and 3. Epsom salt was chosen over castor oil as the purgative agent because of better patient acceptance during repeated administration. An additional benefit of using magnesium sulfate is that magnesium ion directly stimulates bowel motility.[13]

Intraoperative observations during early developmental studies indicated that while many patients achieved complete emptying of the colon with only two or three doses of magnesium sulfate, five purges were necessary to assure complete evacuation of gross feces in all patients. The method

TABLE 1.    Neomycin-Erythromycin Base Colon Preparation

| | |
|---|---|
| *Day 1:* | Low residue diet. |
| | Bisacodyl, one 5 mg. tablet orally at 6 P.M. |
| *Day 2:* | Continue low residue diet. |
| | Magnesium sulfate, 30 ml. 50 per cent solution (15 grams), orally at 10:00 A.M., 2:00 P.M., and 6:00 P.M. |
| | Saline enemas in evening until return clear. |
| *Day 3:* | Clear liquid diet; supplemental intravenous fluids as needed. |
| | Magnesium sulfate, in same dose, at 10:00 A.M. and 2:00 P.M. |
| | No enemas. |
| | Neomycin, 1 gram            ⎫ Orally at 1:00 P.M., |
| | Erythromycin base, 1 gram  ⎬   2:00 P.M., and 11:00 P.M. |
| *Day 4:* | Operation scheduled at 8:00 A.M. |

of mechanical cleansing we recommend reliably yields a colon empty of feces and containing little or no residual fluid content.

## ANTIBIOTIC PREPARATION

In choosing antibiotics for bowel preparation, consideration must be given first to the route of administration and the length of time drugs are to be administered. A choice then must be made among the several antibiotics effective against colon pathogens. Preference is given to drugs for which there are no other widespread uses in hospitalized patients.

Should the drugs be given orally or systemically? Preoperative systemic administration of antibiotics is effective in reducing wound sepsis.[5, 19] However, since the objective of giving antibiotics is to kill bacteria within the lumen of the colon, our thesis is that drugs should be applied as directly as possible to the site of their desired action. Thus, we have chosen to administer antibiotics orally. In choosing antibiotics, we have also given preference to the more poorly absorbed drugs, so that the maximal antibacterial action takes place within the lumen of the bowel.

The length of time over which an antibiotic must be administered obviously falls between the minimal time required for the drug to interfere effectively with bacterial replication and the time at which acquired resistance to the antibiotic becomes a significant factor. Studies have shown that antibiotics administered for 20 to 24 hours are effective in reducing numbers of fecal aerobes.[16] Whether a much shorter period of drug treatment would be as effective is not known. Toward the other end of the time spectrum, resistant strains of bacteria have been found to dominate the fecal flora within 72 hours of the start of antimicrobial therapy.[15, 25]

The development of bacterial resistance to antibiotics is a very complex process.[8, 9] An oversimplified view recognizes two major mechanisms of resistance: genotypic alteration and phenotypic adaptation. Genotypic (chromosomal) alteration involves selection, in the presence of an antibiotic, of spontaneously occurring mutants resistant to the antibiotic. The rate of appearance of genotypically resistant bacteria is relatively slow and is a function of the rate of bacterial replication; antibiotic must be present continuously. Phenotypic adaptation is a much more rapid process, which involves induction in bacteria of extrachromosomal DNA particles, called plasmids, which confer resistance, usually by directing enzyme synthesis. Plasmids may appear in bacteria after very short exposure to low doses of antibiotics. Further, among the Enterobacteriaceae (including *E. coli* and related fecal aerobes), plasmids can be transferred rapidly from one bacterium to another via cytoplasmic processes (pili). As a result, antibiotic resistance among coliforms appears and spreads rapidly; in vitro studies document the dominance of resistant organisms within 24 hours after exposure to an antibiotic.[11, 22]

We administer antibiotics for the shortest time known to be effective and use relatively small doses of drugs at each administration. Arbitrarily, we elected to begin administration of antibiotics together with the last dose of purgative to achieve distribution of the antibiotic in the distal colon. Several hours preoperatively, we administer another dose of antibiotics that act within the proximal colon.

The most important decision, of course, concerns selection of the specific antibiotics to be used. As indicated previously, the desired qualities are effectiveness against fecal pathogens, poor absorption, and lack of use for other purposes in hospitalized patients. Of the antibiotics effective against *E. coli*, the major aerobic fecal pathogen, ampicillin, carbenicillin, and tetracycline were discarded because they are reasonably well absorbed and are widely used in treatment of hospitalized patients. Cephalothin, although poorly absorbed when given orally, was discarded because it too is used to treat serious infections in hospitalized patients. Among the aminoglycosides, kanamycin and gentamicin were rejected for similar reasons. Neomycin, on the other hand, nicely fulfills the required criteria: it is effective against coliforms, is poorly absorbed (less than 2 per cent) when administered orally, and has few other uses in hospitalized patients.

While neomycin also is partially effective against many fecal anaerobes, its activity is incomplete; therefore, an additional drug is required to control anaerobes. Among the antibiotics effective against *Bacteroides fragilis*, the most important anaerobic pathogen in feces, chloramphenicol was excluded for prophylactic use because of its toxicity. Clindamycin was rejected because of its important use systemically in treatment of anaerobic infections. Tetracycline was discarded because it is reasonably well absorbed and also because of the relatively high (about 30 per cent and increasing) incidence of resistance to the drug. Erythromycin remained among the agents effective against *B. fragilis*; it has no widespread uses among in-hospital patients.

Among the several formulations of erythromycin, the base was chosen since it is poorly absorbed (less than 60 per cent) and is active against bacteria in the lumen of the bowel without further metabolism. It should be emphasized that the commonly available erythromycin esters should not be used. Ester formulations were devised to increase absorption of erythromycin from the gut. Because they must be hydrolyzed to the base form by the liver before they are active against bacteria, ester forms of erythromycin have no activity against bacteria in the lumen of the colon. Erythromycin base is not an ideal drug for colon preparation, since there are some (about 15 per cent) strains of *B. fragilis* resistant to it and because significant amounts of the drug are absorbed; nonetheless, among agents presently available, it comes closest to fulfilling the desired criteria.

## Are Oral Antibiotics Effective?

Answering this important question involves obtaining answers to two further questions. First, does preoperative administration of oral antibiotics reduce the concentration of bacteria in the colon? Second, is the reduction of colonic bacteria associated with a reduction in wound infections and other septic complications of colon operations?

Evidence of the effectiveness of oral antibiotics in reducing numbers of bacteria in the colon has been obtained in an extensive study conducted by our group[3, 17, 18] and from studies by other investigators.[1, 2, 10, 18, 20, 21, 24] As illustrated in Figures 1 and 2, preoperative oral administration of a variety of

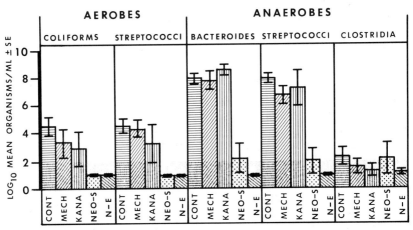

*Figure 1.* Numbers of pathogenic bacteria recovered by intraoperative needle aspiration of the transverse colon after no preparation (*cont*), after vigorous catharsis that removed all feces from the colon (*mech*), and after similar mechanical preparation combined with oral administration of kanamycin (*kana*), neomycin and phthalylsulfathiazole (*neo-s*), or neomycin and erythromycin base (*n-e*). The concentration of microorganisms is indicated on the vertical axis. The shaded area at the bottom of the figure indicates the zone of no growth. Neomycin and erythromycin reduce the concentration of both aerobic and anaerobic pathogens in the transverse colon to levels equivalent to "no growth." (Data from Nichols, R. L., Broido, P., Condon, R. E., Gorbach, S. L., and Nyhus, L. M.: Effect of preoperative neomycin-erythromycin intestinal preparation on the incidence of infectious complications following colon surgery. Ann. Surg. *178*:453, 1973.)

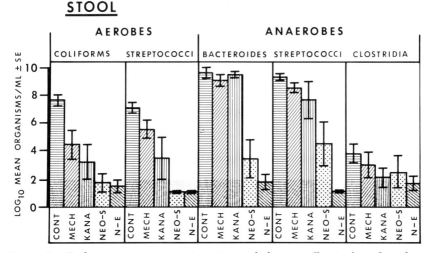

*Figure 2.* Pathogenic microorganisms in stool also are effectively reduced to concentrations approximating "no growth" following administration of neomycin and erythromycin base. (Labels are the same as those used in Figure 1.) The increased concentration of bacteria of unprepared controls as compared with transverse colon controls is due to dehydration and packing of stool in the rectum. (Data from Nichols, R. L., Broido, P., Condon, R. E., Gorbach, S. L., and Nyhus, L. M.: Effect of preoperative neomycin-erythromycin intestinal preparation on the incidence of infectious complications following colon surgery. Ann. Surg. 178:453, 1973.)

common antimicrobial agents is effective in reducing the concentration of colonic aerobes; an appropriate combination of antibiotics, such as neomycin-erythromycin base, is most effective in reducing numbers of fecal anaerobes.

It must be emphasized that the neomycin-erythromycin bowel preparation (or any other regimen of preoperative colon preparation) does not render the colon sterile. Sterility is an impossible objective. However, what can be accomplished is transient reduction in the concentration of organisms residual in the colon at the time of operation. The inevitable intraoperative contamination of tissues from the colon lumen may then be sufficiently reduced so that the incidence of septic complications is lessened. Our experience is that in about half the patients undergoing colon preparation by our method, one or more species of microorganisms may be recovered by intraoperative culture of the colon.[7]

The literature abounds with papers on the subject of antibiotics and wound infections. In answering the second question posed at the beginning of this section, certain conditions must be met. For evidence to be considered reliable, clinical studies must have been conducted under controlled and randomized conditions and antibiotics that reasonably could be expected to affect the colonic microflora must have been utilized. Recent studies that fulfill these conditions are summarized in Table 2. These studies provide a body of reliable information indicating that preoperative oral administration of potent antibiotics reduces the incidence of wound sepsis. In

TABLE 2.  Controlled Studies of Oral Antibiotic Prophylaxis in Colon Surgery

| Author | Antibiotics Used | Wound Sepsis | | | |
|--------|------------------|--------------|---|---|---|
| | | Treated | | Controls | |
| | | Number | Per Cent | Number | Per Cent |
| Everett[10] | neomycin | 8/13 | 62 | 9/16 | 56 |
| Sellwood[21] | neomycin, bacitracin | 4/19 | 21 | 10/16† | 62° |
| Rosenberg[20] | neomycin, phthalylsulfathiazole | 8/40 | 20 | 17/43 | 40° |
| Barker[2] | colistin, phthalylsulfathiazole | 16/50 | 32 | 19/50† | 38 |
| Andersen[1] | neomycin, bacitracin‡ | 5/136 | 4 | 20/104 | 20° |
| Nichols[18] | neomycin, erythromycin | 0/10 | 0 | 3/10 | 30 |
| Washington[24] | neomycin, tetracycline | 3/65 | 5 | 27/63 | 43° |

° Difference is significant ($p < 0.05$).
†Received phthalylsulfathiazole but no other antimicrobials.
‡Some also received topical ampicillin.

addition, extensive, albeit uncontrolled patient experience with the neomycin-erythromycin method of bowel preparation has provided further evidence of its clinical effectiveness in reducing the incidence of wound infections following colon operations to a rate comparable to that of clean operative cases.[7]

In the past, the incidence of certain complications—postoperative enterocolitis, anastomotic leakage, and tumor recurrence at the suture line—was thought to be influenced by use or omission of antibiotics. In 234 personal patients of the author and his colleagues, no cases of enterocolitis have been encountered with the neomycin-erythromycin bowel preparation. Six cases of postoperative diarrhea associated with recovery of *Candida albicans* in the stool have been noted; all patients promptly recovered after resumption of an oral solid diet, although two patients also were given (probably needlessly) single oral doses of nystatin. There have been no cases of chronic diarrhea.

It is our view that anastomotic leakage and suture line tumor recurrence are technical problems not influenced by use or nonuse of antibiotics. We know of no evidence in the literature to sustain or refute our point of view. What controlled data is available in the literature concerning suture line tumor recurrence derives from studies in animals using highly artificial tumor systems. Whether such data is applicable to man remains moot, since no prospective studies in man have provided evidence to support the notion that antibiotics foster tumor implantation. Because the incidence of such problems is so low, our current personal experience with the neomycin-erythromycin preparation provides insufficient patient numbers and an insufficient length of follow-up to resolve this issue.

## Clinical Recommendations for Preparation of the Colon and Rectum

Patients who do not have obstruction of the colon and who are having an elective operation, or a polypectomy via the colonoscope, are prepared following exactly the regimen listed in Table 1. The same method of preparation is used, regardless of whether the bowel segment involved is the distal ileum, right colon, sigmoid, or rectum. Patients needing emergency operations, as well as those with active inflammatory bowel disease and those having partial or complete obstruction, present particular problems requiring modification of the preparation regimen.

In the presence of low-grade obstruction, sufficient to cause cramps or other symptoms but not resulting in dilation of proximal bowel, preparation is begun about a week preoperatively. The first objective is removal of all gross feces; a full liquid diet is begun and a stool softener is administered twice daily. Five days before operation, purgation is begun with single doses of 30 ml. 50 per cent magnesium sulfate solution each morning and saline enemas until clear each afternoon. If symptoms of obstruction do not worsen, once-daily purgation and enemas are continued until the day before operation. Patients then have final purgation and antibiotic preparation as do nonobstructed patients, using the Day 3 instructions listed in Table 1 during the preoperative day. During this week of preparation, if symptoms worsen, the patient becomes distended, or the bowel proximal to the partial obstruction dilates, preparation is stopped, and the patient is managed as are patients with high-grade obstruction.

The presence of a complete or high-grade obstruction makes it impossible to remove all feces from the intact colon. Under such circumstances, oral antibiotics are ineffective. A preliminary colostomy is performed, placing the colostomy as close as possible to the point of obstruction without compromising the future definitive resection. Feces are removed from the bowel proximal to the colostomy by purgation, from the colon segment between the obstruction and the colostomy by repeated irrigation, and from the bowel distal to the obstruction by enemas. When all gross feces have been removed, the patient is scheduled for operation. Systemic antibiotics, as described in the last paragraph of this section, are administered beginning preoperatively.

Patients with toxic megacolon also are prepared with systemic antibiotics as indicated below. Active, but less severe, inflammatory colon disease usually produces hypermotility, so that shifting the patient to a clear liquid diet for 3 to 4 days rids the colon of gross feces. Purgation and enemas usually are not used. Final preoperative antibiotic preparation is carried out orally. Because of increased colonic motility, much drug may be expelled per anum during preparation; more frequent administration of oral antibiotics is therefore required, but the total length of time during which antibiotics are given is not increased. Neomycin, 1 gram, and erythromycin base, 1 gram, are administered together orally at 2 P.M. on the day before operation, repeated at 4 P.M., 8 P.M., and 12 midnight, and a final dose of each drug is given orally at 4 A.M. on the day of operation.

Patients with trauma and other conditions requiring emergency intervention must undergo colon operation without the benefit of preoperative oral bowel preparation. Also included in this group of patients are those with toxic megacolon and those with obstruction who have had a preliminary decompressive colostomy. In such patients, systemic antibiotics are administered intravenously, beginning drugs several hours preoperatively and continuing administration for 36 hours postoperatively. A combination of agents effective against the full aerobic and anaerobic spectrum of fecal microbes is required; our current preference is for gentamicin and clindamycin.

# References

1. Andersen, B., Korner, B., and Ostergaard, A. H.: Topical ampicillin against wound infection after colorectal surgery. Ann. Surg. 176:129, 1972.
2. Barker, K., Graham, N. G., Mason, M. C., DeDombal, F. T., and Goligher, J. C.: The relative significance of preoperative oral antibiotics, mechanical bowel preparation, and preoperative peritoneal contamination in the avoidance of sepsis after radical surgery for ulcerative colitis and Crohn's disease of the large bowel. Br. J. Surg. 58:270, 19711
3. Bentley, D. W., Nichols, R. L., Condon, R. E., and Gorbach, S. L.: The microflora of the human ileum and intra-abdominal colon: results of direct needle aspiration at surgery and evaluation of the technique. J. Lab. Clin. Med. 79:421, 1972.
4. Cohn, I., Jr.: Intestinal Antisepsis. Springfield, Ill., Charles C Thomas, 1968.
5. Condon, R. E.: Rational use of prophylactic antibiotics in gastrointestinal surgery. Surg. Clin. North Amer. To be published December, 1975.
6. Condon, R. E., and Nichols, R. L.: Antimicrobial therapy for surgical gastrointestinal disease. In Kagan, B. M. (ed.): Antimicrobial Therapy. 2nd ed., Philadelphia, W. B. Saunders Co., 1974.
7. Condon, R. E., and Nichols, R. L.: The present position of the neomycin-erythromycin bowel prep. Surg. Clin. North Amer. 55:1331, 1975.
8. Davies, J. E., and Rownd, R.: Transmissible multiple drug resistance in Enterobacteriaceae. Science 176:758, 1972.
9. Davis, B. D., Dulbecco, R., Eisen, H. N., Ginsberg, H. S., Wood, W. B., Jr., and McCarty, M.: Microbiology Including Immunology and Molecular Genetics. 2nd ed. New York, Harper & Row, 1973, pp. 161–165; 1105–1109.
10. Everett, M. T., Brogan, T. D., and Nettleton, J.: The place of antibiotics in colon surgery: a clinical study. Br. J. Surg. 56:679, 1969.
11. Falkow, S., Tompkins, L. S., Silver, R. P., Guerry, P., and LeBlanc, D. J.: The replication of R-factor DNA in Escherichia coli K-12 following conjugation. Ann. N. Y. Acad. Sci. 182:153, 1971.
12. Gorbach, S. L.: Intestinal microflora. Gastroenterology 60:1110, 1971.
13. Harvey, R. F., and Read, A. E.: Effects of oral magnesium sulfate on colonic motility. Gut 14:425, 1973.
14. Kislak, J. W.: The susceptibility of Bacteroides fragilis to antibiotics. J. Infect. Dis. 125:295, 1972.
15. Koonkhamlert, C., and Sawyer, W. D.: Drug-resistant Escherichia coli and Klebsiella-Enterobacter in healthy adults in Thailand and the effect of antibiotic administration. Antimicrob. Agents Chemother. 4:198, 1973.
16. Nichols, R. L., and Condon, R. E.: Preoperative preparation of the colon. Surg. Gynecol. Obstet. 132:323, 1971.
17. Nichols, R. L., Condon, R. E., Gorbach, S. L., and Nyhus, L. M.: Efficacy of preoperative antimicrobial preparation of the bowel. Ann. Surg. 176:227, 1972.
18. Nichols, R. L., Broido, P., Condon, R. E., Gorbach, S. L., and Nyhus, L. M.: Effect of preoperative neomycin-erythromycin intestinal preparation on the incidence of infectious complications following colon surgery. Ann. Surg. 178:453, 1973.
19. Polk, H. C., and Lopez-Mayor, J. F.: Postoperative wound infection: a prospective study of determinant factors and prevention. Surgery 66:97, 1969.
20. Rosenberg, I. L., Graham, N. G., DeDombal, F. T., and Goligher, J. C.: Preparation of the intestine in patients undergoing major large-bowel surgery, mainly for neoplasms of the colon and rectum. Br. J. Surg. 58:266, 1971.
21. Sellwood, R. A., Burn, J. I., Waterworth, P. M., and Welbourn, R. B.: A second clinical trial to compare two methods for preoperative preparation of the large bowel. Br. J. Surg. 56:610, 1969.
22. Smith, H. W.: Observations on the in vivo transfer of R factors. Ann. N. Y. Acad. Sci. 182:80, 1970.

23. Swenson, R. M., Lorber, B., Michaelson, T. C., and Spaulding, E. H.: The bacteriology of intra-abdominal infections. Arch. Surg. *109*:398, 1974.
24. Washington, J. A., II, Dearing, W. H., Judd, E. S., and Elveback, L. R.: Effect of preoperative antibiotic regimen on development of infection after intestinal surgery: prospective, randomized, double-blind study. Ann. Surg. *180*:567, 1974.
25. Winberg, J., Bergstrom, T., Lincoln, K., and Lidin-Janson, G.: Treatment trials in urinary tract infection (UTI) with special reference to the effect of antimicrobials on the fecal and periurethral flora. Clin. Nephrol. *1*:142, 1973.

# Routine Antibiotic Preparation is Unwarranted

FREDERIC P. HERTER

*Columbia University College of Physicians and Surgeons*

The rate of infection following open colon operations is more a reflection of the carefulness and competence of the surgeon than of the state of preparation of the bowel. However, this fact in no way minimizes the importance of bowel preparation; efforts to reduce the size of the bacterial inoculum incurred during operation not only are justified but are critical to the safety of the procedure. The issue is not *whether* the colon should be prepared before operation, but rather *how* this can be done most effectively and safely.

It is my contention, based on the evidence at hand, that the routine use of oral intestinal antibiotics for preparation of the unobstructed colon is unwarranted and that intestinal antibiotics should be reserved for situations in which mechanical preparation is inadequate or in which the anticipated anastomosis is extraperitoneal in location. Support for this position will be developed subsequently.

## Mechanical Preparation

There is no dispute about the necessity for adequate mechanical cleansing of the colon prior to operation. The properly prepared bowel, devoid of particulate stool, does not begin to approach bacterial sterility, but there is evidence that indicates that the total number of enteric organisms is reduced significantly by mechanical measures alone. In studies on the effects of saline irrigation of isolated loops of canine intestine, Gliedman[18] found that there was a linear reduction in the total bacterial count according to the volume of the irrigant. Tyson and Spaulding[40] demonstrated in man a hundred-fold decrease in the bacterial population of the colon after thorough mechanical cleansing, which persisted for 12 to 18 hours after completion of

27

preparation. Despite the contradictory report of Bornside and Cohn,[5] proponents of the use of intestinal antibiotics agree that the desired relative bacterial sterility of the colon cannot be achieved without the concomitant mechanical elimination of particulate stool,[8] and many surgeons would find gross contamination of the operative field by stool or fecal fluid an indication for complementary proximal diversion of the bowel. Hence, the importance of rigorous physical measures to render the colon empty of fecal content would appear to be uncontested.

There are many ways to prepare the bowel mechanically, yet there is general agreement that the essential components of successful preparation of the unobstructed colon include staged reduction of oral food intake and the use of enemas and orally administered purgatives. The schedule I prefer to follow is shown in Table 1.

A degree of individualization is necessary in the application of this schedule, and close supervision by the responsible surgeon is mandatory throughout the preparation to insure effectiveness and to make certain that the outlined measures are not too rigorous. Needless to say, care must be exercised in preparing fragile, elderly, or depleted patients; it may well be prudent to eliminate or reduce the second dose of the purgative in such individuals. The hematocrit and serum electrolytes should be checked on the day prior to operation and deficits restored parenterally, if necessary. When there is evidence of significant volume depletion, intravenous replacement should be started the evening prior to operation and continued throughout the night.

The use of soapsuds enemas should be avoided in the immediate preoperative period; hyperemia, edema, and irritability of the colon have been observed by our colonoscopist after such preparation.[15] In our experience, no such changes are observed following cleansing enemas of physiologic saline.

The preparation suggested in Table 1 applies to the unobstructed colon in which catharsis presents no obvious risk. The totally or almost totally obstructed colon is beyond the effective scope of these mechanical measures; diverting proximal colostomy must be carried out to insure the safety of the later definitive resective procedure. The distal colostomy loop can be irrigated mechanically with some success, and antibiotic solutions can be introduced via this route preoperatively, if necessary.

**TABLE 1.   Schedule for Mechanical Preparation of the Unobstructed Colon**

| Preoperative Day | Diet | Purgative | Enema |
|---|---|---|---|
| 3 | Low residue | Castor oil, 60 ml. | None |
| 2 | Full fluids* | Castor oil, 60 ml. | Soapsuds enema (P.M.) |
| 1 | Clear fluids† | None | Saline enemas until clear (P.M.) |

*Juice, soup, strained cereal, custard, junket, soft-boiled egg.
†Clear broth, tea, water.

The partially obstructed patient presents a more difficult problem in management. Mechanical preparation may or may not be effective in such patients; it generally requires a more prolonged period of preoperative dietary restriction. The use of vigorous purgatives may be contraindicated. When the diagnosis is first made, a low residue diet or, if the patient will tolerate it, an elemental diet of Vivonex or Sustacal should be instituted. Mild purgation should be attempted tentatively; if stimulation of the bowel provokes crampy pain, without corresponding evacuation, or if trial enemas produce no returns, consideration should be given to proximal diversion as a prelude to resection. On the other hand, if these measures are well tolerated and effective, nonoperative preparation can continue. The low residue diet should be replaced by full fluids 4 to 5 days before operation and by clear fluids on the day prior to operation.

During the operative procedure, if particulate fecal material is encountered on division of the bowel, careful irrigation of the divided segments with half-strength Dakin's solution will not only complete the mechanical aspects of preparation, but will also provide a local application of both a bacteriocidal and cancerocidal agent.

## Intestinal Antibiotic Preparation

Intraluminal antibiotics, if chosen carefully and administered in appropriate dosage, will significantly reduce the populations of both aerobic and anaerobic enteric bacteria, provided concomitant mechanical preparation is carried out.[8] Although these populations cannot be eliminated entirely, as evidenced by the rapid repopulation of the colon by the same organisms after cessation of antibiotic therapy, there is no question but that the bacterial inoculum to which the local tissues are subjected on opening the colon is appreciably diminished. It is difficult, then, to argue persuasively against such a laudable and feasible goal, and it is little wonder that the majority of surgeons have employed intestinal antibiotics in various forms since their emergence more than 30 years ago. What must be examined critically, however, is not the issue of whether such antibiotics are effective in eliminating the fecal flora—their effectiveness is well established—but whether this reduction is followed by a corresponding diminution in postoperative infection rates, and whether this potential advantage outweighs the possible complications of antibiotic therapy. These two controversial issues should be considered separately.

### DO INTESTINAL ANTIBIOTICS SIGNIFICANTLY REDUCE INFECTION RATES?

We lack a sizeable, prospective, and randomized study to provide an accurate answer to this question. Existing reports are in conflict. Many studies were retrospective in nature, with all the defects inherent therein, many lacked randomization of study groups and were therefore subject to bias, and some employed inappropriate antibiotic choice and dosage. Gaylor[17] in comparing a randomized group of patients prepared by mechanical measures alone with a group prepared with intestinal antibiotics as well as mechanical measures, found that the postoperative wound infection rate was lower in the former. Antibiotic dosage, however, was less than would now be considered satisfactory. Polacek and Sanfelippo[31] reported a 27 per cent incidence of diarrhea and a 23 per cent incidence of wound infection in a large group of patients undergoing open colon operation after preparation with intestinal antibiotics. Their control group, prepared with mechanical measures only, had no diarrhea and a wound infection rate of only 4 per cent. Grant and Barbara[19] had similar results; they found a lower infection rate and fewer anastomotic leaks in patients prepared by mechanical means only. Altemeier's studies[1] led him to the same conclusions; he continues to avoid intestinal antibiotics and relies instead on perioperative systemic antibiotics. Tyson[40] recommends mechanical cleansing without antibiotics. In 1967, we reported a retrospective comparison of 724 patients prepared for colon operation with a variety of antibiotic regimens as well as with mechanical cleansing and 318 patients prepared with mechanical measures alone.[24] Where the anastomosis was intraperitoneal in location, there was no significant difference between the wound infection rates of the two groups; however, antibiotic preparation appeared to have a definite protective effect in the anterior resection category, in which anastomoses were performed extraperitoneally. Anastomotic leaks occurred in 8 per cent of patients prepared with antibiotics and in 25 per cent of those prepared only by mechanical means. The overall wound infection rates following anterior resection were an appalling 24 and 43 per cent respectively. In contrast, a personal consecutive series of 118 open colorectal operations, including 45 anterior resections, employing a single-layer anastomotic closure of catgut, silk, or Polydek, disclosed an overall infection rate of 11 per cent (nine wound infections, two peritoneal infections, two anastomotic leaks).[22] Antibiotic preparation was used in 33 patients, of whom 5 developed infection (15.1 per cent); of the remaining 85 patients prepared with mechanical measures only, 8 developed infections (9.4 per cent). The number of cases in this study was relatively small and there was no prospective randomization; the results suggest, nonetheless, that one form of preparation has no striking advantage over another.

In an experimental study on cats, Sternberg[38] compared the effects on anastomotic healing and wound infection rates after colon resection in animals receiving preoperative antibiotics (kanamycin and chloramphenicol) and those totally unprepared. Not only was the wound infection rate lower in the unprepared group, but by the fourth postoperative day, there appeared to be morphologic evidence of delay in healing in the antibiotically prepared animals. Dangerous as it is to extrapolate from animal experience, Sternberg concludes that there is no justification for the use of intestinal antibiotics in man.

None of the foregoing studies provide conclusive evidence that mechanical preparation is equal or superior to antibiotic plus mechanical preparation. Nor do the proponents of the use of intestinal antibiotics present irrefutable evidence in their favor. Cohn[8] has been their most active and articulate spokesman. In his study of over 1000 patients prepared for colon operation with oral kanamycin or neomycin and tetracycline, wound infections occurred in only 10 per cent (13.7 per cent for colon resections). He does not, however, have a control group with which to compare results. Poth has been an equally strong proponent of antibiotic preparation; his 1960 study[33] of 170 patients undergoing bowel operation after a variety of preparatory regimens is supportive. Eighteen patients who were prepared by mechanical measures only but received postoperative antibiotics had an 11 per cent mortality and a 77 per cent wound infection rate; in contrast, 58 patients receiving neomycin-phthalylsulfathiazole for preparation had a 3.4 per cent wound infection rate. The study, although suggestive, suffers from inadequate numbers, and the mortality and morbidity rates in the unprepared patients are unacceptably high. Azar and Drapanas[3] cite a 17.9 per cent wound infection rate in 414 patients prepared with neomycin-phthalylsulfathiazole, as opposed to a 36 per cent rate in 31 patients treated by postoperative antibiotics only. There was no randomization, and the control group is obviously too small. The same criticism can be leveled at the study by Haffner.[20] Antibiotic preparation was associated with a 13.5 per cent wound infection rate following 200 consecutive colon resections, but the control group, in which 8 of 13 patients developed infections, is too small for meaningful comparison.

We are left, then, with a mass of conflicting clinical data relating to the efficacy of antibiotic preparation in preventing infection, and we can only conclude that the evidence as presented to date is inconclusive and confers no convincing advantage on either mode of preparation.

## WHAT ARE THE POSSIBLE HAZARDS OF ORAL ANTIBIOTIC PREPARATION?

With suppression by oral antibiotics of the indigenous bacterial flora of the large bowel, yeasts and opportunistic antibiotic-resistant organisms, particularly staphylococci, can proliferate unopposed, producing varying degrees of enterocolitis manifested by diarrhea, severe volume depletion, and systemic toxicity and contributing significantly to wound infection rates. Numerous reports appeared in the early and mid 1950's (after the introduction of broad-spectrum antibiotics) that related the occurrence of pseudomembranous or staphylococcal enterocolitis to intestinal antimicrobial therapy. Although no dominant organism could be isolated from some cases of pseudomembranous enterocolitis, hemolytic *Staphylococcus aureus* was incriminated in most instances of both the membranous and nonmembranous forms of the disease. Hummel[26] cultured S. *aureus* from the stool of 4 of 30 patients prior to the initiation of oral neomycin bowel preparation. Following preparation, stool cultures were positive for S. *aureus* in 23 of the patients; 22 of the cultures were phage-typed as UC-18. Eight patients had postoperative diarrhea, all of whom had positive cultures, and one patient died from fulminant enterocolitis. In a later study,[1] Altemeier, in comparing various combinations of pre- and postoperative antibiotics, found that the combination of preoperative neomycin and phthalylsulfathiazole and post-operative penicillin and tetracycline produced the highest incidence of diarrhea (21 per cent). Azar and Drapanas[3] reported a 10 per cent rate of entero-colitis following 445 elective colon resections; the greatest predisposition to this complication appeared in that group of patients who received oral antibiotics preoperatively and systemic antibiotics postoperatively. Staphylococci were cultured from 44 per cent of the postoperative wound infections, whereas this organism was isolated by culture from only one individual at the time of operation. In Gaylor's double-blind clinical study,[17] *Staphylococcus aureus* was recovered from over 30 per cent of the patients treated with intestinal antibiotics (neomycin and kanamycin); in contrast, no staphylococci were cultured from the stool of patients prepared with mechanical measures only. Vandertoll and Beahrs[41] stressed the seriousness of enterocolitis as a complication; in 766 curative anterior resections done between 1946 and 1957, there were 74 operative (hospital) deaths, 14 of which resulted from enterocolitis. The experience at our institution has been similar. Of the 1042 colorectal resections reported by us,[24] enterocolitis developed in less than 1 per cent; 8 of the 10 patients were prepared with intestinal antibiotics, 2 of whom died. Staphylococcus was recovered from the stool of both. The Massachusetts General Hospital experience was almost identical; Welch and Burke[44] reported three deaths from staphylococcus enterocolitis following over 1300 colorectal operations. Cohn[8] claimed but one instance of enterocolitis in more than 800 patients prepared with either kanamycin alone or a combination of neomycin and tetracycline, and Poth[34] denied a single instance of enterocolitis between 1950 and 1964, despite the routine use of preoperative oral antibiotics.

It is of considerable interest that this form of "superinfection" has not only varied in occurrence from institution to institution but has also virtually disappeared from the surgical literature during the last 10 years. We have not encountered a single case of severe staphylococcal enterocolitis in our hospital during this period, despite relative consistency in the use of broad-spectrum antibiotics. The reasons for this are not altogether clear, but we must assume that the particular strain of resistant staphylococcus responsible for the almost epidemic appearance of enterocolitis 20 years ago has disappeared, at least temporarily. Support for this assumption comes from bacteriologic studies in our department;[14] in 1967, Klebsiella, as well as a strain of methicillin-resistant staphylococcus, were found in a disproportionally high percentage of our wound infections. This phenomenon was short lived and unexplained. More recently, bacteroides have been found with increasing frequency in our surgical infections. Of 46 wound infections following colorectal operations in 1970 reported by this author,[21] 57 per cent were found to contain this organism. This is certainly not a factor of improved anaerobic culture technique alone. It would appear likely that periodic or cyclic variations in the occurrence and pathogenicity of certain organisms can be anticipated, related at least in some degree to the use or abuse of antibiotics.

Experimental work bearing on antibiotic-induced infection is at least suggestive. Following the experiments of Dubos and Schaedler,[11] which showed that mice deficient in normal enteric bacteria were more susceptible than controls to experimentally induced infections, Dineen[10] used neomycin to lower the bacterial population of the colon in mice and then challenged the animals with an intravenous inoculation of hemolytic *S. aureus*. The SD-50 for the control animals was 14 days, and for the neomycin-prepared mice, 5 days.

Beyond the problem of antibiotic-related "superinfection," and also of clinical importance, is the potential danger of suture line tumor recurrence. In 1954, Vink[42] published the results of an experimental study in rabbits in which the implantation and growth of inoculated viable tumor cells at the suture line, following colon resection, appeared to be favored by relative bacterial sterility. This provocative study was duplicated and enlarged upon by Cohn,[9] with essentially the same findings. Our laboratory attempts to document this relationship between bacterial population and tumor implantation were not corroborative,[23] but a subsequent clinical study[25] strongly suggested the validity of Vink's thesis. Twenty-five documented suture line recurrences were encountered following 790 colon resections (an incidence of 3.2 per cent); 15 of the 16 recurrences after anterior resection occurred in patients prepared for surgery with intestinal antibiotics. Although the risks of this type of tumor recurrence are relatively small if assiduous measures are taken to eliminate free tumor cells from the divided bowel prior to anastomosis (bowel ligation above and below the tumor before manipulation, thorough irrigation of the bowel lumen, both proximal and distal, with a cancerocidal solution), it must be kept in mind that the greater the sterility of the bowel, the greater the possibility of successful implantation of cancer cells at any site in which the normal mucosal barrier is violated.

## INDICATIONS FOR THE USE OF ORAL ANTIBIOTICS

Given the aforementioned potential hazards of intestinal antimicrobial therapy, and faced with inconclusive evidence that wound infection rates are substantially lowered by antibiotic bowel preparation, I find it difficult at this time to embrace the routine practice of using preoperative oral antibiotics for uncomplicated colon lesions.

Two exceptions must be noted, however. If the cancer is semi-obstructive in nature, and it is clear that mechanical cleansing of the bowel is not wholly satisfactory, preoperative antibiotics are justified as possible protection against excessive bacterial contamination at operation. The second situation that warrants antibiotic preparation, alluded to previously, is when there is a low sigmoid or rectal lesion in which the anticipated anastomosis is extraperitoneal in location. Normal peritoneal protective mechanisms are absent, and control of contamination during the anastomosis is more difficult to achieve. Thus all anterior resections, in my opinion, should be preceded by antibiotic as well as mechanical preparation.

The choice of antibiotics and the duration of their administration are open to some controversy. Cohn concluded from his exhaustive investigations of 48 different agents or drug combinations[8] that kanamycin was the most effective single antibiotic in ridding the bowel of aerobic enteric organisms. We have found neomycin to have precisely the same antibacterial spectrum as kanamycin, and for many years at our institution, neomycin was the agent of choice in bowel preparation. Because of the lack of effectiveness of both neomycin and kanamycin in suppressing anaerobic growth, and faced with a rising number of bacteroides infections, we concluded that a combination of neomycin and phthalylsulfathiazole (Sulfathalidine) or bacitracin (both combinations of which had been demonstrated by Cohn to be highly effective against both aerobes and anerobes) was more appropriate. During the past two years, I have used clindamycin, which is specifically active against bacteroides, as an adjunct to neomycin. Although no complications have ensued from the use of this combination, the growing number of reports of clindamycin-related colitis probably militate against its continued prophylactic use. Nichols[29] has found the combination of neomycin-erythromycin base to be highly effective, and I have no evidence to suggest that erythromycin, as an adjunct to neomycin, is not the equal of bacitracin or Sulfathalidine.

Our experience with the three-dose, 19-hour preparation, as suggested by Nichols, has not been wholly satisfactory; in roughly half the cultures taken from the bowel at operation, enteric organisms have been recovered in variable number. On the other hand, the 72-hour preparation advocated by Cohn appears excessive and, in theory at least, favors the emergence of resistant organisms. My practice, which represents a compromise on this issue, is to start combination therapy at 1:00 P.M. on the second preoperative day, giving a loading dose of neomycin, 1 gram, and either Sulfathalidine, 1.5 grams, or bacitracin, 40,000 units, at 1:00, 2:00, 3:00, and 4:00 P.M., and every six hours thereafter. This regimen is admittedly arbitrary and perhaps can be shortened somewhat, but it results in absence of growth on bowel culture in a consistently high percentage of cases.

## TOPICAL AND SYSTEMIC ANTIBIOTICS

The topical use of antibiotics during bowel resection has been advocated by many[2, 28, 30] and has an understandable rationale. We routinely use neobacin-soaked sponges (neomycin, 0.5 gram, and bacitracin, 50,000 units, per 100 ml. saline) during the anastomosis, and irrigate the operative field and wound with the same solution prior to closure.

The prophylactic use of systemic antibiotics in the postoperative period is not only unwarranted but may in fact favor the development of wound infection. A clinical study of wound infection carried out by five university hospitals[35] is pertinent in this regard. Infection rates in 4642 wounds of patients to whom prophylactic antibiotics had been given were compared with those in 10,502 untreated wounds. There was more than a threefold difference between the two groups, with 14.3 per cent of the antibiotic-treated population developing infections, in contrast to 4.4 per cent of the control patients. Even adjusting for the large proportion of nonclean wounds in the antibiotic group, the disparity is striking—and, though the precise mechanisms involved are not clearly understood—perhaps important. Chen[7] compared wound infection rates in 331 patients who received pre-, intra-, and/or postoperative antibiotics (both oral and systemic) in conjunction with colon resections with a control group of 326 patients who received no systemic antibiotics after comparable operations. Infection occurred in a significantly higher percentage of those treated with systemic antibiotics postoperatively (11.2 per cent vs. 6.1 per cent); with the elimination from consideration of all emergency, obstructed, or perforated cases, however, the infection rates for the two groups were approximately equal.

The important studies by Burke[6] indicate that tissue defenses are established within one to three hours after the initial injury and that factors influencing the wound response to bacteria are virtually inoperative after that time. In animal experiments, antibiotics given three or more hours after wound inoculation with *Staphylococcus aureus* were without effect. At a clinical level, Bernard and Cole[4] assessed the efficacy of combination antibiotic therapy (penicillin G, methicillin, chloramphenicol) given systemically one to two hours before, during, and within four hours after contaminated operations. This was a double-blind randomized study, with controls receiving a placebo. The infection rate was 5 per cent in the antibiotic-treated group and 25 per cent among the controls. There were more intestinal operations in the control group, but the results are nonetheless significant. Feltis and Hamit[12] conducted a similar clinical study using the same agents (but in different dosages and with different routes of administration), with comparable results. A 1.5 per cent infection rate was noted in the antibiotic-treated group, as opposed to 11 per cent in the controls. Among the colon resections, there were no infections in the treated patients, and a 3.3 per cent rate of infection in the placebo group. This difference may not be significant, but there is clearly statistical importance to the differences in patients undergoing biliary or gastric operations. In a carefully controlled double-blind and randomized study of the effects of cephaloridine given intramuscularly just before operation and at 5 and 12 hours postoperatively, Polk and Lopez-Mayor[32] reported a distinct reduction in wound infections in the treated group; 4 of 54 patients receiving antibiotics in this prophylactic manner developed infections, in contrast to 15 of 50 in the placebo group. The latter infection rate of 30 per cent is distinctly higher than figures reported from other comparable institutions, but the study has validity. Clinical studies of the same nature by Fullen, Hunt, and Altmeier[16] and Stokes[39] are supportive.

Thus there is important, and perhaps incontrovertible, evidence favoring the limited use of antibiotics prophylactically in the perioperative period. The results of this focused and limited form of antibiotic administration stand in sharp contrast to the adverse effects of prolonged prophylactic use of antibiotics during the postoperative period.

## Comments and Conclusions

The issue of whether and how antibiotics should be used in bowel preparation must be viewed in a broader context. The infectious disease epidemiologists are expressing justified concern over the patterns of infection that are emerging against the background of chronic antibiotic abuse. In

1970, Finland[13] described the mounting number of bacteremic patients, particularly those with gram-negative organisms, at the Boston City Hospital, citing an 80 per cent increase between 1957 and 1965. Following the introduction of the sulfonamides, there was a dramatic decline in the fatality rate among bacteremic patients at that hospital; a second, less striking, drop occurred in 1947, after the use of penicillin and streptomycin became widespread. During the ensuing years, however, in spite of the successive introduction of the many broad-spectrum and antistaphylococcal antibiotics, mortality had increased steadily, so that by 1965, the mortality rate of 35 per cent was nearly the same as that observed in 1941 before penicillin first became available! Finland believes that this phenomenon can be attributed to the selective influence of the antibiotics so widely and intensively used in therapy and especially for *prophylaxis.*

Facts relating to the flagrant use of antibiotics for prophylaxis are startling. Simmons and Stolley,[36] in a strong denunciation of antibiotic abuse, refer to a joint hospital survey made in 1972 that reported the use of prophylactic antibiotics in 46 per cent of 331,000 appendectomies for nonperforated appendicitis, 45 per cent of a comparable number of cholecystectomies, and 16 per cent of uncomplicated hernia repairs! In 1972, McCabe[27] estimated that the incidence of gram-negative bacteremia in major hospital centers was 1 case per 100 hospital patients, with a mortality rate of 30 to 50 per cent—and, like Finland, he considered this a factor of drug resistance secondary to injudicious antibiotic therapy. Weinstein[43] pursuing the same theme, reported a "superinfection" rate of 2.2 per cent in more than 3000 patients treated with antibiotics.

Although these reports are general in nature and do not concern themselves specifically with operative infection, the conclusions reached are certainly applicable to the present controversy over the merits of antibiotic bowel preparation. There is little serious doubt about the causal relationship between the widespread prophylactic use of antibiotics two decades ago (both in preoperative intestinal preparation and in postoperative systemic prophylaxis) and the emergence of drug-resistant staphylococcal strains, leading to serious morbidity and mortality from enterocolitis. What has occurred once will inevitably happen again if we continue the same aggressive antibiotic prophylaxis. Depletion of the normal enteric flora, combined with the development of resistant organisms, sets the stage for serious specific bacterial opportunism. Although this may appear to be a theoretical consideration only, particularly at this time when staphylococcal entercolitis is so infrequently encountered, I believe it to be an important one, and I would make the plea that more discrimination be exercised in antimicrobial therapy.

Given the continued high infection rates after colon surgery, indisputable evidence that antibiotic preparation of the bowel significantly lessens the incidence of morbidity and mortality would permit acceptance of risks from "superinfection." However, that evidence is contestable at the present time. The steadily declining septic complication rate following anterior resection that we have experienced[37] is due less to antibiotic preparation than to increased experience and skill in the execution of the procedure. Unfortunately, this is a retrospective impression and it cannot be documented with hard, objective data. Similar fault can be found with the majority of the reports on this subject. What is critically needed is a prospective, randomized study of major size, emanating from a single institution, to help resolve the issue. Not only should mechanical preparation alone be compared with mechanical cleansing plus preoperative oral antibiotics in terms of their effect on postoperative infection rates, but a third arm of the study should include an evaluation of limited perioperative systemic antibiotics.

Until the results of such a study are available, I would favor the use of intestinal antibiotics *only* when the known threat of enteric contamination is high or when local tissue defenses are poor. Inadequacy in the mechanical preparation of the bowel, as when there is partial obstruction, or an anticipated extraperitoneal anastomosis would represent indications for their use. The period of oral antibiotic preparation should be short in order to minimize the dangers of producing drug-resistant bacteria; 24 to 36 hours would appear to be adequate. An antibiotic combination proved to have bacteriocidal activity against both aerobic and anaerobic organisms should be chosen. Neomycin or kanamycin, in combination with erythromycin, bacitracin, or phthalylsulfathiazole, should meet these requirements. There is strong support for the use of topical antibiotics during the operative procedure. The routine administration of prophylactic antibiotics in the postoperative period should be abandoned; if special circumstances call for the use of systemic antimicrobial therapy, there is a convincing argument in favor of its being given just before, during, and immediately after surgery.

# References

1. Altemeier, W. A., Hummel, R. P., and Hill, E. O.: Prevention of infection in colon surgery. Arch. Surg. 93:226, 1966.
2. Andersen, B., Korner, B., and Ostergaard, A. H.: Topical ampicillin against wound infection after colorectal surgery. Ann. Surg. 176:129, 1972.
3. Azar, H., and Drapanas, T.: Relationship of antibiotics to wound infection and enterocolitis in colon surgery. Am. J. Surg. 115:209, 1968.
4. Bernard, H. R., and Cole, W. R.: The prophylaxis of surgical infection: the effect of prophylactic antimicrobial drugs on the incidence of infection following potentially contaminated operations. Surgery 56:151, 1964.
5. Bornside, G. H., and Cohn, I., Jr.: Intestinal antisepsis; stability of fecal flora during mechanical cleansing. Gastroenterology 57:569, 1969.
6. Burke, J. F.: The effective period of preventive antibiotic action in experimental incisions and dermal lesions. Surgery 50:161, 1961.
7. Chen, C., Smink, R. D., Jr., and Shearburn, E. W.: The use or abuse of antibiotics in surgery of the colon. Surg. Clin. North Am. 53:603, 1973.
8. Cohn, I., Jr., Intestinal Antisepsis. Springfield, Ill., Charles C Thomas, 1968, p. 245.
9. Cohn, I., Jr., and Atik, M.: The influence of antibiotics on the spread of tumors of the colon. Ann. Surg. 151:917, 1960.
10. Dineen, P.: Effect of reduction of bowel flora on experimental staphylococcal infection in mice. Proc. Soc. Exp. Biol. Med. 104:760, 1960.
11. Dubos, R. J., and Schaedler, R. W.: Effect of nutrition on the resistance of mice to endotoxin and on the bactericidal power of their tissue. J. Exp. Med. 110:935, 1959.
12. Feltis, J. M., and Hamit, H. F.: Use of prophylactic antimicrobial drugs to prevent postoperative wound infections. Am. J. Surg. 114:867, 1967.
13. Finland, M.: Changing ecology of bacterial infections as related to antibacterial therapy. J. Infect. Dis. 122:419, 1970.

14. Findlay, C. W., Jr.: Personal communication, 1971.
15. Forde, K.: Personal communication, 1975.
16. Fullen, W. D., Hunt, J., and Altemeier, W. A.: Prophylactic antibiotics in penetrating wounds of the abdomen. J. Trauma 12:282, 1972.
17. Gaylor, D. W., Clarke, J. S., Kudinoff, Z., and Finegold, S. M.: Preoperative bowel "sterilization"; a double blind study comparing kanamycin, neomycin, and placebo. In Gray, P., et al. (eds.): Antimicrobial Agents Annual: Proceedings. Conference on Antimicrobial Agents. New York, Plenum Publishing Corp., 1960, p. 392.
18. Gliedman, M. L., Grant, R. N., Vestal, B. L., and Karlson, K. E.: Impromptu bowel cleansing and sterilization. Surgery 43:282, 1958.
19. Grant, R. B., and Barbara, A. C.: Preoperative and postoperative antibiotic therapy in surgery of the colon. Am. J. Surg. 107:810, 1964.
20. Hafner, C. D.: Antibiotics in colon surgery. Am. J. Surg. 121:673, 1971.
21. Herter, F. P.: Preparation of the bowel for surgery. Surg. Clin. North Am. 52:859, 1972.
22. Herter, F. P.: Unpublished data, 1975.
23. Herter, F. P., Santulli, T. V., Terry, S., Buda, J. A., and Beals, R. L.: An experimental study of the influence of the intestinal bacterial flora on suture line recurrence following resection for carcinoma of the colon. Surg. Gynecol. Obstet. 114:267, 1962.
24. Herter, F. P., and Slanetz, C. A., Jr.: Influence of antibiotic preparation of the bowel on complications after colonic resection. Am. J. Surg. 113:165, 1967.
25. Herter, F. P., and Slanetz, C. A., Jr.: Preoperative intestinal preparation in relation to the subsequent development of cancer at the suture line. Surg. Gynecol. Obstet. 127:49, 1968.
26. Hummel, R. P., Altemeier, W. A., and Hill, E. O.: Iatrogenic staphylococcal enterocolitis. Ann. Surg. 160:551, 1964.
27. McCable, W. R., Kreger, B. E., and Johns, M.: Type-specific and cross reactive antibodies in gram-negative bacteremia. N. Engl. J. Med. 287:261, 1972.
28. Nash, A. G., and Hugh, T. B.: Topical ampicillin and wound infection in colon surgery. Br. Med. J. 1:471, 1967.
29. Nichols, R. L., Broido, P., Condon, R. E., Gorbach, S. L., and Nyhus, L. M.: Effect of preoperative neomycin-erythromycin intestinal preparation on the incidence of infectious complications following colon surgery. Ann. Surg. 178:453, 1973.
30. Noon, G. P., Beall, A. C., Jr., Jordon, G. L., Jr., Riggs, S., and DeBakey, M. E.: Clinical evaluation of peritoneal irrigation with antibiotic solution. Surgery 62:73, 1967.
31. Polacek, M. A., and Sanfelippo, P.: Oral antibiotic bowel preparation and complication in colon surgery. Arch. Surg. 97:412, 1968.
32. Polk, H. C., and Lopez-Mayor, J. F.: Postoperative wound infection: a prospective study of determinant factors and prevention. Surgery 66:97, 1969.
33. Poth, E. J.: The role of intestinal antisepsis in the preoperative preparation of the colon. Surgery 47:1018, 1960.
34. Poth, E. J.: Discussion of paper by Hummel, R. P., Altemeier, W. A., and Hill, E. O.: Ann. Surg. 160:551, 1964.
35. Report of an Ad Hoc Committee of the Committee on Trauma, Division of Medical Sciences, National Research Council National Academy of Sciences: The influence of ultraviolet irradiation of the operating room and various other factors. Ann. Surg. 160(Suppl.):1, 1964.
36. Simmons, H. E., and Stolley, P. D.: This is medical progress? J.A.M.A. 227:1023, 1974.
37. Slanetz, C. A., Herter, F. P., and Grinnell, R. S.: Anterior resection versus abdominoperineal resection for cancer of the rectum and rectosigmoid: an analysis of 524 cases. Am. J. Surg. 123:110, 1972.
38. Sternberg, A., Kott, I., Urca, I., and Lurie, M.: Preoperative oral antibiotic treatment: healing of colonic anastomoses in the cat. Arch. Surg. 103:735, 1971.
39. Stokes, E. J.: Short term routine antibiotic prophylaxis in surgery. Br. J. Surg. 61:739, 1974.
40. Tyson, R. R., and Spaulding, E. H.: Should antibiotics be used in large bowel preparation? Surg. Gynecol. Obstet. 108:623, 1959.
41. Vandertoll, D. J., and Beahrs, O. H.: Carcinoma of the rectum and low sigmoid: evaluation of anterior resection of 1766 favorable lesions. Arch. Surg. 90:793, 1965.
42. Vink, M.: Local recurrence of cancer in the large bowel: the role of implantation metastases and bowel disinfection. Br. J. Surg. 41:431, 1954.
43. Weinstein, L., and Musher, D. M.: Antibiotic-induced superinfection. J. Infect. Dis. 119:662, 1969.
44. Welch, C. E., and Burke, J. F.: Carcinoma of the colon and rectum. N. Engl. J. Med. 266:211, 1962.

# 3

# *The Correct Operation for Treatment of Hyperparathyroidism*

THE RATIONALE FOR
SUBTOTAL
PARATHYROIDECTOMY
> *by Edward Paloyan
> and A. M. Lawrence*

PROPHYLACTIC SUBTOTAL
PARATHYROIDECTOMY
SHOULD BE DISCOURAGED
> *by Orlo H. Clark
> and Leon Goldman*

## Statement of the Problem

*Certain students of the subject regard hyperparathyroidism as a generalized disorder of all the glands. The controversy relates to the question of whether removal of an apparently solitary parathyroid adenoma is sufficient treatment.*

*Provide data regarding the frequency of recurrence (or of persistence) of hyperparathyroidism after removal of an apparently solitary parathyroid adenoma. Are these data true: (1) for the chief cell type; (2) for the clear cell type; (3) for those of mixed cellularity; (4) when a rim of normal parathyroid tissue is found adjacent to the lesion?*

*If the concept of hyperparathyroidism as a systemic disease is correct, discuss the possibility that the residual parathyroid tissue left after subtotal parathyroidectomy will undergo hyperplasia and lead to further hyperfunction.*

*Following subtotal parathyroidectomy, what is the frequency of permanent hypoparathyroidism in your series and in others? What is the frequency after simple adenoma removal? What technical method is used to protect function in the fragment of gland left after subtotal parathyroidectomy?*

*If you construe that an adenoma can be solitary and plan to remove it, do you insist on identification and biopsy of the other normal glands?*

# The Rationale for Subtotal Parathyroidectomy

EDWARD PALOYAN
and A. M. LAWRENCE

*Veterans Administration Hospital, Hines, Illinois*

All innovations at one time or other face seemingly blind and irrational resistance on the part of those who have great difficulty in coming to terms with the future.

Alvin Toffler, *Future Shock.*
New York, Random House, Inc., 1970, p. 3.

The current controversy in the surgical treatment of primary hyperparathyroidism is a result of accelerating changes in the character of the population of hyperparathyroid patients. Several centers are reporting an increase in the number of patients being operated on,[1-4] in the incidence of hyperplasia,[1, 3-6] and in the recognition of the disease at an early "chemical" stage when the indications for correction by operation are at best questionable.

These trends are most apparent at centers that have an active group of investigators with a particular interest in calcium metabolism and in hyperparathyroidism. In other centers, the disease may not be recognized or dealt with until it has progressed to the "classic advanced stages"; hence, major discrepancies may develop between observations made at two institutions. Frequently, when a physician known to have a keen interest in hyperparathyroidism joins an institution, a large number of textbook "1930" classic advanced cases of hyperparathyroidism surface during the first year or two. Subsequent cases, however, will have the clinical features characteristic of patients described in the 1960's and 1970's.

The essence of the controversy revolves around the incidence of parathyroid hyperplasia in hyperparathyroidism in 1975. The extent of exploration and of resection is a secondary and technical issue.

41

## *Purpose of This Article*

The purpose of this paper is to show that in patients operated on during the 1960's and 1970's, the incidence of hyperplasia in primary hyperparathyroidism has been rising, and, therefore, that time-honored surgical therapeutic approaches, based on a very low incidence of hyperplasia, must be reappraised and modified.

## *Historical Note*

### *Albert Dies in Vienna . . . of* Recurrent *Hyperparathyroidism*

In 1925, Felix Mandl became the first surgeon to operate successfully on a patient with primary hyperparathyroidism.[7] The fact that he initially removed a large parathyroid "adenoma" from Albert's neck and that Albert's serum calcium plummeted to hypocalcemic levels has been recounted in great detail by Albright[8] and Cope,[5] among many who have reviewed those early days. For obscure reasons, the ensuing events were overlooked: Albert's hypercalcemia *recurred* within a few months.[9] Mandl unsuccessfully *re-explored* the patient in search of other parathyroid "adenomas," and Albert died of the ravages of hyperparathyroidism.[9] Thus, the surgical history of hyperparathyroidism began with an *inadequate* resection in a patient who eventually *died* of *recurrent* hyperparathyroidism.

## *Changing Concepts in Endocrine Pathophysiology*

Cope[5] pointed out in 1966 that:

The apparent incidence of hyperplasias is likely to increase because this has been the history with disease of both the thyroid gland and the adrenal cortex. The first goiters of Graves' disease were called adenomatous goiters. Now we realize that they were the late phase of an initial hyperplasia, and we expect a simple diffuse hyperplasia early in the disease. The first patients with Cushing's disease all had adrenal tumors. It took the surgeons a little time to convince the pathologists that hyperplasia of the adrenal cortex existed at all. Now we know it to be the more frequently encountered type of pathology in Cushing's disease. This is undoubtedly because we are identifying the disease earlier and proceeding with the treatment before the glands have become nodular or "adenomatous."

By analogy, it is to be expected that as we diagnose more and more cases of hyperparathyroidism in the early phase when the disease is mild, more and more of the enlargements will be of a hyperplastic type. The operations for these patients will therefore be increasingly demanding. In a footnote to the same article, Cope pointed out that Drs. Mallory, Albright, and Castleman initially were quite resistant to the idea that hyperplasia could account for primary hyperparathyroidism but that "Castleman eventually agreed with us surgeons regarding the interpretation of the evidence." Finally, Cope stated that chief cell hyperplasia had accounted for hyperparathyroidism in 25 of his last 100 cases.[5] This is already a significantly higher percentage than the 5 per cent quoted so religiously in the literature.[10]

As early as 1948, Albright and Reifenstein[11] stated that:

It seems possible that parathyroid adenomata formation may be connected with the following sequence of events:

1. Some situation tending to lower serum calcium level.
2. Stimulation of all parathyroid tissue.
3. Formation of many circumscribed "germinative centers."
4. Loss on the part of one or more of these centers of their property of being controlled by normal stimuli.

This statement does not require paraphrasing. These concepts, which have long been applied to adenoma formation in the thyroid and adrenals and more recently to the gastrinomas[12] of the pancreatic islets, pertain in general to endocrine glands and in particular to the parathyroids.

## The Incidence of Hyperplasia

### Nomenclature

On the basis of opinions derived from the examination of more than one parathyroid gland from patients with hyperparathyroidism, today's pathologist may have considerable difficulty differentiating adenoma from hyperplasia. For this reason, terms such as "adenomatous hyperplasia," "nodular hyperplasia," "polyglandular disease," and "mixed hyperplasia and adenoma" are gaining in popularity,[4, 13, 14] since they allow the pathologist to straddle the fence or evade the issue altogether. Figure 1 illustrates the coexistence of hyperplasia and adenoma in the same patient; Figures 2 and 3 illustrate the same pathologic findings in the same gland.

To the endocrine surgeon anxious to prevent recurrent disease, only one issue or question is essential: Is there involvement of *more* than one gland? Since treatment will depend upon the answer to this question, the surgeon is interested in distinguishing between three specific categories:

1. polyglandular disease (hyperplasia)
2. adenoma (involvement of only one gland)
3. carcinoma

The incidence of polyglandular disease or hyperplasia in six recent series when more than one gland was examined in each patient is reported in Table 1.

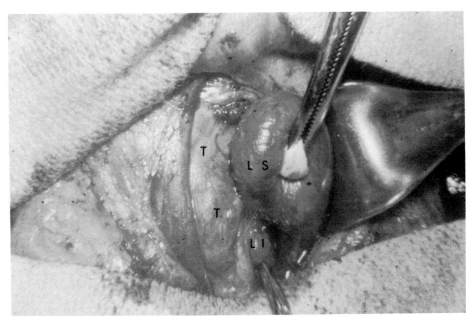

*Figure 1.* This 45-year-old woman was examined for hyperparathyroidism after the diagnosis of chondrocalcinosis was made. Serum calcium was 12.2 mg. per 100 ml. At operation, a very large left superior parathyroid gland weighing 11 grams was found; the cotton pledget points to this tumor *(LS)*. This had all the classic histologic characteristics of an "adenoma." However, the same patient harbored a 200 mg. (five times the normal weight) "hyperplastic" left inferior parathyroid *(LI)*. The parathyroids on the right were "normal" as to size, weight, and histology. The left lobe of the thyroid is shown *(T)*.

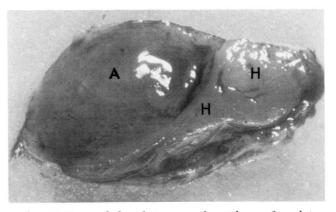

*Figure 2.* This 2000 mg. left inferior parathyroid was found in a 53-year-old woman. The cross section of this tumor shows a darker adenomatous portion *(A)*, which weighed 1600 mg., and a broad rim of hyperplastic parathyroid tissue *(H)* weighing 400 mg. The junction of the adenomatous and hyperplastic zones is shown in Figure 3. The other three glands were hyperplastic and weighed 50, 75, and 90 mg.

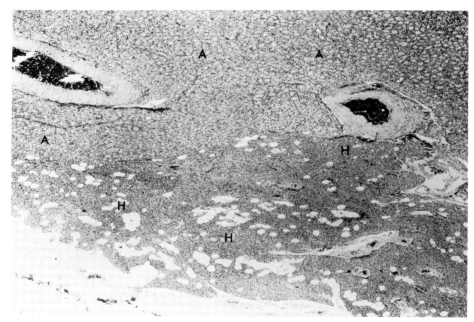

*Figure* 3. The junction of the adenomatous *(A)* and hyperplastic *(H)* zones is shown. It is of interest that 30 to 40 per cent of the hyperplastic zone is composed of signet-ring fat cells, which is considered normal.[13] In spite of its normal fat-parenchymal distribution, this zone must be considered hyperplastic, since it weighed 400 mg. (10 times the normal weight).

# The Rationale for Subtotal Parathyroidectomy

## Definition of Subtotal Parathyroidectomy

Subtotal parathyroidectomy is defined as the resection of a sufficient quantity of parathyroid tissue to achieve long-term normocalcemia. This implies a long-term rate of recurrence of hyperparathyroidism that approaches zero, with an equally low rate of hypoparathyroidism. According to Cope,[5] "In

TABLE 1.  Reported Incidence of Hyperplasia (or Polyglandular Disease)
in Primary Hyperparathyroidism

| Author | Incidence of Hyperplasia | Year Reported |
|---|---|---|
| Cope[5] | 25% | 1966 |
| Straus and Paloyan[13] | 50 | 1969 |
| Haff and Ballinger[14] | 50 | 1971 |
| Johansson et al.[1] | 26 | 1972 |
| Paloyan et al.[6] | 77 | 1973 |
| Haff and Armstrong[3] | 32 | 1974 |
| Esselstyn et al.[4] | 49 | 1974 |

general, with hyperplasia, three glands should be removed and a part of the fourth left." Ballinger's definition is similar.[14] We adopted this approach in 1965,[13] and Block and associates have advocated a similar approach since 1967.[15] The definition of this approach is similar to that of subtotal thyroidectomy for Graves' disease and subtotal adrenalectomy for Cushing's disease. It is noteworthy that subtotal thyroidectomy for Graves' disease has been considered an acceptable therapeutic alternative for many years; subtotal adrenalectomy has yielded to the rather drastic measure of total bilateral adrenalectomy because of unacceptably high recurrence rates.

## Quantity of Parathyroid Tissue Required for Normocalcemia

To determine the quantity required, the following data for normal parathyroids must be considered:

1. Each parathyroid measures approximately $0.5 \times 0.4 \times 0.2$ cm.
2. Each ordinarily weighs in the vicinity of 35 mg.
3. The total mass of all four parathyroids is $135 \pm 15$ mg.[6]
4. There are differences with sex and age. Average total weight is 20 mg. higher in females. The percentage of fat increases with age.
5. By adulthood, 50 per cent of the parathyroid parenchyma is composed of fat cells.[6]
6. In neoplastic glands, chief, water clear, oxyphil,[16] and transitional cells all elaborate parathormone.

From this data, it can be calculated that for normal parathyroid function 70 to 100 mg. of parenchymal tissue will be required in the adult and 100 to 150 mg. in the young. The elderly also seem to require 100 to 150 mg. of parenchyma.

## Diagnosis of Hyperplasia

Difficulties in establishing the diagnosis of hyperplasia, grossly and by frozen section at the time of operation, have led Haff and Ballinger,[14] as well as our group,[17] to generally resect all parathyroid tissue except for a 70 to 100 mg. well-vascularized remnant. This can be achieved by leaving a portion of one or two glands.

## Recurrence of Hyperparathyroidism and Development of Hypoparathyroidism

Recurrence is defined as the return of hypercalcemia and the signs and symptoms of hyperparathyroidism following a period of normocalcemia and remission after parathyroidectomy. This must be distinguished from persistent hypercalcemia following such an operation.

Published reports of recurrence rates following subtotal parathyroidectomy versus excision of the single "adenoma" or less than three glands are summarized in Table 2. The incidence of permanent hypoparathyroidism in similar circumstances is summarized in Table 3. The diagnosis of hypo-

TABLE 2.  Recurrence of Hyperparathyroidism Following Subtotal
Parathyroidectomy (PTHX) vs. Excision of a Single "Adenoma"

| Author | Incidence |
|---|---|
| *Subtotal PTHX* | |
| Paloyan et al.[2] | 0% |
| Haff and Ballinger[14] | 2.5 |
| Bruining[20] | 2.7 |
| *Excision of a Single "Adenoma"* | |
| Johansson et al.[1] | 2% |
| Cope[5] | 5 |
| Paloyan et al.[17] | 15 |
| Haff and Ballinger[14] | 22 |
| Hellstrom[19] | 22 |
| Clark and Taylor[18] | 100* |

*Six cases of osteoclastoma of the jaw.

parathyroidism implies that permanent calciferol therapy is necessary to maintain normocalcemia.

To summarize, the rationale for subtotal parathyroidectomy for primary hyperparathyroidism is based on concepts and therapeutic approaches that have already become well established in the treatment of adenomatous hyperplasia of other endocrine glands. There are sufficient data to allow an estimate of the amount of either normal or hyperplastic endocrine (in this instance, parathyroid) tissue which will be required for normal function. We assume that the etiologic factors which have stimulated hyperplasia of the parathyroids are still present, especially when the disease is diagnosed in young adults. The opponents of subtotal parathyroidectomy may have a valid objection in regard to elderly patients in whom the etiologic factor(s) may have disappeared or when, because of the natural history of the disease, the patient presently has a single adenoma and three atrophic glands. Indeed, one may seriously wonder as to the propriety of leaving 100 mg. of the adenoma in these patients, since there exist a significant risk and incidence of hypoparathyroidism in these patients following excision of the single adenoma.[1, 21]

TABLE 3.  Incidence of Permanent Hypoparathyroidism Following Subtotal
Parathyroidectomy (PTHX) vs. Excision of a Single "Adenoma"

| Author | Incidence |
|---|---|
| *Subtotal PTHX* | |
| Haff and Ballinger[14] | 0% |
| Bruining[20] | 1.2 |
| Paloyan et al.[2] | 2.0 |
| *Excision of a Single "Adenoma"* | |
| Johansson[3] | 8% |

## Technical Notes

The requirements of meticulous technique, patience, optimum hemostasis, and previous experience that are especially applicable to parathyroid surgery have been amply emphasized in numerous articles. The competent, highly respected general surgeon with little, infrequent, or no experience with parathyroid operations may not appreciate the difficulties he may face. Technically, there are a few principles and steps worth outlining:

1. The thyroid should not stand in the way of the dissection. The superior and middle thyroid vessels can usually be divided without impairment of the blood supply to the thyroid gland. However, dissection and division of the vascular supply to the thyroid should be held to a minimum in the region of the parathyroid gland which is chosen as "the remnant."
2. All four glands should be exposed, if possible, before a decision is made as to which are to be excised.
3. The total weight of the remnant(s) should be estimated at about 75 to 100 mg. Sometimes this requires leaving two halves. It is of utmost importance to minimize the dissection and manipulation of the gland chosen as the remnant to avoid injuring its blood supply during biopsy. A metallic clip may be placed across the gland, and the portion distal from the blood supply excised. This assures hemostasis and marks the remnant for future radiologic or operative identification, if necessary.
4. Frozen-section histologic confirmation is obtained on all parathyroid glands, whether excised in toto or left as a remnant. The more experienced the surgeon, the more he appreciates his fallibility. Rarely, even the pathologist may err.

## Proponents of Subtotal Parathyroidectomy

In the following paragraphs, the major flaws in the arguments of the proponents of subtotal parathyroidectomy are noted.

Any single, rigid, and dogmatic approach to such a heterogeneous clinical entity as primary hyperparathyroidism represents a compromise and fails to take into account our ignorance about the pathogenesis of this disease.

Subtotal parathyroidectomy, which seems to be the logical operation for the young adult and middle-aged patients with polyglandular disease, may not necessarily be the operation of choice for the teenager or the elderly patient.

The advocates of a new approach, which is at variance with established precepts, tend to overemphasize the virtues of their concept.

A principal question unanswered by the proponents relates to the long-term (20 to 40 years) physiologic function of the parathyroid remnant. Will it function normally in 40 years, or will it become exhausted, with resulting hypoparathyroidism? There is also the possibility, albeit remote, that this small remnant might become hyperplastic and produce late recurrences.

## *Opponents of Subtotal Parathyroidectomy*

The following paragraphs focus on the weaknesses in the position of the opponents of subtotal parathyroidectomy.

Large series presented for long-term follow-up data are frequently retrospective and include patients who were operated on in the 1930's and 1940's when the diagnosis was made in the late stages of the disease and the single "adenoma" was a prevalent finding.

In these retrospective reports, the criterion for recurrence of disease, or the lack of it, is the serum calcium as determined by the routine clinical laboratory tests. Difficulties with calcium analyses before 1965 have been amply discussed.

The true incidence of multiglandular disease can be ascertained *only* if tissue from each gland is available for the pathologist. The examination of sections of the "adenoma" combined with a visual accounting of the description of structures that the surgeon *thought* were normal glands cannot provide an accurate assessment of the situation.

The pathologist who evaluates the sections of parathyroid tissue must be knowledgeable in endocrinology and experienced in endocrine pathology. Furthermore, he must not be so blinded by dogma that he consciously or unconsciously fails to appreciate and describe the pathology as he sees it.

A report of experience drawn from series of parathyroidectomies done by the same surgeon is far preferable to a report by a resident who performed one operation and reviewed the institution's experience. Advancements in the knowledge of surgery of the parathyroids can only be forthcoming in the former instance.

The fear that subtotal parathyroidectomy will lead to a high incidence of hypoparathyroidism has thus far proved groundless.[2, 14] Actually the incidence may be less than in series in which only the "adenoma" is resected, because the atrophic parathyroid in an elderly patient may not regenerate to a sufficient degree following excision of the adenoma and because proponents of subtotal parathyroidectomy will be extremely careful to leave a well-vascularized remnant. Furthermore, the parathyroid remnant in a young individual may still have considerable regenerative powers.

The argument that if subtotal parathyroidectomy grows in popularity, large numbers of cases of hypoparathyroidism will be created by inexperienced surgeons is a specious one. Should we ban gastrectomy because "inexperienced surgeons" may have difficulties in closing the duodenal stump or performing a Billroth I—technical errors which might well lead to death of the patient? The surgeon who undertakes a parathyroidectomy must have extensive experience with this particular operation, as well as a good background in endocrinology and in the pathology and pathogenesis of hyperparathyroidism. Subtotal parathyroidectomy requires the knowledge and technical skills of the most competent endocrine surgeons. Even though the predicted high incidence of hypoparathyroidism (which can be treated with relative ease) has not materialized, it is difficult to understand the greater consternation about the possibility of that complication than the complication of recurrent hyperparathyroidism. In this regard, one might reflect upon surgeons who create Addison's disease to control Cushing's disease, which at times is a necessary evil.

## Conclusions

It is apparent that the histopathology[4, 13, 14, 22] of hyperparathyroidism in young and middle-aged adults is generally at variance with observations made in the 1930's. Furthermore, the spectrum of histopathology early in the disease is different from that seen in older patients with far advanced disease. We are actually witnessing an apparent increase in "multiglandular" disease or in "adenomatous hyperplasia." This change is probably a result of the recognition and correction of this disease in its early stages and is possibly a result of an increased incidence of the disease itself, produced by new and as yet unrecognized environmental etiologic factors which stimulate all four glands. The questions in the controversy discussed in this article can be answered only with a long-term prospective analysis of data drawn from a large series of patients evaluated by the same surgeon and endocrinologist according to a standard protocol. Specific and sensitive criteria for follow-up evaluation of parathyroid function in these patients must be insured. Reliably accurate total calcium and phosphorus determinations must be carried out in a research laboratory using this protocol. Ionized calcium determinations are desirable. When it becomes available, circulating parathormone immunoassay, with human parathormone as the antigen, may prove to be a very sensitive measure.

## Final Philosophic Note

If there is one statement that can be made with relative impunity about this disease, it is that its clinical characteristics will continue to change. Accordingly, concepts of the pathogenesis and treatment of hyperparathyroidism must be continuously reviewed. The concepts espoused by the authors of this article may well require modification in the near future. Finally, the authors believe that, given a patient with a specific set of clinical and histopathologic findings, most endocrine surgeons today would perform essentially the same operation, no matter with which side of the controversy they ally themselves.

## References

1. Johansson, H., Thoren, L., and Werner, I.: Hyperparathyroidism: clinical experiences from 208 cases. Ups. J. Med. Sci. 77:41–46, 1972.
2. Paloyan, E., Paloyan, D., and Pickleman, J.: Hyperparathyroidism today. Surg. Clin. North Am. 53:211–220, 1973.

3. Haff, R., and Armstrong, R.: Trends in the current management of primary hyperparathyroidism. Surgery 75:715–719, 1974.
4. Esselstyn, C. B., Jr., Levin, H. S., Eversman, J. L., et al.: Reappraisal of parathyroid pathology in hyperparathyroidism. Surg. Clin. North Am. 54:443–447, 1974.
5. Cope, O.: The study of hyperparathyroidism at the Massachusetts General Hospital. N. Engl. J. Med. 274:1174–1182, 1966.
6. Paloyan, E., Lawrence, A. M., and Straus, F. H.: Hyperparathyroidism. New York, Grune & Stratton, Inc., 1973, p. 83.
7. Mandl, F.: Klinisches und Experimentelles zur Frage der lokalisierten und generalisierten Ostitis Fibrosa. Arch. Klin. Chir. 143:1, 1926.
8. Albright, F.: A page out of the history of hyperparathyroidism. J. Clin. Endocrinol. 8:637–657, 1948.
9. Mandl, F.: Zur Technik der Parathyroidektomie bei Osteitis Fibrosa auf Grund Neuer Beobachtungen. Dtsch. Z. Chir. 240:362, 1933.
10. Black, B. M.: The pathology and surgery of the parathyroid glands. In Green, R. O., and Talmage, R. W. (eds.): Proceedings of the Symposium on Advances in Parathyroid Research. Springfield, Ill., Charles C Thomas, 1961, pp. 427–438.
11. Albright, F., and Reifenstein, E. C.: The Parathyroid Glands and Metabolic Bone Disease. Baltimore, The Williams & Wilkins Co., 1948, pp. 47–48.
12. Ellison, E. H., and Wilson, S. D.: The Zollinger-Ellison syndrome: reappraisal and evaluation of 260 registered cases. Ann. Surg. 160:512–530, 1964.
13. Straus, F. H., and Paloyan, E.: The pathology of hyperparathyroidism. Surg. Clin. North Am. 49:27–42, 1969.
14. Haff, R. C., and Ballinger, W. F.: Causes of recurrent hypercalcemia after parathyroidectomy for primary hyperparathyroidism. Ann. Surg. 173:884–890, 1971.
15. Block, M. A., Greenwald, K., Horn, R. C., Jr., et al.: Involvement of multiple parathyroids in hyperparathyroidism. Am. J. Surg. 114:530, 1967.
16. Arnold, B. M., Kovacs, K., Horvath, E., et al.: Functioning oxyphil cell adenoma of the parathyroid gland: evidence for parathyroid secretory activity of oxyphil cells. J. Clin. Endocrinol. Metab. 38:458–462, 1974.
17. Paloyan, E., Lawrence, A. M., Baker, W. H., et al.: Near-total parathyroidectomy. Surg. Clin. North Am. 49:43–48, 1969.
18. Clark, O. H., and Taylor, S.: Osteoclastoma of the jaw and multiple parathyroid tumors. Surg. Gynecol. Obstet. 135:188–192, 1972.
19. Hellstrom, J.: Experience from 105 cases of hyperparathyroidism. Acta Chir. Scand. 113:501, 1957.
20. Bruining, H. A.: Surgical Treatment of Hyperparathyroidism. Springfield, Ill., Charles C Thomas, 1971, p. 65.
21. Paloyan, E., Lawrence, A. M., and Straus, F. H.: Hyperparathyroidism. New York, Grune & Stratton, Inc., 1973, p. 198.
22. Golden, A., Canary, J. J., and Kerwin, O.: Concurrence of hyperplasia and neoplasia of the parathyroid glands. Am. J. Med. 38:562–578, 1965.

# Prophylactic Subtotal Parathyroidectomy Should Be Discouraged

ORLO H. CLARK
and LEON GOLDMAN
*University of California, San Francisco, School of Medicine*

The accepted approach to the treatment of a patient with hyperparathyroidism is to visualize all the parathyroid glands and then to remove the abnormal gland or glands. In the majority of cases, as shown in Table 1, only one gland is adenomatous, and the removal of this gland is all that is required for successful treatment. When multiple adenomas are found, normal glands are also present. In these patients, the enlarged glands should also be removed. Primary hyperplasia, which involves all parathyroids, is treated by subtotal parathyroidectomy, removing all but 50 to 60 mg. of one parathyroid.[17, 21] Everyone agrees that the best time to find a parathyroid tumor or tumors is at the initial operation.

This classical approach to the treatment of hyperparathyroidism has recently been challenged by surgeons who feel that prophylactic subtotal parathyroidectomy should be performed in all instances of hyperparathyroidism because of: (1) histologic or ultrastructural evidence demonstrating that all four glands are or may become involved;[7, 39] (2) the high recurrence rate;[63] and (3) the fact that there is no higher incidence of postoperative hypoparathyroidism with prophylactic subtotal parathyroidectomy.[37, 62] We feel that prophylactic subtotal parathyroidectomy is contraindicated and should be discouraged.

We would like to preface our discussion of the proper treatment of hyperparathyroidism with the following statements: (1) Some of the problems that we are to discuss could be better explained if we understood the etiology of hyperparathyroidism. Unfortunately, despite many hypotheses, the cause of primary hyperparathyroidism remains unknown. (2) Removal of a normal parathyroid gland is of no therapeutic benefit. (3) The disadvantage of subtotal parathyroidectomy is a higher incidence of hypoparathyroidism. (4) One of the major problems concerning the proper treatment of hyper-

TABLE 1. Frequency and Histology of Affected Parathyroid Glands in Hyperparathyroidism

| Author | Year | Institution | Number of Patients | Per Cent Single Adenoma | Per Cent Multiple Adenoma | Per Cent Hyperplasia | Per Cent Carcinoma | Per Cent Unknown |
|---|---|---|---|---|---|---|---|---|
| Norris[58]* | 1947 | Collected | 322 | 94 | 6 | – | – | – |
| Rienhoff[70] | 1950 | Johns Hopkins U. | 25 | 88 | 8 | 4 | – | – |
| Bogdonoff[14] | 1956 | | 27 | 100 | – | – | – | – |
| St. Goar[74] | 1957 | | 45 | 91 | 4 | – | 2 | 2 |
| Cope[21]† | 1958 | Massachusetts Gen. Hosp. | 206 | 76 | 5 | 11 | 4 | 4 |
| McGeown[53] | 1959 | | 73 | 47 | 10 | 30 | 1 | 12 |
| Black[10] | 1961 | Mayo Clinic | 385 | 92 | 2 | 5 | 0.5 | – |
| Hellstrom[40] | 1962 | Karolinska, Stockholm | 138 | 86 | 2 | 9 | – | – |
| Chamberlin[18] | 1963 | Baylor U. | 48 | 88 | 6 | 6 | – | – |
| Pyrah[67] | 1966 | Leeds U., England | 68 | 88 | 6 | 6 | – | – |
| Cope[23] | 1966 | Massachusetts Gen. Hosp. | 343 | 77 | 4 | 15 | 4 | – |
| Schwartz and Hume | 1968 | U. of Rochester and U. of Maryland | 52 | 65 | 6 | 19 | – | – |
| Goldman[37] | 1971 | U. of California, San Francisco | 300 | 92 | 4 | 3 | 1 | – |
| Bruining[15] | 1971 | Rotterdam | 267 | 53 | 24 | 23 | – | – |
| Purnell[65] | 1971 | Mayo Clinic | 171 | 88 | 5 | 6 | 1 | – |
| Krementz[48] | 1971 | Tulane U. | 100 | 96 | – | 3 | 1 | – |
| Haff and Ballinger[39] | 1971 | Barnes Hosp., St. Louis | 74 | 46 | 2 | 43 | 1 | 11 |
| Clark and Taylor[20] | 1972 | Hammersmith, London | 77 | 71 | 6 | 16 | 1 | 13 |
| Friedman[33] | 1973 | Mount Sinai Hosp., New York City | 110 | 80 | 4 | 14 | 2 | – |
| Paloyan[62] | 1973 | U. of Chicago | 84 | 33 | – | 65 | 2 | – |
| Hines[41] | 1973 | Northwestern U. | 51 | 84 | 6 | 4 | 2 | 4 |
| Williams | 1974 | Collected | 751 | 83 | 4 | 11 | 2 | – |
| Myers[55] | 1974 | U. of N. Carolina | 121 | 82 | – | 9 | 1 | – |
| Purnell[66] | 1974 | Mayo Clinic | 475 | 78 | – | 13 | – | 10 |
| Dunegan[29] | 1974 | U. of Pittsburgh | 72 | 74 | – | 24 | – | 2 |

*Only adenomas.

†Chief cell hyperplasia was first described by Cope in 1958; therefore, there are no prior reports of this entity.

TABLE 2. Number of Parathyroid Glands in 527 Autopsy Cases°

| Number of Parathyroids | Number of Patients | Per Cent of Patients |
|:---:|:---:|:---:|
| 6 | 2 | 0.4 |
| 5 | 31 | 5.9 |
| 4 | 419 | 79.5† |
| 3 | 69 | 13.1 |
| 2 | 6 | 1.1 |

°In 1937, Gilmour[35] documented the number of parathyroid glands in 527 autopsy cases.
†It is important to note that approximately 80 per cent of patients have four parathyroid glands. Subtotal parathyroidectomy (three of three and one-half glands) may therefore make 14.2 per cent of patients aparathyroid; in 6.3 per cent more than one half of one gland will remain.

parathyroidism is the difference of opinion among pathologists as to what constitutes a normal or an abnormal parathyroid gland.[13, 71, 72] (5) Recurrent hyperparathyroidism is rare rather than common.

## Number of Parathyroid Glands

According to Gilmour's study of 527 autopsy cases, the number of parathyroid glands is variable (Table 2).[35] In 13.1 per cent of cases, he found only three parathyroid glands, and in 1.1 per cent, only two glands. Alveryd studied 354 autopsy cases and found that 90.6 per cent had four glands, 3.7 per cent, five glands, and 5.1 per cent, three glands.[2] If we assume that these figures are correct, then somewhere between 5 and 14 per cent of patients have fewer than four parathyroid glands. This is especially important for the advocates of prophylactic subtotal parathyroidectomy to consider. If the surgeon advocating subtotal parathyroidectomy removes three parathyroid glands, assuming there is a fourth, between 5 and 14 per cent of his patients will then be aparathyroid. He may also be removing all normal parathyroid glands; therefore, if a parathyroid tumor is missed, the subsequent decision concerning further excision of parathyroid tissue will become even more difficult.

## Histology and Function

Although histologic interpretation in some cases may be difficult, in the majority of patients with hyperparathyroidism, one gland is enlarged and the others are normal or atrophic (Table 1).[24, 32, 72] Parathyroid adenomatous disease is diagnosed by the finding of an enlarged encapsulated parathyroid tumor, with or without a rim of compressed normal or atrophic tissue, in the presence of one or more normal or atrophic parathyroid glands. Parathyroid hyperplasia, however, involves all the parathyroid glands.[21] If one finds enlargement of more than one parathyroid gland, then one must ever so carefully inspect all the parathyroids, since there may be some variance in gland size in hyperplastic parathyroid disease; however, all parathyroid glands are enlarged.[21] In adenomatous parathyroid disease there is generally a positive correlation between increasing tumor size, increasing parathyroid hormone secretion, and increasing levels of serum calcium.[37, 67] Therefore, there is usually a direct relationship between the amount of parathyroid tissue and the severity of the hyperparathyroidism. In a very small proportion of cases, it may be difficult to decide at operation whether a gland is normal; in these instances, biopsy and frozen section examination is essential. We do not routinely biopsy normal glands unless the diagnosis is in doubt or there is some question as to the status of the gland, because random biopsy may jeopardize the survival of normal or atrophic glands.

In our review of the last 100 consecutive patients undergoing parathyroid explorations at the University of California in San Francisco, 91 had solitary adenomas, 4 had multiple adenomas, 3 had primary hyperplasia, and 2 had parathyroid carcinoma.[37] Over 65 per cent of these patients had asymptomatic hyperparathyroidism. We have not found a higher incidence of primary hyperplasia in these patients with asymptomatic hyperparathyroidism, as has been suggested by Paloyan.[63]

The histologic type of parathyroid involvement is important with respect to persistent and recurrent hyperparathyroidism, since patients with multiple endocrine adenomatosis Type I and Type II frequently have multiple parathyroid tumors due to either multiple adenomas or primary chief cell hyperplasia.[21] These patients not only are prone to persistent hyperparathyroidism because of failure to remove all the hypersecreting parathyroid tissue, but also are the ones most likely to develop recurrent hyperparathyroidism.[52]

The advocates of prophylactic subtotal parathyroidectomy state that even though a gland may appear to be normal on routine histologic examination, when it is examined by electron microscopy it is seen to be hyperplastic.[7, 39] However, electron microscopists are not in general agreement that a diagnosis of hyperplasia can be made by this means.[39] It seems that definitive answers to the problems of interpreting parathyroid histology are not as yet available either by routine or electron microscopy.

Hyperfunctioning parathyroid glands have been localized by the preoperative use of selective and highly selective venous catheterization with parathyroid hormone immunoassay. From five reports[31, 64, 69, 76, 78] in which a total of 103 patients were studied by preoperative selective venous catheterization and parathyroid hormone immunoassay, a localized area of increased hormone production was found in 81 per cent of patients. All these patients were found to have solitary parathyroid adenomas at subsequent operation. The incidence of more than one abnormal gland was 18 per cent and that of parathyroid cancer, 1 per cent. These tests, which regularly show localized parathyroid hyperfunction, strongly support the finding that the majority of patients have a single abnormal parathyroid gland.

Perhaps the most appropriate way of determining the best form of treatment for patients with adenomatous parathyroid disease is to document the recurrence rate of hyperparathyroidism after the initial exploration. However, before discussing this point, we will mention another aspect of the controversy, normocalcemic hyperparathyroidism.

## Normocalcemic Hyperparathyroidism

Occasionally, patients with hyperparathyroidism have only intermittent periods of hypercalcemia.[46, 53] Many of these individuals come to a physician's attention because of renal calculi. The percentage of patients with normocalcemic hyperparathyroidism within the larger group of patients having idiopathic hypercalciuria is not known. Magnesium and vitamin D deficiency, as well as excessive phosphate intake, will decrease serum calcium levels in a hyperparathyroid patient.[30, 45] Severe vitamin D deficiency inhibits the calcium-mobilizing action of parathyroid hormone and therefore lowers serum calcium.[68] The mechanism whereby high phosphate intake lowers serum calcium remains a matter of speculation. Theories include a decrease in the excessive bone resorption as well as a decrease in the gastrointestinal absorption of calcium; the latter, at least, occurs with the use of cellulose phosphate.[59]

Although identification of patients with normocalcemic hyperparathyroidism may be difficult, several useful maneuvers are: (1) the serial determination of serum calcium concentrations; (2) determination of the ionized calcium concentration; (3) determination of the serum parathyroid hormone concentration; (4) phosphate restriction; and (5) vitamin D administration. Combinations of these procedures may be helpful. Serum calcium concentrations may fluctuate from normal to high values and back again. Repeated blood tests made over several months may uncover cases of hyperparathyroidism with intermittent hypercalcemia.[46, 53] The combined use of ionized calcium and serum parathyroid hormone concentrations is an excellent method for diagnosing patients with normocalcemic hyperparathyroidism and recurrent renal lithiasis.[54] Unfortunately, these tests, especially the ionized calcium, are difficult to perform. The phosphate deprivation test may also be useful in unmasking hyperparathyroidism in these patients. In normal patients, the serum calcium may rise approximately 1 mg. per 100 ml., while significant hypercalcemia is produced in patients with hyperparathyroidism.[4] The administration of vitamin D may also distinguish the normocalcemic patients from those with idiopathic hypercalciuria. In the hyperparathyroid patients vitamin D administration leads to a significant increase in the plasma calcium concentration, but in normal patients there is no significant increase.[27]

Shieber et al. have described normocalcemic hyperparathyroidism with "normal" parathyroid glands. These patients had recurrent renal calculi and were treated by the removal of three and one-half grossly normal but ultrastructurally abnormal parathyroid glands. No cases of persistent hypoparathyroidism were reported, and the patients were clinically and biochemically improved.[75] Cope et al. found normal parathyroid glands in 17 patients with idiopathic hypercalciuria.[22] The authors feel that in this group of patients parathyroidectomy should not be done indiscriminately but only after the diagnosis of hyperparathyroidism has been substantiated. Parathyroid exploration is seldom a satisfactory method of distinguishing between idiopathic hypercalcemia and normocalcemic hyperparathyroidism.

## Persistent and Recurrent Hyperparathyroidism

In 1971, Haff and Ballinger reported recurrent hyperparathyroidism after 9 of 74 parathyroid explorations.[39] Paloyan et al. in 1969 reported recurrent hyperparathyroidism in 4 of 27 patients having parathyroid operations prior to 1965.[61] In both these reports, the patients did not have *recurrent hyperparathyroidism* but had *persistent hyperparathyroidism* due to failure to remove all the hyperfunctioning parathyroid glands. It seems that both groups did not follow a most important rule in parathyroid surgery, namely, that all parathyroid glands must be visualized before any parathyroid tissue is removed. When patients with persistent hyperparathyroidism have reoperations, even within several days of the failed operation, other enlarged, "missed," parathyroid glands are found.

Persistent hyperparathyroidism may also be the result of an error in diagnosis, since hypercalcemia due to malignancy, vitamin D intoxication, sarcoidosis, milk alkali syndrome, multiple myeloma, or Paget's disease is unlikely to improve with parathyroid exploration or parathyroid removal. Causes of a failed operation that results in persistent hyperparathyroidism are listed in Table 3. The incidence of persistent hyperparathyroidism varies from 1 to 23 per cent (Table 4) and, as might be expected, is highest for the occasional parathyroidectomists. The critical fact is that this persistence is not due to a missed normal-sized hypersecreting gland but to enlarged hypersecreting adenomatous or hyperplastic parathyroid tumors. Careful inspection of all parathyroid tissue can eliminate this problem.

In contrast to persistent hyperparathyroidism, recurrent hyperparathyroidism is unusual. Norris in 1947 did not mention recurrent hyperparathyroidism in his review of 322 cases. He stated that the only effective treatment for primary hyperparathyroidism is operation and that the results of operative removal of an adenoma are generally gratifying.[58] Janelli in 1956 also did not mention this aspect of the disease in his review of 600 cases of

TABLE 3.   Causes of Persistent Hypercalcemia after Parathyroid Exploration

Multiple parathyroid tumors
Error in diagnosis
Ectopic tumor positions
Inadequate exposure
Lack of meticulous dissection in a blood-free field
Confusion with a thyroid tumor
Parathyroid cancer

TABLE 4.  Incidence of Persistent Hyperparathyroidism

| Author | Year | Number of Patients | Per Cent Failed Operations |
|---|---|---|---|
| Hellstrom[40] | 1962 | 138 | 18 |
| Chamberlin[18] | 1963 | 48 | 23 |
| Cope[23] | 1966 | 343 | 15 |
| Bruining[15] | 1971 | 267 | 3 |
| Purnell[65] | 1971 | 171 | 12 |
| Haff and Ballinger[39] | 1971 | 74 (38)* | 12 (1)* |
| Clark and Taylor[19] | 1972 | 77 | 6 |
| Friedman[33] | 1973 | 110 | 21 |
| Paloyan[62]* | 1973 | 84 | 2 |
| Hines[41] | 1973 | 51 | 0 |

*Preventive subtotal parathyroidectomy.

primary hyperparathyroidism collected from the world literature.[44] Paloyan, however, stated that the recurrence rates at his own hospital and those reported by Watanabe are as high as 30 per cent.[63] In his article, Watanabe stated that recurrence of solitary parathyroid adenoma is rare.[77] Black and Zimmer feel that the surgical treatment of hyperparathyroidism is more certain and satisfactory than that of any other surgical endocrinopathy including thyroid disease.[12] Roth and St. Goar have written that in the experience of surgeons and pathologists who are able to distinguish between adenomas and chief cell hyperplasia, recurrent hyperparathyroidism after removal of an adenoma is much too rare to justify exposing patients to the real possibility of hypoparathyroidism that would exist if removal of three and one-half glands was widely adopted.[72]

We define recurrent hyperparathyroidism as the development of hypercalcemia in patients who have been biochemically normal for at least one year after parathyroidectomy. This time interval was chosen because serum calcium may decrease, even if no parathyroid tissue was removed, because of devascularization or traumatization of the tumor.[26] Serum calcium concentration may also decrease slightly after other operative procedures. In both these instances, most patients quickly redevelop hypercalcemia. A thorough collective review of the literature has revealed only 42 patients with recurrent hyperparathyroidism of more than 2000 patients having parathyroid operations.[6, 13, 19, 20, 34, 37, 52] Causes of recurrent hyperparathyroidism are listed in Table 5. Patients with multiple endocrine adenomatosis and those with familial hyperparathyroidism are more likely to redevelop hyperparathyroidism.[52] Subjects who present with osteoclastomas of the jaw also may be

TABLE 5.  Causes of Recurrent Hyperparathyroidism

Multiple parathyroid tumors
Subtotal parathyroid removal
Seeding of parathyroid tumor
Parathyroid cancer
Renal failure

predisposed to recurrent disease.[20] Of interest is the fact that these conditions are associated with a higher incidence of multiple gland involvement due to primary chief cell hyperplasia or multiple adenomas. Even in these cases, however, one usually finds multiple gland involvement at the initial operation. Only two cases have been described in the literature in which a gland that was previously visualized and thought to be normal was subsequently found to be an enlarged parathyroid tumor.[19, 36] One of these patients had familial hyperparathyroidism and the other had multiple endocrine adenomatosis Type I. Kleinfeld has stated that it is impossible to know whether recurrent hyperparathyroidism is due to a new or a missed tumor.[47]

In the last 100 consecutive parathyroid explorations at the University of California, San Francisco, there have been three patients with persistent hypercalcemia due to either an error in diagnosis or a missed tumor. In all three, no abnormal parathyroid tissue was visualized. In our entire series of 400 cervical explorations for hyperparathyroidism, there were nine patients (2.2 per cent) who developed recurrent hyperparathyroidism 2 to 34 years after initial operation. Four of these patients had multiple endocrine adenomatosis Type I and two others had familial hyperparathyroidism.

Both incomplete excision of a parathyroid tumor and seeding of parathyroid tissue at operation may result in recurrent hyperparathyroidism. Burk described a patient who developed recurrent hyperparathyroidism when a piece of parathyroid tumor transplanted into muscle to guard against postoperative hypocalcemia grew into another tumor.[16] Black and Ackerman described a patient who redeveloped hyperparathyroidism seven years after a right lower parathyroid tumor ruptured at the initial operation. At reoperation, numerous small implants of parathyroid tissue were found at the site of the right lower parathyroid tumor, and a normal right upper gland was identified.[8] Even subtotal excision of all but one parathyroid gland would not eliminate this rare complication. Because benign parathyroid tumors can be seeded at operation, careful, gentle, and total removal of a parathyroid tumor is recommended.

Parathyroid cancer may result in persistent or recurrent hyperparathyroidism, but fortunately parathyroid cancer accounts for only about one per cent of all cases of hyperparathyroidism.[42, 51] In some cases, the histologic differentiation of benign and malignant parathyroid tumors is difficult. If there are distant metastases or direct invasion into adjacent structures at the initial operation, then the diagnosis of malignancy is obvious.[17] However, several cases have been described in which a "new invasive growth" causing hyperparathyroidism appeared at the site of a previously removed benign adenoma.[8] Such a residual or new tumor should be treated by en bloc removal including the ipsilateral lobe of the thyroid and regional lymphadenectomy.

## Hypoparathyroidism

Hypoparathyroidism after parathyroidectomy may be due to either decreased parathyroid secretion or increased avidity of the bones for calcium.

The latter situation occurs infrequently today, since we rarely see patients with severe osteitis fibrosa cystica.

The hypocalcemia that results from total removal or destruction of parathyroid tissue is permanent and most unfortunate. The incidence of this complication is reported to be lower for parathyroid operations than for thyroid operations, and the main reason is that the majority of surgeons do not perform prophylactic subtotal parathyroidectomy for adenomatous disease. It seems obvious that the more parathyroid tissue removed, the greater the possibility of hypoparathyroidism.

Prophylactic subtotal parathyroidectomy creates an even more difficult problem when a patient develops persistent or recurrent hyperparathyroidism. At reoperation, should one remove all or part of the residual tumor or tumors? In such cases, is the hypercalcemia due to the parathyroid gland that was biopsied or is it due to another parathyroid tumor? Since these patients may have no other parathyroid tissue, they are even more prone to become hypoparathyroid if they require reoperation after failed prophylactic subtotal parathyroidectomy.

Black has stated that there is always some danger of destroying uninvolved parathyroid glands or their blood supply during a necessarily extensive dissection. He has also written that atrophic glands should never be removed, because the procedure does not influence the hyperparathyroidism and only predisposes the patient to tetany when the adenoma is ultimately found and removed.[9]

Haff and Ballinger reported two instances (5.3 per cent) of "prolonged" hypoparathyroidism in 38 patients having prophylactic subtotal operations (12 of whom had three and one-half glands removed and 26 of whom had three glands removed) for hyperparathyroidism.[39] Despite subtotal excision, hyperparathyroidism recurred within six months after operation in one of their patients. Paloyan described two instances of hypoparathyroidism (2 per cent) and two patients with unsuccessful operations (one with recurrent hyperparathyroidism) in 98 neck explorations for primary and secondary hyperparathyroidism.[62]

Bruining performed prophylactic subtotal parathyroidectomy in 11 patients without regard to local findings.[15] Macroscopically enlarged and sometimes normal glands were removed in the hope of reducing the number of recurrences. Eight patients developed symptoms of hypocalcemia, and in three of these the hypoparathyroidism was prolonged and severe. Bruining viewed the high incidence of severe hypoparathyroidism (27 per cent) after this treatment as a strong argument against removing normal glands. In contrast to this high incidence of hypoparathyroidism in patients having subtotal parathyroidectomy, Bruining found an overall incidence of hypoparathyroidism of only 1.2 per cent in 267 explorations when only the enlarged glands were removed.

One has only to have cared for a patient with severe hypoparathyroidism to know that this is not a minor complication. These patients are anxious and depressed, and long-term complications include eczema, cataracts, calcification of basal ganglia, pseudo-tumor cerebri, and convulsions.[3, 28, 49, 56] Management of the replacement doses of vitamin D and calcium is difficult because the difference between the controlling and an intoxicating dose of vitamin D may be small.[5] Frequent serum calcium determinations are required for years, since a patient's requirements may abruptly change after having previously been well controlled on a maintenance dose of vitamin D.[5]

It seems obvious from reviewing the information available that removal of a parathyroid adenoma is the treatment of choice for the majority of patients with primary hyperparathyroidism. Prophylactic subtotal parathyroidectomy creates more problems than it prevents and results in a higher incidence of hypoparathyroidism. Persistent hyperparathyroidism may be avoided by making sure that the diagnosis of hyperparathyroidism is correct and then by visualizing all the parathyroid glands at operation. Patients with familial hyperparathyroidism, multiple endocrine adenomatosis Type I and Type II or multiple parathyroid tumors are the ones who are most likely to develop either recurrent or persistent hyperparathyroidism. If there is a place for subtotal parathyroidectomy, these are the patients for whom this treatment should be considered, because of the high incidence of multiple gland involvement and the relatively high recurrent rate.[51] If hyperplastic parathyroid disease is present, everyone resorts to subtotal parathyroidectomy. If there is adenomatous parathyroid disease, the authors prefer to remove the enlarged tumor or tumors.

## Conclusions

1. In the majority of patients, hyperfunctioning parathyroid tissue is confined to a single large tumorous gland, the removal of which results in cure.

2. In some patients, abnormal tissue will be present in one or more of the other glands, and therefore all parathyroid glands should be visualized before any parathyroid tissue is removed. If all glands are enlarged, all but approximately 50 to 60 mg. of one parathyroid should be removed.

3. Normocalcemic hyperparathyroidism with or without nephrolithiasis is rare, and methods of unmasking it have been discussed. We have not encountered hyperparathyroidism associated with normal parathyroid glands.

4. Persistent hypercalcemia is due to either failure to remove enlarged hyperfunctioning parathyroid gland(s) or an error in diagnosis.

5. Recurrent hyperparathyroidism is rare and is due to: (1) missed tumors; (2) incomplete resection of the parathyroid tumor; (3) spillage of parathyroid tumor cells upon removal; or (4) parathyroid cancer.

6. The young patient with familial hyperparathyroidism or multiple endocrine adenomatosis has a greater chance of multiple gland involvement. Lifelong follow-up is recommended in this highly select population.

## References

1. Albright, F., and Reifenstein, E. C., Jr.: *The Parathyroid Glands and Metabolic Bone Disease.* Baltimore, The Williams & Wilkins Co., 1948.
   *An original and definitive text on hyperparathyroidism which is well documented and accompanied by an extensive bibliography.*

2. Alveryd, A.: Parathyroid glands in thyroid surgery. Acta Chir. Scand. Suppl. 389:1, 1968.
3. Anderson, J.: The psychiatric aspects of disturbed calcium metabolism. Psychiatric aspects of primary hyperparathyroidism. Proc. R. Soc. Med. 61:1123, 1968.
4. Avioli, L. V.: American College of Physicians, Clinical Endocrinology Course. Ann Arbor, Michigan, 1971.
5. Avioli, L. V.: The therapeutic approach to hypoparathyroidism. Am. J. Med. 57:34, 1974.
6. Balizet, L.: Recurrent parathyroid adenoma. Association with prolonged thiazide administration. J.A.M.A. 225:1238, 1973.
7. Ballinger, W. F., and Haff, R. C.: Hyperparathyroidism: increased frequency of diagnosis. South. Med. J. 63:571, 1970.
8. Black, B. K., and Ackerman, L. V.: Tumors of the parathyroid; review of 23 cases. Cancer 3:415, 1950.
9. Black, B. M.: *Hyperparathyroidism*. Springfield, Ill., Charles C Thomas, 1953.
10. Black, B. M.: The parathyroids. *In* Greep, R. O., and Talmage, R. W. (eds.): *Proceedings of the Symposium on Advances in Parathyroid Research.* Springfield, Ill., Charles C Thomas, 1961, p. 427.
11. Black, B. M.: Difficulties in the treatment of hyperparathyroidism. Surg. Clin. North Am. 43:1115, 1963.
12. Black, B. M., and Zimmer, J. E.: Hyperparathyroidism, with particular reference to treatment; review of 207 proved cases. Arch. Surg. 72:830, 1956.
13. Black, W. C., and Utley, J. R.: The differential diagnosis of parathyroid adenoma and chief cell hyperplasia. Am. J. Clin. Pathol. 49:761, 1968.
14. Bogdonoff, M. D., Woods, A. H., White, J. E., et al.: Hyperparathyroidism. Am. J. Med. 21:583, 1956.
15. Bruining, H. A.: *Surgical Treatment of Hyperparathyroidism.* Springfield, Ill., Charles C Thomas, 1971.
    *A critical review of 267 cases treated for hyperparathyroidism. The author describes the various etiologic theories of hyperparathyroidism and presents a rational approach for treatment.*
16. Burk, L. B., Jr.: Recurrent parathyroid adenoma. Surgery 21:95, 1947.
17. Castleman, B.: Tumors of the parathyroid gland. Sec. 4, Fasc. 15. Washington, D.C., Armed Forces Institute of Pathology, 1952.
18. Chamberlin, J. A., Nicholas, H. O., and Hanna, E.: Experience with hyperparathyroidism. Surgery 53:719, 1963.
19. Clark, O. H., and Taylor, S.: Persistent and recurrent hyperparathyroidism. Br. J. Surg. 59:555, 1972.
20. Clark, O. H., and Taylor, S.: Osteoclastoma of the jaw and multiple parathyroid tumors. Surg. Gynecol. Obstet. 135:188, 1972.
21. Cope, O., Keynes, W. M., Roth, S. I., et al.: Primary chief cell hyperplasia of the parathyroid glands: a new entity in the surgery of hyperparathyroidism. Ann. Surg. 148:375, 1958.
22. Cope, O., Barnes, B. A., Castleman, B., et al.: Vicissitudes of parathyroid surgery: trials of diagnosis and management in 51 patients with a variety of disorders. Ann. Surg. 154:491, 1961.
    *A classic article describing the development at Massachusetts General Hospital of the appropriate surgical treatment for the hypercalcemic patient.*
23. Cope, O.: The study of hyperparathyroidism at the Massachusetts General Hospital. N. Engl. J. Med. 274:1174, 1966.
24. Cope, O., and Goldman, L.: Book review of hyperparathyroidism. J.A.M.A. 228:1038, 1974.
25. Davies, D. R., Ives, D. R., Shaw, D. G., et al.: Selective venous catheterization and radioimmunoassay of parathyroid hormone in the diagnosis and localization of parathyroid tumors. Lancet 1:1079, 1973.
26. Dent, C. E.: Some problems of hyperparathyroidism. Br. Med. J. 5317:1419; 5318:1495, 1962.
27. Dillon, R. S.: Handbook of Endocrinology. Philadelphia, Lea & Febiger, 1973.
28. Dimich, A., Bedrossian, P. B., and Wallach, S.: Hypoparathyroidism: clinical observations in 34 patients. Arch. Intern. Med. 120:449, 1967.
29. Dunegan, L. J., et al.: Primary hyperparathyroidism. Am. J. Surg. 128:471, 1974.
30. Eisenberg, E.: Effects of varying phosphate intake in primary hyperparathyroidism. J. Clin. Endocrinol. 28:651, 1968.
31. Eisenberg, H., Pallotta, J., and Sherwood, L. M.: Selective arteriography, venography and venous hormone assay in diagnosis and localization of parathyroid lesions. Am. J. Med. 56:810, 1974.
32. Fitchett, C. W., and Payne, R. L., Jr.: Surgical treatment of hyperparathyroidism. Va. Med. Mon. 101:101, 1974.

33. Friedman, E. W., et al.: Changing patterns in hyperparathyroidism. Surg. Gynecol. Obstet. *137*:941, 1973.
34. Fulmer, D. H., Rothschild, E. O., and Myers, W. P.: Recurrent parathyroid adenoma. Arch. Intern. Med. *124*:495, 1969.
35. Gilmour, J. R.: The normal histology of the parathyroid glands. J. Pathol. Bacteriol. *48*:187, 1939.
36. Goldman, L.: Unusual manifestations of hyperparathyroidism. Surg. Gynecol. Obstet. *100*:675, 1955.
37. Goldman, L., Gordan, G. S., and Roof, B. S.: The parathyroids: progress, problems and practice. Curr. Probl. Surg. *1*:64, 1971.
    *An excellent monograph presenting information about calcium metabolism, parathyroid hormone, primary and secondary hyperparathyroidism, and pseudohyperparathyroidism.*
38. Haff, R. C., and Armstrong, R. G.: Trends in the current management of primary hyperparathyroidism. Surgery *75*:715, 1974.
39. Haff, R. C., and Ballinger, W. F.: Causes of recurrent hypercalcemia after parathyroidectomy for primary hyperparathyroidism. Ann. Surg. *173*:884, 1971.
40. Hellstrom, J., and Ivemark, B. I.: Primary hyperparathyroidism. Acta Chir. Scand. Suppl. *294*:1, 1962.
41. Hines, J. R., and Suker, J. R.: Some unusual manifestations of parathyroid disease. Surg. Clin. North Am. *53(1)*:221, 1973.
42. Holmes, E. C., Morton, D. L., and Ketcham, A. S.: Parathyroid carcinoma: a collective review. Ann. Surg. *169*:631, 1969.
43. Hume, D. M., and Kaplan, E. L.: Parathyroid. *In* Schwartz, S. I., et al. (eds.): *Principles of Surgery*. 2nd ed. New York, McGraw-Hill Book Co., 1974, pp. 1457–1501.
44. Janelli, D. E.: The parathyroid glands: with special emphasis on surgical aspects. Int. Abst. Surg. *102*:105, 1956.
45. Johnson, R. D., and Conn, J. W.: Hyperparathyroidism with a long period of normocalcemia. J.A.M.A. *210*:2063, 1969.
46. Keynes, W. M., and Caird, F. I.: Hypocalcemic primary hyperparathyroidism. Br. Med. J. *1*:208, 1970.
47. Kleinfeld, G.: A clinical and pathological study of 63 functioning parathyroid tumors. Cancer *12*:902, 1959.
48. Krementz, E. T., Yeager, R., Hawley, W., et al.: The first 100 cases of parathyroid tumor from Charity Hospital of Louisiana. Ann. Surg. *173*:872, 1971.
49. Kyle, L. H., Schaaf, M., and Meyer, R. J.: Unrecognized postoperative hypoparathyroidism. J. Clin. Endocrinol. *14*:579, 1954.
50. Low, J. C., Schaaf, M., Earll, J. M., et al.: Ionic calcium determination in primary hyperparathyroidism. J.A.M.A. *223*:152, 1973.
51. Mallette, L. E., et al.: Parathyroid carcinoma in familial hyperparathyroidism. Am. J. Med. *57*:642, 1974.
52. Marsden, P., and Day, J. L.: Hyperparathyroidism: the risk of recurrence. Clin. Endocrinol. *2*:9, 1973.
53. McGeown, M. G., and Morrison, G.: Hyperparathyroidism. Postgrad. Med. J. *35*:330, 1959.
54. Muldowney, F. P., et al.: Ionized calcium levels in "normocalcemic" hyperparathyroidism. Ir. J. Med. Sci. *142*:223, 1973.
55. Myers, R. T.: Follow-up study of surgically-treated primary hyperparathyroidism. Ann. Surg. *179*:729, 1974.
56. Newton, N. C., and Sumich, M. G.: Hyperfunctioning parathyroid carcinoma. Med. J. Aust. *2*:219, 1968.
57. Nichols, G., Jr., and Flanagan, B.: Normocalcemic hyperparathyroidism. Trans. Assoc. Am. Physicians *80*:314, 1967.
58. Norris, E. H.: The parathyroid adenoma. Int. Abst. Surg. *84*:1, 1947.
59. Pak, C. Y., Wortsman, J., Bennett, J. E., et al.: Control of hypercalcemia with cellulose phosphate. J. Clin. Endocrinol. *28*:1828, 1968.
60. Paloyan, E.: Recent developments in the early diagnosis of hyperparathyroidism. Surg. Clin. North Am. *47*:61, 1967.
61. Paloyan, E., Lawrence, A. M., Baker, W. H., et al.: Near-total parathyroidectomy. Surg. Clin. North Am. *49(1)*:43, 1969.
62. Paloyan, E., Paloyan, D., and Pickleman, J.: Hyperparathyroidism today. Surg. Clin. North Am. *53(1)*:211, 1973.
63. Paloyan, E., Lawrence, A. M., and Straus, F. H.: *Hyperparathyroidism*. New York, Grune & Stratton, Inc., 1973.
    *A controversial book about hyperparathyroidism which should have been titled "Theories about the Etiology and Treatment of Hyperparathyroidism." The value of this book is that it has stimulated thought; however, the authors' recommendation of subtotal parathyroidectomy for all cases of hyperparathyroidism should be condemned.*

64. Powell, D., Shimkin, P. M., Doppman, J. L., et al.: Primary hyperparathyroidism. N. Engl. J. Med. 286:1169, 1972.
65. Purnell, D. C., Smith, L. H., Scholz, D. A., et al.: Primary hyperparathyroidism: a prospective clinical study. Am. J. Med. 50:670, 1971.
66. Purnell, D., et al.: Treatment of primary hyperparathyroidism. Am. J. Med. 56:800, 1974.
67. Pyrah, L. N., Hodgkinson, A., and Anderson, C. K.: Primary hyperparathyroidism. Br. J. Surg. 53:245, 1966.
    *A thorough and well-referenced review of hyperparathyroidism, including pathophysiology, clinical manifestations, and treatment.*
68. Rasmussen, H.: Parathyroid hormone, calcitonin, and the calciferols. *In* Williams, R. H.: *Textbook of Endocrinology.* 5th ed. Philadelphia, W. B. Saunders Co., 1974.
69. Reitz, R. E., Pollard, J. J., Wang, C. A., et al.: Localization of parathyroid adenomas by selective venous catheterization and radioimmunoassay. N. Engl. J. Med. 281:348, 1969.
70. Rienhoff, W. F., Jr.: The surgical treatment of hyperparathyroidism, with a report of 27 cases. Ann. Surg. 131:917, 1950.
71. Roth, S. I.: Pathology of the parathyroids in hyperparathyroidism. Arch. Pathol. 73:495, 1962.
72. Roth, S. I., and St. Goar, W. T.: Book review of hyperparathyroidism. N. Engl. J. Med. 291:109, 1974.
73. Roth, S. I., and St. Goar, W. T.: Book review of hyperparathyroidism. N. Engl. J. Med. 291:913, 1974.
74. St. Goar, W. T.: Gastrointestinal symptoms as a clue to the diagnosis of primary hyperparathyroidism: a review of 45 cases. Ann. Intern. Med. 46:102, 1957.
75. Shieber, W., Birge, S. J., Aviol, L. V., et al.: Normocalcemic hyperparathyroidism with "normal" parathyroid glands. Arch. Surg. 103:299, 1971.
76. Tomlinson, S., et al.: Selective catheterization of the thyroid veins for preoperative localization of parathyroid tumours. Br. J. Surg. 61:633, 1974.
77. Watanabe, M., Baxter, S., and Beck, J. C.: Hyperparathyroidism due to late recurrence of parathyroid adenoma. Am. J. Med. 31:498, 1961.
78. Wells, S. A., Jr., Ketcham, A. S., Marx, S. J., et al.: Preoperative localization of hyperfunctioning parathyroid tissue: radioimmunoassay of parathyroid hormone in plasma from selectively catheterized thyroid veins. Ann. Surg. 177:93, 1973.

# 4

# *The Role of Axillary Node Dissection in the Treatment of Breast Cancer*

THE NECESSITY FOR ROUTINE AXILLARY
NODE REMOVAL IN THE
TREATMENT OF PRIMARY
OPERABLE BREAST CANCER
   *by David V. Habif*

ROUTINE AXILLARY NODE
REMOVAL IN THE TREATMENT
OF BREAST CANCER—AN
ILLOGICAL APPROACH
   *by David P. Krajcovic
   and Leslie Wise*

## Statement of the Problem

*Although concepts of optimal therapy for breast cancer arouse multiple differences of opinion, this controversy focuses only on the question of axillary lymph node dissection in association with removal of the primary lesion. Specifically excluded is the issue of preserving the pectoralis muscles. In analyzing available data, the protagonists necessarily must take into account the questions of extent of removal of the primary lesion and subsequent use of radiation. These are not the main issues, yet much available information confuses the reader with imprecise data concerning these two variables.*

*Examine statistically the question of what fraction of women with breast cancer can potentially benefit from axillary node removal, considering the frequency of negative nodes and the frequency of spread beyond the limits of operation. By what means, if any, can the surgeon select those individuals likely to benefit from axillary node removal?*

*Analyze the data on 10-year survival rates with and without concomitant axillary node dissection. When axillary nodes are removed secondarily (no axillary dissection initially), what are the 5- and 10-year disease-free survival statistics?*

*Discuss morbidity attending axillary dissection with regard to arm swelling or functional disability.*

*Evaluate any data suggesting that axillary dissection actually encourages the spread of breast cancer. Examine evidence suggesting that removal of axillary nodes decreases the lymphatic barrier to tumor spread or that immunologic resistance is altered.*

*Does the size, the location, or the histology of the primary lesion influence the decision to do a concomitant axillary node clearance?*

*What is the frequency of local skin recurrence with and without axillary dissection? What are the 5- and 10-year success rates of operations for local recurrence?*

# The Necessity for Routine Axillary Node Removal in the Treatment of Primary Operable Breast Cancer

DAVID V. HABIF

*Columbia University College of Physicians and Surgeons*

To date, 10-year follow-up studies of 100 or more patients with Columbia Stage A and B or Manchester Stage I and II disease have produced no concrete evidence that any other single operative procedure, or a combination of some type of operation and radiotherapy, or radiotherapy alone is equal to radical mastectomy.

It is well recognized that accurate assessment of the disease in the breast is relatively easy, whereas clinical evaluation of the presence and extent of axillary node involvement is quite difficult. Error in evaluation is greatest when the axilla is "clinically negative" and, particularly, when the nodes are enlarged.[29] The method of evaluating the axillary nodes pathologically varies among institutions, so that it is impossible to compare series. There are differences not only as to the number of nodes recovered but also as to the number involved. At Columbia Presbyterian Medical Center, for example, Dr. R. Lattes and associates of the Surgical Pathology Department continue to clear the fat from the axillary specimens, map out the nodes recovered, and do three level sections through each one. It has been shown[28, 29, 34] that axillae that are characterized as having negative nodes by the single level section do have microscopically positive nodes in more than 20 per cent of cases. Furthermore, it should be borne in mind that patients who have total mastectomy and axillary dissection rarely have the subclavi-

69

cular and Rotter's nodes removed, thus making it more difficult to compare these patients with those having a radical mastectomy.[20, 22, 24]

It is our expectation that with wider use of breast screening clinics and more frequent clinical examinations by physicians more patients will be operated upon whose disease is in Stage A.[30] At the present time, about 60 per cent of women[15] who come for treatment of primary breast cancer have disease in Stage A or B. Of these, about 40 per cent are Stage A and 60 per cent are Stage B. The incidence of positive lymph nodes in the internal mammary chain is directly related to the degree of axillary node involvement in Stage B and the size and the location of the primary lesion.[12] It has been reported[18] that the incidence of internal mammary metastasis in Stage A and B cases is 21 per cent. The percentage of positive nodes found in Level III is directly related to the extent of axillary node involvement.[31] On the basis of this information, it is estimated that approximately 50 per cent of patients who present with primary carcinoma will benefit from an axillary dissection. These patients' cancers should be no larger than 5 cm. in diameter and should be associated with no grave signs. The patients should have either a clinically negative axilla or a clinically positive one with nodes that are movable and lie in the lower or central group only (Level I).

The 10-year survival rate reported for patients who had a radical mastectomy only varies from 54 to 71 per cent in those with Stage A disease and from 28 to 37 per cent in those with Stage B disease.[1, 13, 16, 25, 27] In comparison, one study[7] reported a 41 per cent 10-year survival rate following simple mastectomy in a group of 133 cases which were not staged. A study[13] of simple mastectomy with minimal postoperative radiotherapy reported a 40 per cent 10-year survival rate in those with Stage A disease (115 patients) and a 26 per cent survival rate in those with Stage B disease (34 patients).

If axillary dissection is to be part of the primary operative treatment, it should be done at the time that a total mastectomy or a radical mastectomy is performed. One study[8] reported a 37 per cent 10-year survival rate in a group of 24 patients who had a radical mastectomy following a previous simple mastectomy (the time interval ranged from 25 days to 63 months, with the average being 5 years). The author stated that those patients with "local recurrence after simple mastectomy had a higher incidence of local recurrence and a less hopeful prognosis subsequent to radical mastectomy than patients without local recurrence." Of the eight patients who lived 10 years or more free of disease, six had histologically negative nodes, and the other two had only one node involved.

Patients who have axillary dissections as part of a radical mastectomy or with total mastectomy have little functional disability. Disability is caused by either removal of the pectoral muscles or paralysis of the latissimus dorsi and teres major muscles from dividing the thoracodorsal nerve. The maximum detectable loss of muscle power is usually 5 to 10 per cent, and there should always be a full range of motion. Arm edema (greater than a 3 cm. increase in diameter) develops in about 10 per cent of patients who are operated upon at Presbyterian Hospital, and other authors report about the same incidence.[3, 33] Those patients who have total mastectomy and axillary dissection have a lower incidence of postoperative edema because fewer nodes are removed. Edema is more likely to develop in patients who have obese arms, in those who have postoperative wound complications, particularly flap necrosis and infection, and in those who sustain repeated breaks in the skin of the homolateral hand and arm, which allow bacterial entry and infection.

Axillary dissection should be performed in Stage A and B cases only, because there is a greater likelihood that the operation will be performed through a plane of uninvolved tissue. In Stage C, where there is apt to be more extensive axillary node involvement, there is usually permeating cancer in the lymphatic channels, and there is a higher incidence of local recurrence and, not uncommonly, an earlier demise.[14, 17, 26] The local recurrence rate within 10 years is 7 to 16 per cent in Stage A, 18 to 26 per cent in Stage B, and 29 to 87 per cent in Stage C.[17]

On the basis of information obtained from in vitro studies,[19] the experimental animal,[6, 11] and to some extent, from the human,[10] some investigators have suggested that the regional lymph nodes are immunologically involved in the host response to its tumor. It has been recommended that the axillary nodes not be removed until they are grossly involved with cancer.[6]

It has been demonstrated "that practically all regional lymph node cells from specimens of human mammary carcinoma may be stimulated by phytohemagglutinin which implies immunocompetence."[10] However, others,[21] using a different method of assessment, have shown that regional nodes in humans with mammary carcinoma are not immune competent and possibly are incompetent. This author concludes that there is no concrete evidence to show that removal of axillary nodes in primary operable carcinoma of the breast either decreases the barrier to tumor spread or results in altered immunologic resistance.

When contemplating an axillary dissection for primary operable carcinoma, it is well to keep in mind that large cancers (except for the medullary type) that are greater than 5 cm. in diameter, those that are biologically highly invasive, and those that are located in the central or medial aspect of the breast are associated with a poorer prognosis.[4, 7, 14, 26, 31, 35] Such tumors are more likely to be Stage C.

It is generally agreed that local recurrence following axillary dissection implies a grave prognosis. Such recurrence may be due to the presence of tumor cells in the dermal lymphatics or upgrowth from the internal mammary nodes and from axillary lymphatics or nodes.[9] The majority of patients with local recurrence die within two years from distant metastases. There is complete agreement about the best treatment for local recurrence — namely, radiotherapy. Surgery is employed, when possible, for postradiation recurrence of recurrent tumor in selected cases.

Axillary dissection with total mastectomy or as part of a radical mastectomy is, at present, the best treatment for Stage A and B cases, not only to control local disease but also to achieve the highest survival rate. There is no evidence that axillary dissection is associated with significant morbidity or that it interferes with the patient's immunologic resistance.

# *References*

1. Adair, F., Berg, J., Joubert, L., and Robbins, G. F.: Long-term follow-up of breast cancer patients: the 30 year report. Cancer *33*:1145–1150, 1974.
2. Atkins, H., Hayward, J. L., Klugman, D. J., and Wayte, A. B.: Treatment of early breast cancer: a report after ten years of a clinical trial. Br. Med. J. *2*:423–429, 1972.
3. Britton, R. C., and Nelson, P. A.: Causes and treatment of postmastectomy lymphedema of the arm. J.A.M.A. *180*:95–102, 1962.
4. Christopherson, W. M.: Prognosis of breast cancer based on pathologic type. Cancer *24*:1179–1181, 1969.
5. Crile, G., Jr.: Simplified treatment of cancer of the breast: early results of a clinical study. Ann. Surg. *153*:745–761, 1961.
6. Crile, G., Jr.: A *Biological Consideration of Treatment of Breast Cancer.* Springfield, Ill., Charles C Thomas, 1967.
7. Crile, G., Jr.: Breast cancer: relationship of the size of the tumor and the size of involved nodes to survival. Am. J. Surg. *124*:35–38, 1972.
8. Donegan, W. L.: An evaluation of radical mastectomy following simple mastectomy for carcinoma of the breast. Mo. Med. *61*:1014–1018, 1964.
9. Donegan, W. L., Perez-Mesa, C. M., and Watson, F. R.: A biostatistical study of locally recurrent breast carcinoma. Surg. Gynecol. Obstet. *122*:529–540, 1966.
10. Fisher, B., Saffer, E. A., and Fisher, E. R.: Studies concerning the regional lymph node in cancer. III. Response of regional lymph node cells from breast and colon cancer patients to PHA stimulation. Cancer *30*:1202–1215, 1972.
11. Fisher, B., Saffer, E. A., and Fisher, E. R.: Studies concerning the regional lymph node in cancer. IV. Tumor inhibition by regional lymph nodes. Cancer 33:631–636, 1974.
12. Haagensen, C. D., Bhonslay, S. B., Guttmann, R. J., et al.: Metastasis of carcinoma of the breast to the periphery of the regional lymph node filter. Ann. Surg. *169*:174–190, 1969.
13. Haagensen, C. D., Cooley, E., Miller, E., Handley, R. S., Thackray, A. C., Butcher, H. R., Dahl-Iversen, E., Tobiassen, T., Eilliams, I. G., Stone, J., Kaae, S., and Johansen, H.: Treatment of early mammary carcinoma: a cooperative international study. Ann. Surg. *170*:875–899, 1969.
14. Haagensen, C. D.: *Diseases of the Breast.* 2nd ed. Philadelphia, W. B. Saunders Co., 1971.
15. Haagensen, C. D.: A great leap backward in the treatment of carcinoma of the breast. J.A.M.A. *224*:1181–1183, 1973.
16. Haimov, M., Kark, A. E., and Lesnick, G. J.: Carcinoma of the breast. Thirty years' experience with radical mastectomy. Am. J. Surg. *115*:341–348, 1968.
17. Handley, R. S.: Indications and contraindications for mastectomy. J.A.M.A. *200*:610–612, 1967.
18. Handley, R. S.: Observations and thoughts on cancer of the breast. Proc. R. Soc. Med. *65*:437–444, 1972.
19. Hellstrom, I., Hellstrom, K. E., and Pierce, G. E.: In vitro studies of immune reactions against autochthonous and syngeneic mouse tumors induced by methylcholanthrene and plastic discs. Int. J. Cancer *3*:467–482, 1968.
20. Hultborn, A., Hulten, L., Roos, B., Rosencrantz, M., Bosengren, B., Aohrien, C.: Effectiveness of axillary lymph node dissection in modified radical mastectomy with preservation of pectoral muscles. Ann. Surg. *179*:269–272, 1974.
21. Humphrey, L. J., Barker, C., Bokesch, C., et al.: Immunologic competence of regional lymph nodes in patients with mammary cancer. Ann. Surg. *174*:383–391, 1971.
22. Huvos, A. G., Hutter, R. V. P., and Berg, J. W.: Significance of axillary macrometastases and micrometastases in mammary cancer. Ann. Surg. *173*:44–46, 1971.
23. Johnstone, F. R. C.: Carcinoma of the breast; influence of size of primary lesion and lymph node involvement based on selective biopsy. Am. J. Surg. *124*:158–164, 1972.
24. Kay, S.: Evaluation of Rotter's lymph nodes in radical mastectomy specimens as a guide to prognosis. Cancer *18*:1441–1444, 1965.
25. Leak, G. H., Berg, J., Wesp, E. H., and Robbins, G. F.: Primary treatment of patients with resectable breast carcinoma. Surg. Gynecol. Obstet. *129*:953–959, 1969.
26. Moore, F. D., Woodrow, S. I., Aliapoulios, M. A., et al.: Carcinoma of the breast. N. Engl. J. Med. *277*:343–350, 1967.
27. Payne, W. S., Taylor, W. F., Khonsari, F., et al.: Surgical treatment of breast cancer: trends and factors affecting survival. Arch. Surg. *101*:105–113, 1970.
28. Pickren, J. W.: Lymph node metastasis in carcinoma of the female mammary gland. Roswell Park Bulletin *1*:79–90, 1956.
29. Pickren, J. W.: Significance of occult metastases. Cancer *14*:1266–1271, 1961.

30. Rauscher, F. J.: Special communication. Report to the profession from the Breast Cancer Task Force. Sept. 30, 1974.
31. Robbins, G. F.: Long-term survivals among primary operable breast cancer patients with metastatic axillary lymph nodes at Level III. International Union against Cancer *18*:864–867, 1962.
32. Robbins, G. F.: The rationale for the treatment of women with potentially curable breast carcinoma. Surg. Clin. North Am. *54*:793–800, 1974.
33. Sabiston, D. C., Jr., and Shingleton, W. W.: The surgical management of breast cancer. Surg. Clin. North Am. *46*:1265–1282, 1966.
34. Saphir, O., and Amromin, G. D.: Obscure axillary lymph node metastasis in carcinoma of the breast. Cancer *1*:238–241, 1948.
35. Say, C. C., and Donegan, W. L.: Invasive carcinoma of the breast: prognostic significance of tumor size and involved axillary lymph nodes. Cancer *34*:468–471, 1974.

# Routine Axillary Node Removal in the Treatment of Breast Cancer—an Illogical Approach

**DAVID P. KRAJCOVIC**

*Washington University School of Medicine, St. Louis, Missouri*

and **LESLIE WISE**

*State University of New York at Stony Brook School of Medicine*

One of the earliest papers in the English literature advocating axillary dissection for breast cancer was authored by Banks[2] in 1882 and was entitled "On Free Removal of Mammary Cancer with Extirpation of the Axillary Glands as a Necessary Accomplishment." It is William Halsted, of the Johns Hopkins Hospital, however, who is credited with being the prime advocate of radical mastectomy as we know it today. The procedure reported by him in 1894[16] was a synthesis of what certain of his predecessors and contemporaries had recommended and included complete removal of all breast tissue, the underlying muscles, and the axillary glands.[20]

Radical mastectomy has remained the standard surgical technique for treating potentially curable primary carcinoma of the breast in the United States over the past 80 years. Despite its being the most popular and common procedure, radical mastectomy has been subject to increasing challenges by proponents of both more extensive and more limited procedures. Dissatisfaction with radical mastectomy has been most noticeable in Great Britain, where presently it is used in less than 20 per cent of the potentially curable cases. The basis of the dissatisfaction with radical mastectomy as the method of choice in the treatment of potentially curable breast cancer is that with this mode of therapy nearly 50 per cent of patients eventually die from this disease,[5] and this result is essentially unchanged from what was accomplished 50 years ago. This dismal prognosis and the lack of improvement in survival have led many surgeons to look more critically at the true value of radical mastectomy.[27]

One of the issues that have been most debated is the value of axillary resection. The pioneer in questioning the need for axillary resection in treating breast cancer was McWhirter, who in 1948 suggested that simple mastectomy combined with postoperative radiation therapy might provide long-term results similar to or better than those of radical mastectomy.[21] The rationale of his approach was that radiotherapy could eradicate axillary metastases as effectively as operative excision. Although McWhirter was criticized for comparing results of different modes of therapy from different time periods, his data indicated a 55 per cent 5-year survival rate after simple mastectomy and irradiation as compared to a rate of 44 per cent for patients treated with radical mastectomy alone.

Following McWhirter's lead, authors have filled the literature with numerous studies during the past 25 years, but most of these are of no particular value from our point of view, because they are only retrospective chart reviews of one particular form of treatment. In Table 1, we summarized the results of the studies in which axillary node resection was compared with a method of therapy which did not involve axillary node removal.

As seen from the data presented in Table 1, there is no evidence to suggest that axillary resection is of greater value in the treatment of breast cancer than radiotherapy to the axillary glands. In fact, from the theoretical point of view, radical mastectomy is an illogical operation, and were it not for the influence of Halsted, it probably would have faded into oblivion long ago.

The strongest argument against radical mastectomy is that, while it is purported to be an en bloc cancer resection, it is not. The axillary group of lymph nodes is the major lymph drainage pathway from the breast; however, there is also substantial drainage to the internal mammary chain and from both areas to the supraclavicular lymph nodes. Using dye and colloidal gold injections, Turner-Warwick[25] found that 75 per cent of the lymphatic drainage of the breast is to the ipsilateral axillary nodes, while the remainder is mainly to the ipsilateral internal mammary chain. The classic study on the regional lymph node metastases of breast cancer was done by Handley and Thackray, who performed routine biopsies of the internal mammary group of lymph nodes in a series of patients undergoing radical mastectomy.[17] They concluded that 25 per cent of patients undergoing radical mastectomy had metastases to the internal mammary lymph nodes, and that this figure ranged from 10 per cent to 60 per cent, depending upon the location of the tumor within the breast and whether or not the axillary lymph nodes harbored metastases.

Therefore, to be logical and consistent in the surgical approach for breast cancer, appropriate treatment would have to include resection of the internal mammary lymph node chain. Attempts to extend the operation to include this area by Dahl-Iversen[8] and Cáceres[4] have repeatedly failed to show improved survival and curability. In fact, acceptance of incurability by surgical means in patients with occult metastases at the periphery of the regional lymph node filter for the breast led Haagensen, the most ardent advocate of radical mastectomy, to perform his triple biopsy technique for many years (1951 to 1966). This technique included biopsies of the breast

TABLE 1. Comparison of Survival Rates Following Different Methods of Treatment for Breast Carcinoma

| Author | Stage of Disease (Man-chester) | Number of Patients in Trial Group | Method of Treatment | 5-Year Survival Rate (Per Cent) | 10-Year Survival Rate (Per Cent) |
|---|---|---|---|---|---|
| Porritt[23] | I and II | 107 | Local excision and irradiation | 65 | 45 |
| | I and II | 156 | Radical mastectomy and irradiation | 50 | 34 |
| Peters[22] | I and II | 124 | Local excision and irradiation | 76 | 45 |
| | I and II | 344 | Radical mastectomy and irradiation | 72 | 44 |
| Kaae and Johansen[19] | I | 159 | Simple mastectomy and irradiation | 70 | 50 |
| | | 134 | Extended supraradical mastectomy | 74 | 55 |
| | II | 28 | Simple mastectomy and irradiation | 50 | 32 |
| | | 32 | Supraradical mastectomy | 47 | 34 |
| Wise, Mason, and Ackerman[26] | I | 49 | Local excision and irradiation | 96 | 68 |
| | | 93 | Radical mastectomy | 81 | 69 |
| | II | 47 | Local excision and irradiation | 74 | 53 |
| | | 114 | Radical mastectomy and irradiation | 70 | 59 |
| Brinkley and Haybittle[3] | II | 113 | Simple mastectomy and irradiation | 64 | 46 |
| | | 91 | Radical mastectomy and irradiation | 61 | 49 |
| Atkins et al.[1]* | I | 112 | Local excision and irradiation | 80 | 80 |
| | | 108 | Radical mastectomy | 78 | 78 |
| | II | 70 | Local excision and irradiation | 56 | 28 |
| | | 80 | Radical mastectomy | 72 | 60 |

* Total follow-up was 10 years. At 10 years the number of patients was so small that conclusions should be drawn only with great caution. The dosage of radiotherapy given to these patients would be regarded as inadequate by most radiotherapists.

mass, the lymph nodes in the apex of the axilla, and the internal mammary lymph nodes; if either of the latter two areas demonstrated metastases, the patient was considered unsuitable for radical mastectomy and was treated with irradiation only.[14] Guttmann's results[13] in treating this group (a 54 per cent 5-year survival rate) indicate the relative efficacy of irradiation alone in the treatment of patients with locally advanced breast cancer, none of whom would have been cured by radical mastectomy alone.

Since 1966, Haagensen has reverted to performing radical mastectomy on all patients whose breast carcinomas are classified as Columbia Stage A or B. Of extreme interest also is the statement in his recent publication[15] that postoperative prophylactic irradiation to the internal mammary nodes is given to *all* patients except those with lesions less than 3 cm. in diameter and those with lesions in the outer half of the breast and pathologically negative axillary lymph nodes. Furthermore, he advises that all patients with eight or more positive axillary nodes should receive prophylactic irradiation to the chest wall as well as to the axilla and the supraclavicular region. Such an approach in treatment would suggest that the axillary dissection part of radical mastectomy is simply a means of staging the disease process to indicate both the prognosis and the need for adjunctive therapy. This concept has been previously expressed by Devitt[9] who stated that nodal "metastases are an expression of poor prognosis rather than the determinant of it." Advocates of radical mastectomy should consider the question that if irradiation is considered effective in the treatment of suspected internal mammary node metastases, should it not be equally effective for the treatment of involved axillary nodes?

Another important criticism of axillary dissection is that the the procedure, even theoretically, is beneficial to very few of the women to whom it is applied. An approximation of just how small this figure is can be gained by analysis of the results of previous studies. Using the Manchester Clinical Classification, those women who have potentially curable breast cancer fall into Stage I and Stage II in almost equal numbers. Approximately 40 per cent of women classified clinically as having Stage I cancer (having disease confined to the breast) will be found to have histologic axillary lymph node metastases. For women with Stage II cancer (those with clinically involved axillary nodes), only 60 per cent of specimens will contain histologic lymph node metastases, and 40 per cent will be negative.[26] Therefore, a total of half of all women with potentially curable breast cancer will not have axillary metastases and, in having a radical mastectomy, will have undergone an operation much more extensive than necessary. Axillary dissection contributes nothing to this group except an expected increase in morbidity and cosmetic deformity. Though the operative mortality is virtually the same whether or not the axilla is dissected, there is no question but that the increased morbidity surrounding axillary dissection is real, as shown by the data from our series of 207 radical mastectomies (Table 2).

The problem of cosmetic deformity is ubiquitous and though highly subjective is nevertheless real. Most women view the loss of one or both breasts as a disaster and are understandably afraid of undergoing a mutilating operation. Today, it is probably fear of this loss rather than ignorance of the significance of a lump that is the greatest cause of delay in seeking treatment.

Subjecting one of every two women to an operation more extensive than necessary would be quite acceptable if removing metastatic nodes would be curative. This again, however, is not the case. From data accumulated by Fisher through past National Surgical Adjuvant Breast Project studies,[12] it can be shown that of those women with axillary metastases (who make up 50 per cent of the potentially curable group), approximately one half will have

TABLE 2.    Morbidity Associated with Radical Mastectomies*

| Complications | Percentage of Cases |
|---|---|
| Hematoma or seroma | 22 |
| Edema of arm | 21 |
| Marginal skin necrosis | 14 |
| Wound infection | 12 |
| Shoulder stiffness | 4 |
| Deep vein thrombosis | 2 |
| Bronchopneumonia | 2 |
| Pulmonary embolism | 1 |

*From Wise, L., Mason, A. W., and Ackerman, L. V.: Local excision and irradiation: an alternative method for the treatment of early mammary cancer. Ann. Surg. 174:393, 1971.

three or fewer metastatic lymph nodes in the axillary specimen, and one half will have four or more. Fifty per cent of those with three or less positive nodes will demonstrate evidence of recurrent disease or noncurability within 5 years; for those with four or more, the figure is 85 per cent. Of the combined group of women with axillary metastases, approximately two thirds will not be cured. Therefore, on an overall statistical basis, only one in six women who are thought to have clinically curable breast cancer will have the potential to be cured by including axillary dissection in treatment. This figure is in agreement with the opinion expressed by Sir Hedley Atkins in 1953 that the method of treatment makes a difference in the end result in only approximately 10 per cent of patients.[18] For the five out of six women not potentially benefited by axillary dissection, it has served only as a means of more accurately staging the disease process. Because of these considerations and the fact that modern radiotherapy is probably just as effective therapeutically as operative excision, we feel that routine axillary dissection in the treatment of potentially curable breast cancer is not justifiable. Indeed, the data shown in Table 1 indicate the effectiveness of radiation therapy.

The problem of leaving untreated, possibly involved lymph nodes behind has been considered by Crile[7] and Edwards.[10] Their data suggest that such a delay in treatment is probably not harmful. In fact, what may be harmful is the removal of negative axillary lymph nodes. Though the data are scarce, both theoretical considerations[6] and experimental studies[11] suggest that destruction of regional nodes, where lymphocytes become immunized against cancer, might diminish the immunologic resistance of the host to the implantation and growth of circulating tumor cells. Much work along these lines needs to be done, but the potential for the ultimate control of cancer probably lies in such directions of research.

## Conclusion

On the basis of data accumulated at the present time, we conclude that formal axillary dissection probably has no role in the management of women with primary breast cancer. Axillary dissection must be recognized as being only a means of providing a specimen for the pathologic staging of the disease process. We would argue that the morbidity and cosmetic deformity accompanying the procedure further justify rejecting its routine use. For women with potentially curable breast cancer, the combination of wedge excision (where cosmetically feasible) or simple mastectomy, with postoperative irradiation is probably as adequate as any of the more mutilating procedures. It must be realized that in women with axillary metastases, the disease is usually systemic in nature, and variations in local therapy have little importance. A real advance will be forthcoming only when this group of patients can be studied and treated systemically on an immunologic and chemotherapeutic basis. The acceptance and development of and participation in such studies will be the surgeon's contribution to the effective treatment of carcinoma of the breast in the future.

## References

1. Atkins, H., Hayward, J. L., Klugman, D. J., and Wayte, A. B.: Treatment of early breast cancer: a report after ten years of clinical trial. Br. Med. J. 2:423, 1972.
2. Banks, W. M.: On free removal of mammary cancer with extirpation of the axillary glands as a necessary accomplishment. Br. Med. J. 2:1138, 1882.
3. Brinkley, D., and Haybittle, J. L.: Treatment of Stage II carcinoma of the female breast. Lancet 2:1086, 1971.
4. Cáceres, E.: An evaluation of radical mastectomy and extended radical mastectomy for cancer of the breast. Surg. Gynecol. Obstet. 125:337, 1967.
5. Cancer statistics 1975. CA 25:8, 1975.
6. Crile, G., Jr.: Possible role of uninvolved regional nodes in preventing metastasis from breast cancer. Cancer 24:1283, 1969.
7. Crile, G., Jr.: Results of conservative treatment of breast cancer at 10 and 15 years. Ann. Surg. 181:26, 1975.
8. Dahl-Iversen, E., and Tobiassen, T.: Radical mastectomy with parasternal and supraclavicular dissection for mammary carcinoma. Ann. Surg. 157:170, 1963.
9. Devitt, J. E.: Significance of regional lymph node metastases in breast cancer. Can. Med. Assoc. J. 93:289, 1965.
10. Edwards, M. H., Baum, M., and Magarey, C. J.: Regression of axillary lymph-nodes in cancer of the breast. Br. J. Surg. 59:776, 1972.
11. Fisher, B., and Fisher, E. R.: Studies concerning the regional lymph nodes in cancer. II. Maintenance of immunity. Cancer 29:1496, 1972.
12. Fisher, B., Ravdin, R. G., Ausman, R. K., Slack, N. H., Moore, G. E., and Noer, R. J.: Surgical adjuvant chemotherapy in cancer of the breast: results of a decade of cooperative investigation. Ann. Surg. 168:337, 1968.
13. Guttmann, R. J.: Survival and results after 2 million volt irradiation in the treatment of primary operable carcinoma of the breast with proved positive internal mammary and/or highest axillary nodes. Cancer 15:383, 1962.
14. Haagensen, C. D., Bhonslay, S. B., Guttmann, R. J., Habif, D. V., Kister, S. J., Markowitz, A. M., Sanger, G., Tretter, P., Wiedel, P. D., and Cooley, E.: Metastasis of carcinoma of the breast to the periphery of the regional lymph node filter. Ann. Surg. 169:174, 1969.
15. Haagensen, C. D.: The choice of treatment of operable carcinoma of the breast. Surgery 76:685, 1974.
16. Halsted, W. S.: The results of operations for the cure of cancer of the breast performed at the Johns Hopkins Hospital from June 1889 to January 1894. Ann. Surg. 20:497, 1894.
17. Handley, R. S., and Thackray, A. C.: The internal mammary lymph chain in carcinoma of the breast. Lancet 2:276, 1949.
18. Handley, R. S.: Techniques of surgical treatment. In Atkins, H.: The Treatment of Breast Cancer. Baltimore, University Park Press, 1974, p. 49.
19. Kaae, S., and Johansen, H.: Simple mastectomy plus postoperative irradiation by the method of McWhirter for mammary carcinoma. Ann. Surg. 170:895, 1969.
20. Lewison, E. F.: The surgical treatment of breast cancer: a historical and collective review. Surgery 34:904, 1953.
21. McWhirter, R.: The value of simple mastectomy and radiotherapy in the treatment of cancer of the breast. Br. J. Radiol. 21:599, 1948.
22. Peters, M. V.: Wedge resection and irradiation: an effective treatment of early breast cancer. J.A.M.A. 200:134, 1967.
23. Porritt, A.: Early carcinoma of the breast. Br. J. Surg. 51:214, 1964.
24. Rimsten, A., Johansson, H., and Stenkvist, B.: Preoperative diagnosis of axillary lymph nodes in cancer of the breast. Surg. Gynecol. Obstet. 139:551, 1974.
25. Turner-Warwick, R. T.: The lymphatics of the breast. Br. J. Surg. 46:574, 1959.
26. Wise, L., Mason, A. W., and Ackerman, L. V.: Local excision and irradiation: an alternative method for the treatment of early mammary cancer. Ann. Surg. 174:393, 1971.
27. Wise, L.: Controversies in the management of potentially curable breast cancer. In Nyhus, L. M. (ed.): Surgery Annual, 1974. New York, Appleton-Century-Crofts, 1974, p. 247.

# 5

# Adjunctive Radiotherapy for Breast Cancer

THE ROLE OF RADIATION
THERAPY IN ASSOCIATION WITH
OPERATION IN THE
MANAGEMENT OF BREAST
CANCER
by Ralph R. Weichselbaum
and Samuel Hellman

BREAST CANCER—THE CASE
AGAINST PROPHYLACTIC
RADIOTHERAPY AS A
POSTOPERATIVE MEASURE
by W. H. Bond

## Statement of the Problem

*This controversy deals with the question of when, if ever, radiation should be used after an apparently curative operation for breast cancer. The techniques of radiation are not the central issue, yet they must be examined and identified in assessing results. The data are analyzed with due consideration being given to variations in the operation performed prior to radiation therapy.*

*Primary radiation treatment apparently eliminates breast cancer in some patients, but as an adjunct to operation, the efficacy is sufficiently uncertain that a controversy exists. What is your explanation of this discrepancy? Evaluate the firm data demonstrating that postoperative radiotherapy enhances the likelihood of cures or of long-term survival.*

*Define those patients with breast cancer (potentially cured by operation) who should receive postoperative radiation. Describe fields and dosage of radiation that should be employed.*

*Examine available information indicating that radiation alters morbidity from arm edema and wound infection. Does it reduce the incidence of local recurrence? Discuss potential lung injury. Analyze data suggesting that postoperative radiotherapy adversely affects the course of the disease.*

# The Role of Radiation Therapy in Association with Operation in the Management of Breast Cancer

RALPH R. WEICHSELBAUM
and SAMUEL HELLMAN

*Harvard Medical School*

The first problem to be addressed in evaluating the efficacy of local treatment of breast cancer is that of local control. This is a significant problem in breast cancer management when operation is used alone. The evolution of the modifications of the original Halsted procedure to reduce chest wall and nodal recurrences has reflected the importance of local control. These modifications vary from supraradical operation[1] to special technical modifications, such as meticulous dermal dissection of skin flaps.[2] However, in operable cases, local recurrence rates have remained between 15 and 25 per cent and depend more upon selection of patients than upon the surgical innovations introduced.[1, 4, 8, 10] Delineation of groups at high risk for local recurrence after mastectomy will resolve much of the controversy surrounding postoperative radiotherapy.

An early report of 541 patients with breast carcinoma treated with classical Halsted radical mastectomy between 1899 and 1930 at the Johns Hopkins Hospital describes a local recurrence rate of 26 per cent.[3] In a series of patients treated by radical mastectomy alone during the years 1935 to 1955, Haagensen reports a chest wall recurrence rate at 10 years of 3 per cent in Columbia Stage A patients, 13.7 per cent in Stage B patients, 18 per cent in Stage C patients, and 63 per cent in Stage D patients.[4] These results are among the best in the surgical literature for nonirradiated patients. During these years, Haagensen performed triple biopsy procedures to select favorable patients and developed criteria for operability, making this one of the most highly selective series studied. Supraradical and modified radical procedures, as well as the use of thin skin flaps, have not improved these chest wall recurrence rates.[1,2] Furthermore, patients with large, medial, or central lesions and patients with Stage III and IV lesions (UICC Staging System) are at extremely high risk for local recurrence.[5,6,7] Once chest wall recurrence appears, it can be effectively managed in only 50 per cent of these patients.[8]

A randomized study reported by Paterson showed a decrease in chest wall recurrence rates from 20 to 11 per cent when patients with operable breast carcinoma were treated postoperatively with his quadrate technique.[9] In this study, orthovoltage irradiation was administered at dose levels that were considerably lower than is possible with megavoltage equipment. Furthermore, the supraclavicular region was not included in the treatment portals. Although this study is frequently cited to demonstrate the efficacy of postoperative radiation in reducing the incidence of local recurrences, we would not consider this adequate radiotherapy by present standards.

In our series, patients were divided into three risk groups following radical or modified radical mastectomy.[10] These groups were: patients with upper outer quadrant lesions and negative axillary nodes; patients with medial or central lesions with negative axillary nodes; and patients with positive axillary nodes. The last group was subdivided into patients in whom more or less than 50 per cent of the axillary nodes contained tumor. Since the incidence of local recurrence in patients with small upper outer quadrant lesions and negative axillae is extremely low, these patients were not routinely treated postoperatively unless their disease was Stage III or Stage IV. The second group was treated using a portal that encompassed the internal mammary and supraclavicular nodes alone; the chest wall was not included in the treatment field. A total of 287 patients was included in the third group and was treated with a three-field technique that encompassed the supraclavicular, internal mammary, and chest wall regions. Following this treatment technique, the chest wall recurrence rate at 5 years was 1.5 per cent when the axilla was negative, 1.3 per cent when the axilla was less than 50 per cent positive, and 14.2 per cent when the axillary nodes showed greater than 50 per cent involvement with tumor (see Table 1). The total chest wall recurrence rate for the entire series is 5 per cent. One half of the recurrences appeared within the first year and 83 per cent in the first 2 years. After the second year, the likelihood of recurrence decreases. We realize, of course, that

### TABLE 1.    Chest Wall Recurrences

| Location of Primary Tumor | Axillary Involvement | | |
|---|---|---|---|
| | *None* | *<50 per cent* | *>50 per cent* |
| Medial | 45 (1)* | 15 | 15 (2) |
| Central | 31 (1) | 58 (1) | 42 (7) |
| Lateral | 25 | 79 (1) | 41 (5) |

*( ) = chest wall recurrence.

with further follow-up, more recurrences may appear; however, our data are similar to those of others[9] that indicated that most of the recurrences occur in the first 2 years following treatment. These local recurrence rates are among the lowest in the literature.[11, 12]

We believe that these results are due to several technical modifications. The first is the inclusion of the chest wall in the treatment plan when any axillary nodes are positive for tumor. At the M. D. Anderson Hospital (Houston), a chest wall recurrence rate of 12 per cent was reported in patients with less than 50 per cent of the axilla positive when only the peripheral lymphatics were treated postoperatively. When the axilla showed greater than 50 per cent involvement with tumor, the chest wall recurrence rate was 26 per cent when only the peripheral lymphatics were treated.[12] Thus, irradiation of the chest wall when the axilla was positive for tumor yielded a significant decrease in chest wall recurrence.[10, 12]

A minimum tumor dose of 4500 rads is essential for local control. Fletcher has suggested that studies of chest wall recurrence done before 1959 should be disregarded because of the inadequate dosages delivered by orthovoltage equipment. He further proposed a dose-response curve for the local curability of microscopic breast carcinoma that appears consistent with other human and animal tumor models.[13] We recommend treatment of the peripheral lymphatics with the addition of chest wall irradiation when any axillary nodes are positive. All areas should be treated with a minimum dose of 4500 rads. The adequacy of dose and coverage of potentially involved areas is critical.

Supraclavicular nodal recurrences following classical or extended radical mastectomy occur in 15 to 17 per cent of patients not receiving postoperative radiotherapy.[11, 14] Parasternal recurrences were reported in 10 per cent of patients presenting with medial and central lesions who underwent standard radical mastectomy at the Memorial Hospital (New York) between 1940 and 1945.[15] In Auchincloss' series of 152 patients treated with radical mastectomy, 8 per cent presented with parasternal recurrence as initial evidence of uncontrolled disease.[2] In our series of 352 patients, there were 4 supraclavicular recurrences and no parasternal recurrences.[10] We realize, of course, that since some recurrences manifest themselves late, we may see more with further follow-up; however, these numbers are still quite low. We used a tumor dose of 4500 rads at a depth of 5 cm., and adequate coverage of the medial portion of the ipsilateral supraclavicular region was achieved through application of a single anterior portal. This technique produced a uniform dose across the entire width of the supraclavicular region. The resulting nodal recurrence rate is lower than those of many historical series[11, 14] but is in good agreement with those of centers using similar techniques.[16]

The rates of recurrences on the chest wall and in nodal regions in patients undergoing radical mastectomy give rise to speculation about the curative potential of this procedure. When axillary nodes are involved with tumor, there is as high as a 40 per cent incidence of positive internal mammary nodes.[5] Because these are not treated by a standard radical or modified radical mastectomy, the proportion of patients cured by these operations is smaller. Radical mastectomy is a potentially curative procedure only in patients with disease confined to the breast or in a single subpopulation of patients with lesions confined to the breast (outer quadrant) and axillary nodes. A large group of patients with subclinical disease in the chest wall, internal mammary nodes, or supraclavicular region or with occult distant metastases will not benefit from these operative procedures.

Because of the effectiveness of radiation in decreasing local recurrence with standard mastectomy, one can then ask if more extensive operations are necessary. Perhaps tumor excision is sufficient if it is followed by adequate postoperative radiation. We have seen 39 patients with Stage I or II carcinoma of the breast who were referred because of medical problems restricting the choice of operative procedures or because of patient or referring physician preference.[17] All were treated with radiation following biopsy. The dose planned for external beam was 4500 to 5000 rads over a period of 4½ to 5 weeks. This was followed 2 to 3 weeks later by an additional dose of 1500 to 2000 rads by [192]Ir implantation in those patients felt to have gross residual disease after biopsy. All patients have been followed from 18 months to 7 years; there are as yet no local failures. While our follow-up is shorter than those of most surgical series, Pierquin and other European radiation therapists have had similar results with longer follow-up.[18]

Thus far this discussion has been concerned with local control. This seems appropriate since neither operation nor radiation therapy can control disease outside the field of attention. It has been suggested that postoperative radiation both increases and decreases survival.[19] It is difficult to resolve this issue without a carefully controlled trial using appropriate radiation dosage and having patients appropriately stratified by location of the tumor as well as by nodal status. In terms of survival, the only patients likely to benefit from postoperative radiotherapy are those who have tumor left behind in the chest wall or in regional nodes but whose tumor has not metastasized elsewhere at the time of radiation and in whom the local residual nidus will become the source of metastases before local recurrence is demonstrated and treated. This may be only a small subset of breast cancer patients, which may not be obvious in an overall series unless the patients are carefully stratified. There are some data suggesting such a subgroup.

Roth and Bayat reviewed necropsy data on 23 patients who were treated with a variety of operative, radiotherapeutic, and chemotherapeutic techniques for carcinoma of the breast.[20] Six patients had no clinical evidence of disease during their lifetime, and 17 patients died from active breast carcinoma. Of the six patients clinically free of disease, one patient had disease in the chest wall. Of the 17 patients who died from distant metastases, all 17 had disease in the chest wall. It is of interest that the sole patient treated with chemotherapy (5 Fluorouracil) had no evidence of disease during life; however, at autopsy 2 years after treatment, disease was found to be present, which was confined to the chest wall. The authors hypothesized that perhaps unexcised tumor remnants grow progressively and ultimately give rise to distant metastases. They noted that whenever widespread distant metastases were found, tumor in the chest wall was also found; and when there was no tumor in the chest wall, no distant metastases were observed. These authors concluded that the most likely mode of spread for breast carcinoma is a progression of disease from foci within the chest wall lymphatics. Thus, patients with breast carcinoma confined to this anatomic volume following mastectomy, if given proper postoperative radiation, may have their entire site of persistent disease sterilized.

Another subgroup potentially aided by postoperative radiotherapy is patients with metastases confined to the internal mammary nodes only. These patients do not necessarily have distant metastases. Guttman has shown that 60 per cent of patients with operable disease who demonstrated positive internal mammary nodes by triple biopsy procedure were alive at 5 years, and 30 per cent were alive at 10 years following radical radiotherapy.[21] It is obviously difficult with present diagnostic techniques to identify prospectively the subgroups in which the disease is confined to *only* the chest wall or internal mammary nodes.

It has been postulated that postoperative radiotherapy to the chest wall decreases immunity by suppression of T-lymphocytes following irradiation of the thymus[22] and that leukopenia following postoperative radiotherapy is deleterious to long-term survival. However, once T-cell immunity is established, it is very difficult to destroy with any dose of irradiation employed in clinical medicine.[23] All therapeutic procedures can affect immunity. For example, operation can cause decreased immunologic competence as measured by studies of the ability of blood peripheral lymphocytes to undergo maximal stimulation with phytohemagglutinin.[24] Furthermore, postoperative lymphocyte counts are frequently decreased, and these effects are most pronounced in patients with carcinoma.[25] Profound and lasting leukopenia may be caused by chemotherapeutic agents.[26] The contribution of each therapeutic modality to immunosuppression and their relative effects on long-term survival have yet to be clearly demonstrated.

Stjernsward has interpreted the results of several randomized trials to suggest that survival is decreased when postoperative radiotherapy is administered.[19] Fletcher[30] has carefully reviewed the studies on which Stjernsward based his conclusion. He points out that the Edinburgh and Copenhagen randomized trials compare radical mastectomy to simple mastectomy followed by irradiation[27, 28] and that an evaluation of postoperative irradiation can only be made if the same operative procedures are utilized in both series. Further, he compares failure rates at 5 years, rather than survival rates, in the National Surgical Adjuvant Breast Protocol (NSABP)[29] study. Of the patients who received postoperative irradiation, 49.4 per cent had recurrent disease by 5 years, whereas 54.4 per cent of those who received placebo had recurrences at 5 years. If, instead of comparing mortality rates at 3 years in patients with positive nodes, one compares the percentage of patients who had recurrence of disease by 5 years (Tables 6 and 7 of the NSABP), one sees that the frequency of disease in the placebo treated patients is increased in relation to nodal involvement and menopausal status. These data do not support the contention that radiotherapy is deleterious to survival.[29, 30]

Thus, only the Manchester study[9] is left for consideration, and this study taken alone is not statistically significant. We have previously commented on the inadequate radiotherapeutic techniques employed in the Manchester study. The radiotherapy employed in the National Surgical Adjuvant Breast Protocol study was not appropriate either, because the chest wall was not included in the treatment plan when axillary nodes were positive.

Misinterpretation of the data from the National Surgical Adjuvant Breast Protocol study[29] has implied an increase in distant metastases in the patients treated by irradiation. Patients receiving postoperative radiotherapy had a decreased number of local recurrences; thus, the first site of failure was more frequently a distant metastasis. This alteration in pattern of failure gave the impression of lessened survival in irradiated patients. However, no statistical difference in survival rates was demonstrated, and only the site of failure was altered. The actuarial 5-year survival rates in our postoperative series were 76 and 74 per cent for Stage I and Stage II respectively. In our biopsy plus radiation group, the actuarial 5-year survival rates were 90 per cent and 60 per cent for clinical Stage I and II cases respectively.[10, 17]

Adjuvant chemotherapy has provided an additional dimension to the issue of postoperative radiotherapy and its relationship to long-term survival. Postoperative radiation will not enhance survival following mastectomy procedures in those patients with subclinical metastases outside the treatment field. Such metastases may be sterilized by adjuvant chemotherapy, while the larger residual tumor burden on the chest wall may not and may thus be the major site of local recurrence. Preliminary data from the National Surgical Adjuvant Breast Protocol study[31] indicate that the majority of failures in patients receiving adjuvant chemotherapy are on the chest wall, that is, at the site of gross residual disease. If, with continued observation, adjuvant chemotherapy is shown to be effective, postoperative radiation is even more likely to affect survival, since micrometastases outside the field will be eradicated by chemotherapy; however, the frequency of local recurrences already seen indicates the necessity of radiation to the local area. The effectiveness of adjuvant chemotherapy for subclinical distant metastases in other diseases, such as Wilms' tumor, has highlighted the importance of local control with postoperative radiotherapy for effective cure.[32]

When radiotherapy is properly applied, the complication rate is quite low. In our postoperative series, the radiation complication rate was 3 per cent. Four patients experienced symptomatic radiation pneumonitis but without long-term complications. Six patients developed rib fractures due to radiation osteitis. In the group treated postbiopsy, there were four patients with significant complications; two patients experienced rib fracture and two developed symptomatic radiation pneumonitis. Again, these complications were self-limiting, and no permanent damage resulted. These complications occurred early in our program, prior to significant modification of dose-time relationships, and, with currently employed treatment programs, we believe that these can be reduced. The axilla was rarely treated postoperatively, and thus we know of no cases where radiation increased pre-existing arm edema. In the biopsy alone plus radiation group, there has been no extremity edema so far. Furthermore, these complications seem relatively minor when one compares them to the operative complications of radical mastectomy, as well as the psychologic impact of the loss of a breast.

As patterns of spread of malignant disease are better understood, therapeutic modalities will be altered. This has been most evident in the treatment of the malignant lymphomas and pediatric tumors. In these diseases, an intelligent application of surgery, radiation therapy, and chemotherapy has allowed retention of function and cosmesis, with much improved survival and excellent local control.[6] Even when survival is not lengthened, local control is a desired goal. However, when effective adjuvant therapeutic modalities become available for any malignant disease, local control becomes imperative. This can be achieved with excellent functional and cosmetic results by the combination of conservative operation and properly applied radiation therapy.

## References

1. Dahl-Iversen, E., and Tobiassen, T.: Radical mastectomy with parasternal and supraclavicular dissection for mammary carcinoma. Ann. Surg. 170:889–891, 1969.
2. Auchincloss, H. J. R.: The nature of local recurrence following radical mastectomy. Cancer 11:611–619, 1958.
3. Lewis, D., and Rienhoff, W. F.: A study of results of operation for cure of cancer of the breast. Ann. Surg. 95:336–400, 1932.
4. Haagensen, C. D., and Cooley, E.: Radical mastectomy for mammary cancer. Ann. Surg. 170:884–888, 1969.
5. Moss, W. T., Brand, W. N., and Battifora, H.: Radiation Oncology. St. Louis, The C. V. Mosby Co., 1973, pp. 293–321.
6. Fletcher, G. H.: Textbook of Radiotherapy. Philadelphia, Lea & Febiger, 1973, pp. 457–491, 498–543, 561–580, 783–793.
7. Donegan, W., Perez-Mesa, C., and Watson, F.: Biostatistical study of locally recurrent breast carcinoma. Surg. Gynecol. Obstet. 122:529–540, 1966.
8. Zimmerman, K. W., Montague, E. D., and Fletcher, G. H.: Frequency, anatomic distribution and management of local recurrence after definitive therapy for breast cancer. Cancer 19:67–74, 1966.
9. Paterson, R.: Breast cancer: a report of two clinical trials. J. R. Coll. Surg. Edinb. 7:243–254, 1962.
10. Weichselbaum, R. R., March, A., and Hellman, S.: Postoperative radiotherapy in the management of carcinoma of the breast. Submitted for publication.
11. Robbins, G. F., Lucas, J. C., Fracchia, A. A., and Chu, F.: An evaluation of postoperative prophylactic radiation therapy in breast cancer. Surg. Gynecol. Obstet. 122:979–982, 1966.
12. Fletcher, G. H., Montague, E. D., and White, E. C.: Evaluation of irradiation of the peripheral lymphatics in conjunction with radical mastectomy for cancer of the breast. Cancer 21:791–797, 1968.
13. Fletcher, G. H.: Local results of irradiation in the primary management of localized breast carcinoma. Cancer 29:545–551, 1972.
14. Jackson, S. M.: Carcinoma of the breast. The significance of supraclavicular lymph node metastasis. Clin. Radiol. 17:107–114, 1966.
15. Urban, J. A.: Clinical experience and results of excision of the internal mammary lymph node chain in primary operable breast cancer. Cancer 12:14–22, 1959.
16. Fletcher, G. H., Montague, E. D., and White, E. C.: Evaluation of irradiation of the peripheral lymphatics in conjunction with radical mastectomy for breast cancer. Cancer 21:791–797, 1968.
17. Weber, E., and Hellman, S.: Radiation as the primary treatment for local control of carcinoma of the breast. J.A.M.A. In press.
18. Pierquin, B.: Peut on traiter les cancers de sein de petite taille par la seule radiothérapie. Ann. Med. Interne (Paris) 122:575–579, 1971.
19. Stjernsward, J.: Decreased survival related to irradiation postoperatively in early operable breast cancer. Lancet 2:1285–1286, 1974.

20. Roth, D., and Bayat, H.: The role of residual tumors in the chest wall in the late dissemi-
    nation of mammary cancer. Ann. Surg. *168*:887–890, 1968.
21. Guttman, R.: Radiotherapy in locally advanced cancer of the breast. Cancer *20*:1046–1050,
    1967.
22. Stjernsward, J., Jandal, M., Vanky, F., Wiszell, H., and Sealy, R.: Lymphopenia and changes
    in distribution of human B and T lymphocytes in peripheral blood induced by irradiation
    for mammary carcinoma. Lancet *1*:1352–1356, 1972.
23. Perez, C. A., Stewart, C. C., and Wagner, B.: Role of regional lymph nodes in tumor immu-
    nity. *In* Bond, V. P., Hellman, S., Order, S. E., Suit, H. D., and Withens, H. R. (eds.): *Inter-
    action of Radiation and Host Immune Defense Mechanisms in Malignancy.* (BNL 50418.)
    Upton, New York, Brookhaven National Laboratory, 1974, pp. 225–244.
24. Park, S. K., Brody, J. I., Wallace, H., and Blakemore, W.: Immunosuppressive effect of
    surgery. Lancet *1*:53–55, 1971.
25. Papatestas, A. E., and Kark, A. E.: Peripheral lymphocyte counts in breast carcinoma.
    Cancer *34*:2014–2017, 1974.
26. Holland, J. F., and Frei, E.: *Cancer Medicine.* Philadelphia, Lea & Febiger, 1973, pp. 139–
    859.
27. Bruce, J.: Operable cancer of the breast. Cancer *28*:1443–1452, 1971.
28. Kaae, S., and Johansen, H.: In *Tenovus Symposium. Prognostic Factors in Breast Cancer.*
    Edinburgh, Livingstone, 1968, p. 93.
29. Fisher, B., Slack, N. H., Cavanaugh, P. J., Gardiner, B., and Raudin, R. G.: Postoperative
    radiotherapy in the treatment of breast cancer. Ann. Surg. *172*:711–732, 1970.
30. Fletcher, G. H.: Personal communication.
31. Fisher, B., Carbone, P., Economou, S. G., et al.: L-Phenylalanine mustard in the manage-
    ment of primary breast cancer. N. Engl. J. Med. *292*:117–122, 1975.
32. Wolff, J. A., Krivit, W., Newton, W. A., Jr., and D'Angio, G. J.: Single versus multiple dose
    dactinomycin therapy of Wilms' tumor. N. Engl. J. Med. *279*:290–294, 1968.

# Breast Cancer—the Case Against Prophylactic Radiotherapy as a Postoperative Measure

W. H. BOND

*United Birmingham Hospitals, Birmingham, England*

Radiation therapy of breast cancer can be used as a preoperative measure, as a postoperative adjunct following radical mastectomy, or as the sole measure to control disease. That local control of disease can be obtained by radiation alone is well established; Guttman,[16] in a series of surgically unsuitable cases, achieved a 5-year survival rate that was the equal of the rate in many surgical series and, strangely, was the equal of the rate in similar cases treated by operation in the same institution. It is within the experience of every surgeon that preoperative radiation will shrink the advanced tumor to an extent that radical removal becomes possible, but its value in improving the survival rate is not established by any fully controlled trial.

The greatest controversy, however, concerns the value of postoperative radiotherapy, and indeed it is difficult to establish how its use became popularized to the extent that some would regard its omission as ethically wrong. Undoubtedly, the visible disappearance of recurrent disease on the chest wall impressed surgeons who believed that total eradication of an apparently local disease was a prerequisite of their efforts and thus saw radiotherapy as a valuable adjunct. Radiation could be expected to destroy not only spilled or residual cells but also those cells possibly metastasized to the internal mammary chain and the supraclavicular lymph nodes.

The apparent value of postoperative radiation was reported by Adair,[1] Marshall,[23] and Harrington.[19] In Britain, surgical thinking was strongly influenced by McWhirter[25] when the results of local mastectomy and radiation were claimed to be superior to radical mastectomy, with a lower incidence of local and regional recurrence. However, all these reports were

91

based on uncontrolled trials, which usually compared two groups of cases treated at different times, rather than two groups randomly selected and treated concurrently. While Truscott[39] confirmed McWhirter's findings in a controlled trial, and Kaae[22] showed that McWhirter techniques were the equal of the extended radical mastectomy in a similar trial, never throughout all these trials was radiation regarded as other than beneficial nor was comment made on the morbidity or complications of therapy. Paterson and Russell,[28] Butcher,[9] and Robbins,[31] in reasonably controlled trials, could establish no improvement in survival rates by the use of immediate postoperative radiation.

The technique of postoperative radiation varies from center to center, but common to all is irradiation of the axillary apex and the supraclavicular fossa. In most series, the parasternal region is treated by a separate field, and in the McWhirter technique, which is a popular method employed after radical mastectomy, the chest wall is included. Most centers give a dose equivalent to 3300 to 3500 rads in 3 to 4 weeks, with a maximum tissue or skin dose of 4400 rads. Apart from the skin-sparing effect and reduced absorption in bone, there is no evidence that megavoltage therapy carries any benefit.

Complications are numerous. Radiation sickness, depression or loss of appetite occurs in 50 per cent of patients. With kilovoltage radiation, skin reactions will approach moist desquamation, and many patients show gross late radiation changes within 10 years and risk skin necrosis following minor trauma. With megavoltage radiation, in which advantage is taken of the minimal skin reactions to raise the tissue dose, gross subcutaneous fibrosis may appear, especially in fat laden areas. Edema of the arm is a significant finding when the axillary isthmus receives full dosage, especially when wound complications have arisen. Rubin[34] admitted a 70 per cent incidence of modest edema and a 2 per cent incidence of great edema; Haagensen[17] reported a 30 per cent incidence, and Tough[38] reported an incidence of only 5 per cent when the axilla had not been opened and recurrence was excluded. Injury to the cervical or brachial plexus can occur even when dosage is not enthusiastic, and one of the bravest reports comes from Westling,[41] serving to illustrate the influence of dose level and the closeness of the risk run in therapy. Westling reported 105 cases treated by megavoltage given to relatively small fields covering the axilla, the supraclavicular region, and the parasternal region to a maximum tissue dose of 5400 rads in 23 days. In 90 per cent of patients, subcutaneous induration was apparent within 12 months, and sensory changes appeared during the same period. At 18 months, motor signs appeared, and at 5 years, 60 per cent were affected, the injuries ranging from minor muscle weakness to almost complete paralysis. Such injuries have been seen personally when much lower dosage levels were employed.

Bone injury can occur, including pathologic fractures of the ribs and the scapula and collapse of dorsal vertebrae;[30] osteoporosis, osteonecrosis, and pathologic fractures of ribs and clavicle have also been reported by Bloom,[4] Freid,[13] and Slaughter.[36] Postradiation bone sarcoma has been reported by Hatfield,[20] who in a well-argued article describing 11 cases, showed that survival beyond 10 years increases the risk of sarcoma from 1 in 200,000 to 1 in

500, the disease being lethal in eight of his cases. Fibrosarcoma of the chest wall following radiation was described by Sarrazin[35] and Oberman.[27] Squamous carcinoma of the chest wall has been personally observed in three patients who had been given radiation following mastectomy 20 years previously. In all cases in which the supraclavicular fossa is irradiated, various volumes of the upper lobe will be dosed, and when the chest wall is treated, the periphery of the lung will receive heavy irradiation unless a preliminary pneumothorax is induced. Ross[33] reported pneumonic change in 90 per cent of cases at some time after radiation. Rubin[34] states that 20 to 66 per cent show pulmonary radiation changes, especially with megavoltage therapy; where 5000 rads are given to the periphery of the lung, persistent cough with dyspnea occurs, requiring continuous medication. Other intrathoracic structures are damaged — persistent, but probably benign, changes in the T wave have been reported[3] in 4 of 75 patients treated postoperatively, and Stewart[37] noted an injury rate, mostly to the pericardium, of 5.8 per cent in a larger series of cases.

Not unexpectedly, hematologic changes have been recorded. Meyer[26] noted lymphocyte depression in all treated cases, lasting for 2 to 5 years after therapy. Although in a subsequent paper, McCredie[24] could not show a heightened incidence of a second malignancy at any site, the findings are vitiated by the exclusion of all second breast cancers found within 6 months of treatment of the first. The possibility that tumor spread was facilitated by prophylactic irradiation was considered by Cole[10] in describing cases in which recurrent disease on the chest wall was confined initially to and was sharply demarcated by the treated area, a posterior axillary field even being involved in one instance. Personal experience dictates the reporting of additional and rare complications, including six cases of benign esophageal stenosis requiring regular dilatation and two instances of cordal damage (one patient being paraplegic and the other having a fully developed Brown-Séquard syndrome), apart from numerous instances in which Lhermitte's sign was positive, indicating pial damage.

It is remarkable that with such a list of possible complications, the evidence supporting the use of postoperative radiotherapy should be so tenuous. Indeed, in the literature, there is no single instance of a properly controlled series that shows any improvement in survival when postoperative radiation is employed. Acceptable series confirm a reduction in the incidence of recurrent disease within the treated area, but this difference reduces to much smaller proportions if studied at later years,[6] suggesting that radiation at acceptable dose levels merely delays the reappearance of disease. Over the last 10 years, it has come to be recognized that breast cancer is a generalized disease with a very long preclinical course, possibly as long as 40 years, but on the average 4½ years.[6, 8] During this long prodromal period, dissemination of disease occurs; studies of the early stages in women[15] and in mice[11] reveal that spread into periductal lymphatics occurs when the tumor is at a microscopic stage, rapidly entering the blood stream via intranodal lymphaticovenous channels.[12] The fate of these cells is unknown; Webster[40] found no difference in survival at 5 years when malignant cells were found in the circulation of breast cancer patients. Many cells, however, must become established, because the majority of breast cancer patients die of metastatic disease. The risk falls with time, although in Stage I and II disease only at 13 years postmastectomy does the chance of dying of other disease equal the cancer risk. Even at 25 years, 20 per cent of patients die with active disease present.[6] From this same series, Haybittle[21] deduced that in only 25 per cent of cases was the natural course of the disease changed by the treatment applied. Without operation, half the patients will die within 3.3 years.[5] Since the only factor common to a wide variety of operative procedures all producing approximately the same result is the removal of the breast, the tumor must control the activity of metastatic disease present in virtually all patients. From the known doubling times of breast tumors, there must be a slowing of the activity of metastatic disease when the tumor is removed; such an influence must be via cell-mediated antibodies known to be present in breast cancer patients.[32]

Radiation is immunosuppressive, as is major operation,[18] and an improved immunologic milieu may account for a 2 to 3 week interval between excision biopsy and mastectomy improving results.[29] There are now several series in which a heightened incidence and activity of metastatic disease with a fall in survival rate at 5 years has been observed in those patients given postoperative radiation, and this is possibly attributable to an immunosuppressive process or host defense mechanism damage. The first suggestion of this appeared in Paterson and Russell's series,[28] in which no differences appeared whether the case was "watched" or treated, with a hint of increased visceral disease in irradiated young patients. This series also compared two radiation techniques, one of which included the mediastinum and lymph node areas, and it is this group of patients that showed the lower overall survival rate. Bond[6] demonstrated that in node-negative patients, irradiation reduced the survival rate at 5 years by 9 per cent and increased the incidence of distal metastatic disease from 19.4 to 27.3 per cent. In a later paper,[7] he showed that in node-negative cases, the survival rate in any series fell as an increasing proportion of patients received postoperative radiation, and it was the premenopausal patients who suffered. In 629 patients under the age of 45, the younger the patient, the lower the survival rate when radiation was employed, such that below 30 years of age, those irradiated had a 5-year survival rate half that of those not receiving treatment. Fisher,[12] in his report of the National Surgical Adjuvant Breast Protocol trial, which excluded node-negative cases, revealed similar findings; the metastatic rate increased and the survival rate fell when radiation was employed, and this difference was most marked in premenopausal patients with minimal axillary node involvement. An earlier series, reported by Butcher,[9] of node-positive cases randomly divided into groups receiving mastectomy with and without radiation showed a 5-year result favoring the nonirradiated patients by 41 to 46 per cent. Robbins,[31] in an adequately controlled trial, observed a 13 per cent reduction in the incidence of regional recurrence when postoperative radiation was given but almost equal clinical cures at 5 years, from which it must be deduced that radiation increased the incidence of distal metastatic disease.

On the evidence presented, there can be no case whatsoever for immediate postoperative radiotherapy following mastectomy. To treat a disease of disseminated character in 75 per cent of cases, limited only by operation, by a method carrying high morbidity and possibly disastrous complications capable of reducing host resistance and survival rate is ethically wrong. If the method is to be employed, and its value in controlling local disease is not disputed, techniques must be developed to recognize that extremely small group of patients who are likely to benefit from immediate postoperative radiation. Galasko[14] showed that 24 per cent of early cases and 84 per cent of advanced cases had isotopically demonstrable metastatic disease, so the group must be small; and since over 80 per cent of patients who develop local recurrence also develop active distal metastatic disease within 5 years,[6] a stronger case can be made for systemic therapy than for radiation as the method to control disease residual or recurrent after mastectomy.

As a radiotherapist, one is disheartened by these conclusions, and as a surgeon, one is encouraged to choose more carefully the time and extent of operation, but above all it is important to accept the fact that the correct management of breast cancer is still unknown and that only cooperation in carefully controlled clinical trials will solve the problem.

## References

1. Adair, F. E.: The roles of surgery and irradiation in cancer of the breast. J.A.M.A. *121*:553, 1943.
2. Atkins, H. J. B.: Cancer of the breast. J. R. Coll. Surg. Edinb. *1*:253, 1956.
3. Biran, S., Hochmann, A., and Stern, S.: Therapeutic irradiation of the chest and electrocardiographic changes. Clin. Radiol. *20*:433, 1969.
4. Bloom, H. J. G.: Complications following radiotherapy of the thorax and abdomen. Proc. R. Soc. Med. *52*:495, 1959.
5. Bloom, H. J. G., Richardson, W. W., and Harries, E. J.: The natural history of untreated breast cancer (1805–1933); a comparison of treated and untreated cases according to the histological grade of malignancy. Br. Med. J. *2*:213, 1962.
6. Bond, W. H.: The influence of various treatments on survival rates in cancer of the breast. *In* Jarret, A. S. (ed.): *The Treatment of Carcinoma of the Breast.* Syntex Symposium. Cambridge, Amsterdam, and London; Excerpta Medical Foundation, 1967, pp. 24–39.
7. Bond, W. H.: The prognostic implications of treatment. Proc. R. Soc. Med. *63*:111, 1970.
8. Bond, W. H.: *In* Stoll, B. A. (ed.): *Host Defence in Breast Cancer.* London, William Heinemann Ltd., 1975, pp. 95–110.
9. Butcher, H. R., Jr., Seaman, W. B., Eckert, C., and Saltzstein, S.: An assessment of radical mastectomy and post operative irradiation therapy in the treatment of mammary cancer. Cancer, *17*:480, 1964.
10. Cole, H., and Halnan, K. E.: Facilitation of tumour spread in irradiated tissue after prophylactic postoperative x-ray therapy for breast cancer. Clin. Radiol. *22*:133, 1971.
11. De Ome, K. B.: Formal discussion of: multiple factors in mouse mammary tumorigenesis. Cancer Res. *25*:1348, 1965.
12. Fisher, B., Nelson, H. S., Cavanaugh, P. J., Gardner, B., and Ravdin, R. G.: Postoperative radiotherapy in the treatment of breast cancer: results of the NSABP clinical trial. Ann. Surg. *172*:711, 1970.
13. Freid, J. R., and Goldberg, H.: Post irradiation changes in the lungs and thorax. Am. J. Radiol. *43*:877, 1940.
14. Galasko, C. S. B.: The detection of skeletal metastases from mammary cancer by gamma camera scintigraphy. Br. J. Surg. *56*:757, 1969.
15. Gallagher, H. S., and Martin, J. E.: Early phases in the development of breast cancer. Cancer *24*:1170, 1960.
16. Guttman, R.: Radiotherapy in locally advanced cancer of the breast. Cancer, *20*:1046, 1967.
17. Haagensen, C. D.: *Diseases of the Breast.* 2nd ed. Philadelphia, W. B. Saunders Co., 1971.

18. Han, T.: Postoperative immunosuppression in patients with breast cancer. Lancet, *1*:742, 1972.
19. Harrington, S. W.: Results of surgical treatment of unilateral carcinoma of the breast in women. J.A.M.A. *148*:1007, 1952.
20. Hatfield, P. M., and Schulz, M. D.: Post irradiation sarcoma, including 5 cases after x-ray therapy for breast carcinoma. Radiology 96:593, 1970.
21. Haybittle, J. L.: The cured group in a series of treated breast cancer patients. Br. J. Radiol. *41*:639, 1968.
22. Kaae, S.: Does simple mastectomy followed by radiation offer survival comparable to radical procedures? J.A.M.A. *200*:138, 1967.
23. Marshall, S. F., and Hare, H. F.: Carcinoma of the breast: results of combined treatment with surgery and Roentgen rays. Ann. Surg. *125*:688, 1947.
24. McCredie, J. A., Inch, W. R., and Alderson, M.: Prophylactic postoperative radiotherapy and consecutive primary cancers. Arch. Surg. *105*:297, 1972.
25. McWhirter, R.: Simple mastectomy and radiotherapy in treatment of breast cancer. Br. J. Radiol. 28:128, 1955.
26. Meyer, K. K.: Radiation induced lymphocyte-immune deficiency. Arch. Surg. *101*:114, 1970.
27. Oberman, H. A.: Fibrosarcoma of the chest wall following resection and irradiation of carcinoma of the breast. Am. J. Clin. Pathol. 53:407, 1970.
28. Paterson, R., and Russell, M. H.: Clinical trials in malignant disease. III. Breast cancer: evaluation of postoperative radiotherapy. J. Fac. Radiol. *10*:175, 1961.
29. Peters, V.: *In* Ash, C. L. (ed.): *Cancer of the Breast.* Proceedings of the Tenth Annual Clinical Conference of the Ontario Cancer Treatment and Research Foundation, Nov. 8–9, 1963, Toronto, Canada.
30. Ratzkowski, E., Frankel, M., and Hochman, A.: Bone metastases, osteoporosis and radiation necrosis in breast cancer. Clin. Radiol. *18*:146, 1967.
31. Robbins, G. F., Lucas, J. C., Fracchia, A., Farrow, J. H., and Chu, F.: An evaluation of postoperative prophylactic radiation therapy in breast cancer. Surg. Gynecol. Obstet. *122*:979, 1966.
32. Roberts, M. M., and Bass, E. M.: Studies of the immune response in breast cancer. Br. J. Cancer 28:77, 1973.
33. Ross, W. M.: Radiotherapeutic and radiological aspects of radiation fibrosis of the lungs. Thorax *11*:241, 1956.
34. Rubin, P.: Comment: are metastases and lymphoedema radiation induced? J.A.M.A. *200*:142, 1967.
35. Sarrazin, D., Contesso, G., and Genin, J.: Fibrosarcomas of the chest wall following surgery and irradiation for breast tumour: presentation of 4 cases. Ann. Radiol. (Paris) *15*:667, 1972.
36. Slaughter, D. P.: Radiation osteitis and fracture of the clavicle following irradiation, with report of five cases of fractured clavicle. Am. J. Roentgenol. 48:201, 1942.
37. Stewart, J. R., Cohn, K. E., Fajardo, L. F., Hancock, E. W., and Kaplan, H. S.: Radiation induced heart disease, a study of twenty-five patients. Radiology 89:302, 1967.
38. Tough, I. C.: Oedema of the arm after simple mastectomy and radiotherapy for breast cancer. J. R. Coll. Surg. Edinb. *13*:312, 1968.
39. Truscott, B. McN.: Initial treatment of breast cancer: the controlled trial in East Anglia. Proc. R. Soc. Med. 60:943, 1967.
40. Webster, D. R., and Sabbadini, E.: The prognostic significance of circulating tumour cells—a 5 year follow up study of patients with cancer of the breast. Can. Med. Ass. J. 96:129, 1967.
41. Westling, P., Svensson, H., and Hele, P.: Cervical plexus lesions following post-operative radiation therapy of mammary carcinoma. Acta Radiol. [Ther.] (Stockh.) *11*:209, 1962.

# 6

# Operative Treatment for Duodenal Ulcer

## Statement of the Problem

*In this section, four different operative treatments for duodenal ulcer are considered with respect to selection of patients, immediate operative problems, and long-term results.*

*What diagnostic criteria are necessary to establish the presence of duodenal ulcer disease in a patient under consideration for operative therapy? Are symptoms alone sufficient? Is operative proof of duodenal ulcer essential to accurate analysis of results?*

*List the major criteria you require before advising a patient to undergo an operation. Does the age, sex, or general habitus of the patient make a difference in selecting the procedure?*

*Are preoperative acid secretory values useful in selecting the operation?*

*Indicate the methods used in assessing follow-up data you use as the basis for your decision about the choice of operation. Do they include personal interviews, correspondence, chart reviews, secretory studies, x-rays? Indicate the numbers lost to follow-up. Compare the mortality and causes thereof for the various operations considered.*

*Is your selection of the type of operation influenced by: (1) obstruction; (2) active bleeding; (3) history of previous bleeding; (4) pathologic changes found at laparotomy; (5) age of the patient; (6) sex of the patient?*

*What criteria have you used to establish the presence or absence of postoperative dumping symptoms? Is it possible to predict the likelihood of postgastrectomy symptoms developing in an individual subject?*

*What is the frequency of persistent postoperative anemia?*

*After the various operations, what is the frequency of recurrence of ulcer as established by: (1) symptoms; (2) x-ray studies; (3) endoscopy?*

# Treatment of Peptic Ulcer Disease

**ALTON OCHSNER**

*Alton Ochsner Medical Foundation and Ochsner Clinic*

Peptic ulcer disease, the most common variety of which is duodenal ulcer, can be satisfactorily treated conservatively by medical management. With a few exceptions (usually duodenal ulcer), peptic ulcer results from peptic digestion of the duodenal mucosa in an acid medium. All modalities of therapy, whether medical or surgical, are directed at the control of acid. Because many normal individuals (about 10 per cent of the population) have gastric hyperacidity but no ulceration, it is my conviction that the individual with peptic ulcer, with the exception of those with superficial ulceration, has an inherent predisposition to ulcer genesis and that hydrochloric acid is the precipitating factor.

Operative treatment is indicated only when there is a life-threatening complication, such as massive hemorrhage, perforation, or obstruction, or when severe symptoms persist in spite of adequate medical therapy (intractability). It is impossible to determine what percentage of individuals with duodenal ulcer require operative treatment, unless one follows an entire population for a long period of time. Hospital statistics, and even office practice statistics, are unreliable, because inherent in them is a certain amount of bias by selection, since usually only in the more severe cases do patients consult physicians or enter hospitals. It is probable that no more than one-tenth of one per cent (0.1) require operative treatment.

The operative treatment of duodenal ulcer is less than a hundred years old. The principal methods of operative treatment have been drainage operations (pyloroplasty and gastrojejunostomy), gastric resection, and gastric denervation by vagus resection. Gastroenterostomy was the most widely used procedure throughout the world from the 1890's to the mid 1920's.[1-3] It was easily and safely performed and resulted in a cure in slightly over 50 per cent of cases, but in many cases (approximately 25 per cent) a severe complication, stomal or jejunal ulcer, developed. An advantage of gastroenterostomy, however, was that, if complications developed, it could be taken down.

When I came to Tulane as Professor of Surgery in 1927, for several years the most frequent gastric operation I performed was disconnecting gastrojejunostomies in patients who had developed stomal ulcers. Prior to this, I had been fortunate to serve as an exchange surgical resident under two Continental surgeons who had extensive experience in the operative treatment of peptic ulcer disease, Professor Paul Clairmont in Zurich and Professor Victor Schmieden in Frankfurt am Main. The former had been von Eiselberg's first pupil and contributed much to the development of the operative treatment of ulcer. Both these great gastric surgeons employed gastric resection in intractable peptic ulcer cases with great success, and I, profiting from this tremendous experience, became convinced that this was a valuable, safe method of therapy attended by few sequelae.

After an extensive personal experience (beginning with residency under the two great gastric surgeons mentioned previously, Professor Paul Clairmont, von Eiselberg's first pupil, and Professor Victor Schmieden), nothing has given me greater satisfaction (because of the great relief experienced by the patient) than the treatment of a patient with intractable ulcer disease by wide gastric resection.

Wide gastric resection consists of removal of the distal 70 to 75 per cent of the stomach, including the antrum and the lesser curvature up to the cardia. In patients with duodenal ulcer in whom the operation is usually done for intractability, the duodenum is usually so involved by scarring that a gastroduodenostomy (Billroth I) is not possible. In patients with gastric ulcer in whom less radical gastric resection (60 per cent) is satisfactory and in whom the duodenum is normal, gastroduodenostomy can generally be done. We therefore usually employ a gastrojejunostomy (Billroth II – Hofmeister posterior type) anastomosis, closing the upper portion of the stomach and using the lower end to anastomose (end-to-side) to a short loop of jejunum brought into the lesser sac through an opening in the transverse mesocolon. We are careful to make a small stoma, approximately the size of the jejunal lumen. Wide gastric resection, employed by us, is an operation that can be performed safely only by a well-trained surgeon and is more difficult to perform than most other gastric operations.

We have used wide gastric resection also in the treatment of patients with life-threatening complications. Although the results have been good in the correction of the life-threatening complication, generally, the results in patients who were operated on because of long-term intractable symptoms, or for obstruction, are better than in patients in whom the operation was done as an emergency (massive bleeding or perforation). This may be because the individual with an intractable ulcer has suffered so much that after he is operated on, he is so convinced that any minor postoperative disturbance he might have is of little or no significance that he believes that he has obtained complete and permanent relief. Krause,[4] in discussing postcibal symptoms after gastrectomy, stated, "If patients are operated on with insignificant preoperative subjective symptoms, the incidence of postcibal symptoms is certainly higher. The patient can be said to be 'psychologically immature' for operation." Papo and associates[5] stated, "The longer the history, the more severe the complaints, the older the patients, the better are results of surgery."

In peptic ulcer patients, as in all patients requiring operative therapy, the operation employed should have a high survival rate, the least number of recurrences, and the fewest sequelae. The undesirable sequelae of gastric operation for peptic ulcer disease are dumping, diarrhea, failure to gain weight, and, occasionally, gastric stasis.

Although Exner and Schwarzmann[6] performed vagus resection in 1911 in a patient with tabes dorsalis because of severe gastric crises, and Bircher[2] in 1912 in a patient with gastric hypermotility and hypersecretion, Latarjet[3] in 1922, and several others[7-10] combined vagus resection with gastroenterostomy, the operation never gained any popularity until Dragstedt's[11] splendid investigation of the role of the vagi in the genesis of ulcer, which he and Owens first reported in 1943.

I consider Dragstedt's and his co-workers' physiologic investigation one of the finest contributions ever made. The world will always be indebted to him for this work. Probably because of Dragstedt's great stature and popularity, vagus resection, which he advocated, was quickly adopted by the surgeons of the United States. Moreover, it was easier to perform, required less time, and, in most reported series, had a lower mortality rate than wide gastric resection. Although I was impressed, as were others, by these advantages, I was reluctant to employ vagus resection in the treatment of peptic ulcer disease for two reasons: first, because the results from wide gastric resection were so satisfactory; and second, because I had a vivid recollection of the period when gastroenterostomy was as popular as vagus resection but failed in about half the cases and was followed by a severe complication (stomal ulcer) in about one fourth of the cases. As mentioned previously, gastroenterostomy had the advantage that if it failed or a complication developed, the gastroenterostomy could be taken down and the gastroenteric tube returned to normal. I was concerned that a truncal vagotomy denervated not only the stomach and duodenum but also the biliary tract and the enteric tube down to the mid-portion of the transverse colon when only the stomach and duodenum were involved.

As further experience accumulated, repeated modifications of the procedure were advocated approximately every 5 years — an indication that the previously employed procedures had not produced satisfactory results. At first, vagus resection was performed; then vagus resection combined with gastroenterostomy; then vagus resection plus pyloroplasty; followed by vagus resection plus antral resection; then vagus resection plus 50 per cent gastric resection; and finally, selective vagus resection. Selective vagus resection was more appealing to me, because at least it did not denervate portions of the enteric tube that were uninvolved, and it was less likely to interfere with the intestinal and biliary functions. Although I had through the years been a strong advocate of the wide gastric resection in the treatment of intractable peptic ulcer disease, several of my clinic associates decided that vagus resection should be tried. This was about the time that vagus resection and 50 per cent gastric resection was popular.

At the Ochsner Clinic, peptic ulcer disease is considered, as mentioned previously, to be a condition that should be treated conservatively, and therefore all the patients are admitted to the Department of Gastroenterology, where therapy is undertaken. The surgeons see the patient only if there is failure to control the patient's symptoms or there is a life-threatening complication—in actuality, only cases in which medical treatment has failed. After the patient has completely convalesced from the operation, he again returns to the gastroenterological service for follow-up treatment, although he may be seen from time to time by the surgeon who operated upon him. I believe that gastric ulcer, which frequently is treated by surgical methods, is a different condition from duodenal ulcer. Although it occurs less frequently than duodenal ulcer, more cases require operative treatment. Because of the difficulty in distinguishing a benign from a malignant ulcer, every gastric ulcer must be considered malignant until proved otherwise. With the presently available endoscopic techniques, this can usually be done relatively easily. However, every gastric ulcer treated conservatively must be carefully followed at monthly intervals until the ulcer is completely healed and then at 3-month intervals for a year, because healing of malignant ulcer is possible, as we have repeatedly observed. Although perforation and massive hemorrhage occur less often in gastric ulcer than in duodenal ulcer, they are more lethal.

The Ochsner Clinic experience[12] prior to 1969 consisted of 4489 cases of peptic ulcer—3747 cases of duodenal ulcer (83 per cent) and 742 (17%) gastric ulcer. Five hundred and twenty-eight (14 per cent) of the patients with duodenal ulcers were operated upon, and 253 of the gastric ulcer patients (34 per cent) were operated upon. As emphasized previously, duodenal ulcer is primarily a medical disease, whereas we believe that patients with gastric ulcer should more frequently be operated upon.

Of the 815 patients operated upon, 65 per cent had duodenal ulcer, 31 per cent had gastric ulcer, and 4 per cent had gastrojejunal ulcer. Generally, the gastric ulcer patients had symptoms for relatively short periods of time, whereas those with duodenal and jejunal ulcers had long histories. Conservative therapy was more frequently and consistently used in the last two groups than in those with gastric ulcer. Over half the gastric ulcer patients (56 per cent) had symptoms for less than 6 months, and only 10 per cent had symptoms for over 10 years. Contrariwise, 28 per cent of the patients with duodenal ulcer had symptoms for less than 6 months; 29 per cent, for 2 to 10 years; and 25 per cent, for over 10 years. Eighty-five per cent of jejunal ulcer patients had symptoms for more than 2 years and 44 per cent, for more than 10 years.

The indications for operation in patients with duodenal ulcer were as follows: hemorrhage, 27 per cent; perforation, 6 per cent; obstruction, 26 per cent; intractable symptoms, 52 per cent; fear of possible malignancy, 5 per cent. In the group in which malignant change was considered, the patients were seen before the advent of modern gastroscopy, and it was impossible to tell from roentgenographic examination whether the ulcer was in the duodenum or the pylorus. Of the patients with gastric ulcer, 21 per cent had had hemorrhage; 4 per cent, perforation; 13 per cent, obstruction; 33 per cent, intractable symptoms; and 52 per cent were operated upon because of fear of malignant change. Of those with gastrojejunal ulcer operated upon, 32 per cent had had hemorrhage; 2 per cent, perforation; 11 per cent obstruction; and 76 per cent, intractable symptoms.

The complicating factors at the time of operation that necessitated operation were as follows: of the 528 patients with duodenal ulcer, 28 per cent had obstruction; 13 per cent, massive hemorrhage; and 8 per cent, perforation. Of the 253 patients with gastric ulcer operated upon, 13 per cent had obstruction; 14 per cent, massive hemorrhage; and 7 per cent, perforation. Of the 34 gastrojejunal ulcer patients, 23 per cent had obstruction; 18 per cent, hemorrhage; and 3 per cent, obstruction.

Because gastric resection has been employed for a much longer period of time by our group than has vagus resection, most of our patients had gastric resection. Six hundred and seventy-five (83 per cent) had wide gastric resection; 615 (75 per cent) had gastrojejunostomy (Billroth II), most of which were the Hofmeister posterior type; and 140 (17 per cent) had truncal vagus resection and 50 per cent gastric resection.

Recovery of the patient is the first desideratum after an operative procedure. Wide gastric resection is an extensive operation that requires the experience of a well-trained surgeon if a satisfactory survival rate is to be obtained. Vagus resection is a much easier operation, which requires less skill and time to perform and is associated with a lower mortality rate than wide gastric resection when performed by inexperienced gastric surgeons. In most reported series of ulcer operations, the mortality rate is lower after vagus resection than after wide gastric resection. However, this was not true in our series, in which all operations were performed only by well-trained, highly competent surgeons. The mortality rate following wide gastric resection was 1.4 per cent, whereas the rate following vagus resection plus 50 per cent gastric resection was 4 per cent. The only patients in our series who died postoperatively were those who were operated on because of massive hemorrhage, 57 per cent of whom were treated by wide gastric resection and 43 per cent, by vagus resection. The mortality rate in all patients operated upon for massive hemorrhage was 5.8 per cent. The death rate in those treated by radical gastrectomy for massive hemorrhage was 3.3 per cent and in those treated by vagotomy and partial gastrectomy was 13.6 per cent. This indicates that patients with massively bleeding ulcers are best treated by gastric resection rather than vagus resection.

The lower survival rate in the patients treated by vagus resection was undoubtedly due to the inability of vagus resection and 50 per cent gastric resection to control the massive bleeding; whereas the more difficult procedure — wide gastric resection — was more successful in spite of the greater magnitude of the procedure.

## Results

Our cases have been very carefully followed. In our present series of cases, 21 per cent have been followed for less than a year, 41 per cent for from 1 to 5 years, and 38 per cent for more than 5 years. Only by careful long-term follow-up is true evaluation of any type of treatment of ulcer disease possible. It required a long time to determine that gastrojejunostomy failed to provide relief in over half the ulcer patients, and in approximately one fourth of the patients, results were complicated by a stomal or jejunal ulcer that was worse than the original ulcer. However, as stressed previously, gastrojejunostomy had the advantage that it could be taken down and the normal relations restored.

In evaluation of any operative procedure, three factors are important: a low operative mortality, few sequelae (preferably nondisabling), and complete freedom from symptoms. As already stated, the mortality rate was lower in the patients treated by wide gastric resection (1.4 per cent) than in the patients treated by vagus resection plus 50 per cent gastric resection (4 per cent).

The incidence of recurrent ulcer in patients treated by wide gastric resection was 2.1 per cent and in those treated by vagus resection plus 50 per cent gastric resection, 5.4 per cent. Thus, the mortality rate was over three times greater and the incidence of recurrent ulcer twice as great in the patients treated by vagus resection than in those treated by wide gastrectomy. Other sequelae of operation for peptic ulcer disease are dumping, gastric retention, failure to gain weight, and diarrhea. All may be disabling, but intractable diarrhea is the most frequent disabling sequela. Dumping, although not infrequent immediately after any gastric operation, usually is readily controlled by dietary measures. Gastric retention generally is also easily controlled. Great emphasis has been placed on failure to gain weight, I believe unnecessarily. Although many patients do not gain weight following a gastric operation for peptic ulcer disease, they are free from symptoms and are able to eat and drink anything (especially those who have had wide gastric resection). Obesity is ordinarily considered a health hazard, except, apparently, in a patient who has been operated on for peptic ulcer disease.

Severe diarrhea is the most undesirable sequela and is likely to be the most disabling. In a small number of patients treated by vagus resection, it is so disabling that the most unphysiologic operative procedure imaginable (reversal of a short loop of jejunum) has been employed to control the disabling diarrhea. I know of no case, nor have I found any reported, of such severe diarrhea following wide gastric resection.

The incidence of sequelae in the Ochsner Clinic series was as follows: *dumping*—wide gastric resection, 11 per cent, vagus resection plus 50 per cent gastric resection, 35 per cent; *gastric retention*—wide gastric resection, 1.4 per cent, vagotomy and gastric resection, 3 per cent; *vomiting*—wide gastric resection, 4 per cent, vagotomy and 50 per cent gastric resection, 15 per cent; and *diarrhea*—wide gastric resection, 6.5 per cent, vagotomy plus gastric resection, 44 per cent.

All the sequelae, including recurrence, are undesirable. They vary considerably in their severity, and .although many are amenable to therapy, some may persist for long periods of time. Of the 14 per cent of patients who had dumping following wide gastric resection, it was mild in 11 per cent, moderate in 2 per cent, severe in 0.5 per cent, and persistent in 3.8 per cent.

Of the 35 per cent with dumping following vagus resection and 50 per cent gastric resection, it was mild in 14 per cent, moderate in 15 per cent, severe in 3 per cent, and persistent in 26 per cent.

Dumping is generally less frequent following Billroth I gastric resection than following Billroth II resection, because, I believe, the stoma in the gastroduodenostomy is usually smaller than that generally made in gastrojejunal anastomosis. We have had few patients with dumping following wide gastric resection, even though in most cases a Billroth II type of operation was used, because the gastrojejunostomy stoma initially is purposely made small, approximately the size of or smaller than the jejunal lumen.

Of the 6.5 per cent of patients in our series who had diarrhea following wide gastric resection, it was mild in 3.4 per cent, moderate in 3.4 per cent, severe in 0.4 per cent, and persistent in 4.8 per cent. Of the 44 per cent who had diarrhea following vagus resection and 50 per cent gastric resection, it was mild in 14 per cent, moderate in 27 per cent, severe in 2 per cent, and persistent in 22 per cent. Thus, diarrhea, the most undesirable of all sequelae, was more frequent (44 per cent) and more persistent (22 per cent) following vagus resection than following wide gastric resection.

As mentioned previously, it is our contention that failure to gain weight following an operation for peptic ulcer disease usually is of little significance. In our series of cases, the failure to gain weight was approximately the same in both groups. There was no difference between the patients treated with wide gastric resection (58 per cent lost less than 15 pounds, 25 per cent lost more than 15 pounds, 16 per cent had no change, and 11 per cent gained weight) and those treated by vagus resection plus 50 per cent gastric resection (33 per cent lost less than 15 pounds, 30 per cent lost more than 15 pounds, 15 per cent had no change, and 13 per cent gained weight).

In the final analysis, the patients' evaluations of the results of therapy are probably the most important. Most of the patients were interviewed personally, a few followed by questionnaire. Those who stated that they were well, without symptoms and able to eat and drink normally, were considered to have an excellent result. Some remained well only when observing some dietary discretion; these were considered to have good results. Others were improved but somewhat restricted in their activities even on dietary restriction and were considered to have fair results. Finally, there was a small number who were not benefited at all or made worse by the operation. Their results were considered poor.

Both groups of patients were categorized according to the long-term results. The patients who underwent wide gastric resection classified themselves as follows: excellent, 80 per cent; good, 13 per cent; fair, 4.3 per cent; and poor, 2.5 per cent. Of those who had vagus resection with 50 per cent gastrectomy, the respective percentages were excellent, 21 per cent; good, 48 per cent; fair, 19 per cent; and poor, 12 per cent.

Almost four times as many patients were completely cured by wide gastric resection as were cured by vagus resection (80 per cent vs. 21 per cent). More than four times as many patients had poor results following vagus resection and 50 per cent gastric resection as those treated by wide gastric resection (12 per cent vs. 2.5 per cent).

Surprisingly few of these patients, both those having wide gastric resection and those having vagus resection, developed anemia that required supplemental iron therapy.

As was previously emphasized, the operative treatment of peptic ulcer disease is indicated only in the most severe forms, in patients in whom treatment has failed to relieve symptoms (intractability) and those with life-threatening complications (massive hemorrhage, perforation, obstruction). All forms of therapy are designed to control acidity. A greater percentage of gastric ulcer patients require operative therapy than do those with duodenal ulcer, because the former do not respond to conservative (medical) therapy as well as the latter. Although life-threatening complications are less frequent in gastric ulcer patients, they are more lethal. A less radical gastrectomy (60 per cent) than is necessary in duodenal ulcer patients is usually satisfactory in gastric ulcer patients. In the former group, if gastrectomy alone is used, it should be approximately 75 per cent.

An operation on the gastrointestinal tract is likely to be followed by sequelae. In choosing an operative procedure, it is necessary to employ one with a low mortality rate and the fewest sequelae.

In intractable ulcer disease, 75-per cent gastric resection, which has been employed for over 75 years, has, when properly performed, resulted in a higher success rate with fewer sequelae than any other gastric operation.

Truncal vagotomy is theoretically unsatisfactory because it denervates not only the stomach and duodenum but also the biliary tract and intestinal tract down to the transverse colon, which are not involved in peptic ulcer disease. Their vagal denervation is of no value and may even be detrimental. Truncal vagotomy is also permanent and cannot be corrected, as is possible in patients who develop sequelae following gastrojejunostomy. We have had no experience with selective vagus resection in which denervation is limited to the stomach and duodenum.

In patients undergoing 75 per cent gastric resection for ulcer disease, the best results (usually complete relief) are obtained in those patients whose symptoms are prolonged and have not responded to medical therapy (intractability). On the other hand, patients operated on because of life-threatening complications, usually with a shorter history, have not been as uniformly relieved. One wonders whether the longer suffering of the former group may not motivate them to disregard mild, insignificant manifestations that follow a gastric operation.

As previously emphasized, in my long and extensive experience, no operative procedure that I have performed has been as gratifying to me as 75 per cent gastric resection, because of its complete relief of disabling peptic ulcer disease. Equally important is that the relief is almost invariably permanent.

## References

1. Exner, A.: Ein neues operationsverfahren bei tabischen crises gastriques. Dtsch. Z. Chir. *111*:576–590, 1911.
2. Bircher, E.: Die resektion von aesten der n vagus zur behandlung gastrischer affektionen. Schweiz. Med. Wochenschr. *50*:519–528, 1920.

3. Latarjet, A.: Résection des nerfs de l'estomac. Technique opératoire. Résultats cliniques. Bull. Acad. Med. 87:681–691, 1922.
4. Krause, U.: Long-term results of medical and surgical treatment of peptic ulcer. Acta Chir. Scand. Suppl. 310:5–11, 1963.
5. Papo, I., Bervar, M., Jankuloski, A., Atanasijevic, T., Spasojevic, P., and Smiljanic, T.: Classical gastric resection, a favorite operation for gastroduodenal ulcer. Congr. Soc. Int. Chir. 22:347–352, 1967.
6. Exner, A., and Schwarzmann, E.: Tabische krisen, ulcus ventriculi und vagus. Wien. Klin. Wochenschr. 25:1405–1406, 1912.
7. Podkaminsky, R.: Gastroenterostomie mit prophylaktischer vagotomie. Zentralbl. Chir. 52:568–569, 1925.
8. Schiassi, B.: The role of the pyloro-duodenal nerve supply in the surgery of duodenal ulcer. Ann. Surg. 81:939–948, 1925.
9. Klein, E.: Left vagus section and partial gastrectomy for duodenal ulcer with hyperacidity. Ann. Surg. 90:65–68, 1929.
10. Pieri, G., and Tanferna, V.: Studi sulla fisiologia dell'innervazione viscerale dell'uomo. II. Effetti della resezione del vago sulla secrezione gastrica. Riforma Med. 46:323–326, 1930.
11. Dragstedt, L. R., and Owens, F. M.: Supra-diaphragmatic resection of the vagus nerves in treatment of duodenal ulcer. Proc. Soc. Exp. Biol. (N. Y.) 53:152–154, 1943.
12. Ochsner, A., Zehnder, P. R., and Trammell, S. W.: The surgical treatment of peptic ulcer: a critical analysis of results from subtotal gastrectomy and from vagotomy plus partial gastrectomy. Surgery 67:1017–1028, 1970.

# Truncal Vagotomy with Drainage for the Elective Treatment of Duodenal Ulcer Disease

JACK M. FARRIS

*Veterans Administration Hospital, San Diego, California*

and A. G. GREENBURG

*University of California, San Diego, School of Medicine*

The current wide-ranging reported experience with treatment of duodenal ulcer disease suggests that the results of elective operation for chronic duodenal ulcer are not very different, independent of the operative procedure chosen; thus, safety and ease of performance begin to emerge as decisive factors.

In this article, we have been asked to define the role of truncal vagotomy with drainage as a primary surgical modality in the therapy of chronic duodenal ulcer disease. As the drainage procedure of choice, we are advocating a *Jaboulay gastroduodenostomy* in conjunction with the truncal vagotomy. Recurrent ulcer disease following "vagotomy and drainage" can be due to an incomplete vagotomy, an inadequate drainage procedure, a combination of the two, or some extrinsic mechanism, such as a gastrin-secreting tumor. Although the most critical criterion of success for any operative procedure is its ability to prevent recurrences, there are other factors which must be considered. If one is to compare various operative procedures applied to a specific disease process, it is essential to examine mortality rates and the incidence and severity of early and late complications and sequelae, as well as success in curing the disease. From a patient's vantage point, total rehabilitation time, time lost from work, and time necessary to return to one's usual occupation may be critical. In addition, the chronologic stage of disease must be defined so that a valid comparison can be made, based on patients' experience with the disease.

109

Critics of vagotomy and drainage frequently cite the high ulcer recurrence rate as a reason to abandon this approach. The recurrence rate has variously been reported to range from 3 to 24 per cent.[1] The problem, as we view it, relates to classifying the patients and comparing the operative subgroups prospectively—a massive undertaking. Suffice it to say, all vagotomies and drainages are not the same, for "when two men perform the same task, it is not the same after all." There are at least *four* common variations on the "pyloroplasty." If one assumes that creation of an inadequate gastric drainage can be responsible for recurrent disease, either alone or in concert with inadequate vagotomy, then to obtain significant information, it would be best to compare only that "matched set" of patients who received identical treatment. Such a comparison is not easily attained from a retrospective literature search, because the various forms of drainage are usually lumped together under the heading "pyloroplasty" and, at best, are only differentiated from gastroenterostomy.

There is evidence to support the use of truncal vagotomy and drainage, in the form of a pyloroplasty, if one looks at those clinical series devoted to the elective clinical situation. It is on this group of patients that we should focus our attention, for when the vagaries of emergency and acute stress are eliminated and the elective population is well defined, the recurrence rate is found to be 3 to 7 per cent in those patients followed 5 years or longer.[2-6]

Although the Weinberg modification of the Heineke-Mikulicz pyloroplasty relates more to the method of approximation than the size of the orifice, the Finney and Jaboulay procedures usually create a larger orifice and there is greater opportunity to neutralize residual acid because of the proximity to the ampulla of Vater. In a review of his personal series, Hoerr[18] reported better results with a Finney drainage than with a traditional Heineke-Mikulicz and stated, "The Jaboulay gastroduodenostomy has promise as being perhaps even more effective than the Finney pyloroplasty."

In our previously reported series,[19] a recurrence rate of 3 per cent was obtained for patients with truncal vagotomy and Jaboulay gastroduodenostomy. We attribute this low recurrence rate to the wide drainage afforded the stomach with this procedure and the prevention of gastric stasis, which could play a role, via hormonal mechanisms, in gastric acid secretion and, hence, recurrence. We have also had a lower re-operative rate for late emptying problems than that found after the Heineke-Mikulicz procedure.

Although recurrence rate is a significant factor in assessing the efficacy of an operative procedure, it is but one factor. One of the earlier arguments for the use of truncal vagotomy and pyloroplasty in the treatment of duodenal ulcer disease was the difference noted in mortality rates with this procedure and with resective therapy. Supporters of the nonresective procedure pointed out that their operation was safer and had a shorter convalescence period and was therefore preferable even if it had a higher recurrence rate and a second operation was more frequently required. One could ask why a more formidable procedure should be done if it will be unnecessary in 95 per cent of patients. Over the past 10 to 15 years, it has become apparent that acceptable (i.e., less than 1 per cent) operative mortality rates can be achieved in elective cases, independent of the procedure performed,[7,8] and the occasional gastric surgeon may do best to do the procedure he is most comfortable with.

A variety of arguments have been advanced to support the use of one procedure over another, with particular reference to early or late complications and sequelae that can result in functional impairments. Diarrhea, dumping, and cholelithiasis have been most commonly reported as the major sequelae following various operative procedures for duodenal ulcer disease. In addition, the parameter of *patient satisfaction*, defined by either the Visick classification[9] or some other equally specific categorization, has been increasingly reported. We should note that the Visick classification was originally designed to evaluate postgastrectomy phenomena and therefore may not be directly applicable to evaluation of vagotomies.

After critical evaluation of a series of articles dealing with these problems, one would have to conclude that what little variation exists between the groups treated by various operative procedures is difficult to explain. With regard to "diarrhea," a great deal depends on the definition of this entity. Overall, it would appear that 20 to 25 per cent of patients undergoing truncal vagotomy for duodenal ulcer disease experience an increase in the frequency of stools in the postoperative period, as was well documented by Johnston et al. in 1972.[10] It is interesting to note that the incidence of "diarrhea" is reported in a higher percentage of patients in the various British series than in the United States literature. This, of course, leads to speculation regarding the etiology, and one must search beyond the procedure to adequately define the basis. Is less attention paid to dietary alteration postoperatively? Are the patients instructed in avoidance of hyperosmolar meals? Do these patients ingest more water? Is the mineral content of the local water supply different and thus contributory? Unfortunately these questions are largely unanswered yet are potentially a source of key information. Proponents of vagotomies less extensive than truncal cite this high rate of diarrhea as a reason for performing total gastric or selective proximal vagotomies. They usually then state that their procedure produces less frequent diarrhea, but we don't know the criteria for definition. One must recall that loss of pyloric control may be as contributory to diarrhea as denervation. Clearly, if one denervates the entire gastrointestinal tract, there is an increased possibility of a "diarrhea" complication. However, by the Visick classification, there is no clear evidence to indicate that there is more patient dissatisfaction with a truncal vagotomy and drainage than with other procedures.[8] It should be noted that the population group cited may significantly differ (socioeconomically) from those of other series in which differences were found.[7]

Looking a little further, the incidence of the hypoglycemic syndrome, "dumping," did not differ with the type of vagotomy or type of drainage employed, although the latter was difficult to define. The series generally examined to determine the "incidence" usually randomized the type of vagotomy but failed to standardize the drainage procedure.[6, 11-14] As noted previously, if a procedure has two components, either can be involved as the cause. For the complications discussed here, it is all but impossible to critically sort the factors of significance.

Truncal vagotomy has been said to increase the incidence of cholelithiasis, and thus, procedures to spare the hepatic vagal innervation have been developed and used. Although logically sound, the idea is hardly supported in fact. The fact that the incidence of cholelithiasis is high in the general population raises the question of whether vagotomy causes the development of stones or whether, in fact, there is a predisposition to stone formation. In the large series reviewed by Postlethwait,[8] there were no differences found in the incidence of cholelithiasis following any of the procedures used. Other series noted previously either failed to mention this problem or were nonspecific in describing it. Indeed, few of the "prospective randomized studies" seem to consider preoperative radiographic examination of the biliary tree to be an important factor in evaluation of the patient. Thus, when cholecystitis appears, it is attributed to the operation and not to a pre-existing disease.

The only currently available reliable evidence for altered biliary function following truncal vagotomy is the fine study of Parkin and co-workers describing the gallbladder volume and contractility after various types of vagotomy.[15] They very clearly demonstrate that the gallbladder resting volume increased significantly (49 per cent) following truncal vagotomy as compared with total gastric and selective proximal vagotomies. They noted no contractility impairment; however, the residual volume of the gallbladder was greater in the truncal group, and thus the potential for stasis increased. This may be responsible for stone formation. Although a variety of studies have been performed in experimental animals that purport to demonstrate the "lithogenic" effect of vagotomy, such changes in the bile of man following operation have yet to be demonstrated. The study of Parkin may be significant, but more patients are needed.

The effects of truncal vagotomy on pancreatic function and the development of pancreatic insufficiency and steatorrhea are actually undocumented in man. Steatorrhea may be pancreatic in origin, or it may be related to alterations in bile salts. It has been shown, experimentally, that vagotomy and the resultant achlorhydria produce alterations in the bacterial flora of the upper gastrointestinal tract. These bacterial alterations can produce steatorrhea by deconjugation of bile salts, by metabolism of carbohydrates to short-chain fatty acids which are capable of exerting an osmotic effect, or by conversion of some dietary fat to irritating substances, resulting in diarrhea. Unfortunately, these mechanisms are postulated and demonstrated in dogs, and are only theoretically related to patient experience.[14, 16] In a similar experiment, Crow[17] demonstrated increased stool bulk, fecal fat, and nitrogen following truncal vagotomy; however, the increase in fecal fat was even greater following selective vagotomy.

Thus, in the absence of hard data to demonstrate a true difference in results of the various types of vagotomies and drainage procedures, one is left with personal preference as the deciding factor. Well-planned prospective studies are not readily available to answer the basic questions, and, indeed, retrospective analysis is not sufficient. A few experimental results in animals may offer explanations of the observed phenomena, but demonstration in man is lacking. It is apparent that in most large reviews, prospective or retrospective, the exact type of "drainage procedure" is rarely specified in detail sufficient to allow critical evaluation. Frequently, the Heineke-Mikulicz procedure is grouped with the Weinberg and the Jaboulay with the Finney. Although from a historical point of view, the latter two may be considered to be one and the same, they are today two different procedures. In no prospective series has the stomal size of the "drainage procedure" been standardized, and so comparison is impossible.

We base our preference for truncal vagotomy and Jaboulay gastroduodenostomy in the treatment of chronic duodenal ulcer disease on the following rationale. It is relatively simple to perform the operation in a reasonable period of time. There is no decrease in the gastric reservoir anatomically, although a *functional* decrease may be apparent, as evidenced by decreased gastric emptying time. There is no major risk to the patient in that it is a safe procedure with respect to operative mortality and postoperative morbidity. Of the authors' last 500 patients undergoing elective procedures, 3 died — an operative mortality rate of 0.6 per cent. As noted earlier, there is little hard evidence to indicate differences in long-term complications or sequelae following truncal vagotomy as compared to other vagotomies. At this time, there is no evidence to allow one to speculate on what is the best "drainage" procedure, although the Jaboulay procedure is apparently gaining popularity. In our hands, the rate of recurrent disease in more than 500 patients is approximately 3 per cent. We feel it proper to deal with this small group of patients in a more aggressive manner when recurrent disease becomes intractable and requires a second operation. Prior to that, however, efforts are directed at defining the basis for the recurrence, and if incomplete vagotomy is suspected, a transthoracic vagotomy is performed before gastric secretion therapy. It is imperative to be certain that there are no occult emptying problems contributory to the situation.

Before discussing our criteria for operation and follow-up, let us state that the newer selective proximal gastric vagotomy may be a good operation either without drainage or with gastroduodenostomy. If a more complete vagotomy can be attained by this procedure, then it should be employed. As has been demonstrated with total gastric vagotomy, a more complete denervation is attained when the procedure is more anatomically specific. It is also apparent to us that incomplete vagotomy is less frequently encountered in the patients of surgeons who have performed many operations than in those of surgeons who have done few.

## Diagnostic Criteria

Documented evidence of active or chronic duodenal ulcer disease on radiographic examination of the upper gastrointestinal tract is essential to establish the diagnosis. The presence of an ulcer crater is most significant, while evidence of slow healing or scarring of the duodenal bulb with deformity and loss of normal mucosal patterns are suggestive of chronic disease. Endoscopic examination and photographic documentation of the presence of an ulcer are valuable in documenting and establishing the diagnosis. When associated with a history of recurrent epigastric pain following meals, which is relieved by antacids, these anatomic findings strongly support the presence of chronic inflammatory disease of the duodenum and establish the diagnosis. The symptom complex alone can be misleading and, in the absence of anatomical abnormality, does not establish the diagnosis. Thus, the presence of a symptom complex alone *is not* an indication for operation. Clearly, there is a spectrum between the presence of symptoms and the development of surgically significant complications—obstruction, perforation, or bleeding. At some point in the continuum, essentially for unknown reasons, conservative therapy fails in some patients and operation is advised. By this time, there must exist persistent morphologic evidence of chronic disease, both endoscopically and radiographically as well as at operation. Because there are other disease entities which can produce a symptom complex similar to that of duodenal ulcer, it is essential to make certain that the disease producing the symptomatology is identified. In the event that two diseases are found, for example a hiatus hernia and duodenal ulcer disease, it is almost impossible to state which exerts the greater symptomatology. One could easily be trapped into operating for the duodenal ulcer, only to have a clinical failure because the hiatus hernia persists in giving problems. It is situations like this that may well account for some of the operative failures noted previously.

## Criteria for Operation

We consider intractable pain, gastric outlet obstruction, previous perforation with continued symptoms, and a history of *significant* recurrent bleeding episodes as the primary indications for recommending elective operative intervention in duodenal ulcer disease. Any patient who has bled twice and required multiple transfusions during the hemorrhage or in the immediate posthemorrhage period should be considered a candidate. We define significant bleeds as those requiring 5 or 6 unit replacements.

We advise operative intervention at an earlier time for older patients who have bled, because a major hemorrhage invokes metabolic and physiologic demands for which the patient may be unable to compensate. Similarly, pyloric obstruction with its attendant fluid and electrolyte complications is less well tolerated in the older or more seriously ill patient who may be functioning on the edge of his homeostatic mechanisms and maintaining a delicate balance that is easily upset by a major physiologic insult. Occasionally, sociologic factors, constant stress, a poor home environment, inadequate dietary habits, and inability to adhere to a conservative management program influence our decision, and operation is recommended earlier. We are tending to be more liberal in the use of this less extensive operation. Sex and body build do not influence our decision to operate or choice of procedure.

## Preoperative Studies

Currently, we advocate having and obtain for all patients a set of data regarding the acid secretory capacity of the stomach. We use basal (1 hour)

and Histalog stimulated gastric analysis techniques, as well as 12-hour overnight secretory testing. At this time, we do not use these data to identify
those patients who may require a more extensive (resective) initial procedure. Even if there is evidence of gastric ulcer, the initial procedure would
be a truncal vagotomy and gastroduodenostomy.

## Selection of Operation

In elective cases, there is rarely active bleeding, and thus an incision immediately over the pylorus is unnecessary. In the emergency situation, to
control bleeding, we frequently find it necessary to incise the gastro-pyloro-
duodenum to make a suture ligation of an arterial bleeder. When this is the
case, we assure ourselves of at least an 8 cm. incision and use a Weinberg or
Finney closure. We are not, at the moment, influenced by age, sex, or
amount of disease present, since we are advocating one of the simpler
procedures.

## Postoperative Symptomatology

The postoperative symptomatology associated with rapid gastric emptying (the dumping syndrome, hypoglycemic reaction) is searched for in the
clinical questionnaire, as well as in the verbal interview. We particularly
seek information regarding flushing, feeling of warmth, and tachycardia, but
we never try to lead the patient to an answer. We consider the dumping
"severe" if the patient volunteers all the symptomatology of the entity and
shows weight loss associated with the symptomatology.

The dumping syndrome is associated with an inappropriate peripheral
vasodilatation following ingestion of hypertonic glucose solutions. Using the
facilities of our peripheral vascular laboratory to assess an inappropriate
flow-resistance dissociation, we have evaluated a number of patients preoperatively and postoperatively without any positive findings. Significantly,
although we can demonstrate the phenomenon in an individual known to
have the dumping syndrome, we have not been able to document the phenomenon in any of our patients preoperatively. The fact that the incidence of
dumping is rather slight might preclude finding a case in our recently started
series.

Because of the rather constant reports indicating Visick ratings of group
IV for about 10 per cent of all patients undergoing operation for duodenal
ulcer disease, we have recently begun to define our patients' psychologic
constitution. All patients currently scheduled for operative therapy are
preoperatively given a Minnesota Multiphasic Personality Test for purposes
of assessing psychologic makeup. We hope to correlate the results with
postoperative complaints, particularly for patients classified into Visick
group IV.

## Postoperative Anemia

We are not aware of any major problem with anemia in our patient population undergoing vagotomy and drainage. The vitamin $B_{12}$-related anemias are primarily associated with achlorhydria and folate deficiency, which are usually seen after gastrectomies of greater than 50 per cent. Although truncal vagotomy is effective in reducing basal acid secretion, there is still a sufficient parietal cell mass to produce acid, and achlorhydria does not exist. In the absence of such a mechanism, anemia is rare, assuming that a relatively normal diet is consumed.

## Follow-up Data

We are currently very aggressive in our follow-up, because we consider it critical to the successful evaluation of any procedure. We follow our patients by rehospitalization for 1 to 2 days in the 3-month and 12-month postoperative periods. At this time, gastric motility studies and emptying time, secretory data, and definition of completeness of vagotomy are assessed. In addition, any special projects associated with the effects of vagotomy on gastric physiology are repeated in patients giving consent. Between these periods, for the first year, we call or correspond with all patients in the group in order to obtain answers to a standard clinical questionnaire. This questionnaire serves as the basis for evaluating the patient's response to his illness and postoperative condition and is administered for the first time preoperatively. With it, we can track an unsatisfactory course and possibly identify temporally its onset. The questionnaire allows us to define a Visick category for each patient. All charts are reviewed annually to detect any missed problems that might possibly have been spirited away by other specialists. Prior to 1973, in our personal experience with over 700 patients, follow-up was obtained by mail questionnaires and personal interviews. Only if recurrence was suspected were secretory tests repeated.

## Summary

We feel that truncal vagotomy and Jaboulay gastroduodenostomy is an effective operative procedure in the treatment of complications of duodenal ulcer disease. In our hands, there is an acceptable mortality rate (0.6 per cent) and a low recurrence rate (3 per cent) with an approximately 96 per cent patient follow-up. For the few patients with virulent disease, a second operation of greater magnitude (for example, resective therapy such as antrectomy) may be required. Little hard data support the deficiencies usually attributed to truncal vagotomy, and even less information is available to evaluate the relationship between operative results and the type of drainage procedure used. After a careful analysis, one is left supporting a procedure that has been *personally satisfactory* for the vast majority of patients so treated. We must add, however, that proper evaluation of the various procedures requires a well-designed prospective randomized study that differentiates the procedures and the sequelae, as well as recurrences and clinical results. Such studies are currently underway in many centers, and we anxiously await their critical reports.

# *References*

1. Herrington, J. L., Jr.: Current operations for duodenal ulcer. Curr. Probl. Surg. July, 1972, pp. 1–61.
2. Eisenberg, M. M., Woodward, R. R., Carsan, T. J., and Dragstedt, L. T.: Vagotomy and drainage procedure for duodenal ulcer. Ann. Surg. 170:317, 1969.
3. Evans, R. H., Zatchuk, R., and Menguy, R.: Role of vagotomy and gastric drainage in the surgical treatment of duodenal ulcer. Surg. Clin. North Am. 47:141, 1967.
4. Schofield, P. F., Watson-Williams, E. J., and Sorrell, V. F.: Vagotomy and pyloric drainage for chronic duodenal ulcer. Arch. Surg. 95:615, 1967.
5. Jordan, P. H., and Condon, R. E.: A prospective evaluation of vagotomy-pyloroplasty and vagotomy-antrectomy for treatment of duodenal ulcer. Ann. Surg. 172:547, 1970.
6. Kennedy, F., MacKay, C., Bedi, B. S., and Kay, A. W.: Truncal vagotomy and drainage for chronic duodenal ulcer disease: a controlled trial. Br. Med. J. 2:71, 1973.
7. Goligher, J. C., Pulvertaft, C. N., Irvin, T. T., Johnston, D., Walker, B., Hall, R. A., Willison-Pepper, J., and Matheson, T. S.: Five to eight-year results of truncal vagotomy and pyloroplasty for duodenal ulcer. Br. Med. J. 1:7, 1972.
8. Postlethwait, R. W.: Five-year follow-up results of operations for duodenal ulcer. Surg. Gynecol. Obstet. 137:387, 1973.
9. Visick, A. H.: The study of failures after gastrectomy. Ann. R. Coll. Surgeons England 3:266, 1948.
10. Johnston, D., Humphrey, C. S., Walker, B. E., Pulvertaft, C. N., and Goligher, J. C.: Vagotomy without diarrhea. Br. Med. J. 3:788, 1972.
11. Kraft, R. O., Fry, W. J., Wilhelm, K. G., and Ransom, H. K.: Selective gastric vagotomy: a critical appraisal. Arch. Surg. 95:625, 1967.
12. Mason, M. C., Giles, G. R., Graham, N. G., Clark, C. G., and Goligher, J. C.: An early assessment of selective and total vagotomy. Br. J. Surg. 55:677, 1968.
13. Sawyers, J. L., Scott, H. W., Edwards, W. H., Shull, H. J., and Law, D. H., IV: Comparative studies of the clinical effects of truncal and selective gastric vagotomy. Am. J. Surg. 115:165, 1968.
14. Kronborg, O., Malmström, J., and Christiansen, P. M.: A comparison between the results of truncal and selective vagotomy in patients with duodenal ulcer. Scand. J. Gastroenterol. 5:519, 1970.
15. Parkin, G. J. S., Smith, R. B., and Johnston, D.: Gallbladder volume and contractility after truncal, selective and highly selective (parietal cell) vagotomy in man. Ann. Surg. 178:581, 1973.
16. Broido, P. W., Gorbach, S. L., Condon, R. E., and Nyhus, L. M.: Upper intestinal microfloral control effects of gastric acid and vagal denervation on bacterial concentrations. Arch. Surg. 106:90, 1973.
17. Crow, R. W., Schulte, W. J., Ellison, E. H., and Winship, D. H.: Selective versus truncal vagotomy: a comprehensive study of fecal nitrogen and fat losses. Am. J. Surg. 121:684, 1971.
18. Hoerr, S. O.: Comparative results of operations for duodenal ulcer. Am. J. Surg. 125:3–11, 1973.
19. Farris, J. M., and Smith, G. K.: Appraisal of the long term results of vagotomy and pyloroplasty in 100 patients with bleeding duodenal ulcer. Ann. Surg. 166:630, 1967.

# Proximal Gastric Vagotomy without Drainage for Duodenal Ulcer

GEORGE A. HALLENBECK

*Scripps Clinic, La Jolla, California*

Truncal vagotomy (TV) vagally denervates the abdominal contents, because the vagal trunks are divided proximal to the origins of the gastric, hepatic, and celiac branches. Selective gastric vagotomy (SV) vagally denervates the entire stomach but not the other abdominal viscera, because the branches to the stomach are divided distal to the origins of the hepatic and celiac nerves. Both TV and SV cause unacceptable gastric stasis, which is commonly prevented by adding pyloroplasty, gastrojejunostomy, or antrectomy. Proximal gastric vagotomy (PGV) vagally denervates only the corpus and fundus of the stomach, because the nerves in the lesser omentum that innervate the antrum (nerves of Latarjet) are preserved and because the hepatic and celiac branches are preserved as they are in SV. Some synonyms for PGV found in the literature are: highly selective vagotomy, parietal cell vagotomy, selective vagotomy of the parietal cell mass, selective proximal vagotomy, proximal selective vagotomy, and acid-fundic selective vagotomy. If the operation survives the tests of experience, one name may be adopted by consensus. My choice is proximal gastric vagotomy, because it is precise anatomically and says neither too much nor too little.

Goligher[1] has published a superb description of the operative technique for PGV that should be consulted and carefully read by anyone interested in the operation. PGV differs from other common operations for duodenal ulcer by preserving vagal innervation of the gastric antrum. This makes prevention of gastric stasis by pyloroplasty, gastrojejunostomy, or, of course, antrectomy unnecessary, thereby minimizing interference with the normal control of gastric emptying. To the extent that uncontrolled and usually abnormally rapid gastric emptying, especially of hyperosmolar liquids, causes or helps to cause dumping and diarrhea, and to the extent that uncontrolled regurgita-

119

tion of bile into the stomach causes bile vomiting and distressing gastritis, PGV should be advantageous if it really preserves more nearly normal gastric emptying. If PGV also sufficiently reduced gastric secretion of acid and pepsin so that duodenal ulcers healed and did not recur, and if it were to have the lowest operative mortality rate, it would clearly be the superior operation.

My position in 1976 regarding PGV without drainage for elective treatment of duodenal ulcer without obstruction is as follows: (1) PGV reduces gastric secretion of acid and pepsin to the same degree that TV and SV do. (2) PGV alters gastric emptying less than other operations currently used for duodenal ulcer. (3) In retrospective studies by several authors, PGV has been shown to control the duodenal ulcer diathesis with few undesirable side effects. (4) PGV has been reported by other authors to be followed by an unacceptably high incidence of recurrent duodenal ulcer, but gastric secretory data, where available, indicate that many of these vagotomies were incomplete. (5) Not enough time has yet elapsed for assessment of the permanence of the effects of properly performed PGV. (6) Although several controlled trials of PGV randomized with other elective operations for duodenal ulcer are known to be in progress, none has yet reached the point of decision about the operation.

Let me try to support this position with data.

## Effects of PGV on Gastric Secretion in Humans

The gastric secretory changes caused by PGV, by TV with pyloroplasty (TV + P), or by SV with pyloroplasty (SV + P) are remarkably similar.

Clarke, Allan, and Alexander-Williams[2] conducted a controlled trial in which 40 consecutive male patients with duodenal ulcers proven radiologically and at elective operation underwent either PGV or SV, with the choice selected randomly during the operation by a previously arranged computerized technique. The first 20 patients had no "drainage procedure"; the remaining 20, of whom 10 had PGV and 10 had SV, also had the Weinberg pyloroplasty. Tests of gastric secretion made preoperatively and 3 to 4 months postoperatively showed that reductions in basal acid output (BAO), peak acid output after pentagastrin (PAO$^{Pg}$), and the peak acid output after insulin-hypoglycemia (PAO$^I$) were not significantly different after the two operations whether pyloroplasty was added or not (Table 1). Reduction in pepsin secretion (not shown in the table) was entirely similar.

Kronborg and associates[3] carried out a similar controlled trial, randomizing TV and SV among 81 patients. The Heineke-Mikulicz pyloroplasty was used in most patients, but four with SV and five with TV had gastrojejunostomy. No significant difference in histamine- or insulin-activated gastric acid secretion could be demonstrated 10 days postoperatively. In 1972, Kronborg and Madsen[4] reported results of a controlled trial in which elective PGV was randomized with SV + P (Heineke-Mikulicz) among 60 patients, all under 60 years of age, with duodenal ulcers that were demonstrated radiologically and

TABLE 1. Reduction in Gastric Acid Secretion in Controlled Trials
in which Various Operations for Duodenal Ulcer Were Randomized°

| HCl Secretion (mEq./hr.) | Author | Number of Patients | Per Cent Reduction after: | | |
|---|---|---|---|---|---|
| | | | PGV | TV + P | SV + P |
| BAO | Clarke et al.[2] | 40 | 76 | – | 80 |
| | Kronborg and Madsen[4] | 60 | 83 | – | 84 |
| PAO[Pg or H] | Clarke et al. | 40 | 70 | – | 62 |
| | Kronborg et al.[3] | 81 | – | 59 | 59 |
| | Kronborg and Madsen | 60 | 59 | – | 68 |
| PAO[I] | Clarke et al. | 40 | 96 | – | 92 |
| | Kronborg et al. | 81 | – | 93 | 88 |
| | Kronborg and Madsen | 60 | 90 | – | 95 |

° Differences were not significant statistically.

confirmed during operation. Reduction in BAO, the peak acid output to histamine (PAO[H]), and PAO[I] did not differ significantly 10 days after operation (Table 1). Uncontrolled comparisons of data from other reports[5-8] also indicate that reduction in acid secretion after PGV is substantial and is not significantly different from that after TV + P or SV + P (Table 2).

The BAO after PGV is reduced the most soon after operation: there was a reduction of 86 per cent at 2 to 3 months and 80 per cent after 12 to 24 months in a series of 48 patients reported jointly from Leeds and Copenhagen by Johnston et al.;[9] 80 per cent at 1 month and 70 per cent after 3 years in Hedenstedt's[6] experience; and 81 per cent at 2 to 3 months and 71 per cent after 1 to 2 years in cases reported by Liavag and Roland.[8]

PAO[Pg] was also reduced more at 2 to 3 months (−68 per cent) than at 6 to 12 months (−55 per cent) in the patients reported jointly from Leeds and Copenhagen[9] ($p < 0.01$) and remained at −55 per cent during the second

TABLE 2. Uncontrolled Comparisons of Reduction in Gastric Acid Secretion
after Various Operations Performed for Duodenal Ulcer

| HCl Secretion (mEq./hr.) | Author | Time After Operation | Number of Patients | Per Cent Reduction after: | | |
|---|---|---|---|---|---|---|
| | | | | PGV | TV + P | SV + P |
| BAO | Johnston[5] | >1 yr. | 15–30 | 81 | 75 | 75 |
| | Hedenstedt[6] | 1 mo. | 116 | 80 | | |
| | Jordan[7] | 2 mos. | 32 | 77 | | |
| | Liavag and Roland[8] | 2–3 mos. | >200 | 81 | | |
| | | 1–2 yrs. | | 71 | | |
| PAO[Pg or H] | Johnston | >1 yr. | 15–30 | 55 | 52 | 48 |
| | Hedenstedt | 1 mo. | 116 | 61 | | |
| | Jordan | 6 mos. | 29 | 62 | | |
| | Liavag and Roland | 2–3 mos. | >200 | 61 | | |
| | | 1–2 yrs. | | 56 | | |
| PAO[I] | Johnston | >1 yr. | 15–30 | 89 | 91 | 90 |
| | Jordan | 2 mos. | 32 | 95 | | |

year after operation. Hedenstedt's comparable values were −61 per cent at 1 month and −50 per cent at 3 years; this difference was not significant statistically. Liavag and Roland found a similar trend: −61 per cent at 2 to 3 months and −56 per cent at 1 to 2 years; statistical significance was not given.

PAO[1] was reduced by about 90 per cent 1 year after the three vagotomy operations at Leeds[5] (Table 2). One week after PGV, insulin tests were negative according to Hollander's criteria in 97 of 100 cases. As time passed, the PAO increased, so that from 1 to 2 years after PGV, it averaged 3.9 mEq./hr., about 12 per cent of the average value of 33 mEq./hr. obtained preoperatively in 60 patients in the series.[10] Insulin tests were negative in 89 per cent of 238 patients 2 to 3 months after PGV as reported by Liavag and Roland and in 93 per cent of 116 cases reported by Hedenstedt. Hedenstedt's data also confirm the observation that with time, some responsiveness to insulin-hypoglycemia returns. As the first year passed, a significant increase occurred in secretion during the second hour after insulin was given, and between 1 and 3 years after operation, secretion during both the first and second hours increased. Nonetheless, at 3 years, the first hour response of 1.9 mEq. was not different from the BAO, and the second hour response for 52 patients averaged only 4 mEq. Jordan[7] recorded the acid output for 2 hours after injection of regular insulin, 0.2 U./kg., and found the mean value for 35 patients to be 41.2 mEq. preoperatively. Two months after PGV, the mean value for 32 patients was 2 mEq. (−95 per cent); 6 months postoperatively, the mean for 29 patients was 4.2 mEq. (−90 per cent). Similar results were obtained when the BAO and responses to pentagastrin and to insulin-induced hypoglycemia were compared after PGV and SV + P by Kragelund and co-workers.[11]

These data concerning gastric secretion of HCl should reassure those who fear that after PGV the vagally innervated antrum might cause gastric hypersecretion by liberating gastrin ceaselessly. Through measurements of serum gastrin by radioimmunoassay, the effects of various operations on serum gastrin are known, although interpretation of the data is complicated by the heterogeneity of gastrin peptides in the circulation and because laboratories may use antibodies that differ in specificity. The subject was reviewed in 1974 by Stadil,[12] who began his discussion of the effects of vagotomy with the following: "Assuming a continuous release of gastrin by the vagus, vagotomy might be expected to decrease gastrin concentrations in serum. On the other hand, reduced acidity of the gastric juice, distension and reflux might stimulate gastrin release postoperatively, the net result being unpredictable." His review shows that TV, SV, and PGV all are followed by *increases* in fasting serum gastrin to 1.5 to 2 times the preoperative values. This finding, taken with the reduction in BAO that follows all three kinds of vagotomy, is surprising until one remembers that, except with the Zollinger-Ellison syndrome, there is no positive correlation between BAO and basal serum gastrin. Indeed, some of the highest basal serum gastrin values are found in achlorhydric patients with pernicious anemia.

The data indicate that the reductions in gastric secretion that follow properly performed PGV equal those that follow TV or SV.

## Effects of PGV on Gastric Emptying

After properly performed PGV, stomachs empty without gastric stasis. If the nerves of Latarjet to the antrum are cut inadvertently, the operation becomes SV without drainage; poor gastric emptying occurs, and gastric ulceration has been reported. In the Leeds and Copenhagen series,[13] only 1 per cent of patients have come to need a drainage procedure after PGV.

Gastric emptying is not normal after PGV, but it is more nearly so than after TV or SV with drainage procedures. Clarke and Alexander-Williams[14] measured rates of gastric emptying of 750 ml. of 10 per cent (hypertonic) dextrose before and after operation in the 40 patients whose elective duodenal ulcer operations were randomized among SV, SV + P, PGV and PGV + P and whose gastric secretion was described previously. The first half of the meal was emptied faster after all the operations than preoperatively, but the change was least after PGV. Final emptying times were prolonged after SV, unchanged by PGV, variable after SV + P, and shortened by PGV + P. Eight patients developed dumping during the tests, and seven had diarrhea; none of these had PGV without drainage.

Madsen, Kronborg, and Feldt-Rasmussen[15] studied gastric emptying of 54 patients with duodenal ulcer whose operations were randomized between PGV and SV + P. A "nutritional contrast medium" containing blenderized food and barium was fed, and serial roentgenograms were made. The tests were done 6 months postoperatively. Gastric emptying time and small intestinal transit time were shorter after SV + P than after PGV. Symptoms of dumping occurred in 9 of 27 patients who had SV + P but in none of 27 patients who had PGV. Retrospective studies and uncontrolled comparisons have given the same results; gastric emptying of food-barium meals is slowed and is more nearly normal after PGV than after TV + P or SV + P.[16]

These and similar data show clearly that properly performed PGV without a drainage procedure does not cause gastric stasis, permits emptying of hypertonic liquids at a rate that is more rapid than normal but less rapid than after TV + P or SV + P, and is followed by a more nearly normal rate of emptying of meals of food and barium than these latter two operations.

## Clinical Results after PGV: Retrospective Studies and Uncontrolled Comparisons with other Operations

Amdrup and associates in Denmark and Johnston and colleagues in Leeds have on several occasions published combined data, the last of which describes 271 patients, 212 male and 59 female, who underwent elective PGV for duodenal ulcer without obstruction beginning in 1969.[13] There were no postoperative deaths, and only 8 per cent of the patients had complications of any kind. Poor results occurred in 4.6 per cent of 173 patients followed more than 1 year. They included two patients with gastric stasis requiring reoperation, three instances of ulcer-like symptoms in patients in whom ulcers could not be demonstrated at reoperation, one patient with persistent epigastric pain without radiologic evidence of ulcer, and two patients with gastric ulcers of which one required operative treatment. There was no proven recurrent or persistent duodenal ulcer. Of 180 patients followed 2 to 4 years, 7.4 per cent had a fair result, 22.2 per cent, very good, and 65.8 per cent, "perfect."

Table 3 lists the incidence of several alimentary symptoms as observed by Goligher and associates[13, 17] 2 years after several operations performed electively for duodenal ulcer without obstruction. Only 60 patients had PGV, all of which were done at Leeds. Thus, although only data for truncal vagotomy plus gastroenterostomy (TV + GE), truncal vagotomy plus antrectomy (TV + A), and 66 to 75 per cent gastric resection without vagotomy, Billroth II technique (GR), were derived from a controlled trial with operations randomized, all the assessments were made in the same manner in the same gastric clinic. Inspection of the table shows that, except for epigastric fullness after eating, the data generally favor PGV. Gastric vagotomy has been shown to impair receptive relaxation of the corpus and fundus of the stomach,[18-21] and this may account for the epigastric fullness reported by many patients after vagotomies performed without gastric resection. Note the low incidence of diarrhea after PGV. Another retrospective study[22] showed that passing of liquid or very loose stools with some urgency occurred in 24 per cent of 50 patients after TV + P, 18 per cent of 50 patients after SV + P, and only 2 per cent of 50 patients after PGV. Diarrhea was severe in 6 per cent after TV, in only 2 per cent after SV, and in none after PGV.

Table 4, a comparison similar to that in Table 3, shows Visick scores to be very good after PGV. It would require a large number of randomized

TABLE 3.    Symptoms Two Years after Various Elective Operations for Duodenal Ulcer in Males*

| Symptom | Per Cent of Patients with Each Symptom after: | | | | |
| | TV + GE (110)‡ | TV + P† (158) | TV + A (106) | GR (93) | PGV† (60) |
| --- | --- | --- | --- | --- | --- |
| Nausea | 16 | 26 | 15 | 20 | 8 |
| Vomiting bile | 16 | 11 | 14 | 12 | 2 |
| Vomiting food | 6 | 8 | 5 | 10 | 3 |
| Epigastric fullness p.c. | 28 | 47 | 35 | 40 | 29 |
| Early dumping | 11 | 10 | 11 | 17 | 7 |
| Heartburn | 15 | 18 | 16 | 2 | 12 |
| Dysphagia | 0 | 1 | 0 | 0 | 0 |
| Diarrhea | | | | | |
| mild, moderate | 21 | 20 | 21 | 6 | 3 |
| severe | 5 | 2 | 3 | 1 | 0 |

*Data from Goligher, J. C., Pulvertaft, C. N., De Dombal, F. T., et al.: Clinical comparison of vagotomy and pyloroplasty with other forms of elective surgery for duodenal ulcer. Br. Med. J. 2:787, 1968; and Amdrup, E., Jensen, H.-E., Johnston, D., Walker, B. E., and Goligher, J. C.: Clinical results of parietal cell vagotomy (highly selective vagotomy) two to four years after operation. Ann. Surg. 180:279, 1974.
    †Nonrandom uncontrolled comparison.
    ‡Numbers in parentheses are the number of patients.

TABLE 4.   Results of Various Elective Operations for Duodenal Ulcer
in Males after Two Years°

| Visick Category | Per Cent of Patients in Each Category after: | | | | |
|---|---|---|---|---|---|
| | TV + GE (110)‡ | TV + P† (158) | TV + A (106) | GR (93) | PGV† (108)§ |
| I – Excellent; no symptoms | 54 ⎱ 73 | 37 ⎱ 64 | 58 ⎱ 84 | 60 ⎱ 83 | 66 ⎱ 88 |
| II – Good; few mild symptoms | 19 ⎰ | 27 ⎰ | 26 ⎰ | 23 ⎰ | 22 ⎰ |
| III – Fair; symptoms controlled with care | 22 | 24 | 12 | 15 | 7 |
| IV – Poor | 5 | 12 | 4 | 2 | 5 |

°Data from Goligher, J. C., Pulvertaft, C. N., De Dombal, F. T., et al.: Clinical comparison of vagotomy and pyloroplasty with other forms of elective surgery for duodenal ulcer. Br. Med. J. 2:787, 1968; and Amdrup, E., Jensen, H.-E., Johnston, D., Walker, B. E., and Goligher, J. C.: Clinical results of parietal cell vagotomy (highly selective vagotomy) two to four years after operation. Ann. Surg. 180:279, 1974.

†Nonrandom uncontrolled comparison.
‡Number in parentheses is the number of patients.
§Followed 2 to 4 years after PGV.

operations to determine whether in this respect there are statistically significant differences between results of PGV and other operations. Equally good early clinical results following PGV without drainage have been reported in retrospective studies by Hedenstedt,[6] Jordan,[7] Liavag and Roland,[8] with incidences of recurrent ulcers in the short term of no more than 1 per cent.

These data indicate that properly performed PGV without drainage controls gastric secretion well enough to prevent persistent or recurrent duodenal ulcers during the first few years after operation and that clinical results are in other respects equal to or better than those after the other common operations mentioned. Not enough time has passed for data on long-term results to be available.

## Reported Failures of PGV without Drainage to Prevent Persistence or Recurrence of Duodenal Ulcers

At one point in our experience, we had 32 patients followed one year after PGV, of whom four (12.5 per cent) were proven to have and two (6.3 per cent) were suspected of having recurrent duodenal ulcer. Three months after operation, PAO[1] values were 52, 34, 28, and 13 mEq./hr. in the four patients with proven ulcers and 36 and 7.3 in the two patients with suspected recurrence. Clearly these vagotomies were incomplete. Reduction of gastric secretion generally was not as great in the 72 per cent of our patients who reported Visick I or II results, as was the case in other series cited previously in which recurrences were not proven or were rare. Through the kindness of Professor Goligher and Mr. David Johnston, I compared our technique with that used at Leeds and found that the significant difference was that we had been clearing only the distal 1 to 2 cm. of esophagus of nerves and other tissue, rather than 5 to 7.5 cm. as is done at Leeds. We have not yet accumulated enough data to prove that this change in technique will correct the problem.

Apparently others have had similar experiences. Moberg and Hedenstedt[23] observed three recurrences within a year among 48 patients followed 3 years after PGV. Two were insulin positive and one was insulin negative. These were the only recurrent ulcers Hedenstedt encountered in over 300 cases he reported in 1974, and of them he wrote that "at reoperation vagal branches in the region of the cardia were found to have been overlooked. After this experience more careful attention was paid to the dissection in this area, and since this policy was followed, the insulin test indicated a far better vagotomy. In the later series, no relapses have occurred."

Liedberg and Oscarson,[24] after noting only a 40 per cent reduction of BAO, a 33 per cent reduction of PAO$^{Pg}$ and 17 per cent negative insulin tests 2 months after PGV without drainage, together with four recurrent ulcers in their first 20 cases, changed the technique to include skeletonization of the distal 6 to 8 cm. of esophagus and cardia of the stomach. In the next 60 cases, BAO was reduced by 80 per cent and PAO$^{Pg}$ by 58 per cent and insulin tests were positive in only 31 per cent of patients 2 months postoperatively. No more early recurrences had been recognized during the still short follow-up period.

Failure to prevent recurrence of ulceration has been a problem in several controlled trials that have been started to assess PGV by randomizing its use with standard operations done electively for duodenal ulcer disease without obstruction. Madsen and Kronborg[25] reported better clinical results 12 months postoperatively with PGV than with SV + P, except for recurrent ulceration, which occurred in 3 of 30 patients with PGV and in 1 of 20 with SV + P. Two of those early recurrences after PGV had high PAO$^I$ (15 and 13 mEq./hr.), indicating incomplete vagotomy, and the other had what appears to be adequate vagotomy (PAO$^I$ = 2.6 mEq./hr.). The single recurrence after SV + P had incomplete vagotomy (PAO$^I$ = 28.8 mEq./hr.).

Bombeck et al.,[26] randomizing PGV with TV + A and SV + A, gave results in 21 patients. The usual great reduction in BAO and PAO$^H$ (86 to 94 per cent) followed TV + A and SV + A and persisted through the 1 year of follow-up. One year after PGV, BAO and PAO$^H$ were reduced by only 25 and 20 per cent respectively as compared with preoperative values, and one recurrent ulcer had been confirmed and another suspected.

The role of incomplete vagotomy in causing two proven and one suspected recurrence among 16 patients with PGV randomized with 20 patients having PGV + P, as reported by Wastell et al.,[27] is less certain. Reductions in PAO$^{Pg}$ were 59 and 56 per cent respectively about 10 days postoperatively, but at about the same time, in tests of 35 patients, 5 showed early positive responses and five showed late positive responses to insulin according to Hollander's criteria.

In the Aarhus County (Denmark) vagotomy trial,[28] in which 286 patients have been randomized among SV plus drainage (SV + D), SV + A, PGV + D, or PGV, operations have been done by several surgeons. Amdrup, in presenting the paper, changed the incidence of recurrence from 1 in 38 patients with PGV observed more than a year to 3 in 38 (8 per cent). I do not have gastric secretory data to permit determination of the cause of these recurrences. I did not find other reports of any prospective controlled trials randomizing PGV with other operations that had reached a point at which meaningful comparisons could be made.

To me, the data indicate that when duodenal ulcers recur within the first year or two after PGV, the most probable cause is incomplete vagotomy. To conclude otherwise, one would have to ignore over 800 cases reported by other authors who cite incidences of early recurrent ulcer of 0 to 1 per cent and who provide enough gastric secretory data to show that their vagotomies are more nearly complete.

## Operative Mortality Rate of PGV

Johnston[29] notes that there was no operative mortality among more than 1000 PGV operations reported by ten groups of workers. All operations carry some risk of death, and there has been at least one such case reported;[30] another death after PGV performed for gastric ulcer has been reported.[29] For uncomplicated duodenal ulcer, the mortality rate of PGV is low indeed, probably because there are no suture lines.

## Summary

PGV without drainage, if performed properly, controls the duodenal ulcer diathesis over the short term as well as or better than standard operations, rarely causes gastric stasis or vomiting of bile, prevents "postvagotomy diarrhea," is followed by a low incidence of other unpleasant gastrointestinal symptoms, and carries a very low operative mortality rate. However, more time must elapse before we can know how long the early good results will persist.

Controlled comparisons between PGV and other operations for duodenal ulcer are needed to be certain that the apparently good results are not due to selection of cases; such studies are underway in several parts of the world. The trouble that many surgeons have had in learning to achieve the desired vagal denervation by PGV emphasizes the great importance of adequate preparation before the operation is done, whether in trials or not. If technical failures are common and if tests of gastric secretion are not made to identify them, the data concerning recurrent ulceration will be impossible to interpret. Technical problems are neither unique nor great, but the concept of what has to be done, which is so well explained by Goligher,[1] must be clearly understood.

If the technique of PGV is mastered by surgeons generally and if the good early results persist and are confirmed in controlled trials, PGV will emerge as the best elective operation thus far designed for duodenal ulcer disease without pyloric obstruction. Exploration of its use in other circumstances[31-33] will be most interesting.

## References

1. Goligher, J. C.: A technique for highly selective (parietal cell or proximal gastric) vagotomy for duodenal ulcer. Br. J. Surg. 61:337, 1974.
2. Clarke, R. J., Allan, R. N., and Alexander-Williams, J.: The effect of retaining antral innervation on the reductions of gastric acid and pepsin secretion after vagotomy. Gut 13:894, 1972.
3. Kronborg, O., Malmstrom, J., and Christiansen, P. M.: A comparison between the results of truncal and selective vagotomy in patients with duodenal ulcer. Scand. J. Gastroenterol. 5:519, 1970.
4. Kronborg, O., and Madsen, P.: A comparison of gastric acid secretions after highly selective vagotomy without drainage and selective vagotomy with a pyloroplasty. Scand. J. Gastroenterol. 7:615, 1972.
5. Johnston, D.: A new look at vagotomy. In Nyhus, L. M. (ed.): Surgery Annual. Vol. 6. New York, Appleton-Century-Crofts, 1974, p. 125.
6. Hedenstedt, S.: Experiences of selective proximal vagotomy in 400 cases of uncomplicated and complicated ulcers during 6 years. Presented at Clinical Congress, American College of Surgeons, Oct. 24, 1974.
7. Jordan, P. H.: Parietal cell vagotomy without drainage. Early evaluation of results in the treatment of duodenal ulcer. Arch. Surg. 108:434, 1974.
8. Liavag, I., and Roland, M.: Selective proximal vagotomy in the treatment of gastroduodenal ulcers. (Abstract.) Scand. J. Gastroenterol. Suppl. 20:10, 1973.
9. Johnston, D., Wilkinson, A. R., Humphrey, C. S., Smith, R. B., Goligher, J. C., Kragelund, E., and Amdrup, E.: Serial studies of gastric secretion in patients after highly selective (parietal cell) vagotomy without a drainage procedure for duodenal ulcer. I. Effect of highly selective vagotomy on basal and pentagastrin-stimulated maximal acid output. Gastroenterology 64:1, 1973.
10. Johnston, D., Wilkinson, A. R., Humphrey, C. S., Smith, R. B., Goligher, J. C., Kragelund, E., and Amdrup, E.: Serial studies of gastric secretion in patients after highly selective (parietal cell) vagotomy without a drainage procedure for duodenal ulcer. II. The insulin test after highly selective vagotomy. Gastroenterology 64:12, 1973.
11. Kragelund, E., Amdrup, E., and Jensen, H-E.: Pentapeptide and insulin stimulated gastric acid secretion in patients with duodenal ulcer before and after selective gastric vagotomy and antrum drainage: comparison with results obtained from studies before and after parietal cell vagotomy with no drainage procedure. Ann. Surg. 176:649, 1972.
12. Stadil, F.: Gastrin and insulin hypoglycemia. Scand. J. Gastroenterol. Suppl. 9:23, 1974.
13. Amdrup, E., Jensen, H.-E., Johnston, D., Walker, B. E., and Goligher, J. C.: Clinical results of parietal cell vagotomy (highly selective vagotomy) two to four years after operation. Ann. Surg. 180:279, 1974.
14. Clarke, R. J., and Alexander-Williams, J.: The effect of preserving antral innervation and of a pyloroplasty on gastric emptying after vagotomy in man. Gut 14:300, 1973.
15. Madsen, P., Kronborg, O., and Feldt-Rasmussen, K.: The gastric emptying and small intestinal transit after highly selective vagotomy without drainage and selective vagotomy with pyloroplasty. Scand. J. Gastroenterol. 8:541, 1973.
16. Wilkinson, A. R., and Johnston, D.: Effect of truncal, selective and highly selective vagotomy on gastric emptying and intestinal transit of a food-barium meal in man. Ann. Surg. 178:190, 1973.
17. Goligher, J. C., Pulvertaft, C. N., De Dombal, F. T., et al.: Clinical comparison of vagotomy and pyloroplasty with other forms of elective surgery for duodenal ulcer. Br. Med. J. 2:787, 1968.
18. Jansson, G.: Extrinsic nervous control of gastric motility. Acta Physiol. Scand. Suppl. 326:1, 1969.

19. Jahnberg, T., and Martinson, J.: Gastric receptive relaxation before and after vagotomy. (Abstract.) Scand. J. Gastroenterol. Suppl. 20:15, 1973.

20. Koster, J., and Madsen, P.: The intra-gastric pressure before and immediately after truncal vagotomy. Scand. J. Gastroenterol. 5:381, 1970.

21. Stadaas, J., and Aune, S.: Intragastric pressure/volume before and after vagotomy. Acta Chir. Scand. 136:611, 1970.

22. Johnston, D., Humphrey, C. S., Walker, B. E., Pulvertaft, C. N., and Goligher, J. C.: Vagotomy without diarrhea. Br. Med. J. 2:788, 1972.

23. Moberg, S., and Hedenstedt, S.: Selective proximal vagotomy. A three year follow-up. (Abstract.) Scand. J. Gastroenterol. Suppl. 20:9, 1973.

24. Liedberg, G., and Oscarson, J.: Selective proximal vagotomy—short time followup of 80 patients. (Abstract.) Scand. J. Gastroenterol. Suppl. 20:12, 1973.

25. Madsen, P., and Kronborg, O.: A double-blind trial of highly selective vagotomy without drainage and selective vagotomy with pyloroplasty in the treatment of duodenal ulcer. (Abstract.) Scand. J. Gastroenterol. Suppl. 20:12, 1973.

26. Bombeck, C. T., Condon, R. E., Miller, B., and Nyhus, L. M.: Vagotomy: a prospective randomized study. Surg. Forum 25:327, 1974.

27. Wastell, C., Colin, J. F., MacNaughton, J. I., and Gleeson, J.: Selective proximal vagotomy with and without Finney pyloroplasty. Br. Med. J. 1:28, 1972.

28. Amdrup, E., Andersen, D., and Hostrup, H.: The Aarhus County vagotomy trial. (Abstract.) Third World Congress, Collegium International Chirurgiae Digestivae, Chicago, Oct. 10–13, 1974.

29. Johnston, D.: Progress report. Highly selective vagotomy. Gut 15:748, 1974.

30. Newcombe, J. F.: Fatality after highly selective vagotomy. (Letter.) Br. Med. J. 1:610, 1973.

31. Johnston, D., Lyndon, P. J., Smith, R. B., and Humphrey, C. S.: Highly selective vagotomy without a drainage procedure in the treatment of haemorrhage, perforation, and pyloric stenosis due to peptic ulcer. Br. J. Surg. 60:790, 1973.

32. Hedenstedt, S., and Moberg, S.: Gastric ulcer treated with selective proximal vagotomy (SPV). Acta Chir. Scand. 140:309, 1974.

33. Johnston, D., Humphrey, C. S., Smith, R. B., and Wilkinson, A. R.: Treatment of gastric ulcer by highly selective vagotomy without a drainage procedure: an interim report. Br. J. Surg. 59:787, 1972.

# Truncal Vagotomy and Antrectomy as the Preferred Operation for Treatment of Duodenal Ulcer

JOHN L. SAWYERS

*Vanderbilt University School of Medicine*

Various operations are currently used for the surgical treatment of duodenal ulcer, but none has been more effective in controlling the ulcer diathesis than truncal vagotomy and antrectomy. This operation was specifically designed to eliminate various phases of gastric acid secretion. Follow-up studies on patients subjected to truncal vagotomy-antrectomy for duodenal ulcer are available up to 26 years after operation.

Since it is well established that patients who develop duodenal ulcer sui generis, unrelated to stress of traumatic injury, burns, massive infections, intracranial disease, or steroids or other ulcerogenic drugs, are hypersecretors of gastric acid,[1,2] operations for treatment of duodenal ulcer should be aimed at reducing gastric acid secretion. In 1943, Dragstedt awakened surgeons to the role of vagal section in treating duodenal ulcer.[3] This report brought clinical confirmation of the importance of the cephalic phase of gastric secretion in patients with duodenal ulcer. Experimental work in surgical research laboratories demonstrated the importance of the antrum in stimulating the parietal cells to secrete acid by its hormone, gastrin.[4] The stimulatory phases of gastric acid secretion include: (1) direct vagal — direct stimulation of the parietal cells via the vagus nerves; (2) vagal-antral — release of gastrin from the antrum in response to vagal stimulation; (3) local antral — stimulation of the parietal cells by gastrin release as a result of direct stimulation of the antrum; and (4) intestinal — parietal cell stimulation resulting from a release of hormones by the intestinal mucosa.[5] Truncal vagotomy-antrectomy is designed to remove the first three of these stimulatory phases of gastric acid secretion. In most patients, the intestinal phase is thought to be of the least clinical importance.

131

Truncal vagotomy and antrectomy for duodenal ulcer was performed by Farmer and Smithwick in Boston in 1946 and independently a few months later by L. W. Edwards in Nashville. The Nashville series of patients subjected to truncal vagotomy-antrectomy for duodenal ulcer from January, 1947, to January, 1972, totals 3584 patients. The age range has been from 8 to 94 years; the average age was in the mid-40's. The ratio of men to women was approximately 5:1.

Truncal vagotomy-antrectomy may be used for any of the indications for operation for chronic duodenal ulcer and its complications. The principal indication for operation was intractability to medical therapy in 51 per cent of patients, hemorrhage, either acute or intermittent, in 32 per cent, obstruction in 14 per cent, and acute perforation in 3 per cent (Table 1). The duration of symptoms prior to operation has been as long as 40 years, with an average duration of 12 years. When the indication for operation was intractability, operation was offered only to patients with recurrent duodenal ulcer symptoms and persistent pain refractory to medical management over a long period of time.

The diagnosis of duodenal ulcer has generally been established not only by the patient's symptoms but also by demonstration of the presence of an ulcer crater on upper gastrointestinal roentgenologic studies. In the past 5 years since the fiberoptic flexible gastroscope has been so readily available, many of our patients have had both gastroscopic and roentgenologic demonstration of their duodenal ulcer. All patients with upper gastrointestinal hemorrhage undergo esophagogastroduodenoscopy as soon as their condition permits. This is usually done in the intensive care unit concurrent with whatever supportive or resuscitative measures are needed. Endoscopy is usually more accurate in diagnosing bleeding duodenal ulcers than upper gastrointestinal fluoroscopy and roentgenography, although the latter is also done for diagnostic purposes after the acute bleeding episode subsides. Acute perforation is usually diagnosed by history, physical findings, and roentgenologic demonstration of free air in the peritoneal cavity. In a recent review of 360 patients with perforated duodenal ulcer, pneumoperitoneum was demonstrated in 71 per cent by either chest or abdominal roentgenograms.[6] In all our patients subjected to vagotomy-antrectomy, either a duodenal ulcer crater or a duodenal deformity from scarring secondary to ulcer disease has been present.

Preoperative gastric acid secretory studies are not considered necessary

TABLE 1.  Principal Indications for Vagotomy-Antrectomy
for Duodenal Ulcer

| Indication | Per Cent of Patients |
|---|---|
| Intractability | 51 |
| Hemorrhage (massive or recurrent) | 32 |
| Obstruction | 14 |
| Perforation | 3 |

in all patients. Most of our patients have had acid studies before and after operation, because we want to collect these data for evaluation studies. We have not used preoperative acid studies as a basis for selecting an operation for duodenal ulcer, unless the acid secretions suggest the presence of the Zollinger-Ellison syndrome. In these patients, serum gastrin levels are obtained prior to operation. We formerly used the 12-hour overnight gastric secretory collection as described by Dragstedt,[7] but we now use a 1-hour basal gastric acid secretion analysis followed by a maximum acid secretion test with Histalog stimulation.

## Operative Technique

The technique of vagotomy and antrectomy as it has been performed in the Nashville series of patients is based on a meticulously performed bilateral subdiaphragmatic truncal vagotomy with a resection of the distal 40 per cent of the stomach. The abdomen is usually entered through an upper midline incision, which is carried just to the left of the xiphoid process. The left hepatic lobe is elevated superiorly with the Weinberg retractor, without dividing the suspensory ligament of the liver. Moist laparotomy packs are used to protect the spleen against injury. The stomach is retracted downward, and the peritoneum overlying the abdominal esophagus is incised transversely. A previously placed indwelling nasogastric tube aids in identification of the esophagus. The esophagus is mobilized circumferentially and freed from its areolar attachments. The anterior vagal trunk is identified and elevated from the esophagus by a long nerve hook. Any vagal branches that pass downward toward the esophagogastric junction are divided. A 4 to 6 cm. segment of the anterior vagal trunk is resected, and hemoclips are placed on the ends of the divided nerve trunk. In a similar manner, the posterior vagal trunk is dissected free, elevated, and freed up into the lower mediastinum. A segment of the posterior trunk is excised and the ends secured with hemoclips or ligated with silk. After checking carefully for residual vagal fibers, especially on the anterior wall of the esophagus, the abdominal esophagus is reflected to the patient's left, and the diaphragmatic crura are approximated posterior to the esophagus with a few silk sutures to tighten the hiatus to the width of one finger laid alongside the esophagus.

Attention is now directed to removing the antrum of the stomach. The point for division on the greater curvature is determined by dropping an imaginary line from the incisura straight down to the greater curvature, which is then cleared by dividing the gastrocolic ligament between clamps toward the pylorus. The lesser curvature is divided 1 cm. proximal to the point midway between the gastroesophageal junction and the pylorus. The antrum extends farther up (toward the cardia) on the lesser curvature than on the greater curvature. The extent of distal gastric resection is determined with the aim of removing all antral tissue while preserving an adequate gastric reservoir. Resection of the distal 40 per cent of the stomach satisfactorily accomplishes this purpose.

We prefer to divide the stomach between two straight Allen clamps placed at right angles to the long axis of the stomach at the point selected for division on the greater curvature. These clamps define the size of the gastroenteric stoma, which is usually planned to be identical with the diameter of the duodenum. After this portion of stomach is transected, another pair of clamps is applied from this point of division in a like manner across the gastric wall up to the previously selected point for division on the lesser curvature. After completing the transection of the stomach, the lesser curvature portion of the divided end of the stomach is closed with a continuous hemostatic chromic catgut suture and inverted with interrupted silk sutures. The distal end of the transected stomach may be used as a handle to facilitate mobilization and dissection of the proximal duodenum. We do not think that it is necessary to remove the duodenal ulcer itself, but it is important to excise all antral tissue. Gastrointestinal reconstruction may be accomplished either by gastroduodenostomy or gastrojejunostomy. We prefer the Schoemaker-Billroth I method of gastroduodenostomy and use this in over 90 per cent of our patients. Gastroduodenostomy offers certain physiologic advantages over gastrojejunostomy, since nutritional studies have indicated diminished loss of fecal fat and nitrogen and improved iron absorption with gastroduodenostomy.

## Results

Follow-up study among the entire series has been 98 per cent. Those patients who have subsequently died of disease unrelated to duodenal ulcer have been followed until the time of death, and their results have continued to be tabulated in the clinical study. A critical appraisal has been made of the overall clinical result in each patient available for follow-up. Personal interview, postoperative gastrointestinal roentgenogram series, and acid studies, when possible, have been done in early and late intervals after operation.

Results have been graded as excellent, good, fair, and poor. An excellent result indicates that the patient is in excellent nutritional condition and has no symptoms or manifestations referable to the gastrointestinal tract. A good result is attributed to those patients who have excellent gastrointestinal function with no ulcer symptoms and good nutritional condition but occasionally experience epigastric fullness after meals, mild dumping, or intermittent bouts of mild diarrhea. Except for modest restriction of carbohydrate intake, these patients can follow an unlimited diet. We consider patients in the excellent or good category to have entirely satisfactory results from their operative procedure. Patients judged as having a fair result have obtained benefit from operation and are without residual ulcer symptoms, but dumping, diarrhea, or abdominal fullness have been prominent sequelae. In the poor result category are patients with recurrent ulcer, nutritional difficulties, and postgastrectomy symptoms of such severity that they interfere with their livelihood. This grading system is similar to the Visick classification, in which patients in Visick group I have excellent results, group II, good, group III, fair, and group IV, poor.

According to our criteria, the clinical results have been excellent in 66 per cent of patients, good in 28 per cent, fair in 5 per cent, and poor in 1 per cent. Thus, 94 per cent (3055 patients) in the series are considered to have an entirely satisfactory result after vagotomy and antrectomy (Table 2).

Postoperative weights have been measured in the follow-up of most patients. Ten per cent of patients have lost weight to some degree after operation and have weights below their ideal levels. Another 10 per cent have gained weight and are above their preoperative and ideal weight levels. The remaining 80 per cent have maintained their weights in the preoperative or ideal range.

Anemias have been a rare finding in the postoperative follow-up. Intermittent episodes of diarrhea have occurred in about 10 per cent of patients but have constituted a serious problem in less than 1 per cent. Careful questioning and clinical testing revealed that symptoms suggesting the dumping syndrome were experienced by 25 per cent of patients. These symptoms were usually initiated by high carbohydrate intake and in most instances were readily prevented by a low carbohydrate diet. Severe dumping symptoms occurred in less than 1 per cent of patients. Dumping symptoms occurred with almost equal frequency following Billroth I and Billroth II operations. The hourly basal total acid output was usually 0.1 to 0.5 mEq., and the stimulated total acid output was less than 2 mEq. in those patients subjected to postoperative acid secretion studies.

The operative mortality rate in this series of 3584 patients was 1.6 per cent (55 patients). The majority of deaths (31) occurred in patients undergoing operation as an emergency measure for control of massive bleeding. Many of these patients were elderly and had cardiovascular or renal disease. The causes of death are listed in Table 3.

Vagotomy and antrectomy have been extraordinarily effective in controlling the ulcer diathesis and preventing ulcer recurrence. Only 20 proved recurrent ulcers have developed, an incidence of 0.6 per cent. More than 1500 patients have been followed longer than 10 years. Each of the 20 recurrent ulcers occurred within 24 months of operation. Thirteen patients have been reoperated upon and found to have an incomplete vagotomy. Four patients developed recurrent ulcers because of the Zollinger-Ellison syndrome with

TABLE 2. Results of Truncal Vagotomy and Antrectomy
in 3250 Patients Followed up to 25 Years

| Results | Number of Patients | Per Cent of Patients |
| --- | --- | --- |
| Excellent | 2145 | 66 |
| Good | 910 | 28 |
| Fair | 163 | 5 |
| Poor | 32 | 1 |

TABLE 3.    Causes of Death in 55 Patients (1.6 Per Cent Mortality Rate)
Following Truncal Vagotomy and Antrectomy for Duodenal Ulcer

| Cause | Number of Patients |
|---|---|
| Emergency operation to control bleeding | 31 |
| Duodenal stump leakage | 12 |
| Respiratory failure | 7 |
| Hemorrhagic pancreatitis | 3 |
| Uncontrolled rebleeding | 2 |

a nonbeta islet cell tumor of the pancreas that was present but unrecognized by the surgeon at the time of the initial procedure. A functioning adrenal tumor was responsible for recurrence in one patient. Two additional patients with recurrence probably had an incomplete vagotomy, but this was not proved.

Of the 20 recurrences, 13 followed a Billroth I reconstruction and 7 occurred after a Billroth II, but it should be noted that in this series, the Billroth I was the more frequently used type of anastomosis.

## Discussion

An appraisal of the clinical data in this series of 3584 patients supports the conclusion that vagotomy and antrectomy provides very effective therapy for chronic duodenal ulcer and its complications. This operation appears to be the most dependable method thus far devised for control of the ulcer diathesis. The procedure is based on the sound physiologic concepts of eliminating both cephalic and gastric sources of stimulus to excessive gastric acid secretion while preserving a sufficiently large hypochlorhydric gastric reservoir.

The proponents of other operations for duodenal ulcer have criticized the operative mortality rate. An analysis by Herrington[8] of the etiologic factors influencing the operative mortality after this operation emphasized that the greatest risk of the procedure has been encountered in its application to the management of massive bleeding from duodenal ulcer, especially in elderly debilitated patients. Clearly, the dissection and handling of the diseased duodenum constitute the most hazardous part of operation for duodenal ulcer. In an attempt to reduce the mortality rates, we have tended to use vagotomy and a drainage procedure, usually pyloroplasty, in lieu of antral resection in elderly debilitated patients, especially those with massive bleeding and those who present technical problems that increase the hazards of antral resection. Since adopting this approach in 1964, the operative mortality rate has steadily dropped from a high of 3.1 per cent in 1958 to 1.6 per cent in 1972.

## Other Studies

Reports from other medical centers attest to the efficacy of treating the complications of duodenal ulcer by truncal vagotomy-antrectomy (Table 4). All but one of these studies has been a retrospective analysis, but collectively these groups, together with our patients, include more than 5000 patients. The recurrence rate of less than 1 per cent is far lower than that of any other operation for duodenal ulcer.

The Jordan-Condon study[16] was a prospective randomized study of 200 consecutive patients who required elective operation for treatment of duodenal ulcer. Truncal vagotomy and antrectomy was randomized with truncal vagotomy and drainage. A 5 to 8 year follow-up study of this series since operation has recently been reported.[9] This elegant study confirms the danger of truncal vagotomy and drainage—recurrent ulcer that required reoperation in nine patients (8.3 per cent). Only one recurrent ulcer (1.1 per cent) has developed following vagotomy-antrectomy. This study helps to answer the major criticism of vagotomy-antrectomy, which has been its higher mortality rate as compared to vagotomy and drainage. The Jordan-Condon study suggests that if one abstains from resection in patients in whom technical difficulties with the duodenum can be expected, vagotomy and antrectomy can be performed with a mortality rate as low as that usually reported for vagotomy and drainage. This study concluded that vagotomy and antrectomy is superior to vagotomy and drainage "for the majority of patients because it is associated with fewer recurrent ulcers without a significant difference in the severity of other postoperative gastrointestinal complaints."

Goligher's Leeds/York study[10] is another excellent report based on prospective, randomized studies. Subtotal distal gastrectomy without vagotomy, truncal vagotomy-antrectomy, and truncal vagotomy with drainage were compared. On the basis of their Visick grading after operation, the authors concluded that vagotomy-antrectomy and subtotal gastrectomy were slightly superior to vagotomy and drainage, but the difference was statis-

TABLE 4.  Results from Other Medical Centers Using Truncal
Vagotomy-Antrectomy for Duodenal Ulcer

| Author | Number of Patients | Good to Excellent Results (Per Cent) | Mortality (Per Cent) | Ulcer Recurrence (Per Cent) | Follow-up (Years) |
|---|---|---|---|---|---|
| °Smithwick[11] | 719 | 93 | 1.9 | 1.5 | 1–26 |
| °Thoroughman[12] | 504 | 91 | 1.6 | 0.4 | 2–14 |
| °Palumbo[13] | 510 | 90 | 2.7 | 0.6 | 1–16 |
| °Wolf[14] | 547 | 90 | 1.1 | 0.6 | 1–10 |
| Remine[15] | 223 | 90 | 0 | 1.3 | 7–17 |
| †Jordan[16] | 90 | 89 | 0 | 1.1 | 1–8 |

° Elective and emergency cases
† Elective cases

tically insignificant. As in the Jordan-Condon study, patients were relegated to the vagotomy-drainage group if it was believed that resection could not be performed with reasonable safety. One can conclude from this study that patients can be treated by vagotomy-antrectomy (or subtotal resection) with negligible mortality if vagotomy-drainage is used for patients in whom dissection of the duodenum may be unduly hazardous.

## Summary

Opinions regarding the best operation for duodenal ulcer disease are not unanimous. It would appear that vagotomy has become the keystone of treatment, but there are varying opinions regarding the type of vagotomy (truncal, selective gastric, or parietal cell) and the type of complementary procedure (antrectomy, pyloroplasty, gastrojejunostomy, or none). Our experience in the use of truncal vagotomy with antrectomy in 3584 patients with an ulcer recurrence rate of 0.6 per cent is summarized. Results from other institutions using truncal vagotomy with antral resection for the surgical treatment of duodenal ulcer are tabulated. The two excellent reports of prospective, randomized, well-controlled studies of truncal vagotomy and antrectomy are reported (Leeds/York study and Jordan-Condon study).

The results of all these studies indicate that truncal vagotomy with antral resection affords lasting protection for the patient against the ulcer diathesis and may be used safely in good-risk patients requiring operation for any of the complications of duodenal ulcer. A lesser procedure (pyloroplasty or gastrojejunostomy) should probably be used with vagotomy instead of antral resection in the poor-risk patient in whom immediate salvage of life and not long-range control of ulcer disease is the primary concern.

## References

1. Hollander, F.: Current views on the physiology of the gastric secretions. Am. J. Med. 13:453, 1952.
2. Palmer, W. L.: Causality in peptic ulcer. Arch. Intern. Med. 106:786, 1960.
3. Dragstedt, L. R., and Owens, F. M., Jr.: Supradiaphragmatic section of the vagus nerve in the treatment of duodenal ulcer. Proc. Soc. Exp. Biol. Med. 53:152, 1943.
4. Dragstedt, L. R., Oberhelman, H. A., Jr., and Smith, C. A.: Experimental hyperfunction of the gastric antrum with ulcer formation. Ann. Surg. 134:332, 1951.
5. Nyhus, L. M., Chapman, N. D., DeVito, R. V., and Harkins, H. N.: The control of gastrin release: an experimental study illustrating a new concept. Gastroenterology 39:582, 1960.
6. Sawyers, J. L., Herrington, J. L., Jr., Mulherin, J. L., Whitehead, W. A., Body, B., and Marsh, J.: Evaluation of surgical management of acute perforated duodenal ulcer. Arch. Surg. 110:527, 1975.
7. Dragstedt, L. R., Woodward, E. R., Storer, E. R., Oberhelman, H. A., Jr., and Smith, C. A.: Quantitative studies on the mechanism of gastric secretion in health and disease. Ann. Surg. 132:626, 1950.
8. Herrington, J. L., Jr., Edwards, W. H., Sawyers, J. L., Gobbel, W. G., Jr., and Scott, H. W., Jr.: Etiologic factors influencing the operative mortality after vagotomy and antrectomy for duodenal ulcer. Am. J. Surg. 107:289, 1964.

9. Jordan, P. H., Jr.: A followup report of a prospective evaluation of vagotomy-pyloroplasty and vagotomy-antrectomy for treatment of duodenal ulcer. Ann. Surg. *180*:259, 1974.
10. Goligher, J. C., Pulvertaft, C. N., De Dombal, F. T., Conyers, J. H., Duthie, H. L., Feather, D. B., Latchmore, A. J. C., Harrop-Shoesmith, J., Smiddy, F. G., and Willison-Pepper, J.: Five-to-eight year results of Leeds/York controlled trial of elective surgery for duodenal ulcer. Br. Med. J. *2*:781, 1968.
11. Smithwick, R. H., Farmer, D. A., and Harrower, H. W.: Hemigastrectomy and truncal vagotomy in the treatment of duodenal ulcer. Am. J. Surg. *127*:631, 1974.
12. Thoroughman, J. C., Walker, L. G., Jr., Raft, D.: A review of 504 patients with peptic ulcer treated by hemigastrectomy and vagotomy. Surg. Gynecol. Obstet. *119*:257, 1964.
13. Palumbo, L. T., Sharpe, W. S., Lulu, D. J., Bloom, M. H., and Dragstedt, L. R., II.: Distal antrectomy with vagectomy for duodenal ulcer. Arch. Surg. *100*:182, 1970.
14. Wolf, J. S., Bell, C. C., Zimberg, Y. H.: Analysis of ten years in experience with surgery for peptic ulcer disease. Am. Surg. *38*:187, 1972.
15. Remine, W. H.: Personal communication, 1972.
16. Jordan, P. H., Jr., and Condon, R. H.: A prospective evaluation of vagotomy-pyloroplasty and vagotomy-antrectomy for treatment of duodenal ulcer. Ann. Surg. *172*:547, 1970.

# 7

# Management of the Clinically Solitary Thyroid Nodule

TREATMENT OF THE CLINICALLY SOLITARY
THYROID NODULE WITH THYROID
HORMONE
   *by Carl E. Cassidy*

INDICATIONS FOR EXCISION
OF THE CLINICALLY SOLITARY
THYROID NODULE
   *by Oliver H. Beahrs*

NEEDLE BIOPSY OF THYROID
NODULES
   *by George Crile, Jr.*

## Statement of the Problem

The questions addressed concern the accuracy of diagnosis of the presence of a single nodule, its clinical importance, and noninvasive means of distinguishing benign from malignant lesions.

In distinguishing a truly solitary nodule from a multinodular goiter, how accurate is: (1) physical examination; (2) radioisotope scanning; (3) echogram? What specific characteristics of a nodule, on physical examination, influence the decision to operate?

Does a solitary nodule have a more serious import than multiple nodules? If so, cite the evidence. Cite data comparing the clinical preoperative impression that a solitary nodule is present with the operative and the pathologic findings.

What potential exists for differentiating a malignant from a benign nodule by suppressing thyrotrophic hormone production with oral administrations of thyroid hormone?

Are needle biopsies appropriate for determining the histologic character of thyroid nodules? Comment on the possible risk of "seeding" the needle track with tumor cells and on the accuracy of needle-size samples for ruling out malignancy.

Given a potentially fluid-filled cyst, when is aspiration justified? If fluid is obtained, does this assure that the lesion is benign?

In deciding to observe or to remove a clinically solitary nodule, of what significance are age and gender?

# Treatment of the Clinically Solitary Thyroid Nodule with Thyroid Hormone

CARL E. CASSIDY

*Tufts University School of Medicine*

## *Statement of the Problem*

Throughout the world, and particularly in the United States, operative removal of clinically solitary thyroid nodules is the most widely practiced treatment for this disorder. Most physicians are fearful of a solitary nodule in the thyroid, largely because of the common teaching that a significant percentage of these lesions are cancerous or precancerous and that they must be regarded as malignant until a microscopic section demonstrates otherwise. When a malignant lesion is found at operation, the assumption is made that the best possible initial treatment has been rendered; in spite of the finding of a benign lesion in 80 to 90 per cent of cases, the operative approach is defended on the basis that the operative risk is small.

This rationale for the nearly routine removal of thyroid nodules fails to incorporate into the reasoning several critical factors: (1) the frequency of thyroid nodules in the general population; (2) the incidence and type of carcinoma, based on microscopic sections of the thyroid obtained from surgical specimens; (3) the frequency of death from carcinoma of the thyroid; and (4) the effect of treatment on the outcome of the disease. Furthermore, the limited accuracy of studies to differentiate benign and malignant lesions is seldom considered, and yet the results of such studies are often used to support the decision to operate, a decision that has already been made at the time of the initial examination. Lastly, medical treatment, although gaining in popularity, is not considered seriously often enough, and the published results of such treatment do not appear to be widely known. The author's contention that solitary thyroid nodules for the most part are best treated

143

with thyroid hormone is based upon the factors mentioned previously, coupled with the results of such treatment in a large consecutive personal series.

## Frequency of Thyroid Nodules

The frequency of thyroid nodules, the incidence and type of carcinoma found in these lesions, and the death rate from carcinoma are well documented in the United States and *collectively* provide very meaningful data. Vander et al.[1] have provided the only data available for the incidence of thyroid nodules that can be detected clinically in unselected patients. The study stemmed from the examination of 5127 persons, aged 30 to 50 years, randomly selected from a nongoitrous area. At the beginning of the study, 146 people (2.8 per cent) had nodules thought to be solitary on the basis of clinical examination, but we know that they are even more common. Postmortem examination by Mortensen et al. (Table 1) of 821 clinically normal thyroids demonstrated that half of individuals dying of other causes had single (12.2 per cent) or multiple (37.3 per cent) thyroid nodules that were not detected during life. Beyond that, the study clearly documented the very limited accuracy of even *direct* palpation of the thyroid, which, poor as it is, must exceed by a large margin the accuracy of examination *in situ*. By direct palpation, 649 goiters were classified as diffuse, 101 as multinodular, and 71 as uninodular; sectioning of the glands revealed that only 415 were diffuse, 306 were multinodular, and 100 contained a solitary nodule. Furthermore, the solitary nodule was correctly identified by direct palpation in only 23 of the 100 glands that contained such lesions, and nodules ranging in diameter from 2.0 cm. to 7.5 cm., none of which were detected during the patient's lifetime, were present in 35 per cent of the nodular glands!

## Accuracy of Clinical Designations of Thyroid Nodules

The study of Mortensen and co-workers (Table 1) clearly shows that thyroid nodules that are never detected are very common and that the desig-

TABLE 1. Frequency of Thyroid Nodules in Clinically Normal Thyroid Glands*

| Classification of Thyroid Gland | Direct Palpation | | Pathologic Section | |
|---|---|---|---|---|
| | *Number* | *Per Cent* | *Number* | *Per Cent* |
| Diffuse | 649 | 79.1 | 415 | 50.5 |
| Solitary Nodule | 71 | 8.6 | 100 | 12.2 |
| Multinodular | 101 | 12.3 | 306 | 37.3 |
| Totals | 821 | 100.0 | 821 | 100.0 |

*From Mortensen, J D, Woolner, L. B., and Bennett, W. A.: Gross and microscopic findings in clinically normal thyroid glands. J. Clin. Endocrinol. *15*:1270, 1955.

nation of single or multiple nodules, even when done by direct palpation of the thyroid extracorporeally, is quite inaccurate. Several other studies have confirmed the inaccuracy of the designation of a clinically solitary nodule in living patients. Kambal,[2] Leichty,[3] and Miller[4] have reported that 31.5, 47, and 44 per cent respectively of glands thought to contain a single nodule preoperatively in fact were found to contain more than one nodule at operation. One cannot accurately predict the presence of a solitary nodule clinically, and one cannot therefore apply to a given patient the accepted frequency of carcinoma in a solitary nodule, since that designation may be incorrect in one third to one half of the cases.

Combining the reported incidences of 12.2 per cent for *undetected* solitary nodules and 2.8 per cent for *detectable* single thyroid nodules (realizing the error in such a designation), one must conclude that in a city of a million people, 15 per cent, or 150,000, must have solitary thyroid nodules. The frequency of carcinoma in these common lesions then is of paramount importance.

## Frequency of Thyroid Carcinoma in Surgical Specimens and Death Rate from Thyroid Carcinoma

The reported incidence of carcinoma in excised thyroid nodules varies from 1.3 per cent[2] to 28.7 per cent,[5] with 10 per cent being about the average. In a city of a million, then, 28,000 people should have a detectable thyroid nodule, and were all to receive operative treatment, a diagnosis of cancer of the thyroid would be made in about 2800 patients. It follows that thyroid cancer and death from carcinoma of the thyroid should be common, yet VanderLaan[6] has shown that only carcinoma of the pituitary is a rarer cause of death than carcinoma of the thyroid. Furthermore, Sokal[7] and Sloan and Frantz[8] have demonstrated that carcinoma of the thyroid accounts for only 0.1 per cent of all deaths per year in the United States and for about six deaths per year in a city of a million people. Especially important is the fact that only about one of these deaths is due to a differentiated thyroid tumor and about five are due to anaplastic carcinoma of the thyroid, which rarely, if ever, presents as a thyroid nodule.

## Value of Palpation of the Thyroid

Examination of the thyroid by palpation provides extremely valuable information to experienced individuals. Diffuse enlargement that is not fixed to surrounding tissues and is not accompanied by palpable lymph nodes is clearly a benign disorder. Hyperthyroidism, diffuse nontoxic (simple) goiter, thyroiditis, or goiter and hypothyroidism are the most common disorders which can easily be differentiated by appropriate studies. Few would take issue that medical therapy is indicated in these diseases.

The presence of two or more nodules in a goiter that moves freely with swallowing is again little cause for concern. Sokal[9] has shown that the *cumulative* lifetime risk that a patient with nodular goiter will develop thyroid carcinoma is about 1 per cent and that the risk of nodular goiter being malignant at any one time is even smaller. Firmness of a nodule in itself does not indicate the likelihood of malignancy, but other well-known findings do: progressive growth of a firm or hard mass that is not sharply defined, fixation to the skin and other structures, the presence of palpable nodes, vocal cord paralysis, and obstructive symptoms.

The voluminous literature on thyroid nodules, much of it repetitious, reflects not so much scientific endeavor as failure of the experts to agree upon the factors discussed previously. Zimmerman and Wagner[10] have presented convincing evidence *against* an etiologic relationship between nodular goiter and carcinoma and have discounted the role of thyroid nodules in the genesis of thyroid cancer. Nonetheless, when thyroid nodules are found, the concern that carcinoma is present becomes the first consideration, and a sense of urgency compelling prompt operative treatment seems to prevail. For some reason or other, the accuracy of preoperative diagnosis of cancer is disregarded. For example, Shimaoka et al.[11] and Jackson and Thomson[12] have found only a 2 per cent incidence of unsuspected cancer. One can usually make the diagnosis of anaplastic carcinoma of the thyroid solely on the basis of the history and examination; diagnostic procedures are seldom, if ever, indicated, but some physicians might prefer biopsy prior to palliative operative treatment. Medullary carcinoma of the thyroid can be suspected from concurrent abnormalities of other organs or a family history of thyroid carcinoma, and its presence should be confirmed by measuring thyrocalcitonin in serum. This determination is highly specific and accurate; the other tests are of no diagnostic help. Biopsy is not necessary before thyroidectomy. Papillary, follicular, or mixed tumors then account for the remaining 80 per cent of thyroid carcinomas. These tumors are usually indolent and are only rarely fatal, but the danger they present to the patient, their relationship to thyroid nodules, and the best treatment for them are issues that have never been resolved.

The failure to appreciate or accept the accuracy of the clinical findings in thyroid carcinoma, coupled with the conviction that operative treatment must be instituted promptly, has overshadowed the likelihood that the outcome of thyroid cancer depends on the biologic characteristics of the tumor, rather than on the treatment and the speed with which it is instituted.

## Noninvasive Examinations of the Thyroid

Even though the inaccuracy of the clinical designation of solitary thyroid nodule has been well documented, the concern that carcinoma may exist when such a designation is made persists, and a great deal of effort has been directed toward the development of noninvasive techniques that would differentiate benign from malignant lesions, solitary nodules from multinodular goiter, and, more recently, solid tumors from cysts.

Scintiscans (radioiodine) demonstrate the ability of thyroid nodules to accumulate radioiodine. They have shown that thyroid cancer is present very rarely, if ever, in hot nodules, and operative excision based on the fear of carcinoma in these cases cannot be sanctioned. The hope that the finding of cold or nonfunctioning thyroid nodules would differentiate carcinoma from benign lesions has not been realized.

Scintiscanning of the thyroid gland may demonstrate the location and *relative function* of nodules and other lesions but does not provide even the probable diagnosis of these macroscopic lesions. Fitzgerald and Foote,[13] using radioautography, have shown that many types of nodules that appear inactive on scans do accumulate iodine, although in lower concentrations than normal thyroid tissue. Groesbeck[14] and others have shown that the scan is more accurate than palpation in distinguishing solitary from multiple nodules, but one must keep in mind that a nonfunctioning nodule must measure at least 1 cm. in diameter to be resolved by scanning and that posterior nodules covered by functioning tissue do not change recorded counts, and therefore defects in the thyroid image do not appear.

Cancer accounts for only a minority of the cold nodules, which in fact more often represent functional changes present in benign adenomas or multinodular goiter, cysts, subacute and chronic thyroiditis, hemorrhage, necrosis, and fibrosis. The failure of scintiscans to differentiate between benign and malignant lesions has been documented by Kendall and Condon,[15] who found that 83 per cent of benign nodules were cool or cold, as were 75 per cent of malignant nodules. Shimaoka and Sokal[16] also demonstrated that the interpretations of thyroid scintiscans in 169 patients did not show a significant difference in the frequency of malignant lesions. Most experienced physicians would agree with Miller et al.[17] that "no scintigram should reverse the diagnosis of benignancy made by an experienced clinician."

Several additional studies have been suggested to differentiate benign cold nodules from malignant ones, but none have proved successful. While some cold nodules may disappear from a scintiscan following the administration of thyrotropin,[18] one could not expect cysts and the other lesions mentioned previously to respond. The clinical value of scans using selenomethionine[19] or fluorescence,[20] thermography,[21] and angiography[22] cannot be evaluated at this time.

Echography (sonography), either by the A-mode technique or B-mode scanning, may provide excellent distinction between cystic and solid structures under certain conditions. Blum et al.[23] studied 67 cold nodules measuring 1 to 3 cm. in diameter. All 13 cysts and 54 solid tumors were correctly diagnosed. All lesions over 4 cm. in diameter showed a combination of cystic and solid patterns, and the echogram did not differentiate carcinoma from multinodular goiter, Hashimoto's thyroiditis, benign adenoma, or lymphoma. Lesions less than 1 cm. in diameter escape detection by this method. The value of echography then is in differentiating cystic from solid lesions, provided the diameter is between 1 and 3 cm.

## *Thyroid Cysts*

Identification of a cyst makes malignancy very unlikely, and treatment may be accomplished by aspiration with a needle rather than by operative excision, when treatment is indicated for other reasons. Crile[24] reported the success of such treatment in 47 of 50 patients followed from 4 months to 10 years and noted, as have others, that the coincidental presence of carcinoma in cystic lesions of the thyroid is extremely rare. It is generally felt that cytologic examination of the aspirate, even by the most experienced individuals, is of limited value; for example, Crockford and Bain[25] have pointed out that the diagnosis of well-differentiated thyroid carcinoma may be difficult, because the cells may be indistinguishable from those aspirated from benign thyroid lesions.

## *Biopsy of the Thyroid*

Although Crile reported dissemination of a papillary carcinoma following needle biopsy in 1956,[26] no additional cases have been reported since then, and this possibility is now of minimal concern. Complications from fine needle biopsy, cylinder biopsy, and high-speed pneumatic drill biopsy are said to be very infrequent. The questions of when and if a biopsy of the thyroid should be done and which method is superior have not been resolved. Those who favor open biopsy contend that the diagnostic accuracy is greater and that one need not fear dissemination of the tumor. The latter concern is not valid, since such dissemination occurred only once in more than 2000 biopsies done by Crile;[27] Kirstaedter[27] has had no implants of cancer in the needle tracts of 900 aspiration biopsies of cold thyroid nodules.

Although Crile obtained sufficient material for diagnosis in 92 per cent of cases (81 of 88 patients), others have reported only a 75 per cent success rate.[28] It should be pointed out that the clinical diagnosis without biopsy was correct in 96 per cent of patients with struma lymphomatosis and in 86 per cent of patients with nodular goiter in Crile's series. All suspected cancers were confirmed by needle biopsy, and only four unsuspected cancers were discovered. However, in a recent preliminary study of a small series of fine needle biopsies followed by open biopsy done to determine the value of fine needle biopsy in diagnosing thyroiditis and malignant lesions, Hansen and Kølendorf[29] concluded that it was not valuable in the diagnosis of malignant lesions, in view of the false positives and false negatives obtained. If the technique is unsatisfactory for the major purpose for which it is commonly employed, as suggested by this study, its use for any purpose at all becomes very suspect. Successful biopsies have also been obtained without complications by high-speed pneumatic drill[30] in 93 per cent of 54 cases. Clinical accuracy was not included in this report.

## Age and Sex

Koutras et al.[31] have presented statistical evidence from a study of 408 cold thyroid nodules removed by operation that the probability of malignancy in males was double that in females ($p < 0.05$), and that in all patients 60 years of age or older, the likelihood of malignancy was four times greater than in those 60 years of age or younger ($p < 0.001$). The incidence of malignancy for patients 20 years of age or younger, 21 to 40 years of age, and 41 to 60 years of age was remarkably constant at 10.0, 10.4, and 10.7 per cent respectively. Veith et al.[32] reported their findings in 498 patients *selected* for thyroidectomy because of nodularity of the thyroid and the fear of carcinoma. No statistical analysis was done, but the incidence of malignancy in men with single nodules appeared to be higher than in women. They emphasized that because of the selectivity involved, the data cannot be applied to the population at large. The same restriction applies to the data presented by Koutras.[31]

Data do not exist on the incidence of carcinoma in nodules in children who have never received radiation to the neck. Refetoff et al.[33] have confirmed the relationship between radiation in childhood and the later development of nodules and well-differentiated tumors, as previously pointed out by Winship and Rosvoll[34] and others. Nearly half of the known cases of carcinoma in childhood reported from the world literature occurred in children who received such radiation. Only about 481 cases of thyroid carcinoma in children not known to have received such radiation were reported from 1902 to 1968; at most, this could account for only a few cases per year throughout the world. During a 30-year interval, Exelby and Frazell[35] saw only 46 patients 16 years of age or younger with carcinoma of the thyroid who had not received prior radiation to the head and neck.

The finding of a nodule in a child who has never received radiotherapy and who has no evidence of metastasis is in all likelihood not as serious, nor is treatment as urgent, as is commonly supposed. Winship and Rosvoll[34] reported that 74 per cent of the patients had metastases when first seen, and Exelby and Frazell[35] have pointed out that the prognosis is excellent even when metastases are present.

## Survival Rates

Woolner et al.[36] have shown that the 5- and 10-year survival rates for both sexes in those patients treated by operation in whom the diagnosis of papillary tumor was made before the age of 40 were approximately normal, but that they were significantly lower in those in whom the diagnosis was made after the age of 40. The ratio of females to males was 2.4:1 in the group as a whole, but in the more aggressive and extensive tumors it was 1:1, and the survival rates were no different. Again, these data are based on a group of patients who were highly selected for operation and cannot be applied to the general population. Final assessment of the medical treatment of nodules lacking a pathologic diagnosis and of known papillary and mixed tumors will depend on the demonstration of survival rates that are at least equal to those for cases treated by operation.

The study of Vander et al.[1] provides the only data for untreated clinically solitary nodules and multinodular glands in both sexes in the age group of 30 to 50 years. During a 15-year follow-up, no cases of carcinoma developed. In considering a single patient with a nodule who does not obviously have carcinoma, consideration of these data is far more relevant than the surgical data derived from selected patients. In addition, Bowens and Vander[37] have shown that the risk of delaying operation in asymptomatic lesions is small and that a trial of medical treatment is warranted.

## Treatment of Thyroid Nodules with Thyroid Hormones

The rationale for the treatment of thyroid nodules has been previously summarized by Astwood[38] and Cassidy,[39] and their earlier experience was published 15 years ago.[40] All nodules were treated with thyroid hormone; 54 per cent of the solitary nodules disappeared or became smaller, and 46 per cent did not change in size. The major objection to the study was that since biopsies were not done, benign and malignant lesions were not identified. Such is the case. However, it could not possibly be that only benign lesions were referred to us for therapy; probably, the percentage of cancer in clinically solitary nodules in our series, had they been biopsied or excised, would not differ significantly from those reported by most large surgical clinics.

An analysis of more than 150 consecutive patients with clinically solitary thyroid nodules and more than 250 consecutive patients with multinodular goiter treated with thyroid hormone is underway,[41] and some preliminary data are available. The age groups ranged from the second to ninth decades. About 63 per cent were followed for 5 years or longer, 30 per cent for 10 years or longer, and 7 per cent for 15 years or longer. The experience has been similar to that in the untreated cases of Vander et al.[1] and in addition, about two thirds of the solitary nodules decreased in size or disappeared. Life table analyses are expected to show survival rates equivalent to the normal.

## Summary

Thyroid nodules that can be detected clinically are common, and an even larger number remain undetected in clinically normal thyroid glands. Thyroid carcinoma is a rare cause of death, and its importance in relation to nodular goiter and clinically solitary thyroid nodules has been grossly exaggerated. Treatment of these lesions with thyroid hormone has been condemned because of the fear that medical therapy of undiagnosed well-differentiated tumors is inferior to surgical treatment. No evidence to support this contention has been forthcoming. Failure of a nodule to decrease in size has been regarded as a treatment failure, when morbidity or death would be more appropriate criteria. The author's experience to date indicates that the treatment of thyroid nodules with thyroid hormones is safe and less hazardous than surgical treatment.

## References

1. Vander, J. B., Gaston, E. A., and Dawber, T. R.: The significance of nontoxic thyroid nodules. Final report of a 15-year study of the incidence of thyroid malignancy. Ann. Intern. Med. 69:537, 1968.
2. Kambal, A.: Carcinoma in solitary thyroid nodules. Br. J. Surg. 56:434, 1969.
3. Liechty, R. D., Graham, M., and Freemeyer, P.: Benign solitary thyroid nodules. Surg. Gynecol. Obstet. 121:571, 1965.
4. Miller, J. M.: Carcinoma and thyroid nodules; problem in endemic goiter area. N. Engl. J. Med. 252:247, 1955.
5. Hoffman, G. L., Thompson, N. W., and Heffron, C.: The solitary thyroid nodule. A reassessment. Arch. Surg. 105:379, 1972.
6. VanderLaan, W. P.: The occurrence of carcinoma of the thyroid in autopsy material. N. Engl. J. Med. 237:221, 1947.
7. Sokal, J. E.: Occurrence of thyroid cancer. N. Engl. J. Med. 249:393, 1953.
8. Sloan, L. W., and Frantz, V. K.: Thyroid cancer: clinical aspects. In Werner, S. C. (ed.): The Thyroid. New York, P. B. Hoeber, Inc., 1955.
9. Sokal, J. E.: The incidence of thyroid cancer and the problem of malignancy in nodular goiter. In Astwood, E. B. (ed.): Clinical Endocrinology. Vol. 1. New York, Grune & Stratton, Inc., 1960, p. 168.
10. Zimmerman, L. M., and Wagner, D. H.: Relation of nodular goiter to thyroid carcinoma. In Astwood, E. B. (ed.): Clinical Endocrinology. Vol. 1. New York, Grune & Stratton, Inc., 1960, p. 160.
11. Shimaoka, K., Badillo, J., Sokal, J. E., and Marchetta, F. C.: Clinical differentiation between thyroid cancer and benign goiter. An evaluation. J.A.M.A. 181:179, 1962.
12. Jackson, I., and Thomson, J. A.: The relationship of carcinoma to the single thyroid nodule. Br. J. Surg. 54:1007, 1967.
13. Fitzgerald, P. J., and Foote, F. W.: The function of various types of thyroid carcinoma as revealed by the radioautographic demonstration of radioactive iodine (I$^{131}$). J. Clin. Endocrinol. 9:1153, 1949.
14. Groesbeck, H. P.: Evaluation of routine scintiscanning of nontoxic thyroid nodules. I. The preoperative diagnosis of thyroid cancer. Cancer 12:1, 1959.
15. Kendall, L. W., and Condon, R. E.: Prediction of malignancy in solitary thyroid nodules. Lancet 1:1071, 1969.
16. Shimaoka, K., and Sokal, J. E.: Differentiation of benign and malignant thyroid nodules by scintiscan. Arch. Intern. Med. 114:36, 1964.
17. Miller, J. M., Hamburger, J. I., and Mellinger, R. C.: The thyroid scintigram. II. The cold nodule. Radiology 85:702, 1965.
18. Gibbs, J. C., Halligan, E. J., Grieco, R. V., and McKeown, J. E.: Scintiscanning the thyroid nodule. An aid in its surgical management. Arch. Surg. 90:323, 1965.
19. Thomas, C. G., Jr., Pepper, F. D., and Owen, J.: Differentiation of malignant from benign lesions of the thyroid gland using complementary scanning with $^{75}$ selenomethionine and radioiodine. Ann. Surg. 170:396, 1969.
20. Hoffer, P. B., and Gottschalk, A.: Fluorescent thyroid scanning. Scanning without radioisotopes: initial clinical results. Radiology 99:117, 1971.
21. Samuels, B. I.: Thermography: a valuable tool in the detection of thyroid disease. Radiology 102:59, 1972.
22. Damascelli, B., Cascinelli, N., Terno, G., Dragoni, G., and Saccozzi, R.: Second thoughts on the value of selective thyroid angiography. Am. J. Roentgenol. Radium Ther. Nucl. Med. 114:822, 1972.

23. Blum, M., Goldman, A. B., Herskovic, A., and Hernberg, J.: Clinical applications of thyroid echography. N. Engl. J. Med. 287:1164, 1972.
24. Crile, G., Jr.: Treatment of thyroid cysts by aspiration. Surgery 59:210, 1966.
25. Crockford, P. M., and Bain, G. O.: Fine-needle aspiration biopsy of the thyroid. Can. Med. Assoc. J. 110:1029, 1974.
26. Crile, G., Jr.: The danger of surgical dissemination of papillary carcinoma of the thyroid. Surg. Gynecol. Obstet. 102:161, 1956.
27. Crile, G., Jr., and Hawk, W. A., Jr.: Aspiration biopsy of thyroid nodules. Surg. Gynecol. Obstet. 136:241, 1973.
28. Singh, P., Khanna, S. D., and Manchanda, R. L.: Needle biopsy of the thyroid. Arch. Surg. 91:646, 1965.
29. Hansen, J. B., and Kølendorf, K.: Fine-needle biopsy of thyroid lesions. N. Engl. J. Med. 291:851, 1974.
30. Sachdeva, H. S., Wig, J. D., Kanta, C., and Dutta, B. N.: High-speed pneumatic drill for biopsy of thyroid lesions. Arch. Surg. 108:744, 1974.
31. Koutras, D. A., Livadas, D., Sfontouris, J., Messaris, G., and Statherou, P. K.: A study of 408 cold thyroid nodules in a country with endemic goiter. Nucl. Med. 7:165, 1968.
32. Veith, F. J., Brooks, J. R., Grigsby, W. P., and Selenkow, H. A.: The nodular thyroid gland and cancer. N. Engl. J. Med. 270:431, 1964.
33. Refetoff, S., Harrison, J., Karanfilski, B. T., Kaplan, E. L., DeGroot, L. J., and Bekerman, C.: Continuing occurrence of thyroid carcinoma after irradiation to the neck in infancy and childhood. N. Engl. J. Med. 292:171, 1975.
34. Winship, T., and Rosvoll, R. V.: Cancer of the thyroid in children. Proc. Natl. Cancer Conf. 6:677, 1970.
35. Exelby, P. E., and Frazell, E. L.: Carcinoma of the thyroid in children. Surg. Clin. North Am. 49:249, 1969.
36. Woolner, L. B., Beahrs, O. H., Black, B. M., McConahey, W. M., and Keating, F. R., Jr.: Classification and prognosis of thyroid carcinoma. A study of 885 cases observed in a 30 year period. Am. J. Surg. 102:354, 1961.
37. Bowens, O. M., and Vander, J. B.: Thyroid nodules and thyroid malignancy. The risk involved in delayed surgery. Ann. Intern. Med. 57:245, 1962.
38. Astwood, E. B.: The problem of nodules in the thyroid gland. Pediatrics 18:501, 1956.
39. Cassidy, C. E.: Les raisons d'utiliser l'hormone thyroidienne pour le traitement des nodules thyroidiens. Médecine et Hygiène 994:65, 1972.
40. Astwood, E. B., Cassidy, C. E., and Aurbach, G. D.: Treatment of goiter and thyroid nodules with thyroid. J.A.M.A. 174:459, 1960.
41. Cassidy, C. E.: Unpublished data.

# Indications for Excision of the Clinically Solitary Thyroid Nodule

OLIVER H. BEAHRS

*Mayo Clinic and Mayo Foundation*

The management of nodular goiters and thyroid nodules varies widely and remains a controversial subject. Some physicians believe that such goiters can be managed medically or not treated at all. Moreover, they regard thyroid cancer as being most often so "benign" that it does not require operative treatment. (If the thyroid cancer is of high grade or is anaplastic, operation is again superfluous because any treatment for these lesions is unsuccessful.) Other physicians view nodular goiters as a real hazard for the patient and believe that if a nodule is proved to be malignant, then radical operative treatment is required, just as it is with some other histologic types of cancer in the head and neck. However, in deciding how to manage the problem of nodular goiter, the majority of physicians and surgeons today adopt a position between these extremes.

The incidence of nodular goiter in the adult population is high (about 50 per cent), as demonstrated by Mortensen and associates[12] in an autopsy study. Determining what proportion of the population harbors clinical thyroid nodules probably depends on each physician's definition of nodular goiter, on the consistency and care with which he seeks them, and on his competence in examining the thyroid. Many nodular goiters are present but are not obvious clinically, and others that are clinically evident carry a very small risk of complications. Thus, careful selection of nodular goiters for operative treatment must be based on the many diagnostic factors available to the physician.

In managing nodular goiters, the risk of cancer is the primary unknown hazard to be considered, but risks of hyperthyroidism, pressure on structures in the neck and mediastinum, and cosmetic deformity should also be taken into account. The decision about management must be based on consideration of all these risks; however, in this discussion, only the risk of cancer will be considered.

Cancer of the thyroid gland can be diagnosed with certainty only by studying the suspected lesion histologically. For this reason, any nodule suspected of being a cancer, based on any diagnostic criteria, should be removed for pathologic diagnosis. If the specimen is malignant, the appropriate definitive operative procedure can be carried out. It is possible, based on available criteria, to select lesions for operative therapy fairly efficiently. At our clinic, we operate on about 10 per cent of the patients who have nodular goiters that are sufficiently identified and significant to be indexed. Of this selected group undergoing operation, 14 per cent proved to have one of the several types of cancer of the thyroid gland. (During this time, some goiters were being removed for other causes, such as hyperthyroidism or cosmetic deformity.) We might ask whether a 14 per cent incidence of cancer in patients operated on is not too low a percentage and whether some patients are being operated on unnecessarily. Selection of nodules for operative treatment because of cancer will not approximate 100 per cent until there is a diagnostic test other than histologic study. In the meantime, because thyroidectomy carries a mortality of zero (except in certain emergency conditions, such as airway obstruction) and a minimal morbidity, it seems reasonable to offer any patient operative removal of a nodular goiter that might be malignant.

Errors in clinical examination for thyroid nodules are frequent. For this reason, it has always seemed unreasonable to state definitely that a goiter contains only one nodule when it may be multinodular. In a high percentage of patients operated on for what was considered clinically to be a single nodule, multiple nodules were found at the time of operation or on histologic study. It would seem more reasonable to refer to what clinically appears to be a single or solitary nodule as a *discrete* nodule, felt distinctly and separately from other thyroid tissue, a term that does not eliminate the possibility that other nodules might be present. Because of the substantial potential for error in clinical judgments based on palpation and laboratory studies, we have not separated out a group called "single" or "solitary" nodular goiter, and we do not believe that this should be done. It is not uncommon, when operating on what is considered to be a discrete or single nodule in the thyroid gland, to find that an occult lesion elsewhere in the gland is a cancer.

## Clinical Factors Leading to Selection of Nodular Goiter for Thyroidectomy

### History

The fact that a goiter has been present for a long time without significant change in size reduces the likelihood that cancer is present. On the other hand, the presence of a nodule for a short period or of one not known to be present until the time of examination raises the suspicion that the lesion is more likely to be a neoplasm. If a nodular goiter is known to be increasing in size (especially if the increase is rapid), the assumption should be that it is growing and is likely to be malignant. However, rapid growth associated with pain or the sudden appearance of a nodule not previously known (along with pain and tenderness) almost always denotes hemorrhage into a pre-existing adenoma, which in turn almost eliminates the possibility that the lesion is a cancer.

Unusual hoarseness in the presence of a nodular goiter that is increasing in size is cause for suspicion. A cancer can invade the recurrent laryngeal nerve, paralyzing the ipsilateral vocal cord; a benign goiter rarely interferes with nerve function even if the goiter is large and greatly displaces the nerve. Dysphagia can be a symptom of thyroid cancer, but most often it occurs late in the course of the disease when the diagnosis is already obvious.

A history of x-ray exposure from therapy to the head and neck region early in life raises the suspicion of cancer in any thyroid nodule. Although the incidence of thyroid cancer in children receiving radiation therapy to this anatomic region is unknown, it has been firmly established[6] that about 85 per cent of young patients with thyroid cancer will have had x-ray therapy to this area because of lymphadenitis, enlarged thymic gland, skin pathology, or other reasons. This finding has been substantiated by Hayles and associates.[10]

A family history of thyroid cancer is now recognized as a factor to consider in making a judgment about a nodular goiter. Medullary cancer occurs in family groups and in multiple endocrine adenomatosis (Sipple's syndrome). Anyone who has a nodular goiter and who comes from a family group in which other members are known to have medullary adenocarcinoma of the thyroid must be considered to have a cancer until proved otherwise. Some medullary cancers produce elevation in the serum calcitonin levels. Members of such a family group who have an elevated serum calcitonin, even though a nodule is not palpated, almost always will have an undetected medullary adenocarcinoma of the thyroid gland or, if not, will have "C-cell" hyperplasia.[5] In addition, any patient who has had a pheochromocytoma or parathyroid disease and in whom a thyroid nodule is discovered should have a thyroidectomy because of the risk of cancer.[5]

### Age and Sex

Age and sex are important determinants in deciding for or against thyroidectomy for nodular goiters. In their review of pediatric patients, Hayles et al.[10] found that 50 to 70 per cent of thyroid nodules in patients 14 years of age or less were associated with cancer of the thyroid gland. In the adult, the incidence has been variously reported as from 5 per cent[2] to over 30 per cent.[7] Mortensen and coworkers'[12] figure of 5.3 per cent in nodular thyroid glands seen at autopsy may be a representative percentage for patients in the older age group. Sokal[13] has reported a figure of 1 per cent or less. This figure is lower than that seen in surgical experience, since there is no selection on clinical grounds.

Goiters are seen more frequently in women, as is cancer of the thyroid gland. However, because goiter in general is seen so much less frequently in men, the incidence of cancer in a nodular thyroid gland in men is greater than in women. For this reason, more emphasis should be given to the need to remove a discrete nodule in a man than in a woman.

## *Physical Examination*

Although there are several methods of examining the thyroid gland, there are certain advantages to approaching the patient from the front. First, inspection often is more revealing than palpation. Asymmetry of the neck should be looked for, and a nodule often can be seen easily on swallowing. Inspection should always include the lateral portion of the neck, where significant lymphadenopathy can be seen at times. In our experience, 22 per cent of papillary adenocarcinomas were diagnosed initially because of the presence of metastasis to the lateral cervical nodes, rather than on palpation of a nodule in the thyroid gland itself.

If a discrete nodule is felt, it is reasonable, since most cancers are single lesions, to assume that the risk of cancer is greater than in an obviously multinodular gland, although cancer does occur in the latter. The rationale for not dividing goiters into single and multinodular varieties has been discussed previously.

The consistency of the nodule should be determined carefully. The fact that it is cystic or hard does not signify that cancer is present, but if the nodule is definitely cystic, the chance that it is a cancer is much less than if it is firm, rubbery, hard, infiltrating, or somewhat fixed to adjacent tissues. If the lesion is stony-hard or calcified, it is most likely a calcified adenoma. Some papillary cancers have flecks of calcification within them, but the lesion will not feel like a calcified adenoma. Follicular cancer can be soft or firm and may feel like a benign adenoma.

About 20 per cent of papillary adenocarcinomas and 50 per cent or more of medullary cancers will be multicentric, either in one thyroid lobe or in both. For this reason, the presence of more than one palpable lesion is no guarantee that cancer is not present.

The discovery of lymphadenopathy in the lateral neck frequently can lead to the diagnosis of thyroid cancer. For this reason, examination for goiter should always include palpation for lymph nodes along the jugular chain and in the substernal notch, as well as a search for the Delphian node.

The presence of coexisting known or unknown thyroid pathology does not eliminate the possibility that cancer is also present. For example, 3 per cent of patients who have a firm, diffusely nodular goiter known, or thought, to be Hashimoto's thyroiditis will have a coexisting papillary adenocarcinoma, and another 3 per cent will prove to have lymphosarcoma when the goiter is removed.[4] If Hashimoto's thyroiditis is treated medically, the patient should be followed carefully, and if other glandular changes are noted, thyroidectomy should be done.

Beahrs and Sakulsky[3] found a 2 per cent incidence of coexisting papillary adenocarcinoma in 377 operatively treated cases of exophthalmic goiter. Thus in Graves' disease managed with radioactive iodine or antithyroid drugs, the possibility of a cancer should be kept in mind.

## Laboratory Studies

Needle biopsy or aspiration of thyroid nodules is tried by some physicians, but I oppose this approach for several reasons.[8] First, if the biopsy specimen is positive for cancer, the lesion must be removed, and the risk of seeding the biopsy-needle tract theoretically exists. I believe that the decision for thyroidectomy can be made adequately on other evidence. If the needle specimen shows no evidence of cancer, there is no guarantee that a representative sample of the pathology was obtained. Open inspection of any lesion warranting biopsy seems the best approach, since this permits gross inspection of the lesion. Then the definitive surgical procedure can be carried out immediately, based on the pathologic findings. If a lesion is most likely a cyst, according to all other findings (softness, sudden enlargement, pain, and tenderness), then needle aspiration might be considered. However, this should not be done for a nodule suspected of being a cancer.

Radioiodine scanning of the thyroid establishes whether a nodule is nonfunctioning (cold) or functioning (hot). This information is of value diagnostically, but again the procedure is not pathognomonic. Some hot nodules have been found to be functioning follicular carcinomas. In one review of cases of thyroid cancer in which scans were obtained, the cancer was a cold nodule in 60 per cent, the scan was not helpful in 34 per cent, and the nodule appeared to have increased uptake over the adjacent thyroid tissue in 6 per cent.[1] It has been shown by Gibbs and associates[9] that cold nodules that do not respond to thyroid-stimulating hormone should be removed by operation, because they are more likely to be cancerous than cold nodules that do show function after stimulation.

The echogram gives valuable information, but again it does not definitely determine the histologic character of the lesion.[11] It most likely will differentiate between a cystic and a solid lesion. Some follicular adenocarcinomas are cystic or appear to be cysts by echogram. Thus, this diagnostic aid provides additional information, but it is not essential in making a judgment about managing a particular lesion.

Thyroid suppression of a nodular goiter is believed to be of value. The majority of thyroid cancers are well differentiated and grow slowly. Regression of the thyroid mass after thyroid feeding is more likely caused by atrophy of normally functioning thyroid parenchyma than by regression of any neoplasm that might be present. I have yet to see what I consider a true thyroid nodule or neoplasm disappear after thyroid replacement therapy.

Thyroid function tests are of no value in evaluating the histologic character of thyroid nodules.

## Conclusions

Considering the factors discussed, we can easily identify the two extremes in management of thyroid nodules.

If the patient is a male child who has had x-ray therapy to the head and neck earlier in childhood and has cervical lymphadenopathy and a recently noted discrete firm nodule that is increasing in size, and if the nodule is cold on [131]I scan and not cystic on echogram, the nodule is almost certainly a cancer, and thyroidectomy must be strongly recommended. On the other hand, if the patient is an older woman with an obviously multinodular goiter that is soft and has been present for many years and is not increasing in size, and if the radioiodine scan is normal and the echogram shows a cystic lesion, the goiter is obviously benign and need not be treated unless other complications exist.

Between these extremes, the various factors discussed must be weighed carefully to assure proper management of the particular nodular goiter. It is an unfortunate experience to have operated on what proved to be a benign nodular goiter that was asymptomatic, but a greater error is to overlook a cancer which, in time, would jeopardize the life of the patient.

## References

1. Beahrs, O. H., and Kubista, T. P.: Diagnosis of thyroid cancer. In: *Cancer Management.* Philadelphia, J. B. Lippincott Co., 1968, pp. 573–579.
2. Beahrs, O. H., Pemberton, J., and Black, B. M.: Nodular goiter and malignant lesions of the thyroid gland. J. Clin. Endocrinol. *11*:1157–1165, 1951.
3. Beahrs, O. H., and Sakulsky, S. B.: Surgical thyroidectomy in the management of exophthalmic goiter. Arch. Surg. *96*:512–516, 1968.
4. Beahrs, O. H., Woolner, L. B., and McConahey, W. M.: Struma lymphomatosa (Hashimoto's thyroiditis) and related thyroidal disorders. J. Clin. Endocrinol. Metab. *19*:53–83, 1959.
5. Chong, G. C., Beahrs, O. H., Sizemore, G. W., et al.: Medullary carcinoma of the thyroid gland. Cancer. *35*:695–704, 1975.
6. Clark, R. L.: Surgical treatment of cancer of the thyroid. In: *Cancer Management.* Philadelphia, J. B. Lippincott Co., 1968, pp. 581–583.
7. Cole, W. H., Majarakis, J. D., and Slaughter, D. P.: Incidence of carcinoma of the thyroid in nodular goiter. J. Clin. Endocrinol. *9*:1007–1011, 1949.
8. Crile, G., Jr., and Hawk, W. A., Jr.: Aspiration biopsy of thyroid nodules. Surg. Gynecol. Obstet. *136*:241–245, 1973.
9. Gibbs, J. C., Halligan, E. J., Grieco, R. V., et al.: Scintiscanning the thyroid nodule: an aid in its surgical management. Arch. Surg. *90*:323–328, 1965.
10. Hayles, A. B., Johnson, L. M., Beahrs, O. H., et al.: Carcinoma of the thyroid in children. Am. J. Surg. *106*:735–743, 1963.
11. Miskin, M., Rosen, I. B., and Walfish, P. G.: B-mode ultrasonography in assessment of thyroid gland lesions. Ann. Intern. Med. *79*:505–510, 1973.
12. Mortensen, J. D., Bennett, W. A., and Woolner, L. B.: Incidence of carcinoma in thyroid glands removed at 1000 consecutive routine necropsies. Surg. Forum *5*:659–663, 1954.
13. Sokal, J. E.: Incidence of malignancy in toxic and nontoxic nodular goiter. J.A.M.A. *154*:1321–1325, 1954.

# Needle Biopsy of Thyroid Nodules

GEORGE CRILE, JR.

*Cleveland Clinic Foundation*

For many years, it has been standard practice to confirm the diagnosis of struma lymphomatosa by needle biopsy of the thyroid, but until 1971, we did not routinely take biopsies of thyroid nodules. If we thought a nodule was a cyst, we would not hesitate to aspirate it, and in this way many operations were avoided. However, most nodules were colloid adenomas that were so gelatinous that it was impossible to obtain a good core with a Vim-Silverman needle. Now we no longer try to use the Silverman needle for nodules; instead, we take an aspiration biopsy with an 18- or 15-gauge needle or a needle biopsy with the new Tru-cut needle.*

## Anesthesia

The skin is numbed with a cold spray, and a few drops of Procaine are infiltrated under it and over the most prominent part of the nodule.

## Aspiration of Cysts

If the nodule is thought to be a cyst or a hemorrhage into an adenoma (history of sudden appearance or of discomfort), an 18-gauge needle is inserted into the nodule and the contents are aspirated. If there is no residual mass, it is unlikely that the nodule is malignant, and nothing more need be done. In more than 90 per cent of the cases, one, two, or three aspirations of

---

*Manufactured by Travenol, Deerfield, Illinois 60015.

159

the cyst result in its permanent disappearance or in a striking reduction in size.

Occasionally, 1 ml. of a sclerosing solution widely used for injection of varicose veins (Sotradecol) is introduced into the cyst after aspiration. Since the cysts are part of a nodular goiter, suppressive doses of thyroxin (Synthroid, 0.2 mg.) are given. In this way, about 25 per cent of all thyroid nodules can be successfully removed or controlled. The fluid from the cyst is always examined, but only in one of several hundred cases have we observed abnormal cells.[1]

## Aspiration Biopsy

If there is a residual mass, the needle is inserted into it and a suction biopsy is obtained. The same technique is used to obtain a specimen from a colloid nodule that is so gelatinous that it does not hold together and is therefore not suited to biopsy by Silverman needles.

Strong suction is exerted by pulling on the plunger of the syringe while the point of the needle is run back and forth two or three times through the nodule. The needle is then withdrawn, and the fixative (Zenker's solution) is sucked into the syringe through the needle. The contents of the syringe are then expelled into a small jar of fixative and sent to the laboratory where the material is spun down and a cell block is made. If one tries to remove the fragments of tissue from the syringe by rinsing with saline, they stick to the sides; this is why it is necessary to fix the tissue before trying to expel it.

Usually there is ample material visible in the fixative, but if it seems sparse, one need only substitute a 15-gauge needle for the 18 and, while suction is exerted on the plunger, squeeze the nodule gently. Sometimes most of the nodule is sucked into the syringe. Pressure is applied to the neck for a few minutes to control bleeding. The needle should always be directed away from the trachea to avoid possible injury of the recurrent laryngeal nerve.

## Tru-cut Needle Biopsy

As mentioned before, the Silverman needle obtains an excellent core in patients with cancers or thyroiditis, but it is unsatisfactory for those with colloid adenomas. Here the Tru-cut needle is much better, and it is also better for patients with lymphomas and lymphoid types of thyroiditis, because it does not crush the cells the way the Silverman needle does.

After a nick is made in the anesthetized skin overlying the nodule, the needle is inserted through the capsule. The stilette is then advanced 1 or 2 cm., the sheath advanced over the stylette, and the entire needle withdrawn. The specimen is fixed and sent to the laboratory. In a series of more than 2000 needle biopsies, I have seen only one complication: a symptomless ecchymosis that began at the level of the sternum and spread down over the breasts.

The pathologist classifies about 85 per cent of the adequate biopsies obtained from the thyroid nodules as benign, about 5 per cent as malignant, and about 10 per cent as questionable. Papillary carcinomas and the more malignant and undifferentiated types of cancer are easily recognized. It is the low-grade angioinvasive follicular carcinomas that are indistinguishable from cellular adenomas unless capsular specimens with blood vessels are available for study. For this reason, the pathologist tends to consider many cellular adenomas as potentially malignant. For this group of patients, we advise operation. There have been no mistakes made in the patients whose tumors were diagnosed as cancer.

In several hundred patients who were diagnosed as having benign disease, one mistake was made. Clinically, this tumor was malignant, and on this basis a thyroidectomy was later performed. However, the biopsy showed nothing but a benign nodule, totally different from the anaplastic carcinoma of which no vestige was present in the sections. The biopsy had obtained material from a benign nodule instead of from the malignant one.

## Discussion

The value of needle biopsy in determining whether or not a thyroid nodule is malignant is based on the competence of the pathologist in histocytology. In the days when pathologists depended on the architecture of a tissue to determine its malignant potential, needle biopsy of the thyroid was of limited value, confined chiefly to confirming the diagnosis of thyroiditis. But with increasing experience with the Papanicolaou smear and with aspiration biopsy of tumors, more and more pathologists are able to establish the diagnosis of malignancy by the appearance of individual cells or clusters of them. Fortunately, it is easy to aspirate a large amount of material from a thyroid nodule.

One advantage of needle biopsy of thyroid nodules is that the material aspirated from a nodule is representative of the entire nodule. In the breast, for example, a negative cytologic diagnosis does not mean that no cancer is present; it means that no cancer cells were obtained. However, if benign clusters of cells are obtained from a thyroid nodule, it means that that nodule is benign. Each nodule is either benign or malignant, and there is no mixture of the two within any single nodule.

One of the chief objections to needle biopsy of the thyroid has been the possibility that cancer cells could be implanted in the needle track. Such an occurrence is exceedingly rare, and probably if it did take place could be dealt with easily by excision. In reporting on the results of 900 aspiration biopsies of cold nodules, 5 per cent of which were malignant, Kirstaedter[2] observed no implants. In more than 2000 needle biopsies of the thyroid, I have seen only one implant: a tiny nodule in the skin that was easily excised. At the time of the biopsy the patient had distant metastasis, and no doubt there was little or no concomitant immunity. This experience supports Southam and Brunschwig's study[3] in which they found that the concomitant immunity of patients with cancer caused rejection of implants of cancer in all but 30 per cent of the patients tested. Those who did not reject the implant were in terminal stages or were receiving immunosuppressive drugs.

As clinical experience with needle biopsy in all areas of the body increases, there is mounting evidence that the danger of implantation has been greatly exaggerated. Since 1919, when Wood[4] originally published his work on diagnostic incision of tumors, many laboratory experiments have confirmed this observation. Clinical evidence to the contrary has not been reported.

Since practically all adults have microscopic nodules of the thyroid and nearly 10 per cent of older people have some palpable nodularity of the gland, it is impossible to consider removing all thyroid nodules. Even if the mortality rate of operation were only 1 in 1000, the death rate in a population group would be far higher than that of thyroid cancer, which kills only 1 per 100,000 people.

Scans are of little or no value in diagnosing thyroid cancer, because at least 90 per cent of all thyroid nodules are cold or cool. Only in the rare instance of a hot nodule is the scan worthwhile.

Ultrasonography may be useful in diagnosing a cyst, but aspiration by a fine needle both diagnoses and cures.

Short of biopsy, there are no effective tests for diagnosing cancer of the thyroid. Since needle biopsy is both safe and effective, it should be used more often. When it is used routinely in the diagnosis of disease of the thyroid, thyroidectomy will become exceedingly rare.

## Summary

Needle biopsy of the thyroid, either by aspiration or with the Tru-cut needle, is a safe and effective way of distinguishing between benign and malignant nodules.

When needle biopsy is used there are very few indications for thyroidectomy.

## References

1. Crile, G., Jr.: Treatment of thyroid cysts by aspiration. Surgery 69:200–210, 1966.
2. Kirstaedter, H. J.: Personal communication, 1971.
3. Southam, C. M., and Brunschwig, A.: Quantitative studies of autotransplantation of human cancer. Cancer 14:971–978, 1961.
4. Wood, F. C.: Diagnostic excision of tumors. J.A.M.A. 73:764–766, 1919.

# 8

# Operation for Papillary Carcinoma of the Thyroid

TOTAL THYROIDECTOMY
AND NECK DISSECTION
SHOULD NOT BE DONE
ROUTINELY
   *by George Crile, Jr.*

THE NEED FOR
INDIVIDUALIZED TREATMENT
   *by Edgar L. Frazell*

## Statement of the Problem

*This controversy focuses on how much of the thyroid gland should be removed and the extent of the lymph node dissection in a patient with biopsy-proved papillary carcinoma of the thyroid.*

*With gross papillary carcinoma in one lobe, what is the frequency of occult microscopic foci of tumor in the opposite lobe? What is the clinical significance of the histologic identification of a focus of papillary carcinoma in the opposite lobe? What is the frequency of clinical "recurrence" in the residual, grossly involved gland?*

*Discuss the distribution of spread within the gland when the main lesion arises in the isthmus.*

*Is it routinely possible to preserve adequate parathyroid function and still do an adequate total thyroidectomy and node dissection for cancer? Comment on the value of preserving the posterior aspect of the grossly free lobe to avoid parathyroid excision.*

*When should node dissection be done? If carried out, what nodal chains should be removed? Should the thymus gland or a portion of it be removed during thyroidectomy for papillary cancer?*

*Is it feasible to preserve the jugular vein, sternocleidomastoid muscle, and/or spinal accessory nerve and yet carry out a thorough neck dissection?*

*With what frequency does papillary carcinoma metastasize to nodes lateral to the carotid, to the submandibular area, and to the submental space?*

*What is the clinical behavior of a thyroid malignancy which is mixed papillary and follicular in histology or partially undifferentiated?*

*After total thyroidectomy what is the frequency of these complications: recurrent nerve palsy; permanent hypoparathyroidism?*

*Discuss the magnitude of the clinical problem of permanent hypoparathyroidism. Are there individual patients whose serum calcium cannot be controlled with oral vitamin D and calcium?*

# Total Thyroidectomy and Neck Dissection Should Not Be Done Routinely

GEORGE CRILE, JR.

*Cleveland Clinic Foundatiin*

Five years ago, the treatment of papillary carcinoma of the thyroid was highly controversial. A large number of surgeons, many of whom trained in cancer centers, were convinced that patients with papillary carcinoma should be treated by the same type of radical neck dissection that surgeons specializing in surgery of the head and neck employ routinely in the treatment of squamous cell cancers. They advocated removal of the sternocleidomastoid muscle and jugular vein on the affected side and sacrifice of the eleventh nerve, even if there was no apparent involvement of nodes. Many of these surgeons also advocated total thyroidectomy. Papillary carcinoma commonly affects young women, and the operation produced considerable deformity and even disability. There was also a significant incidence of permanent tetany, with its long-range complications.

An equally large number of surgeons, most of whom had been trained on general surgical services or on services specializing in surgery of the thyroid rather than in cancer hospitals, believed that radical neck dissection and total thyroidectomy were seldom, if ever, indicated in the treatment of papillary carcinoma. They recognized that papillary carcinoma rarely kills as a direct result of its cervical metastases, that there is little if any correlation between the patient's survival and the extent of nodal involvement, and that distant metastasis is not only rare but also does not appear to be related to reappearance of the cancer in nodes. They noted that the conventional radical operation disregarded some of the most common sites of nodal involvement—the paratracheal nodes, the mediastinal nodes, and the midline "Delphian" node. They also realized that in patients under 50 years of age, the tumor is usually endocrine-dependent and can be controlled by feeding

165

suppressive doses of thyroid.[1] They recognized the multicentricity of micro-foci of papillary carcinoma but also realized that when suppressive doses of thyroid are given, it is rare for clinical cancers to appear in the contralateral lobe, and that even without suppression, contralateral recurrence is rare.[2] For these reasons, most surgeons were content to remove all the thyroid on the affected side, the isthmus, and most of the other lobe. Unless there was clinical evidence of contralateral disease, the contralateral posterior capsule was left to protect the parathyroids.

The surgeons who advocated the conservative approach did not remove the sternocleidomastoid muscle or the eleventh nerve but dissected around them, removing the fat and the node-bearing tissue, and they did not routinely remove the jugular vein. The recurrent nerve was not sacrificed unless it was already paralyzed or inseparable from the tumor. Sometimes, especially in men, the operation was done through a hockey-stick type of anterior sternomastoid incision, but more often, and notably in young women, it was done through a high wide thyroidectomy incision, and if the nodes were extensively involved, with a secondary smaller transverse incision high in the neck. Following these operations, the scarring and deformity were minimal, the incidence of tetany was practically nil, and there was no discomfort in the neck or shoulder.

The controversy that raged between these two schools of treatment was both heated and futile. The exponents of the radical operation pointed out that their opponents were violating all the basic principles of cancer surgery. The proponents of the conservative operation responded that their cure rates, at from 5 to 25 years, were just as high as those of the surgeons who performed radical operations and that their operative mortality and morbidity were much lower.[2] However, the surgeons favoring radical operation simply did not accept these results.

Finally, as the basic biology of cancer became better understood, surgeons began to realize that papillary carcinoma of the thyroid is not like other cancers. In most cancers, the more nodes that are involved, the worse the prognosis. In papillary cancer of the thyroid, however, there is no correlation between the extent of nodal involvement and the incidence of cure. Patients with as many as 40 involved nodes often are permanently cured by relatively conservative operations, whereas in no other type of cancer is this the case. In fact, the prognosis in children and young adults, who tend to have small primary tumors and extensive nodal metastasis, is very much better than that of patients over the age of 40, who tend to have bulky tumors and few nodes involved.[3]

In addition, the endocrine-dependence of papillary carcinoma differs from that of such cancers as those of the breast and prostate in that once there had been a regression of distant metastases, the tumor never loses its dependence.[1] It remains controlled indefinitely as long as suppressive doses of thyroid are given.

Until recently, there was little change in the opinions of the two groups. However in 1970 and 1972, two key articles were published in which noted authorities in the field of papillary carcinoma took a position of compromise.[4, 5] They denied the necessity for neck dissection when there was no apparent involvement of nodes and advised total thyroidectomy only in patients with clinical evidence of bilateral involvement.

The data on which these articles were based were so extensive and well-studied that it was nearly impossible to refute the author's conclusions. It seems therefore that the controversy is really over. Even those who routinely performed the conventional radical operation have begun to modify it to save the eleventh nerve and often the sternocleiodmastoid muscle. Surgeons who are still holding out for the routine use of radical operations will almost certainly be forced to modify their positions. I am certain that if they do so, it will not be at the expense of the survival of their patients.

The following list of questions and answers is offered to help to clarify some of the issues in this controversy:

*With gross papillary carcinoma in one lobe, what is the frequency of occult microscopic foci of tumor in the opposite lobe?*
The incidence of microfoci of cancer in the contralateral lobe depends on how many sections of the lobe are made. If many sections are examined, the incidence of microfoci of cancer is as high as 61.7 per cent.[6, 7]

*What is the clinical significance of the histologic identification of a focus of papillary carcinoma in the opposite lobe?*
Usually none. In the Cleveland Clinic series of 307 patients, there were 273 with papillary carcinoma who were treated by lobectomy or subtotal thyroidectomy and followed for from 5 to 33 years. There was only one patient who had clinical evidence of recurrence in the remaining thyroid. Most of these patients were treated by full suppressive doses of desiccated thyroid, which may have played a major role in suppressing the growth of microfoci of cancer.[2]

*Is it possible to perform a total thyroidectomy and still preserve adequate parathyroid function?*
The reported incidence of tetany after total thyroidectomy varies from 3.5 per cent in the series reported by Attie and his associates to 21 per cent in the Cleveland Clinic series (6 of 27 patients).

Note, however, that in Attie's series more than half the patients were treated by total thyroidectomy, whereas in the Cleveland Clinic series only 9 per cent were so treated, these being the patients with clinical evidence of bilateral disease. In such patients, the incidence of tetany is high because it is difficult to differentiate between parathyroids and small capsular nodes involved by tumor. Also, although many surgeons report that they have performed total thyroidectomies, a postoperative scan usually shows that some thyroid was left.[2, 8]

Most surgeons agree that total thyroidectomy performed on patients with obvious bilateral disease is attended by a high incidence of tetany, but I do not doubt that there are some surgeons who have perfected their technique to such an extent that the incidence is as low as that in Attie's series. Since the reported incidence of both tetany and recurrence of cancer in the contralateral lobe is practically nil when a total lobectomy is performed on one side and all but a little of the posterior capsule is removed from the other, it seems that in cases in which there is no clinical evidence of contralateral involvement this is the safest technique.

*When should node dissection be done?*
Node dissection should be done when, at the time of operation, there are nodes that are grossly involved or when frozen section shows cancer in one or more representative nodes.

*What groups of nodes should be removed?*
The most commonly involved are the paratracheal nodes that lie behind the thyroid, along the recurrent nerve, and down into the superior mediastinum. The jug-

ular chain is commonly involved in patients who have tumors of the superior pole. Tumors involving the isthmus tend to metastasize to the midline "Delphian" node above the isthmus and to the superior mediastinal nodes. In advanced disease, the supraclavicular nodes and those of the posterior triangle may be involved. Metastasis is rare in the submaxillary or submental nodes. I have not seen metastasis to the thymus gland.

*Is it possible to perform a thorough neck dissection and still preserve the spinal accessory nerve, the sternocleidomastoid muscle, and the jugular vein?*

Most surgeons have modified the standard radical neck dissection to preserve the spinal accessory nerve and the sternocleiodmastoid muscle. These structures are dissected out and preserved while the node-bearing fat and areolar tissue are removed as in the standard dissection. When there is extensive metastasis, it may be convenient to remove the jugular vein on the affected side, but both veins should not be removed. A much better cosmetic result is obtained if the neck dissection is done through a high wide thyroidectomy incision and, if necessary, a secondary transverse incision high in the neck.

*What is the clinical behavior of a thyroid malignancy which is mixed papillary and follicular in histology, and what if the tumor is partially undifferentiated?*

Mixed papillary and follicular tumors and those that are predominantly follicular with only a few papillary areas behave just like all other papillary carcinomas. The only type that is different, from the standpoint of prognosis, is the tall cell variant of the papillary carcinoma that occurs in people over the age of 50. It is not endocrine-dependent and tends to metastasize to lung and bone.

If there are elements of anaplastic carcinoma in a papillary carcinoma, the prognosis is poor.

*After total thyroidectomy, what is the incidence of recurrent nerve palsy and of permanent hypoparathyroidism?*

In the hands of experienced surgeons, recurrent laryngeal nerve palsy is no more common after total than after subtotal thyroidectomy. Unilateral paralysis occurred 32 times in the Cleveland Clinic series of 307 cases (10.6 per cent), but in almost all these the nerve was sacrificed purposely because of preoperative paralysis or inseparability from the tumor.

In the Cleveland Clinic series, the incidence of hypoparathyroidism was 21 per cent in 27 patients subjected to total thyroidectomy for extensive bilateral disease. It was only 2 per cent in the entire group operated on for papillary carcinoma.

*Is permanent hypoparathyroidism a major problem?*

Usually it is not, but if good control is not maintained complications such as cataracts may occur. There is an occasional patient whose hypocalcemia cannot be controlled by vitamin D and calcium, but usually such patients will respond to treatment with synthesized dihydrotachysterol.

*Which patients respond best to suppression by feeding thyroid?*

The younger the patient, the more apt the cancer is to be endocrine-dependent. It makes no difference whether it is predominantly follicular or mainly papillary. Those patients whose cancers developed after radiation therapy in infancy and childhood almost always have endocrine-dependent tumors. For this reason, major surgical morbidity should not be inflicted on young people until a trial on suppression has been given.

## References

1. Crile, G., Jr.: The endocrine dependency of certain thyroid cancers and the danger that hypothyroidism may stimulate their growth. Cancer 10:119–137, 1957.
2. Crile, G., Jr.: Changing end results in patients with papillary carcinoma of the thyroid. Surg. Gynecol. Obstet. 132:460–468, 1971.

3. Crile, G., Jr., and Hazard, J. B.: Relationship of the age of the patient to the natural history and prognosis of carcinoma of the thyroid. Ann. Surg. 138:33–38, 1953.
4. Hutter, R. V. P., Frazell, E. L., and Foote, F. W., Jr.: Elective radical neck dissection. Cancer 20:87–93, 1970.
5. Tollefsen, H. R., Shah, J. P., and Huvos, A. G.: Papillary carcinoma of the thyroid. Am. J. Surg. 124:468–472, 1972.
6. Clark, R. L., Ibanez, M. L., and White, E. C.: What constitutes an adequate operation for carcinoma of the thyroid? Arch. Surg. 92:23–26, 1966.
7. Clark, R. L., Jr., White, E. C., and Russell, W. O.: Total thyroidectomy for cancer of the thyroid: significance of intraglandular dissemination. Ann. Surg. 149:858–866, 1959.
8. Attie, J. N., Khafif, R. A., and Steckler, R. M.: Elective neck dissection in papillary carcinoma of the thyroid. Am. J. Surg. 122:464–470, 1971.

# The Need for Individualized Treatment

EDGAR L. FRAZELL

*The University of Texas Health Science Center at San Antonio*

## General Considerations

Basically, controversies in the surgical management of papillary thyroid cancer are concerned with the questions of: (1) how much of the thyroid gland should be excised; and (2) whether there is a role for the extended operation in the management of cervical lymph node metastasis. A satisfactory clinicopathologic classification of thyroid neoplasms is now widely accepted,[27] and relatively large numbers of treated patients are now available for extended follow-up studies. Such data plus a recognition of the oddities of clinical behavior inherent in the natural history of these tumors hopefully will provide an answer to the question, "What constitutes an adequate operation for papillary thyroid cancer?"

Formerly, there was some confusion due to the fact that the morphologic pattern in both the primary lesion and in metastatic foci from these well-differentiated tumors often show wide differences in the relative proportion of the papillary component. Although a few tumors exhibit an almost "pure" papillary structure, the more common picture is that of a mixture of papillary and follicular features; at times other histologic traits may be identified. These morphologic variations need not cause confusion in treatment recommendations, however, since there is no well-documented evidence that clinical behavior and treatment response will differ, with the exception of anaplastic foci.[8, 12, 27, 28] It should be noted, however, that papillary cancers of similar or identical morphologic appearance commonly exhibit wide differences in their clinical presentation.[11] For example, the primary lesion may vary in size from occult (the so-called laboratory cancer) to large, and it may be solitary or grossly multinodular. It may mimic a benign lesion, or it may be obviously infiltrative. Regional lymph node metastases may be clinically absent or may be extensive. They may be ipsilateral, contralateral, or bilateral. Pulmonary metastasis is not an uncommon initial finding, and on rare oc-

171

casions a distant focus may be present. Such diverse findings are of paramount importance, since they have a fundamental bearing on what treatment is to be advised.

Although papillary cancer may in a few cases pursue an aggressive course and cause death of the patient within a year or so after diagnosis, this is unusual. Large primary lesions, those in elderly patients, and those in males may be associated with a relatively unfavorable prognosis.[13] Patients with infiltrative growths that involve midline structures (e.g., the larynx, trachea, esophagus, or mediastinum) do poorly. Late involvement at these sites, often after decades of relative quiescence, is the most common cause of death.[11, 16, 23, 25] It is important that these behavior patterns be recognized, since it is questionable whether the ultimate prognosis in such cases would be altered by choosing one or another of the commonly recommended operations. Nothing short of initial massive resection would be effective under these circumstances. Finally, a few patients succumb to the little understood but well-documented phenomenon of transformation of a long-standing well-differentiated papillary tumor into one that is highly anaplastic in nature.[4, 15, 23]

Despite the variation in morphological and clinical manifestations, accumulated data now confirms that, in the majority of patients, papillary cancer runs a slow and protracted course and kills few of its victims.[18] Most patients are clinically "cured" for years or even decades after any and all forms of operative treatment. In others, persistent disease may be present for long periods of time following standard operative measures without causing discomfort or killing the patient. Such oddities pose considerable difficulty for the clinicians who claim the superiority of one treatment method over another. Thus, dogmatic statements about therapy and prognosis in a given patient are risky and must be examined in the light of the natural history of the disease.[5]

## Treatment

The primary treatment for papillary thyroid cancer is operative.[26] As with cancer arising elsewhere in the body, it should be the objective of the surgeon to excise all resectable foci of tumor at the initial operation. Unfortunately, due to the variations in clinical presentation mentioned previously, this sound surgical principle cannot be applied in a routine manner, nor should it be, since survival figures from many sources clearly indicate that considerable lattitude in treatment is permissible without compromising the patient's chance of survival.[5, 8, 17] Thus, depending on the clinical setting, surgeons often employ: (1) wide local excision of the primary tumor; (2) unilateral lobectomy (with or without isthmus excision plus partial removal of the other lobe); or (3) total removal of the gland. Local excision of suspected metastatic lymph nodes is employed by some surgeons, while others advocate neck dissection which may be unilateral, bilateral, classical, or modified in type. There are ample arguments for and against these alternatives.

### Partial Lobectomy

Incomplete excision of a thyroid lobe containing a clinically solitary mass of unknown nature is not advisable. This is particularly true if the mass is "cold" on scan, has increased in size during administration of thyroid medication, or is in a male patient under 40 years of age. Under such conditions and with proper selection of patients, the likelihood that the mass is a cancer is significant.[4] That many thyroid cancers are clinically indistinguishable from benign lesions is common knowledge, but that at least 50 per cent of them are undiagnosed prior to laboratory examination is surprising.[11] Since papillary cancers are unencapsulated and often multinodular, the hazards of incomplete tumor excision or "wound seeding" by tumor cells is diminished by employing complete rather than partial lobectomy as an initial procedure. This operation also provides a dry surgical field, which facilitates isolation and preservation of the recurrent nerve and parathyroid glands. Should the mass prove to be a cancer, either on immediate frozen-section examination or at a later date (as is often the case), the decision as to the need for further operation can then be made in an orderly manner. In view of the high incidence of "stump recurrence,"[2, 20, 21] one must conclude that total extracapsular thyroid lobectomy is the minimal operation for papillary cancer. It is also often curative.[11]

### Extended Thyroidectomy

When the primary lesion is bulky or when there is gross involvement of both lobes, total thyroidectomy is clearly indicated. The risk that the complications often associated with this procedure will develop is then justified in the interest of complete tumor removal. The indications are less clear-cut in the case of lesions arising in the isthmus or when bilateral cervical lymph node metastases are diagnosed.

Once the diagnosis of papillary thyroid cancer has been established by either lymph node biopsy or thyroid lobectomy, some surgeons recommend total thyroidectomy as routine treatment.[3, 6, 24] They cite the high incidence (87 per cent) of multiple microscopic foci of tumor involvement throughout the gland as an indication for such treatment. The argument is persuasive and would be acceptable were it not for the frequency with which the serious complication of permanent parathyroid deficiency is observed. The reported incidence of permanent tetany varies from 0 to 50 per cent following total thyroidectomy for cancer,[1, 3, 19, 22] but even a minimal incidence of this complication is not justified in the absence of gross involvement of both thyroid lobes. There is little doubt that many surgeons are technically able to do total thyroidectomy without the complication of permanent hypoparathyroidism. But is it a good cancer operation to save parathyroids on the side of major involvement, and is it justifiable to remove the remaining few grams of gland parenchyma on the grossly normal side because of the possibility of recurrence at that site? Furthermore, an improved survival rate after total thyroidectomy has not been demonstrated,[5, 8] and the clinical significance of the microscopic foci remains in doubt.[7, 22]

At the present state of our knowledge and depending upon the clinical setting, thyroid lobectomy alone or combined with subtotal removal of the second lobe offers an equal chance of control of disease at the primary site. Ablation of the residue of gland, should it be indicated or desired to facilitate future isotope therapy, may then be accomplished with radioactive iodine without additional risk to the patient.

### Neck Dissection

Metastasis to cervical lymph nodes is one of the most characteristic features of papillary thyroid cancer. Surgical removal of such foci of disease is an integral part of primary treatment, *provided* that the primary lesion can be removed in its entirety. Extended follow-up studies of treated patients now confirm, however, that the finding of cervical metastases, particularly in youthful patients, has limited bearing on the prognosis for long-term survival, provided that the nodes are eventually excised.[8, 14, 26] Furthermore, the degree of involvement is not critical, since surgical excision of either single or multiple nodes is regularly followed by long disease-free intervals. Finally, 20- to 30-year follow-ups in a few untreated patients[10] have raised serious doubts about the role of cervical metastasis in the dissemination of this form of cancer.

In view of these considerations, it would appear that, despite the high incidence of occult metastasis in neck nodes, the routine so-called "prophylactic" neck dissection in the presence of clinically negative findings is not indicated, and neck dissection should be reserved for patients with clinically palpable nodes. Would routine removal of mediastinal nodes yield the same degree of involvement? Although the radical operation is the most efficient method for removal of neck node metastases, more conservative procedures are often advised.[9] These include local excision of nodes and various modifications of the radical operation aimed at minimizing the cosmetic and functional deformities that result from the extended operation. A reasonable solution to this controversy would seem to be that the extent of operation be decided on the basis of the clinical findings at time of operation.[17]

## Conclusions

The term "cure" for papillary thyroid cancer should be used advisedly in view of the demonstrated frequency of occult foci of tumor throughout the thyroid and cervical lymph nodes and the fact that similar involvement of mediastinal nodes seems likely. Despite this pessimistic appraisal, long-term clinical control of disease is achieved in most patients after all types of operations. Contrary to opinions previously held, a high degree of individualization in treatment is permissible, depending upon the clinical findings. In terms of survival, the superiority of an extended operation for eradication of the primary or regional lymph node metastases has not been conclusively demonstrated. It is questionable whether the few patients who die of this disease die because of failure to employ extended operation. Permanent hypoparathyroidism is a serious complication, and its incidence following total thyroidectomy for cancer is significant. The risk of this complication makes total thyroidectomy unacceptable as a *routine* measure in the treatment of papillary cancer.

## References

1. Beahrs, O. H., Ryan, R. F., and White, R. A.: Complications of thyroid surgery. J. Clin. Endocrinol. Metab. *16*:1456, 1956.
2. Black, B. M., Kirk, T. A. Jr., and Woolner, L. B.: Multicentricity of papillary adenocarcinoma of the thyroid: influence on treatment. J. Clin. Endocrinol. *20*:130, 1960.
3. Block, M. A., Horn, R. C., and Brush, B. E.: The place of total thyroidectomy in surgery for thyroid carcinoma. Arch. Surg. *81*:236, 1960.
4. Brooks, J. R.: The solitary thyroid nodule. Am. J. Surg. *125*:477, 1973.
5. Buckwalter, J. A., Soper, R. T., Madaras, J. S. Jr., et al.: The effectiveness of treatment of well differentiated thyroid carcinoma. Surg. Gynecol. Obstet. *113*:427, 1961.
6. Clark, R. L., Ibanez, M. L., and White, E. C.: What constitutes an adequate operation for carcinoma of the thyroid? Arch. Surg. *92*:23, 1966.
7. Crile, G., Jr.: Carcinoma of the thyroid in children. Ann. Surg. *150*:959, 1959.
8. Crile, G., Jr.: Survival of patients with papillary carcinoma of the thyroid after conservative operations. Am. J. Surg. *108*:862, 1964.
9. Crile, G., Jr., Suhrer, J. G., Jr., and Hazard, J. B.: Results of conservative operations for malignant tumors of thyroid. J. Clin. Endocrinol. *15*:1422, 1955.
10. Frazell, E. L.: Personal observations.
11. Frazell, E. L., and Foote, F. W., Jr.: Papillary cancer of the thyroid. A review of 25 years of experience. Cancer *11*:895, 1958.
12. Frazell, E. L., and Foote, F. W., Jr.: Papillary thyroid carcinoma: pathological findings in cases with and without clinical evidence of cervical node involvement. Cancer *8*:1164, 1955.
13. Frazell, E. L., Schottenfeld, D., and Hutter, R. V. P.: The prognosis and insurability of thyroid cancer patients. C.A. *20*:270, 1970; Trans. Assoc. Life Ins. Med. Directors Am. *53*:290, 1969.
14. Hutter, R. V. P., Frazell, E. L., and Foote, F. W., Jr.: Elective radical neck dissection: an assessment of its use in the management of papillary thyroid cancer. C.A. *20*:87, 1970.
15. Hutter, R. V. P., Tollefsen, H. R., DeCosse, J. J., et al.: Spindle and giant cell metaplasia in papillary carcinoma of the thyroid. Am. J. Surg. *110*:660, 1965.
16. Ibanez, M. L., Russell, W. O., Albores-Saavedra, J., et al.: Thyroid carcinoma—biologic behavior and mortality. Postmortem findings in 42 cases, including 27 in which the disease was fatal. Cancer *19*:1039, 1966.
17. Klopp, C. T., Rosvoll, R. V., and Winship, T.: Is destructive surgery ever necessary for treatment of thyroid cancer in children. Ann. Surg. *165*:745, 1967.
18. McKenzie, A. D.: The natural history of thyroid cancer. A report of 102 cases analyzed 10 to 15 years after diagnosis. Arch. Surg. *102*:274, 1971.
19. McKenzie, J. M., and Murphy, S. S.: Treatment of the thyroid nodule. Adv. Intern. Med. *17*:215, 1971.
20. Rose, R. G., Kelsey, M. P., Russell, W. O., et al.: Follow-up study of thyroid cancer treated by unilateral lobectomy. Am. J. Surg. *106*:494, 1963.
21. Rundle, F. F., and Basser, A. G.: Stump recurrence and total thyroidectomy in papillary thyroid cancer. Cancer *9*:692, 1956.
22. Tollefsen, H. R., and DeCosse, J. J.: Papillary carcinoma of the thyroid. Recurrence in the thyroid gland after initial surgical treatment. Am. J. Surg. *106*:728, 1963.
23. Tollefsen, H. R., DeCosse, J. J., and Hutter, R. V. P.: Papillary carcinoma of the thyroid. A clinical and pathological study of 70 fatal cases. Cancer *17*:1035, 1964.
24. Wade, J. S.: Review of thyroid carcinomas in the United Cardiff Hospitals. Proc. Roy. Soc. Med. *62*:812, 1969.
25. Walt, A. J.: Carcinoma of the thyroid. The Cancer Bulletin *19*:102, 1967.
26. Winship, T., and Rosvoll, R. V.: Thyroid carcinoma in childhood: final report on a 20 year study. Clin. Proc. Child. Hosp. D.C. *26*:327, 1970.
27. Woolner, L. B., Beahrs, O. H., Black, B. M., et al.: Classification and prognosis of thyroid carcinoma. A study of 885 cases observed in a thirty year period. Am. J. Surg. *102*:354, 1961.
28. Wychulis, A. R., Beahrs, O. H., and Woolner, L. B.: Papillary carcinoma with associated anaplastic carcinoma in the thyroid gland. Surg. Gynecol. Obstet. *120*:28, 1965.

# 9

# *Aorto-Coronary Bypass in Ischemic Heart Disease*

THE CORONARY ARTERY BYPASS
OPERATION IN THE TREATMENT
OF ANGINA PECTORIS

*by M. Terry McEnany,
Eldred D. Mundth,
and W. Gerald Austen*

CORONARY ARTERY BYPASS
OPERATION REQUIRES FURTHER
THERAPEUTIC EVALUATION

*by G. E. Burch
and T. D. Giles*

## Statement of the Problem

*The controversy is whether this operation improves cardiac function, alleviates angina or heart failure, and prolongs life.*

*Discuss data dealing with prolongation of life by coronary bypass operations, indicating techniques used—vein graft, arterial graft, direct arterial anastomoses.*

*Summarize pertinent published facts on operative mortality, graft patency rates, and relief of symptoms. Where wide variability exists, analyze these differences. Discuss patient selection as a determinant of success or failure rates.*

*Discuss coronary arteriographic findings as a predictor of success or failure. Evaluate other methods as determinants of success in myocardial revascularization.*

*Analyze objective data which demonstrate improved cardiac function following bypass grafts. This could include coronary sinus lactate values, end diastolic ventricular pressures, ejection fractions, cardiac output, and myocardial oxygen consumption.*

# The Coronary Artery Bypass Operation in the Treatment of Angina Pectoris

M. TERRY McENANY,
ELDRED D. MUNDTH,
and W. GERALD AUSTEN

*The Massachusetts General Hospital*

Pain as a manifestation of cellular ischemia is well recognized in obstructive disease of the mesenteric, axillobrachial, and iliofemoral arterial system.[1] Operative procedures utilized to increase blood flow to ischemic limbs and intestine have resulted in excellent physiologic and symptomatic improvement.[2,3] Angina pectoris, long thought to be a concomitant of coronary atherosclerosis,[4] has become a public health problem of major proportion, disabling tens of thousands of persons yearly. Its status as a clinical precursor of myocardial infarction and death has been lucidly delineated in recent years in large-scale clinical and angiographic studies.[5-9] Angina pectoris, without any angiographic corroboration, is associated with a mortality rate of about 4 per cent per year. Angiographic examination of patients with angina has clearly demonstrated that mortality increases with the degree of coronary atherosclerosis to a yearly mortality rate of 10 to 11 per cent for patients with either three-vessel narrowing or major stenosis of the main left coronary artery. A repeatedly high percentage (10 to 33 per cent) of patients with typical or atypical angina pectoris have no coronary arterial disease on coronary arteriographic examination. This fact, together with the good prognosis for these patients in terms of nonprogression of symptoms and near absence of myocardial infarction, makes comparison of surgical and medical therapy difficult, except in those series with total angiographic substantiation of the extent of coronary arterial disease.[10-12]

Selective coronary arteriography, introduced by Sones and Shirey[13] and

179

expanded by Judkins,[14] has allowed specific anatomic correlation between coronary atherosclerosis and symptoms of myocardial ischemia. The first direct operative procedure performed to treat localized atherosclerosis was coronary endarterectomy.[15] Endarterectomy or endarterotomy and patch angioplasty were performed extensively during the mid-1960's,[16] but the high mortality rates in series of patients with left coronary arterial lesions and the frequent absence of relief from symptoms in right coronary arterial disease,[17] in many instances associated with occlusion of the endarterectomized artery, stimulated a search for more effective and safer techniques of direct myocardial revascularization. Sabiston performed a saphenous vein-aortocoronary artery interposition in 1962,[18] and in 1968, Favaloro reported on venous interposition in 55 patients, with only two deaths.[19] However, of these cases, 52 involved only the right coronary artery; direct intervention on the left coronary arterial system was still considered too hazardous. Favaloro extended the early experimental work of Sauvage et al.[20] and utilized autologous venous bypass grafts to treat lesions of the left coronary arterial system and, ultimately, all stenotic lesions.[21]

## Risk of Operation

Since 1970, aortocoronary arterial bypass grafting has become the most prevalent cardiac surgical procedure in the United States. The operation has been of considerable benefit in alleviating disabling angina pectoris[22] and in treating the complications of myocardial infarction.[23] Coronary arterial bypass grafts have been utilized in more than 100,000 patients with low mortality and morbidity rates, excellent palliation of debilitating symptoms, measured improvement in cardiac function, and, probably, increased life expectancy.[24, 25]

Many investigators have demonstrated a drastically increased mortality risk associated with left ventricular dysfunction. Cohn et al.[26] reported an operative mortality rate of 80 per cent in patients with ejection fractions less than 0.30, 28 per cent in patients with ejection fractions from 0.30 to 0.50, and only 3 per cent in patients with both coronary and valvular heart disease and ejection fractions greater than 0.50. Oldham et al.[27] experienced a mortality rate of 55 per cent in coronary artery bypass patients with ejection fractions less than 0.25 and only 4 per cent in patients with ejection fractions greater than 0.25. They also demonstrated significant increase in risk with a left ventricular end-diastolic pressure greater than 18 mm. Hg or an arteriovenous oxygen difference greater than 6 vol. per cent. Kouchoukos et al.[28] pointed out the great discrepancy between mortality risk in those patients with angina only (1.9 per cent) and those with congestive heart failure (29 per cent). Hammermeister and Kennedy[29] confirmed the importance of the ejection fraction (0.33 or less) and left ventricular end-diastolic pressure (18 mm. Hg or more) and also pointed out the predictive value of an end-diastolic volume greater than 103 ml. per meter$^2$ (mortality rate of 19 per cent vs. 2.6 per cent). The differences in results related to ventricular function can be appreciated from an examination of the data in Table 1.[26-31] Long-term results in survivors with preoperative left ventricular dysfunction are few; the experience reported by Spencer et al.,[32] in which a good clinical result was obtained in only 20 per cent of patients, has been reproduced by many groups, but *careful* selection of patients, which includes only those with coexistent severe angina pectoris, can contribute to much more acceptable results, as reported from the Massachusetts General Hospital by Mundth et al.[33] ·The association of angina with ventricular failure implies that a significant amount of ischemic (angina-producing) myocardium, amenable to reversal by revascularization, is contributing to the ventricular dysfunction, rather than fibrotic, scarred muscle being the sole factor. Most surgical groups are circumspect regarding coronary arterial bypass graft procedures in patients whose only symptom is congestive heart failure without an attendant left ventricular aneurysm, mitral regurgitation, or ventricular septal defect.[34]

In early experiences with coronary artery bypass grafting, a marked difference was noted between survival rates in patients with single and multiple vessel involvement.[35, 36] As experience has accumulated, the mortality rate for coronary artery bypass graft procedures has equilibrated, and at present no consistent difference in risks exists between single and multiple grafts[25, 27, 28, 37-41] (Table 2). The reasons for this are several: (1) technical facility increases with experience, and multiple grafts now require shorter periods of cardiopulmonary bypass; (2) greater realization that *all* significant stenotic lesions should be bypassed has led to an increasing number and percentage of multiple grafts, providing more complete revascularization for patients with multiple vessel involvement; and (3) better selection of patients tends to exclude those with multiple vessel disease *and* severe left ventricular dysfunction, thereby reducing the mortality rate in patients with

**TABLE 1.  Determinants of Operative Risk in Coronary Artery Bypass Operation**

| Authors | Determinant of Left Ventricular Function | Mortality Rate "Good Risk" (Per Cent) | "Poor Risk" (Per Cent) |
|---|---|---|---|
| Cohn et al.[26] | Ejection fraction >0.50 | 3.0 | 35 |
| Hammermeister and Kennedy[29] | End-diastolic volume <103 ml./m.² | 2.6 | 19 |
| | Ejection fraction >0.33 | 3.1 | 33 |
| | LVEDP° <18 mm. Hg | 3.3 | 19 |
| Kouchoukos et al.[28] | Clinical failure | 1.9 | 29 |
| McRaven et al.[31] | Angiographic assessment of ventricular contractility | Normal 5.0 | Localized double wall impairment 30 |
| Oldham et al.[27] | Ejection fraction >0.25 | 4.0 | 55 |
| | A-VO₂† <6 ml./100 ml. | 8.0 | 26 |
| | LVEDP <18 mm. Hg | 9.0 | 30 |
| Siderys et al.[30] | LVEDP <25 mm. Hg | 4.0 | 31 |

°LVEDP = left ventricular end-diastolic pressure.
†A-VO₂ = arteriovenous oxygen difference.

TABLE 2. Mortality Risk for Single and Multiple Bypass Grafts
for Stable Angina Pectoris

| Authors | Single Graft (Per Cent) | Mortality Rate Double Graft (Per Cent) | Triple Graft (Per Cent) |
|---|---|---|---|
| Anderson et al.[25] | 0.9 | 2.8 | 5.4° |
| Bricker and Dalton[39] | 2.1 | 1.3 | 3.0 |
| Cheanvechai et al.[40] | – | – | 2.5 |
| Cooley et al.[41] | 5.1 | 7.1 | 8.8 |
| Kouchoukos et al.[28] | 5.4 | 2.3 | 4.0 |
| Tector and McNabb[37] | 0 | 0 | 0 |
| Oldham et al.[27] | 0 | 1.2 | 2.1 |
| Wisoff et al.[38] | 0 | 0 | 0 |

° Significant difference from single bypass but not from double.

multiple vessel involvement. Several groups have established limits of ejection fraction below which they will not accept a patient for operation.[42] This certainly contributes to the spectacular results of large numbers of bypass procedures without mortality.[37, 38]

The most frequent causes of operative death are myocardial infarction and ventricular failure.[43] Better revascularization has been demonstrated to reduce the number of postoperative myocardial infarctions. A bypass of each ischemia-producing lesion is important in relieving symptoms and in protecting against perioperative infarction.[25]

## Graft Patency

Relief of angina is inferential proof of the merit of graft-generated myocardial blood flow, and there is a striking parallel between symptomatic improvement and vein graft patency.[40] Early vein graft patency (less than 6 months) at 75 to 90 per cent and 1-year patency at 70 to 85 per cent have been readily achieved.[40, 44–47] (Table 3). This compares well with patency rates for femoropopliteal venous bypass grafts.[48] As in other anatomic locations, few venous grafts fail after 1 year. Flemma et al.[44] noted a graft closure rate of only 9 per cent between 13 and 32 months. The factors contributing to graft patency are both technical (perfect anastomoses, appropriate length, position, and quality of vein) and biologic (status of native distal circulation ["run-off"], progress of distal coronary arterial disease, and degenerative changes in arterialized venous segments). Intraoperative measurement of flow through the graft serves as a single focus for many of these contributing elements and has been shown to be a significant prognosticator of graft patency, as has been the experience with femoropopliteal venous grafts.[49] Grondin et al.[50] noted a mean intraoperative flow rate of 44 ml. per minute in 16 grafts that later occluded and a mean flow of 74.8 ml. per minute in 70 grafts that maintained patency. Walker et al.[47] reported a rate of early graft failure of 50 per cent with flow less than 20 ml. per minute and a late patency rate of 90 per cent with basal

TABLE 3.   Venous Graft Patency

| Authors | Early | | Late | |
| | Patency Rate | Interval | Patency Rate | Mean Follow-up |
| --- | --- | --- | --- | --- |
| Cheanvechai et al.[40] | 76.7% | <6 mos. | 82.2% | 7–31 mos. |
| Flemma et al.[44] | 87.0% | 0–3 mos. | 85.0% | 13–32 mos. |
| Grondin et al.[45] | 88.6% | 11–23 days | 77.5% | 12 mos. |
| Sheldon et al.[46] | 86.4% | 0–6 mos. | 83.3% | 25–36 mos. |
| Walker et al.[47] | 87.0% | <3 mos. | 74.0% | 4–31 mos. |

flow greater than 41 ml. per minute. The results of Grondin et al. agreed with those of Walker et al. in that all grafts with flow less than 20 ml. per minute or that did not respond to papaverine failed, while all grafts with flow greater than 45 ml. per minute remained patent 10 to 21 days postoperatively. This coincides well with the previously mentioned fact that most graft closures occur early; therefore, they are likely to be related to technical or "run-off" factors that are most accurately exposed by intraoperative flow recordings.

Adhesions occurring after pericardiotomy have been associated with increased graft failure,[51] and the syndrome of postoperative fever, lymphocytosis, pericardial pain, and rub should be treated with indomethacin or other anti-inflammatory agents.

The *major* cause of *late* graft failure is an intimal proliferative reaction seen in as many as 10 per cent of all venous grafts[29] and in 1 of 8 patients[52] with functioning venous grafts. Flemma et al.[44] implicate this reaction in essentially all late closures and point out that 5 per cent of veins have fibrous intimal proliferation at the time of coronary arterial grafting. Intimal changes can be seen immediately after insertion of venous bypass grafts and are thought to be secondary to infiltration of blood elements into increasingly permeable endothelium.[53] Electron microscopic evidence of intimal thickening is seen as early as 19 days postoperatively, and macroscopic thickening is evident within 1 month. Recent elucidation of the deleterious effect of saline on vascular intima[54] has prompted many surgeons to use heparinized blood rather than saline to distend the vein, and it is hoped that close monitoring of such distention pressures will reduce hydraulic damage to the intima.

Demonstration by Fuchs et al.[55] of acute lipid influx into arterialized veins and chronic alterations in lipid constituents of grafts may help in clarifying the cause of this transformation, which results in occlusion of only a *small* proportion of venous grafts. That occlusion does not seem to be time-related or inevitable is supported by the data of Flemma et al.[44] and by the recent report of Garrett et al.[56] of a venous graft functioning 7 years after insertion.

Green[57] and Loop et al.[58] have advocated the use of direct internal mammary-coronary artery anastomoses to improve on the patency rate of 75 to 85 per cent seen with venous grafts. Use of the internal mammary artery is advocated for the following reasons: (1) one less anastomosis is necessary; (2) less discrepancy occurs between diameters of the mammary artery and coronary artery than between diameters of the saphenous vein and coronary artery, thereby contributing to faster flow and less turbulence in the arterial graft; and (3) the proliferative changes seen in venous grafts are precluded by the arterial nature of the graft. The internal mammary artery is infrequently involved with atherosclerotic lesions, and its potential flow and histologic integrity are closely scrutinized before an anastomosis is fashioned. (The distal saphenous vein has been used to avoid the discrepancy in diameter that usually occurs when larger, proximal veins are used.[59]) A patency rate of 90 to 95 per cent is feasible for internal mammary arterial grafts on repeated angiographic examinations.

## Relief from Symptoms

Symptomatic relief from angina pectoris has been uniformly good after bypass grafting and has been clearly shown to be closely related to graft patency[36, 40, 46, 60-64] (Table 4). Of patients with triple vessel disease, Cheanvechai et al.[40] reported that 42.8 per cent returned to an asymptomatic state with only one graft patent, 74.2 per cent did so with two functioning grafts, and 87.8 per cent did so with all three bypass grafts functioning. Balcon et al.[62] also demonstrated a close correlation between graft patency and relief from anginal symptoms. The experience of the Stanford[61] and Alabama[28] groups confirmed this.

A placebo effect definitely occurs in a small number of patients who have significant reduction of or relief from symptoms in the absence of functioning grafts to oligemic myocardium. In a large proportion of these patients, relief of pain is thought to be secondary to perioperative myocardial infarction that has been well tolerated by the patient. Matlof et al.[63] reproduced the results of Cheanvechai et al.[40] and Balcon et al.[62] but also reported on four patients with completely patent vein grafts and no relief from symptoms; however, each patient had coronary arterial stenoses that had not been bypassed. Matlof et al. also cited perioperative infarction as a cause of symptomatic relief without a patent graft in the ischemic area.

### TABLE 4. Relief from Anginal Symptoms in Survivors of Operation

| Authors | Total Relief from Pain (Per Cent) | Improvement in Symptoms (Per Cent) |
|---|---|---|
| Adam et al.[60] | 78 | 16 |
| Alderman et al.[61] | 69 | 14 |
| Balcon et al.[62] | 72 | 24 |
| Cheanvechai et al.[40] | 79 | 17 |
| Matlof et al.[63] | 64 | 17 |
| Morris et al.[36] | 75 | 17 |
| Mundth et al.[64] | 61 | 31 |
| Sheldon et al.[46] | 71 | 21 |

## *Improvement in Ventricular Function*

Functional improvement of the left ventricle relies on two factors: (1) preoperative impairment must be a concomitant of muscular ischemia, not fibrous scar, so that there remains a potential for normal or improved mechanics; and (2) the ischemic area of the ventricular wall must be satisfactorily revascularized. Coronary vasodilation is a reproducible response of the myocardium to ischemia, and this physiologic attempt at homeostasis can be used both as a guide in determining the appropriateness of revascularization and, like basal graft flows, as a prognosticator of increasing muscle function. To elicit and to measure this response, a functioning bypass graft is occluded for 10 to 30 seconds after baseline flows are determined. After flow is reinstated, measured flow through the graft usually increases substantially. This "reactive hyperemia" response indicates that the bypass graft is supplying *ischemic*, not fibrotic, myocardium (coronary vasodilation during graft occlusion-caused ischemia leads to increased flow following release), and the basal flow through the graft is necessary to prevent ischemia. Grafts that do not demonstrate a reactive hyperemia response are not considered to be supplying myocardium with an ischemia-preventing amount of blood flow.[65]

Improvement in ventricular function after bypass has been demonstrated by many groups, using angiographic, hemodynamic, and electrocardiographic methods. Campeau et al.[66] reported significant improvement in left ventricular end-diastolic pressure and stroke work index during exercise in patients with preoperative hypokinesia and patent grafts 1 year after operation. No improvement occurred in patients with significant preoperative akinesia or normal function. In intraoperative studies, Anderson[67] demonstrated marked impairment in ventricular function, as measured by a reduction in left ventricular contractility and an increase in left ventricular end-diastolic pressure with momentary occlusion of functioning grafts. Using a direct measurement of myocardial contractility, Moran et al.[68] showed that bypass flow contributes significantly to myocardial contractile force, for when grafts were temporarily occluded, the contractility of the myocardium in the distribution of graft perfusion decreased an average of 23 per cent. Their results are different from those of most investigators, in that they observed a highly significant correlation between bypass flow before occlusion and the decrease in contractility during occlusion. This is to be expected, but it had not been so well demonstrated previously. Rees et al.[69] demonstrated postoperative improvement measured by increased ejection fraction, increased rate of circumferential fiber shortening, and decreased end-systolic volume, when compared with preoperative values. These changes were not seen in patients with occluded grafts; indeed, ventricular function deteriorated measurably in patients with incomplete revascularization. Chatterjee et al.[70] observed marked improvement in ventricular asynergy in patients without a previous infarction and with patent venous grafts. In patients with previous infarction, segmental wall motion was still abnormal in the area of prior infarction but was improved in noninfarcted segments. They also recorded improvement in the hemodynamic parameters of ventricular function. Johnson et al.[71] confirmed this inability to improve the contractility of akinetic myocardium by comparing dynamic indices of contractility before and after bypass. Hamby et al.[42] recorded these improvements and also demonstrated that relief of asynergy by bypass grafting is common, but akinetic areas are infrequently returned to normal function. By careful observation of preoperative ventricular contraction patterns and electrocardiographic changes, predictions as to the probability of mechanical improvement following bypass grafting can be easily made. A previous myocardial infarction is tantamount to preclusion of a return to totally normal ventricular function, either angiographically or manometrically, even with excellent relief from angina. This implies that areas of viable myocardium juxtaposed or interspersed with fibrotic segments of ventricular wall can become ischemic and angina-producing and that even if they are revascularized and ischemia-free, they do not afford enough *contractile* muscle mass to provide demonstrable improvement in ventricular function.

Demonstrations by Guiney et al.[72] and Amsterdam et al.[73] of functional improvement in postoperative stress testing in most patients support the claim that a functioning bypass alters ventricular function. Neither angina nor ST segment changes could be elicited in 50 per cent of patients after coronary arterial bypass when they were exercised to fatigue, and the rate-pressure product at fatigue was increased 48 per cent. Angina or ST segment changes did develop in one fourth of patients but at a higher rate-pressure product than preoperatively.[72] Comparison of the angiographic status of venous grafts and stress electrocardiogram by Dodek et al.[74] clearly showed a significant correlation between a negative stress electrocardiogram and increased exercise ability and patent grafts. The converse was also (and perhaps more significantly) true: when the stress electrocardiogram after bypass was positive and the patient was unable to achieve greater exercise or heart rate, there was either graft occlusion or significant unbypassed coronary arterial disease. The response to successful bypass grafting was also dramatically demonstrated by Knoebel et al.,[75] who showed normal myocardial blood flow reserve as measured by coincidence counting with rubidium chloride in patients with patent coronary arterial bypass grafts.

## *Improved Life Expectancy*

It is generally agreed that coronary arterial bypass grafting is a successful and appropriate method of treating intractable angina pectoris. The studies described previously have proved that blood flow through the graft participates in the mechanical function of the ventricle and may lead to improved ventricular function for a protracted period, but the question of whether bypass grafting prolongs life has yet to be answered to everybody's satisfaction.[11] As has been pointed out, the major difficulty in determining the life-extending capability of coronary arterial surgery is that of achieving comparable groups for medical and surgical treatment. Several authors have conceded the benefits of operating on patients with multiple vessel involvement but have questioned the propriety of bypassing single vessel lesions.[28] Risk of operation in patients with single vessel disease is generally lower, and the long-term survival of these patients must be measured against that of patients with single vessel disease treated medically. The mortality rate at the Cleveland Clinic for patients unoperated upon and with single vessel lesions varies from 1.0 to 7.5 per cent yearly, depending on the severity (stenosis vs. obstruction) of the major lesion and the presence of associated noncritical stenoses.[7] This sophisticated and detailed study of a large group of patients points out the extreme difficulty in comparing disparate experiences. The in-depth analysis of survival following coronary arterial bypass operation by Anderson et al.[25] does, however, show a 4-year survival rate of 96 per cent for single vessel bypass patients. This is equal to or better than the results achieved by any group with medical therapy and has the added benefit of significant relief from anginal symptoms. Sheldon et al.[46] reported improvement in survival following operation in patients with involvement of only the left anterior descending artery. This result was not achieved when the right coronary artery or circumflex coronary artery was the predominant single vessel involved and bypassed. No deaths occurred in a 2-year follow-up of 105 patients with a single bypass involving the left anterior descending artery. The increasing number of reports of mortality-free surgical series will also help in delineating the long-term differences in medical and surgical therapy for single vessel disease.[37, 38] That the successful coronary arterial bypass operation prolongs life in patients with multiple vessel lesions appears to be likely. Anderson et al.[25] reported 4-year survival rates of 89 and 84 per cent for two-vessel and three-vessel involvement respectively. Excluding operative mortality, Sheldon et al.[46] showed a yearly attrition rate of 2.5 per cent for all coronary arterial bypass procedures as opposed to a yearly loss of 9.3 per cent in the nonsurgical group.

## Summary

Coronary arterial bypass is the most frequently performed cardiac operative procedure. Its benefits are: (1) relief from symptoms of angina pectoris; (2) mechanical improvement in left ventricular function; and (3) protection from myocardial infarction with probable prolongation of life. Excellent relief from angina pectoris has been achieved in about 75 per cent of patients followed for more than 1 year, with significant improvement in symptoms in another 15 per cent. Clinical improvement is closely correlated with graft patency, which remains about 75 to 80 per cent after 1 year for venous grafts and more than 90 per cent for internal mammary arterial bypass grafts. Bypass grafts have been shown to contribute significantly to the mechanical function of the left ventricle, and marked improvement in ventricular performance has been noted in late postoperative studies. Functioning bypass grafts lend a degree of protection from myocardial infarction and have been shown in some series to extend significantly the life expectancy of patients with multiple vessel disease.

In the well-chosen patient, therefore, coronary arterial bypass operation can be offered with a realistically low mortality risk, an excellent chance of relief from symptoms and return to a normal life, and the hope of increased life expectancy, if there is satisfactory revascularization of ischemic myocardium. Further experience with coronary arterial surgery and better understanding of the pathologic changes of venous intimal hyperplasia and coronary atherosclerosis should transform the prospect of such results into a certainty in the near future.

# References

1. Eastcott, H. H. G.: *Arterial Surgery.* Philadelphia, J. B. Lippincott Co., 1969.
2. Morris, G. C., Jr., DeBakey, M. E., and Bernhard, V.: Abdominal angina. Surg. Clin. North Am. 46:919, 1966.
3. Darling, R. C., Linton, R. R., and Razzuk, M. A.: Saphenous vein bypass grafts for femoropopliteal occlusive disease: a reappraisal. Surgery 61:31, 1967.
4. Osler, W.: *Lectures on Angina Pectoris and Allied States.* New York, D. Appleton and Co., 1897.
5. Kannel, W. B., and Feinleib, M.: Natural history of angina pectoris in the Framingham study: prognosis and survival. Am. J. Cardiol. 29:154, 1972.
6. Richards, D. W., Bland, E. F., and White, P. D.: A completed twenty-five-year follow-up study of 456 patients with angina pectoris. J. Chronic Dis. 4:423, 1956.
7. Bruschke, A. V. G., Proudfit, W. L., and Sones, F. M., Jr.: Progress study of 590 consecutive nonsurgical cases of coronary disease followed 5–9 years. I. Arteriographic correlations. Circulation 47:1147, 1973.
8. Bruschke, A. V. G., Proudfit, W. L., and Sones, F. M., Jr.: Progress study of 590 consecutive nonsurgical cases of coronary disease followed 5–9 years. II. Ventriculographic and other correlations. Circulation 47:1154, 1973.
9. Oberman, A., Jones, W. B., Riley, C. P., Reeves, T. J., Sheffield, L. T., and Turner, M. E.: Natural history of coronary artery disease. Bull. N.Y. Acad. Med. 48:1109, 1972.
10. Bemiller, C. R., Pepine, C. J., and Rogers, A. K.: Long-term observations in patients with angina and normal coronary arteriograms. Circulation 47:36, 1973.
11. Russek, H. I.: The "natural" history of severe angina pectoris with intensive medical therapy alone: a five year prospective study of 133 patients. Chest 65:46, 1974.
12. Neill, W. A., Judkins, M. P., Dhindsa, D. S., Metcalfe, J., Kassebaum, D. G., and Kloster, F. E.: Clinically suspect ischemic heart disease not corroborated by demonstrable coronary artery disease: physiologic investigations and clinical course. Am. J. Cardiol. 29:171, 1972.
13. Sones, F. M., Jr., and Shirey, E. K.: Cine-coronary arteriography. Mod. Concepts Cardiovasc. Dis. 31:735, 1962.
14. Judkins, M. P.: Selective coronary arteriography. I. A percutaneous transfemoral technic. Radiology 89:815, 1967.
15. Bailey, C. P., May, A., and Lemmon, W. M.: Survival after coronary endarterectomy in man. J.A.M.A. 164:641, 1957.
16. Effler, D. B., Groves, L. K., Suarez, E. L., and Favaloro, R. G.: Direct coronary artery surgery with endarterotomy and patch-graft reconstruction: clinical application and technical considerations. J. Thorac. Cardiovasc. Surg. 53:93, 1967.
17. Favaloro, R. G.: Direct myocardial revascularization. Surg. Clin. North Am. 51:1035, 1971.
18. Sabiston, D. C., Jr.: The coronary circulation. Johns Hopkins Med. J. 134:314, 1974.
19. Favaloro, R. G.: Saphenous vein autograft replacement of severe segmental coronary artery occlusion: operative techniques. Ann. Thorac. Surg. 5:334, 1968.
20. Sauvage, L. R., Wood, S. J., Eyer, K. M., and Bill, A. H., Jr.: Experimental coronary artery surgery: preliminary observations of bypass venous grafts, longitudinal arteriotomies, and end-to-end anastomoses. J. Thorac. Cardiovasc. Surg. 46:826, 1963.
21. Favaloro, R. G.: Saphenous vein graft in the surgical treatment of coronary artery disease: operative technique. J. Thorac. Cardiovasc. Surg. 58:178, 1969.
22. Effler, D. B., Favaloro, R. G., Groves, L. K., and Loop, F. D.: The simple approach to direct

coronary artery surgery: Cleveland Clinic experience. J. Thorac. Cardiovasc. Surg. 62:503, 1971.
23. Mundth, E. D., Buckley, M. J., Daggett, W. M., Sanders, C. A., and Austen, W. G.: Surgery for complications of acute myocardial infarction. Circulation 45:1279, 1972.
24. Ullyot, D. J., Wisneski, J., Sullivan, R. W., and Gertz, E. W.: Coronary surgery improves survival in patients with extensive coronary artery disease. J. Thorac. Cardiovasc. Surg. 70:405, 1975.
25. Anderson, R. P., Rahimtoola, S. H., Bonchek, L. I., and Starr, A.: The prognosis of patients with coronary artery disease after coronary bypass operations: time-related progress of 532 patients with disabling angina pectoris. Circulation 50:274, 1974.
26. Cohn, P. F., Gorlin, R., Cohn, L. H., and Collins, J. J., Jr.: Left ventricular ejection fraction as a prognostic guide in surgical treatment of coronary and valvular heart disease. Am. J. Cardiol. 34:136, 1974.
27. Oldham, H. N., Jr., Kong, Y., Bartel, A. G., Morris, J. J., Jr., Behar, V. S., Peter, R. H., Rosati, R. A., Young, W. G., Jr., and Sabiston, D. C., Jr.: Risk factors in coronary artery bypass surgery. Arch. Surg. 105:918, 1972.
28. Kouchoukos, N. T., Kirklin, J. W., and Oberman, A.: An appraisal of coronary bypass grafting. Circulation 50:11, 1974.
29. Hammermeister, K. E., and Kennedy, J. W.: Predictors of surgical mortality in patients undergoing direct myocardial revascularization. Circulation 50(Suppl. II):112, 1974.
30. Siderys, H., Pittman, J. N., and Herod, G.: Coronary artery surgery in patients with impaired left ventricular function. Chest 61:482, 1972.
31. McRaven, D. R., Walker, J. A., Friedberg, H. D., and Johnson, W. D.: Survival experience in saphenous vein bypass graft surgery. (Abstract). Am. J. Cardiol. 29:277, 1972.
32. Spencer, F. C., Green, G. E., Tice, D. A., Wallsh, E., Mills, N. L., and Glassman, E.: Coronary artery bypass grafts for congestive heart failure: a report of experience with 40 patients. J. Thorac. Cardiovasc. Surg. 62:529, 1971.
33. Mundth, E. D., Harthorne, J. W., Buckley, M. J., Dinsmore, R., and Austen, W. G.: Direct coronary arterial revascularization: treatment of cardiac failure associated with coronary artery disease. Arch. Surg. 103:529, 1971.
34. Kouchoukos, N. T., Doty, D. B., Buettner, L. E., and Kirklin, J. W.: Treatment of postinfarction cardiac failure by myocardial excision and revascularization. Circulation 45:(Suppl. I):72, 1972.
35. Mitchel, B. F., Adam, M., Lambert, C. J., Sungu, U., and Shiekh, S.: Ascending aorta-to-coronary artery saphenous vein bypass grafts. J. Thorac. Cardiovasc. Surg. 60:457, 1970.
36. Morris, G. C., Jr., Reul, G. J., Howell, J. F., Crawford, E. S., Chapman, D. W., Beazley, H. L., Winters, W. L., Peterson, P. K., and Lewis, J. M.: Follow-up results of distal coronary artery bypass for ischemic heart disease. Am. J. Cardiol. 29:180, 1972.
37. Tector, A. J., and McNabb, P. E.: Direct coronary artery surgery for one year without an operative death: 196 consecutive cases. Ann. Thorac. Surg. 17:345, 1974.
38. Wisoff, B. G., Hartstein, M. L., Aintablian, A., and Hamby, R. I.: Risk of coronary surgery—200 consecutive patients without hospital mortality. (Abstract.) Chest 66:339, 1974.
39. Bricker, D. L., and Dalton, M. L., Jr.: Cardiac surgery in the community hospital. Ann. Thorac. Surg. 17:450, 1974.
40. Cheanvechai, C., Effler, D. B., Groves, L. K., Loop, F. D., Navia, J., Grinfeld, R., Sheldon, W. C., and Sones, F. M., Jr.: Triple bypass graft for the treatment of severe triple coronary vessel disease. Ann. Thorac. Surg. 17:545, 1974.
41. Cooley, D. A., Dawson, J. T., Hallman, G. L., Sandiford, F. M., Wukasch, D. C., Garcia, E., and Hall, R. J.: Aortocoronary saphenous vein bypass: results in 1,492 patients, with particular reference to patients with complicating features. Ann. Thorac. Surg. 16:380, 1973.
42. Hamby, R. I., Tabrah, F., Aintablian, A., Hartstein, M. L., and Wisoff, B. G.: Left ventricular hemodynamics and contractile pattern after aortocoronary bypass surgery: factors affecting reversibility of abnormal left ventricular function. Am. Heart J. 88:149, 1974.
43. Brewer, D. L., Bilbro, R. H., and Bartel, A. G.: Myocardial infarction as a complication of coronary bypass surgery. Circulation 47:58, 1973.
44. Flemma, R. J., Johnson, W. D., Lepley, D., Jr., Tector, A. J., Walker, J., Gale, H., Beddingfield, G., and Manley, J. C.: Late results of saphenous vein bypass grafting for myocardial revascularization. Ann. Thorac. Surg. 14:232, 1972.
45. Grondin, C. M., Castonguay, Y. R., Lespérance, J., Bourassa, M. G., Campeau, L., and Grondin, P.: Attrition rate of aorta-to-coronary artery saphenous vein grafts after one year: a study in a consecutive series of 96 patients. Ann. Thorac. Surg. 14:223, 1972.
46. Sheldon, W. C., Rincon, G., Effler, D. B., Proudfit, W. L., and Sones, F. M., Jr.: Vein graft

surgery for coronary artery disease: survival and angiographic results in 1,000 patients. Circulation 48(Suppl. III):184, 1973.

47. Walker, J. A., Friedberg, H. D., Flemma, R. J., and Johnson, W. D.: Determinants of angiographic patency of aortocoronary vein bypass grafts. Circulation 45(Suppl. I):86, 1972.

48. DeWeese, J. A., and Rob, C. G.: Autogenous venous bypass grafts five years later. Ann. Surg. 174:346, 1971.

49. Little, J. M., Sheil, A. G. R., Loewenthal, J., and Goodman, A. H.: Prognostic value of intraoperative blood-flow measurements in femoropopliteal bypass vein-grafts. Lancet 2:648, 1968.

50. Grondin, C. M., Lepage, G., Castonguay, Y. R., Meere, C., and Grondin, P.: Aortocoronary bypass graft: initial blood flow through the graft, and early postoperative patency. Circulation 44:815, 1971.

51. Urschel, H. C., Jr., Solis, R. M., Miller, E. R., Razzuk, M. A., and Wood, R. E.: Factors influencing flow through aortocoronary artery saphenous vein bypass grafts. (Abstract.) Am. J. Cardiol. 29:295, 1972.

52. Kennedy, J. H., in discussion of Hammermeister, K. E., and Kennedy, J. W.: Predictors of surgical mortality in patients undergoing direct myocardial revascularization. Circulation, 49 and 50(Suppl. II):112, 1974.

53. Unni, K. K., Kottke, B. A., Titus, J. L., Frye, R. L., Wallace, R. B., and Brown, A. L.: Pathologic changes in aortocoronary saphenous vein grafts. Am. J. Cardiol. 34:526, 1974.

54. O'Connell, T. X., Sanchez, M., Mowbray, J. T., and Fonkalsrud, E. W.: Effects on artieral intima of saline infusions. J. Surg. Res. 16:197, 1974.

55. Fuchs, J. C. A., Hagen, P. O., Oldham, H. N., Jr., and Sabiston, D. C., Jr.: Lipid composition in venous arterial bypass grafts. Surg. Forum 23:139, 1972.

56. Garrett, H. E., Dennis, E. W., and DeBakey, M. E.: Aortocoronary bypass with saphenous vein graft: seven-year follow-up. J.A.M.A. 223:792, 1973.

57. Green, G. E.: Internal mammary artery-to-coronary artery anastomosis: three-year experience with 165 patients. Ann. Thorac. Surg. 14:260, 1972.

58. Loop, F. D., Spampinato, N., Siegel, W., and Effler, D. B.: Internal mammary artery grafts without optical assistance: clinical and angiographic analysis of 175 consecutive cases. Circulation 48:(Suppl. III):162, 1973.

59. Furuse, A., Klopp, E. H., Brawley, R. K., and Gott, V. L.: Hemodynamics of aorta-to-coronary artery bypass: experimental and analytical studies. Ann. Thorac. Surg. 14:282, 1972.

60. Adam, M., Mitchel, B. F., Lambert, C. J., and Geisler, G. F.: Long-term results with aorta-to-coronary artery bypass vein grafts. Ann. Thorac. Surg. 14:1, 1972.

61. Alderman, E. L., Matlof, H. J., Wexler, L., Shumway, N. E., and Harrison, D. C.: Results of direct coronary-artery surgery for the treatment of angina pectoris. N. Engl. J. Med. 288:535, 1973.

62. Balcon, R., Honey, M., Rickards, A. F., Sturridge, M. F., Walsh, W., Wilkinson, R. K., and Wright, J. E. C.: Evaluation by exercise testing and atrial pacing of results of aortocoronary bypass surgery. Br. Heart J. 36:841, 1974.

63. Matlof, H. J., Alderman, E. L., Wexler, L., Shumway, N. E., and Harrison, D. C.: What is the relationship between the response of angina to coronary surgery and anatomical success? Circulation 48(Suppl. III):168, 1973.

64. Mundth, E. D., Harthorne, J. W., Buckley, M. J., Daggett, W. M., and Austen, W. G.: Direct coronary artery surgery for coronary artery occlusive disease. Am. J. Surg. 121:478, 1971.

65. Reneman, R. S., and Spencer, M. P.: The use of diastolic reactive hyperemia to evaluate the coronary vascular system. Ann. Thorac. Surg. 13:477, 1972.

66. Campeau, L., Elias, G., Esplugas, E., Lespérance, J., Bourassa, M. G., and Grondin, C. M.: Left ventricular performance during exercise before and one year after aortocoronary bypass surgery for angina pectoris. Circulation 50(Suppl. II):103, 1974.

67. Anderson, R. P.: Effects of coronary bypass graft occlusion on left ventricular performance. Circulation 46:507, 1972.

68. Moran, S. V., Tarazi, R. C., Urzua, J. U., Favaloro, R. G., and Effler, D. B.: Effects of aortocoronary bypass on myocardial contractility. J. Thorac. Cardiovasc. Surg. 65:335, 1973.

69. Rees, G., Bristow, J. D., Kremkau, E. L., Green, G. S., Herr, R. H., Griswold, H. E., and Starr, A.: Influence of aortocoronary bypass surgery on left ventricular performance. N. Engl. J. Med. 284:1116, 1971.

70. Chatterjee, K., Swan, H. J. C., Parmley, W. W., Sustaita, H., Marcus, H. S., and Matloff, J.: Influence of direct myocardial revascularization on left ventricular asynergy and function in patients with coronary heart disease: with and without previous myocardial infarction. Circulation 47:276, 1973.

71. Johnson, P. E., Jr., Buggs, H., Ishikawa, K., Printup, C. A., Jr., Penido, J. R. F., Cotton, B. H., and Gordon, L. S.: Evaluation of the immediate effect of aortocoronary saphenous vein bypass surgery on myocardial contractility. Chest 66:50, 1974.
72. Guiney, T. E., Rubenstein, J. J., Sanders, C. A., and Mundth, E. D.: Functional evaluation of coronary bypass surgery by exercise testing and oxygen consumption. Circulation 48:(Suppl. III):141, 1973.
73. Amsterdam, E. A., Iben, A.. Hurley, E. J., Mansour, E., Hughes, J. L., Salel, A. F., Zelis, R., and Mason, D. T.: Saphenous vein bypass graft for refractory angina pectoris: physiologic evidence for enhanced blood flow to the ischemic myocardium. Am. J. Cardiol. 26:623, 1970.
74. Dodek, A., Kassebaum, D. G., and Griswold, H. E.: Stress electrocardiography in the evaluation of aortocoronary bypass surgery. Am. Heart J. 86:292, 1973.
75. Knoebel, S. B., McHenry, P. L., Phillips, J. F., and Lowe, D. K.: The effect of aortocoronary bypass grafts on myocardial blood flow reserve and treadmill exercise tolerance. Circulation 50:685, 197

# Coronary Artery Bypass Operation Requires Further Therapeutic Evaluation*

G. E. BURCH
and T. D. GILES

*Tulane University School of Medicine*

Arteriosclerotic heart disease remains one of the major causes of death and suffering in the United States. Thus, the importance of coronary arteriosclerosis as a health problem is well accepted. Yet, despite enormous expenditures of research money and professional time in attempting to learn the cause and means of prevention of atherosclerotic and arteriosclerotic disease states, the incidence of coronary heart disease has not changed. People continue to suffer from arteriosclerotic heart disease, and there is no evidence of expected change in incidence in the near future. It is therefore evident that physicians will continue to treat coronary heart disease in thousands of patients for many years to come.

Arteriosclerosis is a diffuse disease involving, to an extremely variable extent, the arteries throughout the body, including the heart. Heart disease is produced by obstruction to coronary blood flow to a variable degree to different parts of the heart. The resultant heart disease is associated with disturbances in exchange of many kinds of substances across nutrient blood vessels.

Coronary arteriosclerosis rarely, if ever, involves only a single arterial site, even though one site is usually more extensively diseased than other sites. Although coronary arteriosclerosis is commonly thought of as a disease of the large coronary arteries, there is no reason to assume that the small blood vessels are necessarily functioning normally. Even though obstruction

*Supported by Grant HL-14789 from the National Heart and Lung Institute of the U.S. Public Health Service, the Rudolph Matas Memorial Fund for the Kate Prewitt Hess Laboratory, the Rowell A. Billups Fund for Research in Heart Disease, and the Feazel Laboratory.

193

to large coronary arteries results in more extensive myocardial disease than does obstruction to a small branch, impairment of blood flow through a small vessel can still cause angina pectoris with fatal and nonfatal arrhythmias and conduction defects.

The ultimate solution of the problem of arteriosclerotic heart disease is prevention. Presently, prevention is not possible, and it will not become possible until the cause is known. Therefore, it is obvious that, until it is possible to prevent arteriosclerosis, patients with ischemic heart disease must be treated.

The *medical* management of coronary arteriosclerosis consists primarily of attempting to prevent progression of the disease (e.g., by reducing elevated arterial blood pressure, discontinuing cigarette smoking, reducing psychic stress, achieving a desirable body weight, eating a prudent diet, engaging in prescribed physical exercise, and managing infections) as well as treating the complications of the disease (e.g., angina pectoris, myocardial infarction, serious arrhythmias and conduction disturbances, and congestive heart failure). The patient is persuaded to reduce the demands placed upon his diseased myocardium to a level that can be supplied by his existing coronary arterial blood flow. Coronary vasodilators are employed to open collateral vessels and partially occluded arteries—those that are still able to respond—to improve the myocardial blood supply. These and other related principles of medical therapy for arteriosclerotic heart disease have been applied for decades with considerable established merit and success. However, these measures have not cured or even helped all patients. The results of medical therapy for arteriosclerotic heart disease are well known to some physicians and are readily available for those who wish to learn what they are.

Despite medical therapy, however, patients continue to die of coronary heart disease. Cardiologists readily admit that the medical management of patients with coronary arteriosclerosis is not ideal, even though it has much to offer the cooperative patient. Therefore, cardiologists are always prepared to introduce into the management of patients with coronary heart disease any established new therapeutic or prophylactic measure. Unfortunately, there is no therapeutic panacea on the horizon.

The *surgical* treatment of coronary arteriosclerosis with bypass operation evolved over a number of years. Operative methods for relieving or bypassing arterial segments in obstructive disease of the lower extremities were developed first. However, in spite of bypass procedures, neither gangrene of the lower extremities nor the need for amputation was eliminated, so that endarterectomy, sympathectomy, resection of arterial segments with replacement, and other operative procedures and medical measures are still employed. The results of bypass operation have been good under certain circumstances in some patients with peripheral arterial disease, in spite of the fact that the procedure has its limitations.

Fairly recently, the same concept of bypassing obstructive arterial lesions has been introduced for the management of coronary arteriosclerosis.[1] The concept is an excellent one for sclerotic obstructive arterial states. However, such operative methods possess intrinsic difficulties. As indicated in previous publications, the coronary artery bypass procedure has not been properly evaluated.[2, 3] That this is true is supported somewhat by the fact that the subject of the bypass procedure is discussed in this book on controversies; were the method fully accepted and well established, its position in the management of coronary heart disease would not be controversial. Yet, in spite of the lack of proper therapeutic evaluation, approximately 20,000 to 30,000 coronary artery bypass operations are performed annually.

Satisfactory therapeutic evaluation of coronary bypass operation is difficult to obtain from reviewing only the medical literature, for there is a natural human tendency to not report unfavorable results, and furthermore, the results of all operations are not reported. In addition, most medical literature emanates from large medical centers; results obtained in small and medium-sized community hospitals are usually not reported. It should be noted that in no series yet reported for this operative procedure have the therapeutic standards of the FDA used for the evaluation of new drugs been employed for the evaluation of the efficacy of coronary bypass operation. Therefore, a critical physician finds it difficult to accept without question the therapeutic claims from published reports. This attitude is supported subsequently by a comparison of medical and surgical treatments of coronary arteriosclerosis.

## Relief of Angina Pectoris

Angina pectoris is one of the main indications for coronary bypass operation. It is reported that following bypass operation, approximately 85 per cent of patients experience relief of pain. Certainly, the relief of pain is a satisfying experience to the patients; however, the significance of the relief of pain is poorly understood. The relief of pain following coronary bypass procedure is generally attributed to improvement of myocardial blood flow; yet, relief of pain occurs even when the venous bypass graft is occluded.[4] The placebo effect of operation has not been closely examined.[5] Other factors responsible for the relief of pain must be considered. For example, all physicians are aware of the excitement that followed the introduction of simple left internal mammary artery ligation[6] for the treatment of angina pectoris. This procedure is physiologically indefensible, yet many patients had the procedure performed, with claims and testimonies of great relief of angina pectoris. Indeed, 68 per cent of 92 patients in one series were found to be either asymptomatic (36 per cent) or immeasurably improved (32 per cent) after the procedure.[7] However, it was soon noted that relief of angina pectoris could be obtained equally well by merely incising the skin over the internal mammary artery without even exposing the artery, much less ligating it.[8]

The placebo effect of operation concerns all physicians and patients. The possible placebo effect of operation may be evident from a series of 56 patients[9] who underwent aortocoronary bypass for angina pectoris. Twelve of these patients had a return of angina pectoris after an initial postoperative pain-free interval. However, the clinical and coronary angiographic findings in the patients in whom angina recurred were no different from those in the group of patients who remained pain free.[9] In another series of 392 patients who underwent aortocoronary bypass procedures, the "completeness" of revascularization was not closely related to 2-year survival or relief of anginal pain.[10]

Another factor to consider when evaluating the reasons for relief of pain by aortocoronary bypass operation is the production of myocardial infarction by the procedure. In one series of 37 patients who underwent aortocoronary bypass operation, the electrocardiograms showed that abnormal Q waves developed postoperatively in 11 patients (29.7 per cent).[11] In several series, the incidence of myocardial infarction that developed postoperatively ranged from 9 to 53 per cent.[12-15] Angina pectoris disappeared in five patients whose bypass grafts had occluded, possibly because of myocardial infarction.[16] The relief of anginal pain in some patients following coronary bypass operation may be associated with the conversion of a partially ischemic area of the myocardium into an area of infarction. Myocardial infarction means permanent loss of heart muscle, a permanent partial loss of the "pump," and therefore must not be considered a salutary result of aortocoronary bypass operation.

If the relief of pain in angina pectoris is the sole surgical therapeutic objective of coronary bypass operation, then one need only incise the skin over the left internal mammary artery.[8] Clearly, in most instances, one must expect a great deal more of the operative procedure than the relief of anginal discomfort to justify the associated operative mortality, morbidity, and expense. After all, the physician must not forget that relief of anginal discomfort can be achieved in most patients with medical methods.[4]

## Influence of Bypass Grafts on Ventricular Function and Congestive Heart Failure

Since it is clear that relief of anginal pain is not the sole objective of coronary artery bypass operation, possible improvement of heart function has been investigated in patients postoperatively. Improvement in heart function is difficult to demonstrate graphically. The significance of studies showing favorable changes in left ventricular end-diastolic pressure and stroke work index obtained in the early postoperative state has been seriously questioned.[17, 18] It is recognized that, in the early postoperative state, many physiologic changes occur which might improve cardiac function independent of the venous graft, such as an increase in circulating catecholamines, psychic improvement, and benefits from bed rest, sedatives, nursing care, cardioactive drugs, and diet. However, no improvement could be found in left ventricular end-diastolic pressure or stroke work index during exercise in a group of 31 patients who had undergone aortocoronary bypass operation for angina pectoris, regardless of whether the bypass grafts were open (23 patients) or completely occluded (8 patients).[19] In this study, the 8 patients with occluded grafts served as a control series. Cine-ventriculographic studies of 51 patients performed prior to and 1 year after aortocoronary bypass operation revealed no improvement in left ventricular volumes or ejection fractions in the patients with patent grafts, whereas deterioration in myocardial function was observed in some of the patients with occluded grafts.[20] These postoperative studies are particularly significant, because they were performed after a fairly long interval following operation.

It is now evident that coronary bypass operation itself produces little or no benefit for patients with chronic congestive heart failure. Forty patients with chronic congestive heart failure underwent aortocoronary bypass operation with virtually no improvement.[21] Of importance, however, was the immediate mortality of 37 per cent of patients in this group.[21] Of another group of 9 patients with severe arteriosclerotic heart disease and ischemic cardiomyopathy with chronic congestive heart failure who underwent coronary bypass operation, 3 patients (33 per cent) died at operation.[22] Four (67 per cent) of the remaining 6 patients died within 4 months of the operation, and the 2 survivors showed no improvement in symptoms or myocardial function. The vein graft was patent in 6 of the 9 patients. In still another group of 40 patients, left ventricular volumes and ejection fractions were measured before and 4 months after aortocoronary bypass operation for chronic angina and showed no improvement in left ventricular performance.[23] One study of 66 patients with ischemic cardiomyopathy that compared the results of medical management (42 patients) with those of coronary bypass operation, ventricular plication, or both (24 patients) showed that the operative treatment was associated with a high mortality rate (33 per cent immediately) and a 6-month survival rate of only 54 per cent.[24] The symptoms in the survivors were not significantly altered, and the patients fared worse than those managed medically.

## Influence on Longevity

All current therapeutic regimens for coronary artery disease and angina pectoris are palliative. Coronary arteriosclerosis is not presently curable. Thus, to offer significant advantages over medical treatment under most circumstances, operative treatment should extend the period of life.

The natural history of patients with coronary artery disease who are treated medically must be known in order to evaluate properly surgical methods of therapy. In this regard, it is interesting that all physicians are considered to be equally capable of providing effective medical treatment to patients with coronary disease, whereas it is well accepted that only surgeons with special technical skills and with proper facilities are capable of instituting surgical treatment of this same disease.[25] Thus, one should compare only the results of medical treatment by a master cardiologist with those of surgical treatment by the master cardiac surgeon. For proper evaluation and comparison of medical and surgical care, the qualifications and facilities of the physicians and surgeons must receive serious, comparable, and proper consideration. It is not acceptable merely to lump all clinical reports and data available throughout the country together with the hope of balancing out the good and the not-so-good.

Several studies are available concerning the life expectancy of patients with angina pectoris with and without myocardial infarction. In one statistical study of 1700 patients with angina pectoris and coronary occlusion treated medically and observed over a period of 25 years, 679 (40 per cent) were dead at the end of the study in 1951.[26] This is approximately an 8.5 per cent annual mortality rate at the end of 10 years. Of 393 patients for whom the cause of death was ascertainable, 16.5 per cent had died from diseases other than coronary artery disease. In another study, published in 1952, of 6882 patients with angina pectoris treated medically and followed for a period of 10 years, the annual mortality rate was approximately 6.3 per cent.[27] The actual causes of death were not determined, but surely all these patients did not die of ischemic heart disease. In a study published in 1956 of 456 patients with angina pectoris treated medically, the mortality rate was 4.1 per cent per year for a mean follow-up of 10 years.[28] Among these patients, 76 per cent of deaths were attributed to cardiac causes, but not all were caused by ischemic heart disease itself. An extremely low annual mortality rate of 2 per cent was found in another study of 690 patients who received medical treatment.[29] All these patients did not die of ischemic heart disease. The exact causes of death were not reported in this study, and in fact, all such studies failed to follow through adequately to clarify the exact causes of death. In a study of 102 "good risk" patients[30] the annual mortality rate with medical treatment over a 5-year period was only 1.2 per cent. In the same study, the "poor risk" patients had a mortality rate of 13.4 per cent annually.

The mean annual mortality rate for all these studies of "medically" treated patients with coronary heart disease was approximately 5 per cent per year. This is the mean annual mortality rate for 10,208 patients, most of whom were followed for a mean period of 10 years, yet relatively few of them apparently were managed entirely by experienced or master cardiologists. These studies have been criticized because of the lack of angiographic data to "confirm" the anatomic distribution of the coronary vascular disease. Nevertheless, considering the limitations of coronary arteriography, these findings, crude as they are, are important. These studies indicate the life span of patients in the United States with coronary heart disease treated medically by North American physicians—that is, without surgical intervention. These data should be considered in conjunction with other reports discussed subsequently in which angiographic data are available.

Long-term studies of patients with angina pectoris who received medical treatment and for whom angiographic data are available are summarized in Table 1.[31-37] One of the largest groups of patients studied were those with "single-vessel" disease. The annual mortality rate for 459 such patients was low, ranging from 0.0 to 6.6 per cent. The mean annual mortality rate was 3.7 per cent.

The other large group of patients was composed of patients with "two-vessel" disease. The annual mortality rate for 473 such patients who received medical treatment ranged from 0.0 to 15.4 per cent, with a mean annual mortality rate of 8.7 per cent (Table 1).

The smallest group of medically treated patients for whom angiographic data are available was composed of patients with "three-vessel" disease (Table 1). As expected, the annual mortality rate in this group was the highest, ranging from 9.6 to 20.0 per cent. The mean annual mortality rate for these 381 patients was 14 per cent.

The highest mortality rate yet reported among the patients who received medical treatment was for patients with obstructive lesions of the left main coronary artery.[38] In those patients, there was a 2-year survival rate of 50 per cent. However, this represents a small group of patients.

It must be realized, when interpreting these data, that coronary arteriography has limitations. Even the methods of estimating severity and grading of obstructive lesions of the coronary arterial system are not uniform. To refer to "single-vessel," "two-vessel," and "three-vessel" disease is misleading. As mentioned before, coronary artery disease is diffuse. It is apparent from Table 1 that the mortality rate among patients with disease "angiographically" confined to a single vessel and treated medically was extremely low, and the annual mortality rate for patients with "two-vessel" disease was not much higher. When three vessels were involved, the mortality rate averaged approximately 14 per cent. It must also be remembered that the longer a follow-up study lasts, the greater is the mean rate of survival.

Interestingly, the mortality rate recorded for patients for whom angiographic data are available was not greatly different from that reported for patients for whom such information is not available. It is likely that the former group represents patients with "more symptoms," which caused their physicians to refer them for angiography. Thus, the true mortality rate from coronary arteriosclerosis and angina pectoris probably lies somewhere between the rates reported for these two groups (those with and those without angiographic data).

Table 2 indicates the influence of coronary bypass operation on patient survival. [39-59] The reported operative mortality for coronary bypass operation ranged from 2.3 to 12.0 per cent for 10,897 patients. It should be recognized, however, that these data represent the results from some of the best surgical centers. Reported results of coronary bypass operation from a large metropolitan area support the contention that the mortality rate from operation may actually be much higher than one would ascertain from the literature.[60] This latter study[60] revealed an operative mortality of 5.0 to 31.0 per cent. These data suggest that the number of patients who die from coronary bypass operation alone equals the mortality rate experienced over 1 to 2 years or more by patients with angina pectoris managed medically. In a study not included in Table 2,[61] the total in-hospital mortality rate for 100 patients undergoing coronary artery bypass operation was 9 per cent. For 33 patients having a single bypass graft, the operative mortality was 11.7 per cent; for 43 patients having two bypass grafts, the operative mortality rate was 4.7 per cent; and for patients having three grafts, the operative mortality rate was

TABLE 1. Mortality Rates in Patients with Angina Pectoris Treated Medically
(Based upon Coronary Artery Disease Determined Angiographically)

| Author | "Single Vessel" Involved | | | "Two Vessels" Involved | | | "Three Vessels" Involved | | |
|---|---|---|---|---|---|---|---|---|---|
| | Number of Patients | Average Follow-up (Months) | Annual Mortality (Per cent) | Number of Patients | Average Follow-up (Months) | Annual Mortality (Per cent) | Number of Patients | Average Follow-up (Months) | Annual Mortality (Per cent) |
| Oberman et al.[31] | 46 | 20 | 2.6 | 50 | 22.7 | 13.7 | 52 | 19.3 | 16.7 |
| Lichtlen and Moccetti[32] | 83 | 32 | 3.6 | 62 | 32.0 | 6.7 | 86 | 32.0 | 12.6 |
| Slagle et al.[33] | 20 | 15 | 4.0 | 26 | 15.0 | 15.4 | 48 | 15.0 | 20.0 |
| Bruschke et al.[34] | 202 | 84 | 3.4 | 233 | 84.0 | 6.4 | 118 | 84.0 | 9.6 |
| Moberg et al.[35] | 84 | 84-108 | 5.8 | 82 | 84.0-108.0 | 6.3 | 34 | 84.0-108.0 | 10.0 |
| Amsterdam et al.[36] | 21 | 26 | 6.6 | 11 | 26.0 | 12.5 | 34 | 26.0 | 13.5 |
| Basta et al.[37] | 3 | 33 | 0.0 | 9 | 33.0 | 0.0 | 9 | 33.0 | 12.0 |

TABLE 2. Operative and Late Mortality Rates Associated with Coronary Artery Bypass Operation

| Author | Number of Patients | Mean Time of Follow-up (Months) | Operative Mortality (Per cent) | Late Mortality (Per cent per Year) |
|---|---|---|---|---|
| Favaloro[39] | 1697 | – | 3.5 | – |
| Cooley et al.[40] | 1492 | 30.0 | 7.1 | 2.4 |
| Effler et al.[41] | 1323 | – | 3.2 | – |
| Hall et al.[42] | 1276 | 3.0–27.0 | 6.6 | 2.3 |
| Sheldon et al.[43] | 1000 | 22.0–60.0 | 4.0 | 2.5 |
| Kouchoukos et al.[44] | 548 | 12.0 | 3.5 | – |
| Morris et al.[45] | 480 | 25.0 | 6.2 | 2.6 |
| Hutchinson et al.[46] | 476 | 12.0 | 2.3 | 1.5 |
| Manley and Johnson[47] | 368 | 12.0 | 6.0 | – |
| Adam et al.[48] | 350 | 6.0–43.0 | 10.0 | 3.0 |
| Kaiser et al.[49] | 242 | 25.0 | 8.7 | 0.8 |
| Anderson et al.[50] | 200 | 9.7 | 6.5 | – |
| Collins et al.[51] | 180 | 8.9 | 5.5 | 4.3 |
| Alderman et al.[52] | 102 | 12.0 | 3.9 | 5.1 |
| Lawrence et al.[53] | 100 | 6.0–24.0 | 5.6 | – |
| Najmi et al.[54] | 100 | 4.0–12.0 | 12.0 | – |
| Favaloro[55] | 300 | 24.0–36.0 | – | 2.0 |
| McRaven et al.[56] | 309 | 6.0–34.0 | – | 6.0 |
| Spencer et al.[57] | 178 | 1.0–34.0 | 7.9 | 3.9 |
| Mitchel et al.[58] | 128 | – | 11.7 | – |
| Mundth et al.[59] | 48 | 3.0–30.0 | 10.0 | 0.0 |

12.5 per cent. In another series[62] of 400 consecutive patients subjected to aortocoronary bypass operation, 12 per cent either were not benefited or incurred major late complications. The operative mortality rate alone was 6.5 per cent.

The late mortality following coronary bypass operation is not yet known. The operative results listed in Table 2 represent data collected over a relatively short period of time. In some studies, the late annual mortality following coronary bypass operation was extremely low (0.8 to 1.5 per cent), whereas other studies showed mortality rates of 5.1 to 6.0 per cent. These late annual mortality rates tend to be similar to those of medically managed patients mentioned previously.

As will be discussed, there is a real need to randomize patients to study the results of medical and surgical management of coronary artery disease. One such study is in progress by a Veterans Administration cooperative group to learn the relative merits of medical and surgical therapy for coronary artery disease. A progress report from this investigation[63] reveals an initial operative mortality rate of 16 per cent for coronary artery bypass operation. The operative mortality rate later declined to 4 per cent. However, no statistically significant difference in survival at the eighteenth month was noted between medical and surgical cases when observations were made on randomized groups of patients with single left main coronary artery lesions. Operation did not modify the overall survival of 2 years in a study in which 402 patients were treated medically and 379 patients were treated with coronary bypass operation and in which 110 items of information were analyzed for comparison.[64]

A careful and critical review of these reports of the rates of survival of patients with coronary heart disease reveals difficulties associated with such investigations. For example, such factors as the precise nature of care, the patient's attention to the physician's instructions, and the detailed nature of continuing medical management of all patients, including those who survive operation, are not reported. Careful and meticulous autopsy and coronary artery investigations are lacking. The variables are numerous and are not limited to findings at angiography. Nevertheless, considering the operative mortality and the unimpressive impact on long-term survival, the advantage of coronary artery bypass operation, at this stage of its evolution, in the treatment of coronary heart disease is not apparent.

## Changes in the Coronary Circulation Following Aortocoronary Bypass

Coronary bypass procedures influence the state of the natural coronary circulation. For example, it was recognized that following aortocoronary bypass, the coronary artery proximal to the bypassed obstruction frequently occluded.[65-68] Such progression to stenosis of the proximal and main channel of a bypassed coronary artery occurred in 40 to 50 per cent of bypassed arteries. It has been suggested that the reduction in flow in the bypassed segment is responsible for the occlusion of this proximal segment. When the main segment of the bypassed coronary artery becomes occluded and the venous bypass later also becomes occluded, it is difficult to consider the operation successful, and one cannot help but wonder what influence these changes have on the myocardial blood supply.

Arteriosclerotic changes may occur at the point of anastomosis of coronary artery and bypass venous segments.[69, 70] Such changes occur in approximately 6 to 8 per cent of anastomoses. Aortocoronary bypass may also adversely influence the coronary arteries distal to the bypass anastomosis.[69, 70] The reported incidence of these latter changes varies widely (2 to 27 per cent).[69, 70] New total coronary occlusion occurs 16 times more frequently in grafted coronary artery segments than in nongrafted, previously normal segments. There is also a total rate of progression of occlusion 3.5 times greater in the grafted segments.[71] It has been suggested that progression of arteriosclerosis, operative trauma, and changes in pattern of arterial flow may all contribute to the development of new myocardial and arterial lesions.[72] Because of these and other changes, a great deal more experience is necessary to learn the true value of coronary bypass operation.

Therefore, it is the responsibility of the entire medical profession to determine in a deliberate, well-planned, scientific manner the therapeutic value of coronary bypass operation before this hazardous and expensive procedure is applied generally. The same stringent protocol must be insisted upon for the study of this therapeutic agent as is demanded for the study of new drugs.

## Fate of the Venous Bypass Graft

Following coronary bypass operation, a large number of the venous bypass grafts occlude. The published incidence of graft occlusion is based mainly on angiographic data from patients who survive the operation. One report of postoperative angiographic findings in 317 patients revealed that 12 per cent of vein grafts became occluded soon after operation, with 10 to 15 per cent more becoming occluded at a later date, constituting at least a 22 to 27 per cent closure rate.[73] Another study of 205 patients (320 grafts) revealed that, at an average of 7 months postoperatively, 19 per cent of the grafts had occluded.[74] In another late study for patency of aortocoronary vein grafts in 88 patients, 32 per cent were found to be occluded.[75] Early postoperative occlusion of the bypass grafts may occur in at least 15 per cent of patients.[76]

Occlusion of the aortocoronary vein grafts may be due to several factors, such as sluggish rates of blood flow through the venous segment, intimal thickening of the vein,[77] operative technique, and, perhaps, the state of the coronary circulation in the grafted artery. Furthermore, veins are not functionally or morphologically designed to sustain high intraluminal pressure. Incidentally, the occlusion rate for internal mammary artery bypass segments appears to be lower than the occlusion rate for venous segments.

## Complications of Coronary Arteriography

Although this discussion is not concerned directly with coronary arteriography, the use of this procedure must be considered, since it is an integral part of coronary bypass operation, even though it is not required for the medical management of patients with ischemic heart disease. Coronary arteriography has a significant morbidity and some mortality.[78] Mortality and morbidity may result from myocardial infarction secondary to dissection of coronary arteries, trauma to the arteries, coronary embolism, fatal arrhythmias, systemic embolism, and peripheral arterial complications associated with coronary angiography. Hypersensitivity to the contrast materials accounts for further mortality and morbidity. However, it is not possible to know the true incidence of mortality and morbidity from coronary angiography, since such data are not usually reported.

It has been suggested that the mortality is small, 0.2 per cent. But when, at the same time, it is suggested that we be prepared to do 80,000 coronary angiograms a day,[79] this would mean that 160 Americans would die each day from a diagnostic procedure, or about 58,400 per year—more deaths per year from a diagnostic procedure than the total of American deaths* from the entire 12 years of the Vietnam war. Furthermore, this figure does not include nonfatal but serious reactions, accidents and damage to arteries and veins, infections, embolism, thrombosis, and other complications.

## Conclusions

When one considers the operative mortality of coronary bypass operation, the early occlusion of 12 to 15 per cent of venous grafts, with later occlusion of as many as 32 per cent, the high incidence of induced myocardial infarction, the risks of coronary angiography, the uselessness of coronary angiography in patients with diffuse myocardial disease, the relatively low impact of bypass operation on the longevity of patients with coronary artery disease, the expense and psychic trauma of coronary bypass operation, and the lack of evidence establishing its advantage over medical management of patients with coronary artery disease, the role of coronary artery bypass operation in the management of ischemic heart disease appears limited at the present time.

It will be difficult to establish the true value of coronary artery bypass operation because of the moral and ethical aspects of double blind studies, sham operations, and the numerous important variables to consider in randomization of patients, particularly if the latter involves the performance of sham operations. Nevertheless, the same rigorous standards employed in the evaluation of new drugs should be applied to the evaluation of coronary bypass operation. It is a therapeutic agent just as a drug is.

Nonintentional "sham" operations provide useful control data, and the collection of these cases should be encouraged and studied. We have had four such nonintentional "sham" operative experiences to date, and all patients had clinically "excellent" results, with relief of their anginal pain. For example, one man developed serious anesthetic problems while undergoing operation for coronary bypass, necessitating discontinuance of the operation when the heart was exposed without performance of the bypass procedure. Yet postoperatively, the patient was completely relieved of angina pectoris. Another man had a large posteroseptal infarct followed by rupture of the interventricular septum. Severe angina pectoris and congestive heart failure ensued. Operative closure of the ruptured septum was performed without coronary bypass operation, and his angina pectoris completely disappeared postoperatively. Yet, no coronary bypass procedure had been performed. Certainly, these inadvertent "sham" operations should be collected and studied carefully.

The present wave of enthusiasm for and the extent to which coronary bypass operation is recommended and employed demand that a reliable an-

---

*Statistics from *The World Almanac*, 1974 edition, New York, Newspaper Enterprise Association, Inc., 1973, p. 48.

swer be obtained soon to the question of what is the proper role of coronary bypass operation in the treatment of patients with coronary arteriosclerosis. Until an answer is available, and like any new therapeutic agent to be introduced for general use in the practice of medicine, coronary bypass operation should not be employed except in certain surgical centers which are designed and designated for study and evaluation of the procedure.

In a controversy of this nature, it is not who is right but what is right that matters. What is right cannot be determined by performing more and more operations in all sorts of hospitals under all sorts of conditions. Coronary heart disease is a serious health problem. If 80,000 coronary angiograms were performed per day,[79] an estimated 58,400 Americans would die annually from coronary angiography only, with many more experiencing all sorts of complications; and if 50 per cent of those studied angiographically had bypass operation, with 10 per cent dying, the death rate would be more than 4000 per day. This is a serious problem which needs unbiased evaluation. As indicated previously[3] and as shown in Table 3, there are economic, mortality, morbidity, and other factors which must be carefully investigated to learn the relative merits of medicine and surgery in the management of coronary heart disease. Any physician can produce a "case" or a testimonial in favor of his opinion, but this is not the way the problem will be solved. As Table 3 indicates, surgical rather than medical therapy should be employed only if the advantages of operation justify the risks, costs, and psychic stress to the patient. But where are the data?

Finally, regardless of whether or not operation is employed, medical care must always be of high quality, for even those patients who undergo operation will require continuing medical care. These patients are *not cured;* medical care must be continued postoperatively. It is not possible to "cure" arteriosclerosis at present.

TABLE 3.   Comparisons of Operative Risks of Medical and Surgical Management of Ischemic Heart Disease[*]

| | Treatment | |
|---|---|---|
| | *Surgical* | *Medical* |
| Operative mortality | 4 to 25+% | Zero |
| Operative complications, early and late (myocardial infarction, hemorrhage, infection, thromboembolism, etc.) | 25% | Zero |
| Total cost of operation | $8,000 to $35,000+ | Zero |
| Closure of shunt | 25% in 2 years | Zero |
| Cures | Zero | Zero |
| Operative pain and suffering | 100% | Zero |
| Operative psychic stress to patient and family | 100% | Zero |
| Chronic adhesive pericarditis | 100% | Zero |
| Survival time | Unknown | Known |

*From Burch, G. E.: Surgical versus medical management of coronary heart disease. Am. Heart J. 86:846, 1973. Reproduced by permission of the American Heart Association, Inc.

## *References*

1. Favaloro, R. G.: Saphenous vein autograft replacement of severe segmental coronary artery occlusion: operative technique. Ann. Thorac. Surg. 5:334, 1968.
2. Burch, G. E.: Coronary artery surgery—saphenous vein bypass. Am. Heart J. 82:137, 1971.
3. Burch, G. E.: Surgical versus medical management of coronary heart disease. Am. Heart J. 86:846, 1973.
4. Dunkman, W. B., Perloff, J. K., Kastor, J. A., and Shelburne, J. C.: Medical perspectives in coronary artery surgery—a caveat. Ann. Intern. Med. 81:817, 1974.
5. Spodick, D. H.: Revascularization of the heart—numerators in search of denominators. Am. Heart J. 81:149, 1971.
6. Battezzati, M., Tagliaferro, A., and Cattaneo, A. D.: Clinical evaluation of bilateral internal mammary artery ligation as treatment of coronary heart disease. Am. J. Cardiol. 4:180, 1959.
7. Glover, R. P., Kitchell, J. R., Kyle, R. H., Davila, J. C., and Trout, R. G.: Experiences with myocardial revascularization by division of the internal mammary arteries. Dis. Chest 33:637, 1958.
8. Dimond, E. G., Kittle, C. F., and Crockett, J. E.: Comparison of internal mammary artery ligation and sham operation for angina pectoris. Am. J. Cardiol. 5:483, 1960.
9. Benchimol, A., Fleming, H., Desser, K. B., and Harris, C. L.: Postoperative recurrence of angina pectoris after aortocoronary venous graft bypass. Am. Heart J. 88:11, 1974.
10. McNeer, J. F., Conley, M. J., Starmer, C. F., Behar, V. S., Kong, Y., Peter, R. H., Bartel, A. G., Oldham, H. N., Young, W. G., Jr., Sabiston, D. C., Jr., and Rosati, R. A.: Complete and incomplete revascularization at aortocoronary bypass surgery: experience with 392 consecutive patients. Am. Heart J. 88:176, 1974.
11. Espinoza, J., Lipski, J., Litwak, R., Donoso, E., and Dack, S.: New Q waves after coronary artery bypass surgery for angina pectoris. Am. J. Cardiol. 33:221, 1974.
12. Brewer, D., Bilbro, R., and Bartel, A.: Myocardial infarction as a complication of coronary bypass surgery. Circulation 45 and 46 (Suppl. II):69, 1972.
13. Hultgren, H. N., Miyagawa, M., Buck, W., and Angell, W. W.: Ischemic myocardial injury during coronary artery surgery. Am. Heart J. 82:624, 1971.
14. Kansal, S., Roitman, D., Sheffield, L. T., and Kouchoukos, N. T.: Acute myocardial injury following aortocoronary bypass surgery. (Abstract.) Am. J. Cardiol. 31:140, 1973.
15. Williams, D., Iben, A., Hurley, E., Bonanno, J., Massumi, R. A., Zelis, R., Mason, D. T., and Amsterdam, E. A.: Myocardial infarction during coronary artery bypass surgery. (Abstract.) Am. J. Cardiol. 31:164, 1973.
16. DiLuzio, V., Roy, P. R., and Sowton, E.: Angina in patients with occluded aortocoronary vein grafts. Br. Heart J. 36:139, 1974.
17. Hammermeister, K. E., and Kennedy, J. W.: Myocardial revascularization and ventricular performance. (Letter to the Editor.) Circulation 48:450, 1973.
18. Bourassa, M. G.: Left ventricular performance following direct myocardial revascularization. (Editorial.) Circulation 48:915, 1973.
19. Campeau, L., Elias, G., Esplugas, E., Lespérance, J., Bourassa, M. G., and Grondin, C. M.: Left ventricular performance during exercise before and one year after aortocoronary bypass surgery for angina pectoris. Circulation 50(Suppl. II):103, 1974.
20. Arbogast, R., Solignac, A., and Bourassa, M. G.: Influence of aortocoronary saphenous vein bypass surgery on left ventricular volumes and ejection fraction: comparison before and one year after surgery in 51 patients. Am. J. Med. 54:290, 1973.
21. Spencer, F. C., Green, G. E., Tice, D. A., Walsh, E., Mills, N. L., and Glassman, E.: Coronary artery bypass grafts for congestive heart failure: a report of experiences with 40 patients. J. Thorac. Cardiovasc. Surg. 62:529, 1971.
22. Kouchoukos, N. T., Doty, D. B., Buettner, L. E., and Kirklin, J. W.: Treatment of postinfarction cardiac failure by myocardial excision and revascularization. Circulation 45(Suppl. I):72, 1972.
23. Hammermeister, K. E., Kennedy, J. W., Hamilton, G. W., Stewart, D. K., Gould, K. L., Lipscomb, K., and Murray, J. A.: Aortocoronary saphenous-vein bypass: failure of successful grafting to improve resting left ventricular function in chronic angina. N. Engl. J. Med. 290:186, 1974.
24. Yatteau, R. F., Peter, R. H., Behar, V. S., Bartel, A. G., Rosati, R. A., and Kong, Y.: Ischemic cardiomyopathy: the myopathy of coronary artery disease. Natural history and results of medical versus surgical treatment. Am. J. Cardiol. 34:520, 1974.
25. Kosowsky, B. D.: Coronary surgery outside medical centers. (Letter to the Editor.) Circulation 48:223, 1973.
26. Sigler, L. H.: Prognosis of angina pectoris and coronary occlusion: follow-up of 1,700 cases. J.A.M.A. 146:998, 1951.

27. Block, W. J., Jr., Crumpacker, E. L., Dry, T. J., and Gage, R. P.: Prognosis of angina pectoris: observations in 6,882 cases. J.A.M.A. *150*:259, 1952.
28. Richards, D. W., Bland, E. F., and White, P. D.: A completed twenty-five-year follow-up study of 456 patients with angina pectoris. J. Chronic Dis. *4*:415, 1956.
29. Zukel, W. J., Cohen, B. M., Mattingly, T. W., and Hrubec, Z.: Survival following first diagnosis of coronary heart disease. Am. Heart J. *78*:159, 1969.
30. Russek, H. I.: Prognosis in severe angina pectoris: medical versus surgical therapy. Am. Heart J. *83*:762, 1972.
31. Oberman, A., Jones, W. B., Riley, C. P., Reeves, T. J., Sheffield, L. T., and Turner, M. E.: Natural history of coronary artery disease. Bull. N.Y. Acad. Med. *48*:1109, 1972.
32. Lichtlen, P. R., and Moccetti, T.: Prognostic aspects of coronary angiography. (Abstract.) Circulation *45* and *46* (Suppl. II):7, 1972.
33. Slagle, R. C., Bartel, A. G., Behar, V. S., Peter, R. H., Rosati, R. A., and Kong, Y.: Natural history of angiographically documented coronary artery disease. (Abstract.) Circulation *45* and *46* (Suppl. II):60, 1972.
34. Bruschke, A. V. G., Proudfit, W. L., and Sones, F. M., Jr.: Progress study of 590 consecutive nonsurgical cases of coronary disease followed 5–9 years. I. Arteriographic correlations. Circulation *47*:1147, 1973.
35. Moberg, C. H., Webster, J. S., and Sones, F. M.: Natural history of severe proximal coronary disease as defined by cineangiography (200 patients, 7 year followup). Am. J. Cardiol. *29*:282, 1972.
36. Amsterdam, E. A., Most, A. S., Wolfson, S., Kemp, H. G., and Gorlin, R: Relation of degree of angiographically documented coronary artery disease to mortality. Ann. Intern. Med. *72*:780, 1970.
37. Basta, L. L., and Kioschos, J. M. (introduced by January, L. E.): Results of medical management of angina pectoris in candidates for saphenous vein bypass graft. (Abstract.) J. Lab. Clin. Med. *78*:794, 1971.
38. Cohen, M. V., Cohn, P. F., Herman, M. V., and Gorlin, R.: Diagnosis and prognosis of main left coronary artery obstruction. Circulation *45* and *46* (Suppl. I):57, 1972.
39. Favaloro, R.: Direct and indirect coronary surgery. Circulation *46*:1197, 1972.
40. Cooley, D. A., Dawson, J. T., Hallman, G. L., Sandiford, F. M., Wukasch, D. C., Garcia, E., and Hall, R. J.: Aortocoronary saphenous vein bypass: results in 1,492 patients, with particular reference to patients with complicating features. Ann. Thorac. Surg. *16*:380, 1973.
41. Effler, D. B., Favaloro, R. G., Groves, L. K., and Loop, F. D.: The simple approach to direct coronary artery surgery: Cleveland Clinic experience. J. Thorac. Cardiovasc. Surg. *62*:503, 1971.
42. Hall, R. J., Dawson, J. T., Cooley, D. A., Hallman, G. L., Wukasch, D. C., and Garcia, E.: Coronary artery bypass. Circulation *47* and *48*(Suppl. III):146, 1973.
43. Sheldon, W. C., Rincon, G., Effler, D. B., Proudfit, W. L., and Sones, F. M., Jr.: Vein graft surgery for coronary artery disease: survival and angiographic results in 1,000 patients. Circulation *48*(Suppl. III):184, 1973.
44. Kouchoukos, N. T., Kirklin, J. W., and Oberman, A.: An appraisal of coronary bypass grafting. Circulation *50*:11, 1974.
45. Morris, G. C., Jr., Reul, G. J., Howell, J. F., Crawford, E. S., Chapman, D. W., Beazley, H. L., Winters, W. L., Peterson, P. K., and Lewis, J. M.: Follow-up results of distal coronary artery bypass for ischemic heart disease. Am. J. Cardiol. *29*:180, 1972.
46. Hutchinson, J. E., III, Green, G. E., Mekhjian, H. A., Gallozzi, E., Cameron, A., and Kemp, H. G.: Coronary bypass grafting in 476 patients consecutively operated on. Chest *64*:706, 1973.
47. Manley, J. C., and Johnson, W. D.: Effects of surgery on angina (pre- and postinfarction) and myocardial function (failure). Circulation *46*:1208, 1972.
48. Adam, A., Mitchel, B. F., Lambert, C. J., and Geisler, G. F.: Long-term results with aorta-to-coronary artery bypass vein grafts. Ann. Thorac. Surg. *14*:1, 1972.
49. Kaiser, G. C., Barner, H. B., Willman, V. L., Mudd, J. G., Westura, E. W., and Alves, L. E.: Aortocoronary bypass grafting. Arch. Surg. *105*:319, 1972.
50. Anderson, R. P., Hodam, R., Wood, J., and Starr, A.: Direct revascularization of the heart. Early clinical experience with 200 patients. J. Thorac. Cardiovasc. Surg. *63*:353, 1972.
51. Collins, J. J., Jr., Cohn, L. H., Sonnenblick, E. H., Herman, M. V., Cohn, P. F., and Gorlin, R.: Determinants of survival after coronary artery bypass surgery. Circulation *47* and *48* (Suppl. III):132, 1973.
52. Alderman, E. L., Matlof, H. J., Wexler, L., Shumway, N. E., and Harrison, D. C.: Results of direct coronary-artery surgery for the treatment of angina pectoris. N. Engl. J. Med. *288*:525, 1973.
53. Lawrence, G. H., Riggins, R. C. K., Hipp, R., and Johnston, R. R.: Status of one hundred patients after coronary artery bypass surgery. Am. J. Surg. *126*:277, 1973.

54. Najmi, M., Ushiyama, K., Blanco, G., Adam, A., and Segal, B. L.: Results of aortocoronary artery saphenous vein bypass surgery for ischemic heart disease. Am. J. Cardiol. 33:42, 1974.
55. Favaloro, R. G.: Surgical treatment of coronary arteriosclerosis by the saphenous vein graft technique: critical analysis. Am. J. Cardiol. 28:493, 1971.
56. McRaven, D. R., Walker, J. A., Friedberg, H. D., and Johnson, W. D.: Survival experience in saphenous vein bypass graft surgery. Am. J. Cardiol. 29:277, 1972.
57. Spencer, F. C., Green, G. E., Tice, D. A., and Glassman, E.: Bypass grafting for occlusive disease of the coronary arteries: a report of experience with 195 patients. Ann. Surg. 173:1029, 1971.
58. Mitchel, B. F., Adam, M., Lambert, C. J., Sungu, U., and Shiekh, S.: Ascending aorta-to-coronary artery saphenous vein bypass grafts. J. Thorac. Cardiovasc. Surg. 60:457, 1970.
59. Mundth, E. D., Harthorne, J. W., Buckley, M. J., Daggett, W. M., and Austen, W. G.: Direct coronary artery surgery for coronary artery occlusive disease. Am. J. Surg. 121:478, 1971.
60. Richter, M. A., Dhurandhar, R. W., O'Meallie, L. P., Rosenberg, M., and Glancy, D. L.: Results of all aortocoronary bypass operations in the community hospitals of Greater New Orleans. Circulation 50(Suppl. III):67, 1974.
61. Hammond, G. L., and Poirier, R. A.: Early and late results of direct coronary reconstructive surgery for angina. J. Thorac. Cardiovasc. Surg. 65:127, 1973.
62. Cannom, D. S., Miller, D. C., Shumway, N. E., Fogarty, T. J., Daily, P. O., Hu, M., Brown, B., Jr., and Harrison, D. C.: The long-term follow-up of patients undergoing saphenous vein bypass surgery. Circulation 49:77, 1974.
63. Hultgren, H. N., Takaro, T., Fowler, N., and Wright, E. C.: Evaluation of surgery in angina pectoris. Am. J. Med. 56:1, 1974.
64. McNeer, J. F., Starmer, C. F., Bartel, A. G., Behar, V. S., Kong, Y., Peter, R. H., and Rosati, R. A.: The nature of treatment selection in coronary artery disease: experience with medical and surgical treatment of a chronic disease. Circulation 49:606, 1974.
65. Aldridge, H. E., and Trimble, A. S.: Progression of proximal coronary artery lesions to total occlusion after aorta-coronary saphenous vein bypass grafting. J. Thorac. Cardiovasc. Surg. 62:7, 1971.
66. Bourassa, M. G., Goulet, C., and Lespérance, J.: Progression of coronary arterial disease after aortocoronary bypass grafts. Circulation 47 and 48 (Suppl. III):127, 1973.
67. Malinow, M. R., Kremkau, E. L., Kloster, F. E., Bonchek, L. I., and Rösch, J.: Occlusion of coronary arteries after vein bypass. Circulation 47:1211, 1973.
68. Bousvaros, G., Piracha, A. R., Chaudhry, M. A., Grant, C., Older, T. M., and Pifarre, R.: Increase in severity of proximal coronary disease after successful distal aortocoronary grafts: its nature and effects. Circulation 46:870, 1972.
69. Glassman, E., Spencer, F. C., Krauss, K. R., Weisinger, B., and Isom, O. W.: Changes in the underlying coronary circulation secondary to bypass grafting. Circulation 49 and 50 (Suppl. II):80, 1974.
70. Levine, J. A., Bechtel, D. J., Gorlin, R., Cohn, P. F., and Herman, M. V.: De novo obstructive coronary disease (CAD) following direct revascularization surgery (DRS). (Abstract.) Clin. Res. 21:433, 1973.
71. Maurer, B. J., Oberman, A., Holt, J. H., Jr., Kouchoukos, N. T., Jones, W. B., Russell, R. O., Jr., and Reeves, T. J.: Changes in grafted and nongrafted coronary arteries following saphenous vein bypass grafting. Circulation 50:293, 1974.
72. Griffith, L. S. C., Achuff, S. C., Conti, C. R., Humphries, J. O'N., Brawley, R. K., Gott, V. L., and Ross, R. S.: Changes in intrinsic coronary circulation and segmental ventricular motion after saphenous-vein coronary bypass graft surgery. N. Engl. J. Med. 288:589, 1973.
73. Walker, J. A., Friedberg, H. D., Flemma, R. J., and Johnson, W. D.: Determinants of angiographic patency of aortocoronary vein bypass grafts. Circulation 45 and 46 (Suppl. I):86, 1972.
74. Bonchek, L. I., Rahimtoola, S. H., Chaitman, B. R., Rosch, J., Anderson, R. P., and Starr, A.: Vein graft occlusion: immediate and late consequences and therapeutic implications. Circulation 49 and 50 (Suppl. II):84, 1974.
75. Bourassa, M. G., Lespérance, J., Campeau, L., and Simard, P.: Factors influencing patency of aortocoronary vein grafts. Circulation 45 and 46 (Suppl. I):79, 1972.
76. Wilson, W. S.: Aortocoronary saphenous vein bypass: a review of the literature. Heart and Lung 2:90, 1973.
77. Johnson, W. D., Auer, J. E., and Tector, A. J.: Late changes in coronary vein grafts. (Abstract.) Am. J. Cardiol. 26:640, 1970.
78. Adams, D. F., Fraser, D. B., and Abrams, H. L.: The complications of coronary arteriography. Circulation 48:609, 1973.
79. Does the U.S. need 80,000 coronary angiograms a day? Med. World News 15(No. 34):14, 1974.

# 10

# *Lymph Node Removal for Malignant Melanoma*

ADJUNCTIVE TREATMENT FOR
MALIGNANT MELANOMA
   *by Hiram C. Polk, Jr.*

OPERATIVE TREATMENT OF
MALIGNANT MELANOMA OF THE
LIMBS
   *by Walter Lawrence, Jr.*

## Statement of the Problem

*This controversy centers largely on the question of en bloc regional lymph node dissection at the time the primary lesion is removed. Also discussed are the character of the local excision with respect to extent of skin and contiguous soft tissue excision and the merits of amputation versus wide local excision.*

*For a malignant melanoma, examine the data which determine the breadth and width of skin removed and the depth of excised subcutaneous tissue, fascia, and muscle. Does extent of excision relate to size or histology of the primary lesion or is the proper margin the same for all cases?*

*With a melanoma located on the limb, should regional node dissection be included as primary therapy? Should it be included as a secondary procedure? What are the criteria? What are the data?*

*Evaluate data regarding excision of skin in continuity between the site of the melanoma and the regional lymph nodes.*

*If the melanoma closely approximates or seems fixed to bone, should a primary amputation be performed?*

*Are there data supporting the use of adjunctive systemic chemotherapy at the time of or soon after a potentially curative operation?*

# Adjunctive Treatment for Malignant Melanoma

HIRAM C. POLK, JR.

*University of Louisville School of Medicine*

## Introduction

For at least two reasons, malignant melanoma conjures up a dire prognosis in the minds of most physicians. The first is its relative rarity, and the second is the often impressive visual evidence of metastatic disease. Indeed, a survey of practicing physicians in North Carolina concerning end results of common cancers showed that only melanoma, lymphoma, and carcinoma of the larynx were perceived with inappropriate pessimism as to the likelihood of survival.[1] As a matter of fact, the overall survival rate at 5 years for all patients with malignant melanoma exceeds 60 per cent and often surpasses 70 per cent.

The first consideration is to establish a diagnosis. Although the visual characteristics of the various forms of malignant melanoma are not germane to this discussion, biopsy and histologic study should be the order for any suspicious lesion. There are data suggesting that whether biopsies are incisional or excisional does not influence outcome; ultimately, adequate, prompt treatment, no matter what the technical nature of the biopsy itself, is the critical factor.[2]

Similarly, the treatment of the primary tumor itself does not warrant substantial discussion. An adequately excised margin is required, but what is adequate to preserve function on the face of a young girl and what is adequate on the interscapular portion of the back of an elderly male are obviously dissimilar. Depending on the area and the site, one may choose primary closure or skin graft. No data exist that show that either of these methods of reconstruction influence the outcome significantly.[13] Although the en bloc concept of adequacy of local excision has a sound basis in the surgical attack upon localized neoplastic disease, when applied to melanoma even this thesis is questionable. For example, Olsen has reported that

211

removal of the underlying fascia with the melanoma increases the likelihood of regional metastases.[3]

While such minor debates continue, adequate local excision for the given site and type of tumor remains the keystone of successful treatment of melanoma. Indeed, it is the very high success rate of this particular method that sets the stage for the argument to follow: What are the values and virtues of adjunctive methods of treatment in addition to local excision?

## Statement of the Problem

The problem to be debated is the role of treatment *in addition* to adequate local excision for primary intact melanoma. In a typical clinical setting, the primary tumor itself is either intact or has recently been excised; there is no evidence of satellitosis, and the regional lymph nodes on palpation do not appear to contain metastatic melanoma. The bulk of this discussion will pertain to the utilization of discontinuous elective regional lymph node dissection for melanoma, but there are obvious parallels to the frequent utilization of isolated chemotherapeutic perfusion of the extremity under similar circumstances.

To say that such questions can best be answered by a prospective, truly randomized trial is trite. As a matter of act, such a trial is indeed approaching an end, although it has been collected internationally and cooperatively in many centers. The preliminary results indicate that its conclusion will be consistent with the thesis to be developed here.

Worse than the lack of a prospective, randomized study on the addition or withholding of elective regional lymphadenectomy for melanoma is that the great majority of published comparisons are based upon clinically specious assumptions. It is common practice to report survival in terms of the microscopic state of lymph nodes when the nodes have already been excised, for better or for worse as the case may be. However, the information required is a comparison of results based upon the *clinical* status of the regional lymph nodes. Meaningful comparisons can only be made on the basis of clinical (preoperative) staging.

A valid comparison should proceed as follows, given the clinical setting just described:

1. The primary tumor is treated by adequate local excision, and the regional lymph node group, along with the overall health of the patient, is observed at reasonable intervals over the next few years. Should clinical signs suggesting possible regional metastatic melanoma be identified, the patient would then undergo a so-called "therapeutic" regional lymph node dissection. Analyses of outcome for the patients would be made at periods of 5 and 10 years.

2. Similarly, clinically staged melanoma should be treated alternately by adequate local excision and elective regional lymph node dissection performed simultaneously. The ultimate outcome of that therapeutic encounter would be similarly determined.

# Biologic Behavior of Melanoma

The true biologic behavior of malignant melanoma must be considered in some detail. Many malignant melanomas may be adequately treated and cured by the primary biopsy procedure. Unquestionably, local treatment does cure a significant majority of malignant melanomas. Those patients not cured by adequate local excision often die of disseminated disease without ever having gone through a clinically obvious stage of regional lymphatic metastasis. In other words, some patients initially have an isolated primary melanoma and subsequently appear with disseminated cerebral, pulmonary, or hepatic metastases without ever having shown clinical indications of regional lymph node metastases.

Two explanations are obvious: (1) Melanoma may metastasize widely, bypassing lymph nodes. Careful studies have shown that tumor cells may bypass lymph nodes, even when they are injected into the afferent lymphatics.[4,5] (2) Subclinical metastases to the regional lymph nodes occur but are never apparent to the examiner.

As is true with so many tumors, we find a bimodal distribution with respect to biologic behavior. First, a substantial majority of melanomas (60 to 70 per cent) are cured by virtually any kind of adequate local therapy. By contrast, the biologically unfavorable melanoma (20 to 30 per cent) cannot be cured by any measures presently available.

The remaining group of melanomas, representing 5 to 20 per cent, depending upon the study and the population sampled, is the only conceivable group in which the outcome could be influenced by treatment more aggressive than adequate local excision. At the same time, one must realize that only 50 per cent or less of these individuals (with nodes clinically normal and histologically positive) are salvaged by elective lymphadenectomy. Even in terms of the data most favorable to routine node dissection, only an additional 10 per cent can be cured, and this benefit is counterbalanced by the morbidity and mortality resulting from the node dissection in the full 100 per cent of patients who must be so treated.

On the basis of an older concept of primary cancer metastatic first to regional lymph nodes and only then mechanically capable of wider dissemination, Ackerman and Del Regato incisively stated that the period of lymph node "arrest" for malignant melanoma is very brief indeed.[6] This concept is clinically useful: very few patients with malignant melanoma are likely to be seen by the clinician at the precise time when melanoma has metastasized from the primary tumor to the immediate regional lymph nodes *but not beyond.* Under such unusual circumstances, the disease is potentially curable by adequate local excision plus elective regional lymph node dissection, whereas any lesser treatment would at best incur the risk of leaving those lymph node metastases in place until clinically palpable disease was apparent. Another biologic factor often ignored in consideration of melanoma is that even when a patient develops signs of clinical lymph node metastases, particularly if some time has passed since treatment of the primary tumor, he still has a reasonably good prognosis following node removal. As a whole, such individuals have a 5-year survival rate which exceeds 25 per cent, reflecting some degree of biologic selection in that these patients have manifested their nodal metastases well *after* the primary tumor has been treated and at the subsequent time have no evidence of disseminated disease.

## The Old Arguments

Patients who have undergone adequate local excision and elective regional lymph node dissection and who have no microscopic melanoma in those excised lymph nodes are said to have a better prognosis than patients who have undergone adequate local excision alone. Isn't this only logical? Indeed, patients having the lymph node dissection and having nodes that are microscopically free of melanoma are a clinically *and* pathologically selected group very likely to do well. On the contrary, those patients who have been treated by adequate local excision inevitably include some patients (±20 per cent) who have an adverse determinant of survival—clinically occult metastatic deposits in their regional nodes.

One might even argue that this rate or incidence of clinically occult metastases is in itself sufficient reason for aggressive treatment of clinically normal regional nodes. However, fewer than half the patients with occult lymph node metastases occurring simultaneously with the clinical appearance of their melanoma are then salvaged, even when treated most aggressively (Table 1). Indeed, one may look at this group as one with a biologically relatively poor prognosis.

A similarly specious comparison is that which arises when one of the compared groups (patients having adequate local excision and elective regional lymphadenectomy for nodes proving to be microscopically normal on pathologic examination) proves to have a better prognosis than the group of patients who are treated by adequate local excision, observed, and thereafter found to have metastatic melanoma in the regional lymph nodes and are then treated by delayed therapeutic lymphadenectomy. Here again, the latter group is entirely noncomparable (and bears a poorer prognosis) to the extent that the patients' regional nodes are likely to harbor occult melanoma. In either case, lymph node dissection serves more as an indicator of the extent of disease than as an agent influencing the outcome of the illness. Of course, one must always ask whether obtaining that information is worthwhile in and of itself. Because such adjunctive treatments of melanoma have to date not been shown to be unequivocally effective, one must weigh the mortality and the morbidity resulting from the additional isolated lymph node dissection against the value of such information about outcome.

A further serious criticism of the proponents of routine elective lymph node dissection is that there are so few data available concerning the early and late morbidity and mortality associated with such undertakings. Two arguments are often proposed by individuals who support the frequent use of elective lymph node dissection for cancer. The first is that morbidity is minimal and mortality is absent. Having been privileged to work at the side

TABLE 1. Collected Data Regarding Objective Comparison of the Value of Elective Regional Lymphadenectomy*

| Parameter | Site of Primary Melanoma | | |
| --- | --- | --- | --- |
| | All Excluding Eye | Extremities | Lower Extremity |
| $N_x$ — remain well after local excision alone | 0.66 386/644 patients | 0.70 146/207 patients | 0.70 113/161 patients |
| $N_y$ — develop operable regional nodal metastases without further dissemination | 0.25 123/487 | 0.19 12/62 | 0.19 12/62 |
| $N_z$ — develop unresectable regional node metastases without further dissemination | 0.04 1/125 | No data | No data |
| $N_{dm}$ — develop disseminated metastases without clinical regional metastatic lymphadenopathy | 0.15 — | 0.16 16/101 | 0.14 9/62 |
| $N_{total}$† | 1.00 | 1.05 | 1.03 |
| $S_e$ — survival at 5 years for patients undergoing elective regional lymphadenectomy with microscopic metastatic melanoma | 0.48 113/233 | 0.39 9/23 | 0.44 4/9 |
| $S_d$ — survival at 5 years for late (metachronous metastases) therapeutic lymphadenectomy | 0.39 105/271 | 0.29 31/107 | 0.29 24/83 |
| $M_t$ — hospital deaths, elective lymphadenectomy | — | — | 0.015 12/791 |
| $M_b$ — early and late morbidity, elective lymphadenectomy | — | — | 0.33 |

*Modified from Polk, H. C., Jr., and Linn, B. S.: Selective regional lymphadenectomy for melanoma: a mathematical aid to clinical judgment. (Table I.) Ann. Surg. *174*:402, 1971.

†May exceed 1.00 because of data derived partially from different reports and the small numbers of patients in some groups.

of many superior surgeons over a long period, I have never yet been fortunate enough to encounter any surgeon who can do anything to anyone with any frequency without the ultimate occurrence of mortality or morbidity in some form or other. As a matter of fact, if one studies the collected data regarding certain kinds of isolated elective regional lymph node dissections, one notes a measurable hospital mortality rate of about 1.5 per cent (Table 1) as well as substantial early and late morbidity for dissection of some regional lymph node chains.[7]

The second thesis often promulgated by the dissectionists is that melanoma is a rapidly aggressive malignant disease, justifying any form of operative treatment. The available data do not support this, and in view of current knowledge of tumor biology, this is an unacceptable attitude.

TABLE 2.   Calculation of Net Benefit for Lower Extremity

| Harmed by Regular Practice of Regional Lymphadenectomy | Benefited by Regular Practice of Regional Lymphadenectomy |
|---|---|
| $N_x(M_t + f \times M_b)$[*] <br> $0.70(0.015 + 0.1 \times 0.33)$ <br> $0.0336$ | $N_y(S_e - S_d) + N_z(S_e)$ <br> $0.19(0.44 - 0.29) + 0.004(0.44)$ <br> $0.0303$ |
| 34/1000 patients | 30/1000 patients |

[*] Parameters defined in Table 1.

## *Objective Comparison of Clinical Stages*

Some years ago, we attempted to develop a valid comparision of clinical variables for melanoma, trying to define data from the literature which would allow us to develop a reliable method of outcome prediction.[8, 9] Both of these undertakings were handicapped by the fact that in the great majority of papers published, *clinical* staging of melanoma is so often sacrificed for microscopic staging that valid observations have to be made on a relatively small number of individuals (i.e., less than 2000). This work is summarized in Tables 1, 2, and 3. As published previously, this material indicates that the *net benefit* of the routine practice of elective regional lymph node dissection for primary malignant melanoma is negligible in light of the outcome of primary treatment by adequate local excision with subsequent treatment of clinically detected regional lymph node metastases.

Even if one considers different substitutional values for certain subjectively determined factors, the effect, whether beneficial or detrimental, of elective regional node dissection is still negligible (Table 3). For example, if one chooses to ignore morbidity, holding that any conceivable kind of morbidity is acceptable in order to treat a malignant neoplasm effectively, the net benefit is to 2 of 100 individuals, with the other 98 patients undergoing the treatment with no net effect on the disease beyond that achieved by adequate local excision.

TABLE 3.   Substitution of Extremes of Data[*]

| Data Referable to Regular Elective Lymphadenectomy | $N_x$ | $N_y$ | $N_z$ | $M_t$ | $M_b$ | $f$[‡] | $S_e$ | $S_d$ | Net Effect per 1000 Patients |
|---|---|---|---|---|---|---|---|---|---|
| Most Favorable | 0.6 | 0.19 | 0.1 | 0.0 | 0.0 | 0.01 | 0.48 | 0.29 | 96 Helped |
| Least Favorable | 0.7 | 0.25 | 0.0 | 0.015 | 0.33 | 0.2 | 0.45 | 0.39 | 70 Harmed |

[*] Modified from Polk, H. C., Jr., and Linn, B. S.: Selective regional lymphadenectomy for melanoma: a mathematical aid to clinical judgment. (Table II.) Ann. Surg. *174*:402, 1971.

[†] Parameters defined in Table 1.

[‡] Relative weighting or importance of morbidity with respect to hospital death; e.g., 0.01 implies that 100 complications are required in order to equal the significance of one death.

We assumed that there must be some place for elective lymph node dissection for melanoma. Indeed, we tried clinically to delineate further that group of patients, no matter how small, who were in the stage of "lymph node arrest" at the time melanoma was discovered. For this purpose, based on a multivariate analysis of variance of our experience at the University of Miami, we tried to define whether any characteristics would indicate the clinical likelihood of lymph node metastatic disease with such frequency as to allow the selection of those patients for elective lymphadenectomy. Although the statistical techniques were powerful and took into consideration most of the known parameters (age, sex, coexisting disease, and diameter, depth, and cellular aggressiveness of the melanoma), no parameter by itself was an adequate indicator. However, it was possible to predict an adverse outcome in terms of *ultimate death* from melanoma and to develop, based on discriminant function analysis, weighting factors for each of the six variables just described which produced a prediction accuracy of 95 per cent in terms of survival or death from melanoma. These data proved accurate when applied to the Miami population from which they were derived, but subsequent application to patients at the University of Louisville under the supervision of Condict Moore and at the Queensland Melanoma Project under the direction of Davis and MacLeod were not satisfactory.[10] Indeed, these differing patient populations would require changes in the coefficients to retain applicability.

Stated another way, these coefficients were quite accurate for the patient population studied, but they cannot be applied with the same precision (95 per cent) to other populations. Perhaps all the patient groups could be pooled together and more powerful and meaningful coefficients developed so that one could make a prospective and objective assessment of the probability of an adverse outcome for each melanoma patient. Given the patient with an extremely good prognosis, regional node dissection would appear contraindicated; those few patients with modest-to-poor prognoses would be prime candidates for as aggressive a treatment as could be tolerated.

Better yet, these six parameters possibly could be improved by the substitution of the Clark method of histologic staging of melanoma and perhaps strikingly so by the assessment of some immunologic variable(s). That malignant melanoma is most susceptible to immunologic manipulation has become abundantly clear in the last 4 years.[11, 12] Therefore, some expression of the immunologic responsiveness of the host is perhaps one of the missing links preventing more nearly uniform application of this concept.

Regardless of the reservations expressed, the consensus of a recent international symposium on melanoma[13] and the opinions of other thoughtful investigators[14] were strongly in favor of observation rather than routine dissection on an elective basis of seemingly normal regional lymph nodes after adequate local primary treatment of the melanoma. Indeed, only the American groups seem to be well represented among those who felt that there was a place for the so-called prophylactic or elective lymphadenectomy. Increasing rationality is apparent among even the Americans when more recent studies are considered.[15]

## *Special Local Considerations*

We would be remiss to close this discussion without pointing out some very special local considerations. For example, of all the regional nodal sites for elective dissection for melanoma, the axilla is associated with the lowest figures for early and late morbidity and for mortality. However, data in virtually every series show that melanomas of the upper extremity are those which are associated with the most favorable prognosis. Conversely, the elective treatment of such lymph node groups would be least beneficial. Again we have the paradox: the adjunctive treatment is safer but seemingly less necessary biologically. By contrast, elective groin dissection, even when confined to the superficial lymph node group, is associated with measurable mortality and significant early and late morbidity.

The decision against routine elective lymph node dissection with some truncal melanomas is, of course, even easier. In many situations, this would require, in terms of reasonable probability of metastases, the dissection of two or more lymph node groups. Because the morbidity is additive and because of the mortality associated with such undertakings, the only rational choice for patients so afflicted with melanoma in this particularly adverse site is apparently to watch and wait. However, should the primary tumor overlie or be extremely close to a regional lymph node unit, elective dissection would have a sounder basis, particularly in view of the poorer over-all prognosis for truncal melanoma. Although we can readily accept true en bloc, in-continuity dissection, the ludicrous selection of a 2-inch strip of skin from the shin to the groin as the pathway of choice for intracutaneous melanoma is a travesty of both biology and common sense. Fortunately, this concept has not recently been revived!

## *In-Transit Metastases*

Another point carefully excluded from this evaluation has been the role of the so-called in-transit metastases (those trapped between the primary site and the proximate lymph node area). One may view in-transit disease as a beneficial or adverse outcome. Consider the situation for which we are often asked to see patients for possible chemotherapeutic perfusion: The individual has had adequate local excision of his primary tumor and an elective lymph node dissection with no demonstrable metastases; two years later he develops a rash of in-transit intracutaneous metastases between the primary site and the dissected lymph node chain. Many would argue that the in-transit melanoma would have never developed had the nodes not been dissected and that one would have been capable of dealing with this situation by delayed therapeutic regional node dissection, with an anticipated cure rate in excess of 25 per cent. This argument is based, of course, on the premise that in-transit melanomas represent a failure of the primary treatment. An alternative interpretation is that by virtue of the lymph stasis produced in the extremity, the regional lymph node dissection will have trapped the melanoma within the extremity and delayed widespread dissemination — a beneficial effect.

In-transit metastases are infinitely more common among individuals who have undergone elective node dissection and are strikingly less common in patients who have been treated without such adjunctive measures. It is my perception that in-transit disease represents a failure of treatment and is an additional reason for not performing routine or regular elective regional lymphadectomy for melanoma.

## *Perfusion*

Chemotherapeutic perfusion is an example of another form of adjunctive treatment, probably subject to the same kind of analysis. The problem here is defining the changing nature of the treatment. Unlike dissections, which are for all intents and purposes the same, changing insight and technology with respect to perfusion have precluded its "standardization." For example, chemotherapeutic perfusion at normothermic levels with a single drug and good isolation is associated with minimal adverse effects.[16, 17] In a series of slightly more than 100 patients receiving such treatment, the author observed only *four serious* complications and no deaths. However, there is reliable evidence emerging from the continuing studies of McBride[18] and Stehlin and co-workers[19] that hyperthermic perfusion with two or three drugs is infinitely more effective and therefore more beneficial. However, the early data from the application of these methods indicate a respective increase in morbidity and mortality over the simpler form of therapy. There appears to be very strong evidence that perfusion chemotherapy reduces the frequency of in-transit metastases.

Without going through the same type of analysis for isolated chemotherapeutic perfusion for malignant melanoma, we have found it a safe and useful method (often in lieu of amputation) for the palliative and possibly the curative treatment of individuals who develop extensive in-transit disease. Objective regression after "therapeutic" perfusions have been frequent but of short duration when single-drug perfusion was accomplished. We have opted not to employ this treatment in the elective adjunctive management of a primary intact melanoma. Believing that the same biologically based objections to routine dissection apply to perfusion, we have concluded that for so-called Stage I disease, particularly of relatively superficial levels of invasion (e.g., Clark level I and II), the adverse effects of vigorous perfusion chemotherapy in our hands will ultimately be greater than its benefits.

A study of its overall effects, however, makes perfusion appear somewhat more beneficial. Early morbidity is probably increased in the perfused patient as compared to the individual undergoing groin dissection, but late morbidity is reduced strikingly in the perfused patient. Although neither adjunctive technique seems routinely indicated for superficial Stage I melanoma, perfusion may prove to be the better choice. on balance.

## *Other Considerations*

We have deliberately avoided a critical imponderable in this consideration of treatment directed toward regional lymph nodes: the seemingly critical role of such tissues in the genesis of an immune tumor-specific response to the primary melanoma.[20, 21] Current concepts would indicate that routine excision of nonmetastatic regional nodes might unfavorably alter host immune responsiveness, representing a further indictment of elective node dissections.

Yet another consideration is the several gradations of surgical aggressiveness, many of which apply to other forms of cancer. Clearly, it would be interesting to see what treatment would be recommended were the more extensive operations not associated with substantially greater "allowable" physicians' fees. Indeed, the treatment of a melanoma by adequate local excision, even with a skin graft, warrants a small-to-modest fee, whereas a major lymph node dissection itself commands a several-fold greater fee. Even in situations in which fees may not prejudice individual decisions, one must consider the extent to which professional identities and reputations are staked upon championing a particular adjunctive method of therapy. It may be that either or both of these factors influence the surgeon's decision to opt for elective node dissection more often than might be the case were his actions not so influenced.

## *Precis*

Adequate local excision is the keystone of melanoma management. We do alter adequacy when we consider the function of the body part afflicted; length and width of margin need not exceed 5 centimeters, and less is often satisfactory. In regard to depth, the excision of fascia has been a common practice, but based upon Olsen's data,[3] it is presently being avoided in the extremities.

Elective node dissection should seldom, if ever, be applied in the treatment of a patient with Stage I disease. It is, however, a beneficial palliative and therapeutic maneuver in some patients with advanced stages of melanoma. Deep groin or iliac node dissection is never beneficial and is a questionable triumph of technique over rationale.

Incontinuity excision of the primary melanoma with elective dissection of clinically normal lymph nodes *remote* from the primary site is a biologic farce.

Minor amputations are justifiable in the treatment of melanoma; major ones, almost never!

Adjunctive isolated chemotherapeutic perfusion at present is probably not warranted for superficial Stage I disease but should be a cornerstone of the management of more advanced melanoma of the extremities.[22]

The prime objective in current clinical research on melanoma should be the identification, by means such as we have initiated, of patients likely not to be cured by local excision alone. These individuals should then undergo aggressive operative treatment, including all adjunctive modalities presently under study. By not subjecting the 70 per cent of patients cured by local excision alone to the morbidity and mortality of the adjunctive methods, we will achieve the fundamental surgical goal for most illnesses — true biologic individualization of treatment.

## References

1. Newsome, J. F.: Physician Concepts of Survival of Various Cancers. Scientific Exhibit, Tenth International Union against Cancer Meeting, Houston, Texas, May 22–29, 1970.
2. Epstein, E., Bragg, K., and Linden, G.: Biopsy and prognosis of malignant melanoma. J.A.M.A. 208:1369, 1969.
3. Olsen, G.: The malignant melanoma of the skin. Acta Chir. Scand. Suppl. 365:1, 1966.
4. Pressman, J. J., and Simon, M. B.: Experimental evidence of direct communications between lymph nodes and veins. Surg. Gynecol. Obstet. 113:537, 1961.
5. Fisher, B., and Fisher, E. R.: The interrlationship of hematogenous and lymphatic tumor cell dissemination. Surg. Gynecol. Obstet. 122:791, 1966.
6. Ackerman, L. V., and Del Regato, J. A.: Cancer, Diagnosis, Treatment and Prognosis. St. Louis, The C. V. Mosby Co., 1947, pp. 126–181.
7. Knutson, C. O., and Spratt, J. S.: Unpublished data.
8. Polk, H. C., Jr., Cohn, J. D., and Clarkson, J. G.: An appraisal of elective regional lymphadenectomy for melanoma. Curr. Top. Surg. Res. 1:121, 1969.
9. Polk, H. C., Jr., and Linn, B. S.: Selective regional lymphadenectomy for melanoma: a mathematical aid to clinical judgment. Ann. Surg. 174:402, 1971.
10. Polk, H. C., Jr., and Linn, B. S.: Letter to the Editor. Ann. Surg. 180:257, 1974.
11. Seiger, H. F., Shingleton, W. W., Metzgar, R. S., Buckley, C. E., III, and Bergoc, P. M.: Immunotherapy in patients with melanoma. Ann. Surg. 178:352, 1973.
12. Morton, D. L., Eilber, F. R., Holmes, E. C., Hunt, J. S., Ketcham, A. S., Silverstein, M. J., and Sparks, F. C.: BCG immunotherapy of malignant melanoma: summary of a seven-year experience. Ann. Surg. 180:635, 1974.
13. McCarthy, W. H. (ed.): Melanoma and Skin Cancer: Proceedings of the International Cancer Conference. Sidney, Australia, March 13–17, 1972, pp. 367–451.
14. Regional lymph nodes in malignant melanoma. (Editorial.) Lancet 1:1412, 1966.
15. Fraser, D. G., Bull, J. G., Jr., and Dunphy, J. E.: Malignant melanoma and coexisting malignant neoplasms. Am. J. Surg. 122:169, 1971.
16. Creech, O., Jr., Krementz, E. T., Ryan, R. F., and Winblad, J. N.: Chemotherapy of cancer: regional perfusion utilizing an extracorporeal circuit. Ann. Surg. 148:616, 1958.
17. Krementz, E. T., Creech, O., Jr., and Ryan, R. F.: Evaluation of chemotherapy of cancer by regional perfusion. Cancer 20:834, 1967.
18. McBride, C. M.: Advanced melanoma of the extremities: treatment by isolation-perfusion with a triple drug combination. Arch. Surg. 101:122, 1970.
19. Stehlin, J. S., Jr., Smith, J. L., Jr., Jing, B. S., and Sherrin, D.: Melanomas of the extremities complicated by in-transit metastases. Surg. Gynecol. Obstet. 122:3, 1966.
20. Crile, G., Jr.: Rationale of simple mastectomy without radiation for clinical stage I cancer of the breast. Surg. Gynecol. Obstet. 120:975, 1965.
21. Mitchison, N. A.: Passive transfer of transplantation immunity. Proc. R. Soc. (Biol.) 142:72, 1954.
22. McBride, C. M., Sugarbaker, E. V., and Hickey, R. C.: Prophylactic isolation-perfusion as the primary therapy for invasive malignant melanoma of the limbs. Ann. Surg. 182:316, 1975.

# Operative Treatment of Malignant Melanoma of the Limbs

WALTER LAWRENCE, JR.
*Medical College of Virginia*

Therapeutic decisions in the management of malignant melanoma are often difficult because of limited clinical data to support a choice among the various options that are available to us. Unfortunately, opinions must be developed on the basis of retrospective evaluations of heterogeneous clinical populations with malignant melanoma, and the clinical and pathologic staging processes utilized in these series have been far from uniform. In view of the fact that this neoplasm is relatively infrequent, this lack of reliable resource data is not too surprising. Despite these limitations, an attempt will be made to address the most commonly raised questions regarding the surgical management of malignant melanoma of the limbs.

## The Role and Nature of the Biopsy

Biopsy to establish the diagnosis of malignant melanoma is essential before embarking on operative therapy since most of the lesions clinically suspicious of being melanoma require less aggressive operative excision than melanoma itself. The temptation to carry out wide excision of a "suspicious" lesion for diagnosis should definitely be avoided since the margins obtained will usually be less than desired if the lesion does prove to be a malignant melanoma and unnecessarily radical if the lesion proves to be something other than melanoma. As with most cancers, the appropriate treatment is best administered after a precise diagnosis has been made.

It is generally considered preferable to completely excise a suspicious skin lesion for biopsy if the possibility of melanoma exists. However, in a few patients, the actual size of the lesion might make this neither feasible nor practical, and despite frequently expressed opinions to the contrary, there is no strong evidence that a preliminary partial biopsy is prejudicial to the patient's prognosis.[1] The major problem with a limited biopsy is the distinct possibility that the judgment regarding the depth of the melanoma will be uncertain. This is a cause for concern since depth of invasion has a great effect on prognosis, making this limitation a significant one. We have even seen patients in whom biopsy of a portion of a lesion failed to reveal the area of malignant change that was present, but appropriate and careful selection of the biopsy site will usually prevent this error. If the diagnosis of melanoma is established, definitive treatment can be planned if the depth of invasion is more than "superficial" by one of the various classifications,[2, 3, 4, 5, 6] but a melanoma involving only the papillary dermis on partial biopsy may require additional sections after total excision of the primary lesion before all the necessary therapeutic decisions are made.

## The Character of the Local Excision After Diagnosis is Established

It is generally agreed that wide operative resection of the primary cutaneous melanoma is preferable to other means of aggressive local ablation since operative repair of the resulting defect, usually by skin graft procedures, is so easily accomplished. If other means of local ablation for control (such as irradiation, laser therapy, cryotherapy, or electrocoagulation) had a beneficial systemic effect, immunologic or otherwise, the choice of operative excision for the primary lesion would be in doubt. However, since at this time there are no convincing data to establish such additional advantages for other local therapies, "adequate" operative excision appears to be the treatment of choice.

### PRACTICAL GUIDELINES FOR ADEQUACY OF LOCAL EXCISION

For a specific lesion proved to be malignant melanoma, a minimal gross margin may indeed be "adequate," whereas a much wider and deeper excision might be required for another very similarly appearing lesion to avoid a local treatment failure. The extent of local spread is often difficult to determine by gross examination. However, the disability and the cosmetic defect produced by the scar of wide excision with split thickness graft for wound closure on an extremity is a limited "cost" for the patient in comparison to the gravity of the later "recurrence" occurring in some patients who are treated by a more limited margin. The result of what eventually proves to be an inadequate excision is generally so disastrous, from the standpoint of the limited effectiveness of secondary attempts to control the disease, that some degree of "over-treatment" of the local lesion seems justified.

Another argument for a wider margin of excision for malignant melanoma than we find acceptable for many other malignant skin neoplasms stems from the findings of Wong.[7] This microscopic study of the clinically unaffected epidermal surface surrounding some malignant melanomas demonstrated, using the dopa reaction, an increase in melanocytes, some of which were quite bizarre in both shape and size. These observations may well represent premalignant manifestations of melanoma. Local lymphatic extension of the primary lesion into the tissue immediately surrounding it is also a factor encouraging a "wide" margin, since this mode of spread is usually not clinically detectable and is only apparent on later histologic study of the final specimen.

### Size and Depth of Lesion

If one accepts wide excision as a reasonable concept for the local therapy for invasive malignant melanoma, how *wide* is actually "wide enough"? Clearly, this must be an arbitrary decision that for practical reasons cannot be made on histologic grounds prior to excision, but a 4 to 5 cm. margin in all lateral directions from the periphery of the lesion is generally accepted as a good "rule of thumb" for invasive melanoma on an extremity. Compromise regarding this arbitrary margin is both reasonable and necessary in some anatomic locations (such as a lesion on the digit or on the face), but this recommended margin is an appropriate strategy for most primary melanomas on the extremities, since the actual size of the skin graft is of minimal practical importance. A skin graft is actually required for closure after excision in most locations on the extremity anyway, since primary closure is not feasible, even with smaller margins, without extensive and usually undesirable rotation of skin flaps.

How *deep* should the excision be to be considered adequate? It has been frequently noted that the spread of invasive melanoma is usually limited to the integument and subcutaneous tissue and invades the underlying fascia only in rare instances. Removing the fascial layer underlying the lesion itself may assist in accomplishing containment of the depth of invasion, particularly with larger, deeply ulcerating melanomas, but excision of the underlying fascia can hardly be considered a necessary requirement for all such lesions. The report by Olsen[8] addressed itself to this point, and this study actually appeared to demonstrate more difficulty with subsequent lymphatic spread when the deep fascia underlying the lesion was excised. Although Olsen's interpretation of the data might be open to question on the basis of pathologic stage rather than operative procedure (vis-à-vis cause and effect), these data do demonstrate that the underlying fascia can be safely preserved in many instances unless the melanoma infiltrates deeply.

The relationship of a more precise histologic classification of the depth of invasion (such as that described by Clark[4] and Breslow[5]) to the extent of local excision required is difficult to establish at this time. The depth of excision will normally be to, or through, the underlying fascia in any case, but it is conceivable that a more limited width of excision might be justifiable for a more "superficial" lesion, on the basis of a lower frequency of lymphatic extension. On the extremity, however, the same arbitrary skin margin described for invasive lesions seems indicated for the more superficial lesions for the theoretical and practical reasons outlined previously.

There are a few locations, particularly on the digits, where underlying soft tissue or bone may be involved in close proximity to the melanoma. Amputation serves as an appropriate excision in these specific instances.

## Elective Primary Regional Lymph Node Dissection in the Treatment of Invasive Malignant Melanoma of the Extremity

Malignant melanoma has demonstrated distal spread by both hematogenous and lymphatic routes. Although this is well recognized, most questions regarding surgical management of melanoma center around the regional lymphatics, since control of hematogenous spread is currently beyond our therapeutic ability.

### Presence of Clinically Palpable Nodes

If clinically palpable nodes are present in the lymph node basin draining the primary site of the melanoma at the time of initial diagnosis, most surgeons favor operative excision of these lymph nodes. It is noteworthy, however, that long-term survival after regional lymph node dissection in this clinical setting is extremely low (approximately 10 per cent) if the clinical diagnosis is histologically confirmed[9, 10] (Table 1). This could be interpreted as an indication that the synchronous finding of regional lymph node involvement is a clue that there is distant metastatic disease present, that local lymph node dissection is inadequate when lymphatic involvement is so grossly apparent, or both. At any rate, clinically apparent regional lymph node involvement present at the time of diagnosis of melanoma is surely an indication for careful "staging" procedures designed to detect the spread of melanoma beyond the limb itself. In addition to standard laboratory and radiographic studies, a meticulous search for distant disease, including the use of bone marrow biopsy and laparotomy, is probably indicated before application of aggressive local therapy to the primary site and the regional lymph node basin. Lymphangiography has not been useful for this purpose,

TABLE 1.  Prognosis of Cutaneous Malignant Melanoma in Terms of Regional Lymph Node Status*

| Clinical Examination | Microscopic Examination | 5–Year Survival |
|---|---|---|
| Not palpable | No metastasis | 71% |
| Not palpable | Metastasis | 53% ⎫ 19% |
| Clinically "positive" | Metastasis | 10% ⎭ |

*From McNeer, G., and Das Gupta, T.: Prognosis in malignant melanoma. Surgery 56:512, 1964.

as the findings are misleading and the technique is certainly less precise than direct examination at the time of laparotomy.

If regional lymph nodes are clinically involved, and if more proximal spread of disease has not been detected by a careful search of the type described, operative excision of the regional lymph nodes is indicated in most instances. However, other factors, such as the age and general condition of the patient, play a role in this decision since the very low 5-year survival rates achieved by conventional regional lymph node dissection in this clinical situation lead us to favor lymph node excision by major amputation if both patient status and disease status allow this consideration. This approach would naturally require confirmation of involvement of the clinically enlarged node or nodes. Data obtained from a major amputation experience in a highly selected series at Memorial Hospital for Cancer and Allied Diseases (New York)[11] demonstrate reasonable survival rates (approximately 33 per cent) under these special circumstances and they are the basis for this approach in a small number of patients (Table 2).

## Regional Lymph Node Dissection Without Apparent Clinical Involvement of Regional Lymph Nodes

Whether regional lymph node dissection should be performed if there is no apparent clinical involvement of regional lymph nodes in a patient with malignant melanoma of the extremity is the most frequently raised question in regard to the surgical management of malignant melanoma and is a very difficult one to answer to everyone's satisfaction. Major factors affecting the surgeon's decision for elective lymph node dissection include: (1) whether the yield of histologically positive lymph nodes is worthwhile in terms of the morbidity and potential mortality associated with the procedure and (2) whether or not the prognostic advantage of an elective dissection is sufficiently great to choose it over a later therapeutic dissection after palpable lymph nodes appear.

If the primary lesion is "superficial" (i.e., levels I and II in Clark's classification),[4] the incidence of lymphatic spread is certainly too low to warrant the morbidity produced by regional lymph node dissection. Earlier reports[2] demonstrate less than 5 per cent incidence of lymphatic spread with malignant melanomas having dermal invasion limited to the upper one third of the corium (or less than 1 mm. invasion). More complete clinicopathologic data

TABLE 2. Major Amputations for Recurrent and Metastatic Melanoma*

| Extremity | Number of Cases | Survival at 5 Years with No Evidence of Disease |
|---|---|---|
| Lower | 46 | 16 |
| Upper | 8 | 2 |
| Total | 54 | 18 (33%) |

*From McPeak, C. J., McNeer, G. P., Whiteley, W. H., and Booher, R. J.: Amputation for melanoma of the extremity. Surgery 54:426, 1964.

presently being accumulated by the Melanoma Cooperative Group and others will probably substantiate this range with even greater precision. This yield of involved nodes would not appear to justify the morbidity that is associated with standard regional lymph node dissections in either the axilla or the groin.

If the primary malignant melanoma is not "superficial" and is truly invasive by most histologic means of classification (i.e., involvement of reticular dermis or deeper), the incidence of histologic regional lymph node spread is considerably higher than noted in patients with the more superficial lesions. Retrospective data from Memorial Hospital for Cancer and Allied Diseases (New York)[12] demonstrate a 25 per cent incidence of histologic melanoma in patients thought to have no neoplastic involvement on clinical examination of the regional lymph nodes. The incidence of nodal involvement is essentially equal in the upper and lower extremities (Table 1). Further review of these data demonstrate a 5-year survival rate of approximately 50 per cent in this group with clinically negative, histologically positive lymph nodes treated by standard elective regional lymph node dissection. Retrospective data from results of later therapeutic, rather than elective, lymph node dissection were less favorable (i.e., 20 per cent 5-year survival from the time of initial diagnosis). Admitting the vagaries of retrospective examination of nonrandomized patient populations, one can still estimate the potential advantage of regional lymph node dissection from this information. In more simple terms, 4 of 16 patients with nonpalpable nodes will have a possible advantage from elective lymph node dissection, and the particular patients with these clinical and histologic findings will have 5-year survival rates approximately twice that which would have been achieved by a later therapeutic dissection. Using these approximations we can predict that 1 of 16 patients in the original elective node dissection group will have benefited in terms of survival, in that this patient would not have survived if lymph node dissection had been deferred until nodes were clinically palpable. However, 12 of the 16 will have had regional lymph node dissections without real therapeutic benefit since they would have only histologically negative nodes in the specimen. Elective regional lymph node dissection does have a therapeutic advantage, then, in terms of the potential of the modest increase in survival rate, but this is not as striking an advantage as has been implied by some proponents of elective node dissection.[10, 13, 14] More recent data using levels of invasion by Clark's classification tend to diminish the likelihood of therapeutic advantage from elective dissection for level III and increase this advantage over the previously mentioned estimates for levels IV and V.[15]

Are the morbidity and mortality associated with elective regional lymph node dissection justifiable on the basis of this small potential increase in survival rate for this selected group of patients? The mortality associated with regional lymph node dissection is not a real deterrent. The morbidity associated with axillary lymph node dissection is so low that it would clearly appear to be worthwhile if these treatment results outlined are true estimates of the situation. I personally believe that a therapeutic advantage of elective regional lymph node dissection in this range also justifies wide superficial groin dissection in the young or middle-aged and otherwise healthy patients as well, but the added morbidity associated with groin dissection makes this a more marginal choice, particularly in the older patient or the patient disabled by other problems. I do not include the extraperitoneal iliac portion of the node dissection above Cloquet's node in elective node dissection for lower extremity melanoma since this extension of the procedure for lower extremity lesions is prognostic but rarely, if ever, therapeutic, and morbidity is slightly increased without apparent benefit in terms of survival. The majority of surgeons probably favor this general approach, but it is difficult to fault the surgeon who argues that the morbidity associated with an adequate elective groin dissection outweighs the therapeutic advantages, on the basis of the statistics that have been available to us.[16] As histologic staging of malignant melanoma becomes generally employed, elective node dissection will probably be reserved for levels IV and V by most surgeons.

## Excision of the Skin and Subcutaneous Tissue Between the Primary Malignant Melanoma and the Regional Lymph Nodes

Although it might seem a sound theoretical concept to include the tissues containing the intervening lymphatic channels at the time of excision of a malignant melanoma and the regional lymph nodes, there are no data to substantiate the necessity for this. The "negative" data of Shah and Goldsmith[17] from Memorial Hospital for Cancer and Allied Diseases (New York) are convincing. From a retrospective comparison of discontinuous and incontinuity procedures (whether the node dissection was simultaneous or delayed), they could show no benefit from incontinuity procedures in patients with Stage I or II melanoma of the skin (Table 3). Nevertheless, individual patients treated by discontinuous lymph node dissection who sub-

TABLE 3.   Lack of Benefit from Incontinuity Lymph Node Dissection for Malignant Melanoma*

| Type of Dissection | Simultaneous | | Delayed | |
|---|---|---|---|---|
| | *Number of Patients* | *5-Year Survival* | *Number of Patients* | *5-Year Survival* |
| Stage I | | | | |
| Incontinuity | 63 | 48(76%) | 165 | 128(78%) |
| Discontinuous | 15 | 11(73%) | 53 | 40(75%) |
| Stage II | | | | |
| Incontinuity | 53 | 22(42%) | 167 | 70(42%) |
| Discontinuous | 20 | 7(35%) | 195 | 80(41%) |

*From Shah, J. P., and Goldsmith, H.: Incontinuity versus discontinuous lymph node dissection for malignant melanoma. Cancer 26:610, 1970.

sequently develop satellite nodules in the intervening tissue between the two operative incisions are often presented as examples of the need for incontinuity procedures. However, to include all the lymphatic channels present in this specimen of intervening tissue would usually require a much wider resection of tissue than is usually considered anatomically feasible unless the primary lesion is in very close proximity to the lymph node basin. Being realistic, we should probably reserve the incontinuity approach for melanomas that are very close to the regional lymph nodes, particularly if the regional nodes are not clinically involved.

For some operative procedures, the incontinuity procedure may actually have a technical advantage, even if the distance is too great to really envisage a total excision of the intervening lymphatics between the two sites. This should not be misinterpreted by the surgeon as a therapeutic curative advantage, however, unless he is prepared to remove a massive segment of intervening skin and subcutaneous tissue or perform total integumentectomy as has been described by Hueston.[18] The author has no experience with this approach, but it may have merit in selected patients with clinically involved regional lymph nodes. If the regional lymph nodes are clinically involved and the primary lesion is on the distal part of the extremity, the statements made earlier about major amputation are also worthy of consideration. Amputation is truly an incontinuity procedure for melanomas more distally located on the extremity, but data are insufficient to establish its superiority over the procedures in which only the skin and subcutaneous tissues of the extremity are excised.

## Additional Indications for Consideration of Amputation for Melanoma of the Extremity

Subungual lesions are in close proximity to bone and primary digital amputation is the only way to achieve an adequate local resection. This may also be true of other sites on the digits, but melanoma is rarely in close enough proximity to bone at other sites on the extremity to raise the consideration of amputation.

Another group of patients in whom amputation should be considered are those who develop recurrent melanoma on the extremity following local excision with regional lymph node dissection. Lymphatic dissection often seems to temporarily localize the recurrence and delay more proximal spread of the disease. Major amputation is justified for this clinical problem in carefully selected patients if a clearly adequate operative margin can be accomplished by this approach. Obviously, a patient with gross nodules anywhere near the proposed amputation site is clearly unsuitable for this approach. A meticulous search for distant metastasis, using bone marrow biopsy and laparotomy if necessary, is also essential prior to embarking on amputation in such patients. Other factors such as age, general condition of the patient, time interval since treatment of the primary lesion, and the presence or absence of distant metastases all play a role in this decision.

With some care in patient selection, approximately one third of these patients subjected to major amputation will survive 5 years without recurrence
or metastasis.[11] This statistical result is clearly better than that achieved by
palliative treatment with either regional or systemic chemotherapy and these
are the only other options that are available for this clinical problem, with
the possible exception of the integumentectomy approach mentioned previously.[18]

## Adjunctive Chemotherapy for Primary Treatment of Malignant Melanoma of the Limb

In 1959, Creech and his associates[19] first described regional chemotherapy using extracorporeal perfusion for the management of recurrent malignant melanoma of the extremities. In view of previously disappointing
results with systemic chemotherapy at that time, this method of palliative
treatment became quite popular for recurrent melanoma clinically limited
to the extremity. Some patients have had striking responses to this short-
term high concentration of chemotherapeutic agent, the most frequently
employed and dependable agent being phenylalanine mustard (PAM).
(Combinations of drugs are said to be even more effective.) Early striking
results with palliative perfusion for melanoma then led to the application of
this technique as an adjuvant to the primary operative therapy of curable
melanoma on the extremity. Extensive experience with this approach by
Stehlin[20] and by Rochlin[21] has failed to yield data that demonstrate results
from this approach that are superior to operative treatment alone.[21] Although
some surgeons use perfusion as an adjuvant to primary excisional therapy, I
do not believe that the data available at this time substantiate this approach.
There has been no prospective clinical trial completed which could definitively answer this question, and this approach cannot be recommended for
routine surgical use at this time.

Systemic chemotherapy as an adjuvant to local operative therapy (with
or without lymph node dissection) is an appealing concept for the improvement of treatment results in melanoma, just as it is for many other "solid
tumors" in man. The same is true for nonspecific immunotherapy (i.e.,
bacille Calmette Guérin [BCG], Corynebacterium parvum [C. parvum]) for
"curable" melanoma. The only convincing evidence of benefit thus far from
such adjuncts to "curative" therapy is limited to those cancers in which recurrent disease also has a high response to systemic chemotherapy, particularly tumors in the pediatric age group. Benefit must be demonstrated on
prospective, well-planned, randomized clinical trials before this approach
can be recommended for general use in the treatment of melanoma. On the
other hand, these or other adjunctive approaches are currently the major
hope for improvement in our results from the standard surgical approach that
has been presented. Surgeons should follow ongoing, well-controlled clinical trials of adjuvant therapy with great interest but should adopt these new
methods only when they are proved to be beneficial.

# References

1. Epstein, E., Bragg, K., and Linden, G.: Biopsy and prognosis of malignant melanoma. J.A.M.A. *208*:1369, 1969.
2. Peterson, R. F., Hazard, J. B., Dykes, E. R., and Anderson, R.: Superficial malignant melanomas. Surg. Gynecol. Obstet. *119*:37, 1964.
3. Mehnert, J. H., and Heard, J. L.: Staging of malignant melanomas by depth by invasion—a proposed index to prognosis. Am. J. Surg. *110*:168, 1965.
4. Clark, W. H., Jr.: A classification of malignant melanoma in man correlated with histogenesis and biologic behavior. *In* Montagna, W., et al. *Advances in Biology of Skin and the Pigmentary System*. Vol 8. London, Pergamon Press, 1967, pp. 621–647.
5. Breslow, A.: Thickness, cross-sectional areas and depth of invasion in the prognosis of cutaneous melanoma. Ann. Surg. *172*:902, 1970.
6. McGovern, V. J., Mihm, M. C., Jr., Bailey, C., Booth, J. C., Clark, W. H., Jr., Cochran, A. J., Hardy, E. G., Hicks, J. D., Levine, A., Lewis, M. G., Little, J. H., and Milton, G. W.: The classification of malignant melanoma and its histologic reporting. Cancer *32*:1446, 1973.
7. Wong, C. K.: A study of melanocytes in the normal skin surrounding malignant melanomata. Dermatologica *141*:215, 1970.
8. Olsen, G.: Removal of fascia—cause of more frequent metastases of malignant melanomas of the skin to regional lymph nodes? Cancer *17*:1159, 1964.
9. McNeer, G., and Das Gupta, T.: Prognosis in malignant melanoma. Surgery *56*:512, 1964.
10. Gumport, S. L., and Harris, M. N.: Results of regional lymph node dissection for melanoma. Ann. Surg. *179*:105, 1974.
11. McPeak, C. J., McNeer, G. P., Whiteley, W. H., and Booher, R. J.: Amputation for melanoma of the extremity. Surgery *54*:426, 1964.
12. Das Gupta, T., and McNeer, G.: The incidence of metastasis to accessible lymph nodes from melanoma of the trunk and extremities—its therapeutic significance. Cancer *17*:897, 1964.
13. Southwick, H. W., Slaughter, D. P., Hinkamp, J. F., and Johnson, F. E.: The role of regional node dissection in the treatment of malignant melanoma. Arch. Surg. *85*:63, 1962.
14. Mundth, E. D., Guralnick, E. A., and Raker, J. W.: Malignant melanoma: a clinical study of 427 cases. Ann. Surg. *162*:15, 1965.
15. Wanebo, H. J., Fortner, J. G., Woodruff, J., McLean, B., and Binkowski, E.: Selection of the optimum surgical treatment of Stage I melanoma by depth of microinvasion. Ann. Surg. *182*:302, 1975.
16. Polk, H. C., Jr., and Linn, B. S.: Selective regional lymphadenectomy for melanoma: a mathematical aid to clinical judgement. Ann. Surg. *174*:402, 1971.
17. Shah, J. P., and Goldsmith, H.: Incontinuity versus discontinuous lymph node dissection for malignant melanoma. Cancer *26*:610, 1970.
18. Hueston, J. T.: Integumentectomy for malignant melanoma of the limbs. Aust. N.Z. J. Surg. *40*:114, 1970.
19. Creech, O., Jr., Ryan, R. F., and Krementz, E. T.: Treatment of melanoma by isolation-perfusion technique. J.A.M.A. *169*:339, 1959.
20. Stehlin, J. S., and Clark, R. L.: Melanoma of the extremities: experience with conventional treatment and perfusion in 339 cases. Am. J. Surg. *110*:366, 1965.
21. Rochlin, D. B., and Smart, C. R.: Treatment of malignant melanoma by regional perfusion. Cancer *18*:1544, 1965.

# 11

# *Choledochoduodenostomy versus Sphincteroplasty*

CHOLEDOCHODUODENOSTOMY
*by John L. Madden*

SPHINCTEROPLASTY (NOT
SPHINCTEROTOMY)
VERSUS LATERAL
CHOLEDOCHODUODENOSTOMY
*by S. Austin Jones*

## Statement of the Problem

*Given the clinical circumstances in which operative elimination of sphincter of Oddi function is desirable, the dispute relates to the preferred procedure for accomplishing this end.*

*In contrasting sphincteroplasty and sphincterotomy, the major difference is an attempt to approximate duct mucosa to duodenal mucosa. What suture material should be used? If absorbable, what data are available regarding durability of the suture? If permanent sutures are used, what is the potential for secondary stone formation?*

*Examine data which compare persistent patency — of sphincteroplasty versus sphincterotomy. Is there information comparing sphincteroplasty and sphincterotomy results in which the precise length of incision in the ampulla and duct is provided?*

*Indicate the frequency of pancreatitis due to operative injury of the pancreatic duct orifice in sphincteroplasty.*

*An indication for dividing the sphincter is retained intraoperative stones. Does the procedure solve the problem? Cite available information regarding the frequency with which the stones actually pass through the opened sphincter.*

*Does choledochoduodenostomy decompress the pancreatic ductal system?*

*What facts indicate that choledochoduodenostomy should be of a side-to-side or end-to-side conformation?*

*Analyze published data and your own results regarding mortality and morbidity, leaks, fistulas, abscesses, and ascending cholangitis, comparing the sphincter-dividing operation with choledochoduodenostomy.*

# Choledochoduodenostomy

JOHN L. MADDEN

*St. Clare's Hospital and Health Center, New York, New York*

For the elimination of a functional sphincter of Oddi, my preference is an external side-to-side choledochoduodenostomy. My position in favor of this operation is pragmatic, being based on the results obtained with its use. The preference given to it, however, should not be construed as an indictment of sphincteroplasty. The decision not to use sphincteroplasty was made on the basis of a priori reasoning, which admittedly may often prove fallacious. However, as experience with choledochoduodenostomy accumulated, a more compelling factual basis (a posteriori reasoning) for this decision emerged.

There are two main objections to external side-to-side choledochoduodenostomy. One is that it permits reflux of the duodenal contents into the biliary tract and thereby predisposes to the occurrence of an "ascending" cholangitis. The second objection is that it creates a "blind" segment of common duct between the site of the anastomosis and the papilla of Vater. It has been stressed repeatedly that this bypassed segment acts as a nidus for the accumulation of biliary-intestinal stasis debris which may cause either an "ascending" cholangitis or an obstruction of the anastomotic stoma. On the other hand, in performing a sphincteroplasty, the "blind" segment is eliminated.

I would initially like to comment on the first objection, that choledochoduodenostomy causes a reflux or "ascending" cholangitis. If one stresses this objection in favor of sphincteroplasty, then one also expresses a denial of fact. Reflux or "ascending" cholangitis following sphincteroplasty is rarely emphasized, yet if the operation is properly performed (in which case it is truly a transduodenal internal choledochoduodenostomy), reflux of the duodenal contents into the biliary tract is a natural consequence. One should not stress reflux as an objection to choledochoduodenostomy, and by so doing imply that it does not occur following sphincteroplasty. It occurs after both operations, and accordingly, the presence of reflux cannot logically be used as an argument in favor of sphincteroplasty.

235

In regard to reflux, I should like to deny that it causes "ascending" cholangitis (which is a misnomer). It is not reflux that causes cholangitis but obstruction at the site of the anastomosis. As long as there is free ingress and egress of the intestinal contents through the stoma, difficulties should not ensue. In fact, barium meal roentgenographic studies are obtained in the early postoperative period to demonstrate reflux. Its absence, rather than its presence, is a cause for concern. Interestingly, the first patient in the series herein reported, who is now asymptomatic 23 years postoperatively, had a follow-up barium roentgenogram 19 years after operation which showed ready filling and emptying of the biliary radicles.

It has been argued that the reason why reflux or "ascending" cholangitis does not occur more frequently after choledochoduodenostomy is that the anastomosis is made with the duodenum, the contents of which are relatively sterile. It is stated, however, that the lower one goes in the intestinal tract in making the biliary-intestinal anastomosis, the greater is the contamination, and therefore the more frequent is the complication of cholangitis.

To confirm or negate the logic of this reasoning, an experimental study was performed, which has been cited in detail in a previous publication.[7] In this study, the animals (dogs) were separated into two groups. In one group, the gallbladder was used for the anastomosis to the "unprepared" transverse colon, and in the other group, the common duct was used. One animal demonstrated "ascending" cholangitis, and stenosis of the anastomosis was shown on necropsy. The other animals, which were asymptomatic, were sacrificed 2 to 3 months postoperatively, and boluses of formed feces were found to be present within a widely patent anastomosis. Yet there were no antemortem symptoms of "ascending" cholangitis. This experimental study confirms the frequent clinical observation that it is obstruction of the stoma and not reflux that is the cause of cholangitis. Therefore, this condition should be referred to as obstructive or "descending" cholangitis, as suggested by Bernhard,[2] rather than reflux or "ascending" cholangitis.

In considering these findings, it is of interest that the first biliary-intestinal anastomosis, done in 1882 by von Winiwarter,[11] was an elective anastomosis of the gallbladder to the transverse colon. Similar operations were subsequently reported by Courvoisier,[4] Chavasse,[3] and Robson,[9] all with satisfactory clinical results and no "ascending" cholangitis!

In regard to the second objection to choledochoduodenostomy, I will not deny that it effects the formation of a "blind" segment of common duct, caudad to the anastomosis. In fact, several reports have presented documentary evidence to substantiate the claim that this "blind" segment may be the cause of major delayed postoperative complications. Unfortunately, these reports are of isolated instances and are not based on a large experience by any one surgeon in the use of the procedure. My only reply to this objection is a factual one based on an individual experience in the performance of choledochoduodenostomy in a series of 128 patients during the past 23 years. I can only state that to date none of the patients has had any difficulties relative to the "blind" segment. It would appear that as a source of later complications, it has been overemphasized.

The prime, and most common, indication for choledochoduodenostomy is a primary or stasis stone in the common duct. In fact, when such stones are found, the operation is considered to be mandatory. In a series of 110 patients in whom choledochoduodenostomy was done for benign lesions, the true indication for operation in 65 (59.1 per cent), or approximately 2 in every 3 patients, was common duct stones. Furthermore, in 55 (84.6 per cent) of these patients, or 4 in every 5, the stones were of the primary or autochthonous variety, having been formed where they were found—in the common duct. The fact that 1 in every 4 such patients had no stones in the gallbladder lends further credence to the theory that they originate in the common duct. In 26 (47.3 per cent) of these 55 patients with stasis stones, a concomitant stenosis of the papilla of Vater was present.

There are many who do not believe that in patients with common duct stones, the incidence of primary or stasis stones is as high (84.6 per cent), as stated here. This disbelief only serves to emphasize the importance of establishing a classification of gallbladder and common duct stones to serve as a universal standard. Then and then only will surgeons have a basis for comparative study and be able to "talk the same language." The classification proposed by Aschoff[8] is ideal for general use. Since it is based on the gross morphologic characteristics of the stones, it permits their immediate classification and does not require the performance of sophisticated biochemical assays.

In the surgical management of a patient with a stasis stone or stones in the common duct, a definitive corrective procedure is believed mandatory, precluding simple catheter or T-tube drainage after their removal. If a definitive operation is not done, 1 in every 3 patients will subsequently require a re-operation. Since most of these patients are advanced in age, a re-operation should be avoided because of the potentially high operative risk. To obviate such risks, either an external choledochoduodenostomy or a sphincteroplasty is advised.

Preference is given to choledochoduodenostomy because of: (1) the ease of performance; (2) the low incidence of complications and the concomitant low mortality rate; and (3) the absence of recurrences and the long-term beneficial results obtained. Theoretically, the operative risks are greater in the performance of a sphincteroplasty because technically it is a more difficult operation and because the potential for the occurrence of postoperative complications such as pancreatitis, serious hemorrhage, and fistula formation, either anastomotic or duodenal, is greater.

In reference to the ease of operation, the discussion by Lahey[6] of the presentation by Sanders,[10] who was the first in America to advocate choledochoduodenostomy, is pertinent. Lahey stated that he would prefer to do a sphincterotomy and use a long-armed T-tube which extended across the transected sphincter into the duodenum. In response, Sanders stated that in performing a sphincterotomy in preference to a choledochoduodenostomy, the surgeon was making an easy operation difficult and was unnecessarily predisposing the patient to numerous and serious complications.

A frequently asked question concerns the use of choledochoduodenostomy in the treatment of chronic pancreatitis and whether or not it decompresses the pancreatic ductal system. Although the operation is not done for chronic pancreatitis per se, if the chronic pancreatitis has caused an obstructive jaundice, a choledochoduodenostomy is done for the relief of the jaundice, provided the common duct is dilated. One would not anticipate any decompression effect on the pancreatic ductal system unless there was an obstruction of the duct caused primarily by tissue edema rather than intrinsic obstruction. Under such circumstances, the decompression of the biliary system and the subsequent resolution of the surrounding tissue edema would have a beneficial decompressive effect on the pancreatic ductal system.

The technique for the performance of external side-to-side choledochoduodenostomy has been described previously.[7] An excellent survey of the various other techniques employed has also been published.[5] In doing the anastomosis, interrupted sutures of 5–0 silk are used throughout and the importance of mucosa to mucosa apposition is stressed. Furthermore, the operation should not be done unless the common duct is dilated to a measured 10 mm. or more in its external diameter. In the insertion of the posterior layer of sutures the knots are tied on the inside of the lumen, a procedure to which many object. The objection is based on the belief that the knots of the nonabsorbable sutures serve as a nidus for foreign body encrustations and complications therefrom. Suffice it to say, in our experience with the use of silk sutures in the performance of choledochoduodenostomy or in end-to-end reconstructions of the common duct in which similar sutures are employed, complications relating to their use have not occurred.

Another question pertains to what facts would indicate the preference for a side-to-side or an end-to-side anastomosis? A side-to-side union is preferred because it is technically easier to perform and less likely to be associated with postoperative complications. In patients with obstructions of the terminal portion of the common duct secondary to malignant tumors, transection of the common duct and end-to-side choledochojejunostomy are frequently done for technical expediency and to place the anastomosis at a distance from the expanding tumor in order to lessen the likelihood of recurrent obstruction. An end-to-side anastomosis, again using the jejunum rather than the duodenum, is also advised for treatment of acute accidental injuries to the common duct when the duct is of normal diameter. In one such patient, the caliber of the diameter of the common duct was such that only four 5–0 sutures anteriorly and posteriorly could be used for the anastomosis. However, 4 months later a barium roentgenogram showed excellent reflux and emptying through the anastomotic stoma in the asymptomatic patient.

In reference to sphincterotomy, I have found two indications for its use: (1) in patients with fibrosis of the sphincter of Oddi in whom the common duct is not dilated and in whom, therefore, a choledochoduodenostomy would be contraindicated; and (2) in patients with a stone impacted in the sphincter of Oddi. Characteristically, the impacted stone is a primary or stasis stone. Because of its soft consistency, it is easily impacted in the sphincter, which, in the presence of primary common duct stones, is commonly dilated. In fact, it is this patency of the papilla that facilitates the impaction of the stasis stone. Frequently, the stone has a "dumbbell" constriction in its center, conforming to its location within the sphincter. One end of the stone protrudes into the common duct and the other into the duodenum.

Using the combined transduodenal and transcholedochal approach, the stone is removed. Many times, because of the patency of the papilla, the stone can be removed by instrumental manipulation without the necessity for transection of the sphincter.

Invariably in these patients the common duct is widely dilated (measuring 20 to 24 mm in diameter). After closure of the duodenotomy incision, which is always transverse and never longitudinal, a side-to-side choledochoduodenostomy is done in the usual manner since the simple removal of the impacted stone is not the surgical solution to the problem. One may question the rationale of doing a bypass procedure when the papilla is so widely patent. The fact remains that stasis stones occurred despite the patency, and the operation, done empirically, has proved most satisfactory as prophylaxis for recurrent stone formation.

What then are our clinical results with the use of choledochoduodenostomy? In our series, during the 23-year period between December 9, 1951, and December, 1974, 128 patients have had the operation performed. Eighteen patients had obstruction of the distal end of the common duct secondary to malignant tumors, and the remaining 110 patients had obstructions secondary to benign lesions. There were 45 (35.1 per cent) men and 83 (64.9 per cent) women. Their ages ranged from 35 to 90 years, with an average age of 63.6 years. Eighty-five (66.4 per cent) patients, or 2 of every 3, were over 60 years of age, and 45 (35.1 per cent), or about 1 in 3, were more than 70 years old. Complications occurred in 21 (16.4 per cent) patients. Three (2.3 per cent) patients had wound infections, two (1.5 per cent) had intraperitoneal bleeding, and one (0.8 per cent) had a fatal pulmonary embolus. In four (3.1 per cent) patients there was leakage of bile and in each it stopped spontaneously. The other complications were: wound dehiscence (two patients), thrombophlebitis (two patients), incisional hernia, pulmonary edema, atelectasis, and hepatic coma. None of the patients had intraperitoneal abscesses, fistulas, or "ascending" cholangitis.

Four (3.1 per cent) patients died. Three had benign lesions and one a malignant tumor. One patient, a 72-year-old woman, died of a pulmonary embolus 14 days postoperatively. The cause of death was confirmed on necropsy. A second patient, a 44-year-old man with cirrhosis of the liver and chronic pancreatitis, died in hepatic coma 12 days after operation. The third patient, a 90-year-old woman, whose early postoperative recovery was satisfactory, died of a cerebral thrombosis 29 days after the operation. The fourth patient, an 85-year-old woman with a cancer of the head of the pancreas, had a wound dehiscence on the eighth postoperative day and died 3 weeks postoperatively.

The value of a given operative procedure may be judged by a critical evaluation of the results of a long-term follow-up study. In each of the 128 patients mentioned previously, the operation was performed by the same surgeon. Of the 18 patients with malignant lesions, one died 3 weeks postoperatively and another, lost to follow-up, is presumed dead of disease. Fifteen of the remaining 16 patients died of disease. The average duration of survival was 12 months. None had complications in relation to the choledochoduodenostomy. The remaining patient is alive 6 months postoperatively.

Of the 110 patients with benign lesions, 3 (2.7 per cent) died and 8 (7.2 per cent) were lost to follow-up. The remaining 99 (90.0 per cent) patients have been followed for a minimum period of 1 month and a maximum of 23 years. The average duration of follow-up approximates 10 years. Seventy-two (72.7 per cent) patients, or about 3 in every 4, have been followed longer than 5 years and 41 (41.4 per cent), for more than 10 years.

In 98 (99.0 per cent) of the 99 patients available for long-term study, the results are classified as excellent. The one failure occurred in a 69-year-old woman who, at the age of 61, had had a choledochoduodenostomy for multiple secondary stones in the common duct. The patient had been without symptoms for 8 years when jaundice suddenly appeared. Six months previously, barium roentgenographic studies had shown excellent function of the biliary intestinal anastomosis and normal biliary radicles. The patient was re-operated upon and a patent anastomotic stoma was demonstrated. Exploration of the common duct was "negative" for stones, but a stenosis of the papilla of Vater was present. A transduodenal sphincterotomy was performed and now, 5 years later, the patient is asymptomatic. I should again like to emphasize that none of the 128 patients had "ascending" cholangitis and none had complications related to the caudal "blind" segment of common duct.

It is concluded that external side-to-side choledochoduodenostomy is of proved clinical merit as a curative as well as a palliative operation in the treatment of patients with obstructive lesions of the lower portion of the common duct. Sphincteroplasty, and in a more limited way, sphincterotomy, are similarly suitable procedures, but for the reasons presented, choledochoduodenostomy is generally preferred.

## References

1. Abbe, R.: The surgery of gall-stone obstruction. M. Rec. 43:548, 1893.
2. Bernhard, F.: Über moderne Gesichtspunkte in der chirurgischen Behandlung der Erkankungen der Leber und der Gallenwege. Dtsch. Med. Wochenschr. 75:760, 1950.
3. Chavasse, T. F.: Cited in Abbe, R.: The surgery of gall-stone obstruction. M. Rec. 43:548, 1893.
4. Courvoisier, L. G.: Cited in Abbe, R.: The surgery of gall-stone obstruction. M. Rec. 43:548, 1893.
5. Degenshein, G. A., and Hurwitz, A.: The techniques of side-to-side choledochoduodenostomy. Surgery 61:972, 1967.
6. Lahey, F.: Discussion. In Sanders, R. L.: Indications for and value of choledochoduodenostomy. Ann. Surg. 123:847, 1946.
7. Madden, J. L., Gruwez, J. A., and Tan, P. Y.: Obstructive (surgical) jaundice: an analysis of 140 consecutive cases and a consideration of choledochoduodenostomy in its treatment. Am. J. Surg. 109:89, 1965.
8. Madden, J. L., Vanderheyden, L., and Kandalaft, S.: The nature and surgical significance of common duct stones. Surg. Gynecol. Obstet. 126:3, 1968.
9. Robson, A. M. M.: Cited in Abbe, R.: The surgery of gall-stone obstruction. M. Rec. 43:548, 1893.
10. Sanders, R. L.: Indications for and value of choledochoduodenostomy. Ann. Surg. 123:847, 1946.
11. Von Winiwarter, A.: Ein Fall von Gallenretention bedingt durch impermeabilitat des Ductus choledochus. Anlegung einer Gallenblasen-Darmfistel. Prag. Med. Wochenschr. 7:201, 1882.

# Sphincteroplasty (not Sphincterotomy) versus Lateral Choledochoduodenostomy

S. AUSTIN JONES

*University of California, Irvine, California College of Medicine*

A comparison of sphincteroplasty and lateral choledochoduodenostomy presents two controversial problems rather than a single one. The first is to establish clearly what we mean by sphincteroplasty and in so doing to point out that anatomically and physiologically this procedure is entirely different from sphincterotomy. It is only too obvious that reports in the literature use the terms "sphincterotomy" and "sphincteroplasty" indiscriminately and interchangeably. Sphincteroplasty has been called a "papillostomy" and has even been confused with lateral choledochoduodenostomy.[1] It has been stated that the major difference between sphincterotomy and sphincteroplasty is that sphincteroplasty involves suture approximation of the duodenal wall and common duct mucosa while sphincterotomy does not. *As all of these concepts are entirely incorrect, it is obvious that the first step which must be taken is to describe precisely what we mean by sphincteroplasty and to furnish anatomic and physiologic proof that this procedure is not a sphincterotomy.* Having established this point, we can then proceed objectively to the second problem, that of comparing sphincteroplasty with lateral choledochoduodenostomy, and discuss the relative indications, contraindications, merits, and disadvantages of the two operations.

In approaching the first problem, I should like to begin with a description of the anatomy of the distal ends of the common and pancreatic ducts. Next, we will define sphincterotomy and sphincteroplasty and point out how they differ anatomically. Studies demonstrating the physiologic differences between sphincterotomy and sphincteroplasty will then be presented. At that point, we will have separated the apples from the oranges and will be in

241

a position to compare sphincteroplasty with lateral choledochoduodenostomy.

## Anatomy of the Distal Common and Pancreatic Ducts

In 1681, Glisson[2] described a sphincteric muscular mechanism at the lower end of the common duct. His observations were so remarkable in their accuracy that today, almost three hundred years later, they are difficult to improve upon. He stated in part:

> All return into the ductus communis is prevented by annular fibers which block not only the opening itself, but the whole slanting tract. For just as these annular fibers easily extend themselves as often as the bilious fluid, held back for a little while and now augumented in quantity, hastens to the outlet, so also once that superfluous fluid has flowed out, these same fibers close completely and block all passage until some more fluid again accumulates to force an opening.

In 1887, Oddi[3] described a sphincter in the region of the papilla of Vater at the terminal end of the common duct. He noted that this structure would contract after mechanical irritation, vagal stimulation, or when dilute hydrochloric acid was applied to gastric or duodenal mucosa. Both the sphincteric mechanisms described by Glisson and Oddi were associated with duodenal wall muscle. In 1936, Boyden[4] amplified our knowledge of this area by describing a submucosal muscular sheath which surrounds both the common and pancreatic ducts as they pass obliquely, parallel to one another, through the duodenal wall. The musculature demonstrated by Boyden develops some 5 weeks later in fetal life than does the muscle of the duodenal wall. Ono[5] has shown that the sphincter of Boyden and the muscle of the duodenal wall can contract independently or separately.

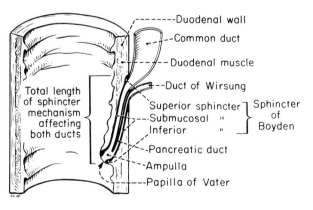

Labels:
- Duodenal wall
- Common duct
- Duodenal muscle
- Duct of Wirsung
- Superior sphincter
- Submucosal "
- Inferior "
- Sphincter of Boyden
- Pancreatic duct
- Ampulla
- Papilla of Vater
- Total length of sphincter mechanism affecting both ducts

NORMAL ANATOMY

*Figure 1.* The submucosal sphincter of Boyden and the duodenal wall muscle, acting separately or together, can compress the common and pancreatic ducts in their oblique intramural course through the bowel wall.

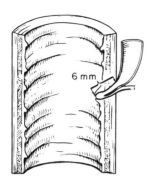 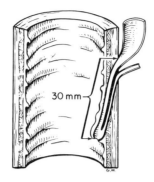

LENGTH OF INTRAMURAL COURSE MAY VARY
FROM 6 to 30 mm

*Figure 2.* The length of the incision required to destroy the sphincteric mechanism depends upon the length of the intramural course, which varies greatly. Therefore, an incision of a "standard length" may be inadequate or excessive. *The incision must be continued until the opening created is as large as the widest part of the common duct.* Only then can one be certain that the sphincteric mechanism *in that particular individual* has been totally ablated.

In Figure 1, the normal oblique course of the ducts as they pass through the duodenal wall is diagrammed. At the point of entry of the common duct into the outer surface of the duodenal wall, the lumen decreases abruptly, changing from 6 to 10 mm. to 2 to 3 mm. in diameter. This diagram also depicts the superior sphincter of Boyden, where the common duct begins its course through the duodenal wall, and the inferior sphincter of Boyden in the region of the papilla. In both these locations, the fibers of the submucosal sheath blend with those of the duodenal wall muscle.

Figure 2 emphasizes that the length of the intramural course of the ducts is not constant. In 50 dissections done by Dr. Louis L. Smith and myself, it varied from 8 to 24 mm., and in other dissections, from 6 to 30 mm. Multiple cross sections through varying levels of the intramural course of the ducts demonstrated that the muscle fibers which encircled the common duct also surrounded the pancreatic duct[6] (Fig. 3). These findings have been confirmed by others.[7, 8]

In summing up the anatomical aspects of this area which are important to the surgeon, let me emphasize two major points:

1. There is a complex of muscular sphincters which, working together or separately, can compress the common and pancreatic ducts in their intramural course.

2. Total elimination of these muscular sphincters requires an incision which extends through the entire length of the intramural course of the common duct. This would result in the apex of the incision being outside the duodenal wall at the point where the common duct enters its outer aspect. Any lesser incision cannot eliminate completely the constricting ability of the sphincters.

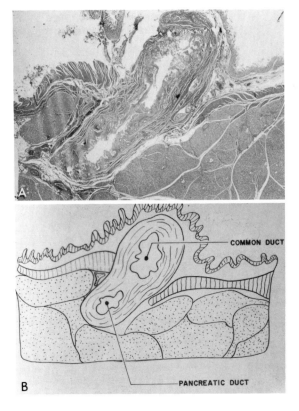

*Figure 3.* Cross sections through the bile and pancreatic ducts in their intramural course demonstrate that the muscle fibers encircle both ducts. *A*, Microscopic section; *B*, diagram of section.

## Sphincterotomy

A sphincterotomy is an incision through the muscular sphincter of the papilla of Vater and the inferior sphincter of Boyden. The lower or distal portion of the sphincteric mechanism is thus divided, leaving the upper proximal segment of the sphincters intact (Fig. 4, *A*). This operation was first performed by McBurney in 1891, who stated that "no sutures were used [to approximate the duodenal and common duct walls] unless the incisions made were of considerable length."[9] It is clear that anatomically such an incision cannot eliminate the entire sphincteric structure. If the incision were extended far enough to accomplish this, it would, as previously stated, extend to the outside of the duodenal wall. *Therefore, if the objective is to totally and permanently destroy the sphincters, sphincterotomy is an incomplete operation.*

## Sphincteroplasty

Sphincteroplasty is a transduodenal method of producing an *end-to-side terminal choledochoduodenostomy with a stoma equal in size to the largest*

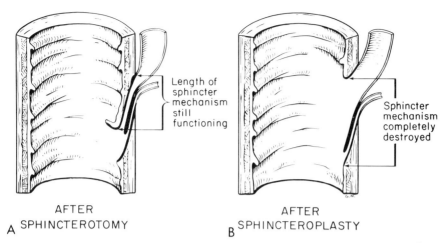

*Figure 4.* After sphincterotomy, a functioning segment of sphincter mechanism remains. This is completely eliminated by sphincteroplasty.

*part of the common duct. Such an opening is noncontractile and permanent, and the entire sphincteric mechanism is completely ablated* (Fig. 4, *B*).

The technique of sphincteroplasty has been described in other publications,[10, 11] and will not be discussed in detail here. Suffice it to say that the duodenum, after mobilization by the Kocher maneuver, is opened longitudinally. In most cases, the common duct has already been explored from above. However, if it has not, and if *the slightest difficulty is encountered in identifying the papilla of Vater from below, the common duct is opened supraduodenally and a No. 10 (3 mm.) rubber catheter is passed downward into the duodenum to make identification of the papilla certain.* Two small clamps are then placed side by side into the papilla, incorporating the common duct and duodenal walls. The tissue between them is divided and the clamps are oversewn with 5-0 arterial silk, which is tied as the clamps are removed. The first pair of clamps is always placed at 10 o'clock in order to avoid injury to the pancreatic duct, which, in our dissections, was always medial to the common duct (Fig. 5). As soon as the pancreatic duct is visualized, subsequent pairs of clamps are placed in an anterior position and the process is continued until the diameter of the stoma is equal to that of the largest part of the common duct (Fig. 6). As this is, in essence, a one layer end-to-side anastomosis, we feel more secure using nonabsorbable suture, and to date we have seen no contraindications to its use. Autopsy studies done several years after sphincteroplasty have shown no evidence of stone encrustation.[12] When the sphincteroplasty is completed, the duodenal wall is closed in the same direction in which it was opened. Longitudinal opening and transverse closure is *not* advised, because the medial side of the duodenum cannot be mobilized and tension would result.

*How does one know how far to continue this incision, and how can the surgeon be certain that he has destroyed all of the sphincteric mechanism?* By referring to Figure 2, we can recognize that the required length of the in-

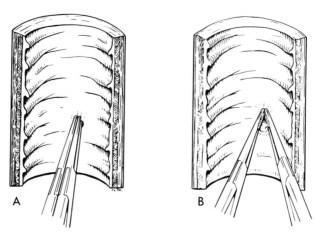

*Figure 5.* A, The first pair of clamps is placed at 10'oclock to avoid pancreatic duct injury. B, After the tissue between the first pair of clamps is divided, the pancreatic duct can be seen and avoided.

cision depends upon the anatomical configuration of each individual patient. It is not possible to use an arbitrary figure of "1 cm. or 1½ cm." as is often done, because in any given case, such an incision may be either inadequate or excessive. The answer is to *continue the clamping, division, and suture of the common duct and duodenal walls until the opening created is as large as the largest part of the common duct. This is the only way in which the surgeon can be assured that the entire sphincteric mechanism has been*

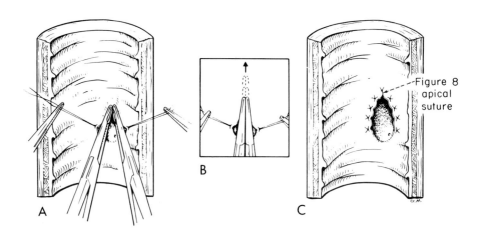

*Figure 6.* A, The second pair of clamps is placed anteriorly. B, Successive clamping, division, and suture are continued upwards until the stoma created equals the diameter of the widest part of the common duct. C, At the upper part of the completed sphincteroplasty, the incision has extended through the duodenal wall, and careful suture approximation, especially at the apex, is mandatory.

*eliminated in that particular patient.* As the procedure progresses, very gentle sounding from below is performed using Bakes dilators, until the bulbous tip passes easily into the common duct with no evidence of narrowing and with the dilator fitting snugly in the supraduodenal portion of the common duct. When this has been accomplished, *it must be recognized that the incision has passed through the entire thickness of the duodenal wall and that meticulous suture approximation, especially at the apex, is mandatory to avoid a leak.*

## Physiologic Differences Between Sphincterotomy and Sphincteroplasty

Up to this point, these two procedures have been compared on an anatomical basis only. Objective evidence must be furnished to prove that sphincterotomy and sphincteroplasty are physiologically separate and distinct operations. The methods we have used to compare the two procedures have been reported previously[10, 11, 12] and will be outlined briefly in this discussion.

I. *Postoperative T-tube pressure studies*

Beginning with our first sphincteroplasty in September, 1951, Dr. Louis L. Smith and I studied the T-tube pressure levels in postoperative patients both before and after the administration of intravenous morphine sulphate, a smooth muscle constrictor. Three groups were included, as shown in Figure 7. When morphine was given to a patient who had had *simple common duct exploration* alone, the drug produced a rapid pressure rise which was sustained

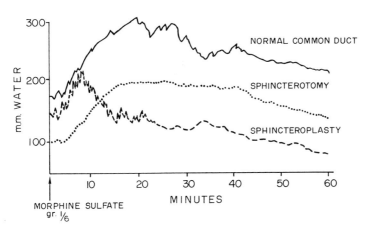

*Figure 7.* Comparison of postoperative T-tube pressure studies after intravenous morphine administration. The initial rise in the sphincteroplasty group is due to duodenal contraction forcing fluid upwards through the wide-open sphincteroplasty stoma.

for more than 1 hour. *Postsphincterotomy patients* so studied developed a gradual pressure rise, reaching a maximum in 15 minutes and maintaining a pressure plateau which was still above the baseline at the end of 1 hour. *Postsphincteroplasty patients* demonstrated a sudden rise in pressure following administration of morphine, reaching a peak in 9 minutes. This was followed by an abrupt fall to the baseline level in 14 minutes, and a gradual reduction to *below* baseline level within 1 hour. The reason for the sudden pressure rise in the postsphincteroplasty patients was confusing. By injecting a colored dye into the duodenum prior to administering the morphine, we found that when the drug was given it produced duodenal contraction which forced the dye upwards through the wide sphincteroplasty opening into the common duct and T-tube, thus explaining the transient pressure elevation.

II. *Postoperative T-tube cholangiography*

   A. Standard postoperative T-tube cholangiography, before and after morphine injection

      1. *Postsphincterotomy patients*

         Dye injected into the T-tube flowed freely into the duodenum, and the remaining narrowed intramural portion of the duct unaffected by the sphincterotomy was clearly delineated. When morphine was given and the cholangiogram repeated, the remaining sphincteric musculature contracted and completely occluded the distal common duct (Fig. 8).

      2. *Postsphincteroplasty patients*

         This study was repeated in patients who had been subjected to sphincteroplasty. The initial injection demonstrated a wide connection between the duodenum and the common duct, with no evidence of intramural narrowing. Following morphine, there was no evidence of constriction, the stoma remaining the same size as the largest portion of the common duct. Both before and after morphine administration, the flow of dye was so free and rapid that it was necessary to place the patient in a deep Trendelenburg position to obtain satisfactory visualization of the distal ductal system (Fig. 9).

   B. *Postoperative T-tube cineradiography*

      Cineradiographic T-tube studies in postsphincterotomy and postsphincteroplasty patients were obtained before and after morphine administration. The previously described results obtained with routine T-tube cholangiography were confirmed. Other subjective and objective differences observed are outlined in Table 1. It was interesting to note that postsphincterotomy patients given morphine would develop complete occlusion of the distal duct which would be followed by dilatation of the proximal duct, nausea, and epigastric pain despite the analgesic effect of the morphine. From time to time, small "squirts" of dye would enter the duodenum with temporary relief of the nausea and pain.

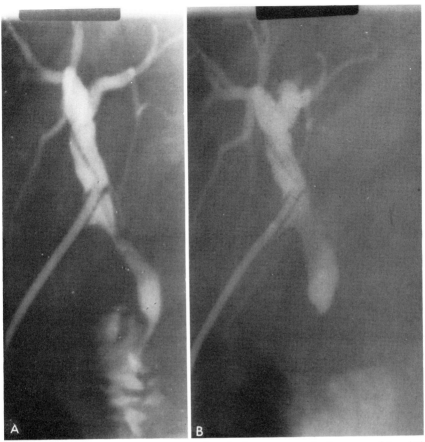

*Figure 8. Postsphincterotomy.* T-tube cholangiograms before morphine *(A)* and after morphine *(B)*. In the premorphine film, the remaining narrowed portion of the duct is visible. After morphine, the remaining sphincteric mechanism occludes the distal duct. (From Jones, S. A., Steedman, R., Keller, T. B., and Smith, L. L.: Transduodenal sphincteroplasty (not sphincterotomy) for biliary and pancreatic disease. Am. J. Surg. *118*:292, 1969.)

III. *Postoperative barium reflux into the biliary tree on upper gastrointestinal studies*

Upper gastrointestinal studies on postsphincterotomy patients demonstrated no reflux of barium into the biliary tree. This finding confirmed those of Doubilet, who considered the absence of reflux to be a protective mechanism against "ascending" cholangitis.[13]

*In contradistinction, every patient who has had a proper sphincteroplasty must demonstrate free barium reflux into the ductal system or we consider the operation to have been inadequately performed.* Cholangitis is the result of intermittent obstruction of the distal duct with a subsequent *descending* infection due to the stasis of the ductal contents. As long as free flow exists, cholangitis will not occur. Madden demonstrated this effectively by showing that even choledochocolostomy performed in the dog would not result in cholangitis unless obstruction of the anastomosis developed.[14]

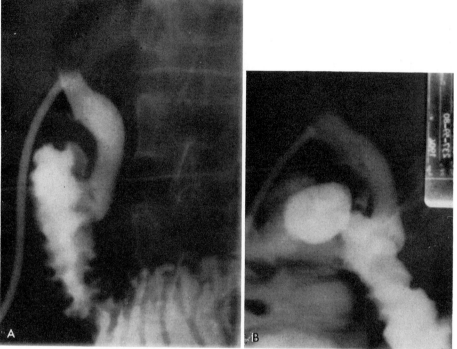

*Figure 9. Postsphincteroplasty.* T-tube cholangiograms before morphine *(A)* and after morphine *(B)*. The distal ductal narrowing is not present, and morphine produces no constriction, the sphincters having been completely destroyed. (From Jones, S. A., Steedman, R., Keller, T. B., and Smith, L. L.: Transduodenal sphincteroplasty (not sphincterotomy) for biliary and pancreatic disease. Am. J. Surg. *118*:292, 1969.)

IV. *Permanence of the sphincteroplasty stoma*

It has been well documented that sphincterotomy will not result in a permanent lowering of resistance of fluid flow through the papilla. Eiseman demonstrated, in both dogs and humans, that common duct pressures would return to preoperative levels and that dogs sacrificed after single cut, double cut, and quadrant excision of the papilla, with or without a long-limbed Cattell tube

TABLE 1.  Postoperative T-Tube Cineradiography

|  | Sphincterotomy | Sphincteroplasty |
|---|---|---|
| Position of patient | Supine | 45° Trendelenburg |
| Rate of Hypaque infusion | 15–30 drops per minute | 150 drops per minute |
| Amount of Hypaque | 30–60 cc. | 180–240 cc. |
| Following intravenous morphine: |  |  |
|   Distal duct | Occluded | Wide open |
|   Proximal ducts | Dilated | Normal size |
|   Pain | Marked | None |
|   Nausea | Marked | None |
|   Reflux from duodenum | None | In all cases |

splint, uniformly developed eventual scarring and a return to pre-sphincterotomy pressure levels.[15]

After sphincteroplasty, however, the stoma properly created according to the procedure described appears to remain open permanently. This conclusion is based upon our findings at late autopsy studies, the absence of evidence of postsphincteroplasty cholangitis in any of our cases, and the fact that free barium reflux on upper gastrointestinal studies has been demonstrated repeatedly long after the sphincteroplasty. The longest interval we have recorded during which free reflux has been demonstrated is 12½ years (Fig. 10).

It is not difficult to understand why sphincterotomy produces only a temporary reduction in ductal pressure, since it follows the basic surgical principle that a single incision through any muscular sphincter will not produce long-term incontinence. However, we have been asked why patency should be more persistent after sphincteroplasty than after implantation of a divided proximal common duct end into a segment of bowel. In the latter situation, there is a definite incidence of stricture formation, regardless of the care with which the anastomosis is performed. We believe that this disparity is due to the fact that with an end-to-side choledochoenterostomy, the sutures must encompass the entire circumference of

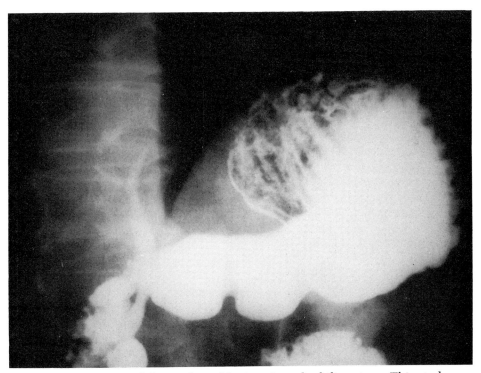

*Figure 10.*   Desired free reflux of barium into the biliary tree. This study was made 12½ years after sphincteroplasty.

the anastomosis. With a sphincteroplasty, only the anterior portion of the stoma requires suture closure, and the posterior aspect is left undisturbed.

To summarize, I believe that the data given answer our first problem, defining sphincteroplasty and distinguishing it from sphincterotomy. We are now in a position to compare sphincteroplasty and lateral choledochoduodenostomy.

## Sphincteroplasty Versus Lateral Choledochoduodenostomy

In the treatment of certain problems producing obstruction of the distal common duct, lateral choledochoduodenostomy — a side-to-side anastomosis between the anterior wall of the common duct and the posterior-superior wall of the duodenum — has definite points in its favor. This operation is technically much simpler than sphincteroplasty. If the common duct is of adequate size, the anastomosis should remain open. Madden emphasizes that a ductal diameter of 12 mm. is the minimum, but in the operations we have done to bypass malignant obstructions, the ducts were at least 18 mm. in width, and I have had no experience in anastomosing smaller ducts to the duodenum. It is certainly true that no cholangitis will develop if there is no anastomotic obstruction and, as with sphincteroplasty, reflux of ingested barium into the biliary tree is a favorable rather than an ominous finding. Lateral choledochoduodenostomy offers a rapid and effective method of palliation in bypassing malignant disease obstructing the distal end of the common duct when the tumor is not large enough to make duodenal obstruction imminent. If such obstruction is expected, A Roux-en-Y choledochojejunostomy and gastroenterostomy would be indicated. In the management of long strictures of the bile duct, as may be seen in some cases of advanced fibrotic chronic pancreatitis, lateral choledochoduodenostomy can be a very safe and effective method of relieving the biliary obstruction.

Controversy arises in regard to the optimum method for relieving ductal obstruction due to either ampullary stenosis or multiple calculi in the common or hepatic ducts. If ampullary stenosis is diagnosed only by failure to pass a 3 mm. Bakes dilator from above, an occasional carcinoma of the papilla of Vater will be overlooked. If ampullary stenosis is suspected, we believe that it should be confirmed by transduodenal exploration, and if no tumor is found, it is best treated by a sphincteroplasty. *I might state here that there is no indication, in our opinion, for a sphincterotomy, whether or not sutures are used.* We have seen three deaths occur when an incomplete operation was performed and fatal pancreatitis followed. *Once a sphincteroplasty is begun it should be completed.*

We believe that sphincteroplasty is superior to lateral choledochoduodenostomy in the prevention and treatment of residual common duct stones and as an approach to the problem of irremovable hepatic duct calculi. On numerous occasions we have seen common ducts filled with calculi but not dilated, making a lateral anastomosis inadvisable. In addition, if a side-to-side anastomosis is made above the normally narrow distal portion of the common duct, a blind pouch or "sump" is created. Overlooked calculi, mud, or sludge may collect in this distal segment, as shown in Figure 11. Such material may occlude the pancreatic duct either by mechanical obstruction or by irritation which contributes to sphincter spasm, resulting in pain or pancreatitis. Further, the duodenum is a strong muscular organ and the common bile duct is elastic, able only to alternately dilate and then resume its normal caliber. If the lateral choledochoduodenostomy stoma is widely patent, the duodenum can force vegetable debris into the common duct, which being less muscular, is unable to expel it. This material can become impacted and occlude the anastomosis.

In Madden's reported cases he had no complications related to the "blind" segment of the common duct. This is not a universal experience when lateral choledochoduodenostomy is done for benign disease and long-term patency is required. Since in our area, this operation is usually used to bypass malignant obstructions, we have seen only three cases in which accumulation of vegetable debris caused occlusion of the stoma, resulting in cholangitis. One of these cases is illustrated in Figure 12. Wilson reported one case in which calculi produced colic requiring transduodenal removal and another case in which stones and sludge obstructed the anastomosis.[16] Silen stated that he had seen stones collect in the distal "pouch" and produce pain, pancreatitis, or stomal obstruction.[17] Sir Rodney Smith of London operated upon 25 patients who were sent to him after lateral choledochoduodenostomy had been performed. In each case, the "sump" was filled with vegetable debris, obstructing the anastomosis and producing

THE "SUMP" SYNDROME

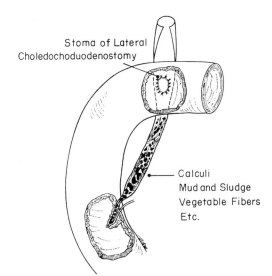

Stoma of Lateral
Choledochoduodenostomy

Calculi
Mud and Sludge
Vegetable Fibers
Etc.

*Figure 11.* Various debris may fill the blind pouch or "sump" following lateral choledochoduodenostomy.

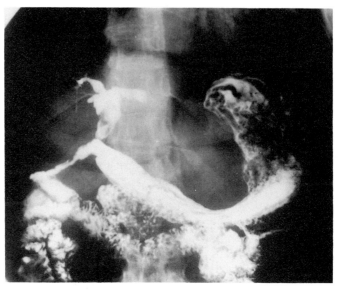

*Figure 12.* Upper gastrointestinal study on a patient who had cholangitis following lateral choledochoduodenostomy. The "sump" was packed with vegetable debris, causing intermittent obstruction at the anastomosis.

cholangitis. Some of these patients also had jaundice and pancreatitis. His treatment was a wide sphincteroplasty. He did not disturb the initial lateral anastomosis, relying upon the distal gravity drainage produced by sphincteroplasty to maintain free bile flow. There was no mortality and the obstruction was relieved in all patients.[18]

Averaged statistics have shown that residual stones are found in 10 per cent of patients who undergo choledocholithotomy and in 5 per cent of patients whose duct explorations are negative. Patients operated upon for residual stones have a 25 per cent chance of having a stone or stones left behind. Numerous recently developed techniques designed to improve the efficacy of ductal exploration have only slightly improved these figures, and sphincterotomy has proved unsatisfactory in the prevention of residual stones. Ampullary dilatation, in our opinion, should never be employed.[12]

Considering these factors, we perform a sphincteroplasty whenever we operate for residual stones or when irremovable hepatic duct calculi, which may eventually reach the common duct, are present. Sphincteroplasty is used at primary duct exploration when mud and sludge, ampullary stenosis, or multiple calculi are present. We consider ampullary stenosis to be present if a No. 10 French (3 mm.) catheter cannot be passed through the papilla after efforts are made from above and below and from both sides of the table. The term "multiple calculi" admittedly presents a gray area and to us implies that a sufficient number of calculi are present to make complete clearing of the ducts doubtful. Too often the surgeon is satisfied with a "normal" completion cholangiogram only to find 8 days later that a T-tube study demonstrates the presence of a stone or stones. The type of calculus does not alter our indications for sphincteroplasty, since stones that either originate in the gallbladder or develop in the duct from stasis can be left behind. We believe that the wide-open distal drainage produced by sphincteroplasty makes it more effective than lateral choledochoduodenostomy in treating ampullary stenosis and in the prevention and treatment of residual common duct stones.

As lateral choledochoduodenostomy has not been advocated as a method of treatment for acute recurrent pancreatitis, the limited but definite indications for sphincteroplasty in this disease will not be discussed here, having been described elsewhere.[6, 10, 12]

Sphincteroplasty is contraindicated at primary duct exploration when the bile is clear, when only a few large stones are present, when the papilla is at least 3 mm. in diameter, and when the completion cholangiogram done with dilute dye is normal. It should not be performed when there is a long stricture such as one may see occasionally with chronic pancreatitis, when a peri-Vaterian diverticulum is found, when there is acute pancreatitis, or when there is any inflammatory disease of the distal duct. With gross dilatation of the common duct, depending upon the cause and level of the obstruction, either a lateral choledochoduodenostomy or a Roux-en-Y choledochojejunostomy is a better choice. The latter operation is advised when the large multiple intrahepatic calculi seen in Oriental cholangiohepatitis are present. Finally, in an elderly and severely ill patient with multiple common duct stones and a dilated duct, we would prefer the simpler and quicker lateral choledochoduodenostomy as a method of drainage, rather than sphincteroplasty.

## Results of Sphincteroplasty

Our conclusions are based on 293 sphincteroplasties performed since September, 1951. In 191 cases, the primary indication for operation was biliary ductal obstruction, as outlined in Table 2. Five patients had irremovable hepatic duct calculi and 21 were sent to us with residual common duct stones. There were four patients in whom overlooked calculi were found in the common duct following sphincteroplasty on a routine postoperative T-tube cholangiogram. In these cases, the ducts were cleared immediately by simple saline irrigation. While it cannot be proved, I am sure that the number of patients with overlooked stones was greater than four, but that in the interval between operation and the postoperative T-tube study the stones had passed into the duodenum through the wide opening created by the sphincteroplasty. Including the four patients in whom overlooked stones were immediately eliminated by T-tube irrigation, *there have been no residual stones demonstrated by roentgenograms or clinical evidence following sphincteroplasty.*

Four of the 293 patients died, three from acute postoperative pancreatitis. In two the cause was technical error, and one late death followed reoperation upon a duodenal fistula 23 months after the sphincteroplasty. The fistula was closed successfully, and a distal pancreatectomy was per-

TABLE 2. Indications for Sphincteroplasty
in Biliary Ductal Obstruction

| Indications | Number of Patients | | |
|---|---|---|---|
| | University | Private | Total |
| *Multiple Common Duct Stones* | | | |
| Alone | 6 | 11 | 17 |
| With hepatic duct stones | 1 | 4 | 5 |
| With gallbladder stones | 16 | 71 | 87 |
| After sphincterotomy | 0 | 1 | 1 |
| With congenital absence of gallbladder | 1 | 0 | 1 |
| With ampullary stenosis | 4 | 10 | 14 |
| With ampullary stenosis with gallbladder stones | 2 | 4 | 6 |
| Sent to us with residual stones | 4 | 17 | 21 |
| Total | 34 | 118 | 152 |
| | | | |
| *Miscellaneous* | | | |
| Gallbladder and hepatic duct stones | 1 | 1 | 2 |
| Ampullary stenosis with gallbladder stones | 1 | 1 | 2 |
| Ampullary stenosis and septal obstruction of common hepatic duct | 0 | 1 | 1 |
| Ampullary stenosis alone | 4 | 21 | 25 |
| Possible ampullary malignancy | 1 | 0 | 1 |
| Ampullary stenosis and ductal hypoplasia | 0 | 1 | 1 |
| Blood clots and sludge in common duct | 0 | 2 | 2 |
| Duodenal diverticulum with obstruction | 0 | 1 | 1 |
| Sent to us with postcholecystectomy syndrome: | | | |
| 1. ampullary stenosis with incomplete cholecystectomy | 0 | 1 | 1 |
| 2. ampullary stenosis with acute recurrent pancreatitis | 0 | 1 | 1 |
| 3. duodenal diverticulum and common duct stones | 0 | 1 | 1 |
| Probable sclerosing cholangitis; stones on operative cholangiogram not found at duct exploration | 1 | 0 | 1 |
| Total | 8 | 31 | 39 |
| | | | |
| Total number of patients operated upon for biliary ductal obstruction | | | 191 |

formed. The patient died from peritonitis and sepsis. The overall morbidity rate was 5.8 per cent, as shown in Table 3.

Recognizing that the mortality rate reported is unusually low for an operation of this magnitude performed in a delicate and potentially dangerous area, I should like to quote from a report presented by Dr. Louis L. Smith and myself in 1971.[10] In this paper we stated:

These results are, in our minds, not representative. It is bizarre that none of this group succumbed to coronary occlusion, congestive heart failure, pulmonary embolism, or comparable postoperative problems which are usually seen in a series of this size. However, while we are certain that the eventual overall mortality rate will be higher than our present one, we are convinced that if the technique given is followed in detail, it will remain acceptable.

Ductal obstruction was relieved in all but two patients noted in Table 3 in whom reoperations demonstrated that grossly incomplete sphincteroplasties had been performed. *None of the sphincteroplasty patients has shown any evidence of cholangitis.*

TABLE 3.   Morbidity in a Series of 293 Patients Undergoing Sphincteroplasty

| Morbidity | Number of Patients |
|---|---|
| *Immediate* | |
| Wound infection | 6 |
| Mild postoperative pancreatitis | 3 |
| Electrolyte imbalance | 2 |
| Excessive T-tube drainage | 1 |
| (probable hematoma at operative site, resolved postoperative day 16) | |
| Postoperative pneumonia | 1 |
| Questionable pulmonary embolism | 1 |
| Duodenal fistula | 1 |
| | 15 |
| *Delayed* | |
| Incomplete sphincteroplasty proved at reoperation | 2 |
| Overall morbidity rate | 5.8% |

# *Conclusion*

In choosing between sphincteroplasty and lateral choledochoduodenostomy to relieve distal common duct obstruction, we favor lateral choledochoduodenostomy only if the common duct is large enough to produce a 2 cm. stoma and for the following purposes: (1) to bypass a malignant obstruction; (2) to treat benign ductal strictures where applicable; (3) to treat aged and infirm patients unable to tolerate a more extensive procedure; (4) when inflammation or anatomic abnormality of the distal common duct is present; and (5) when biliary ductal obstruction and acute pancreatitis coexist.

We advocate transduodenal sphincteroplasty at primary ductal exploration when multiple calculi, mud, sludge, or ampullary stenosis are encountered. Sphincteroplasty is advised whenever one is operating for residual stones or when irremovable hepatic duct calculi are found. It has been used successfully in ducts of normal size packed with small calculi.

We believe that there is evidence to show that the "sump syndrome" is a true entity, especially in long-term survivors operated upon for benign disease. If the contraindications for sphincteroplasty are observed, this operation can be performed with acceptable rates of morbidity and mortality. It has given us excellent long-term results when employed for the indications given. Finally, we should like to re-emphasize that there is *no place in our armamentarium for a sphincterotomy,* which we consider an inadequate and often dangerous operation.

ACKNOWLEDGMENTS:   Gratitude is expressed to Dr. George Gregory, Dr. Thomas B. Keller, and Dr. Louis L. Smith, previous co-authors, for permitting the inclusion of their cases in this series.

# References

1. Thomas, C. G., Jr., Nicholson, C. P., and Owen, J.: Effectiveness of choledochoduodenostomy and transduodenal sphincterotomy in the treatment of benign obstruction of the common duct. Ann. Surg. 173:845, 1971.
2. Glisson, F.: In Hendrickson, W. F.: A study of the musculature of the entire extrahepatic biliary system, including that of the duodenal portion of the common bile duct and of the sphincter. Johns Hopkins Hosp. Bull. 9:223, 1898.
3. Oddi, R.: Sulla tonicita dello sfintere del coledoco, Arch. Sci. Med. 12:333, 1888.
4. Boyden, E. A.: The pars intestinalis of the common bile duct, as viewed by the older anatomists. Anat. Rec. 66:217, 1936.
5. Ono, K., Watanabe, N., Suzuki, K., and Tsuchida, H.: Electrophysiologic and cinefluorographic observations of bile flow mechanism in man. Surg. Forum 18:416, 1967.
6. Jones, S. A., Smith, L. L, and Gregory, G.: Sphincteroplasty for recurrent pancreatitis—a second report. Ann. Surg. 147:180, 1958.
7. Hand, B. H.: An anatomical study of the choledochoduodenal area, Br. J. Surg. 50:468, 1963.
8. Jones, S. A., Smith, L. L., Keller, T. B., and Joergenson, E. J.: Choledochoduodenostomy to prevent residual stones. Arch. Surg. 86:1014, 1963.
9. McBurney, C. L.: Section of the intestine for the removal of a gallstone. N.Y. State J. Med. 53:520, 1891.
10. Jones, S. A., and Smith, L. L.: A reappraisal of sphincteroplasty (not sphincterotomy). Surgery 71:565, 1972.
11. Jones, S. A.: Sphincteroplasty (not sphincterotomy) in the treatment of biliary tract disease. Surg. Clin. North Am. 53:1123, 1973.
12. Jones, S. A., Steedman, R., Keller, T. B., and Smith, L. L.: Transduodenal sphincteroplasty (not sphincterotomy) for biliary and pancreatic disease. Am. J. Surg. 118:292, 1969.
13. Doubilet, H., and Mulholland, J. H.: Etiology and treatment of pancreatitis N.Y. State J. Med. 49:2938, 1949.
14. Madden, J. L., Chun, J. Y., Kandalaft, S., and Parekh, M.: Choledochoduodenostomy, an unjustly maligned surgical procedure. Am. J. Surg. 119:45, 1970.
15. Eiseman, B., Brown, W. H., Virabutr, S., and Gottesfeld, S.: Sphincterotomy—an evaluation of its physiological rationale. Arch. Surg. 79:294, 1959.
16. Wilson, H.: Discussion. In Madden, J. L., Chun, J. Y., Kandalaft, S., and Parekh, M.: Choledochoduodenostomy, an unjustly maligned surgical procedure. Am. J. Surg. 119:45, 1970.
17. Silen, W.: Editor's discussion of reappraisal of sphincteroplasty (not sphincterotomy) by S. A. Jones and L. L. Smith. Year Book of Surgery. Chicago, Year Book Medical Publishers, Inc., 1973, p. 438.
18. Smith, R.: Personal communication, 1973.

# 12

# *Management of the Small Aortic Aneurysm*

SMALL AORTIC ANEURYSMS
SHOULD BE TREATED BY
OPERATION
*by W. Andrew Dale*

CONSIDERATIONS IN THE
MANAGEMENT OF POOR-
RISK PATIENTS WITH SMALL
ASYMPTOMATIC ABDOMINAL
ANEURYSMS
*by Eugene F. Bernstein*

## Statement of the Problem

This controversy concerns the management of the abdominal aortic aneurysm less than 6 cm. in diameter in an asymptomatic normotensive patient. Data regarding operative mortality, late morbidity, and death from ruptured aneurysm are discussed.

Define aneurysms for which early operation is recommended and those for which continuing observation is indicated. How accurately can size be estimated? Cite data to support this judgment.

What is the natural history of a small aneurysm? Compare 5 and 7 cm. lesions. To what degree does arterial blood pressure influence the natural history? Analyze data with respect to the statistical probability of the rupture of a small aneurysm (less than 6 cm. in diameter) per unit time in a normotensive person.

For the operative group, analyze data for in-hospital mortality and late mortality due to aortoenteric fistula, pseudoaneurysm, infected grafts, and other types of graft failure. Outline information on life expectancy in a patient with a small aneurysm which never does rupture.

# Small Aortic Aneurysms Should Be Treated by Operation

W. ANDREW DALE

*Vanderbilt University School of Medicine*

Elective graft replacement of abdominal aortic aneurysms has been stand-ardized to the extent that it is recommended as a safer course than non-operative management for most patients.[5,9] Because of the availability of modern vascular instruments, precise angiographic techniques, blood, and improved anesthesia, repair of an abdominal aortic aneurysm has be-come a much more simplified procedure.

The following features of the procedure are worthy of comment: (1) complete excision of the aneurysm with attendant danger to the nearby ve-nous structures, ureters, and duodenum has been abandoned. The anterior portion only of the aneurysm is removed without any attempt to dissect the adjacent structures from the lateral aspects. (2) It has been recognized that an inlay graft can be placed without the necessity for complete encirclement of the proximal and distal arteries and the blood loss and risks that often ac-company these maneuvers. (3) There is an awareness that a straight tube graft is feasible in many instances and that the more complicated placement of a Y-graft is not always necessary. (4) Intraoperative heparin is used to reduce the likelihood of intravascular thrombosis during the period of arte-rial occlusion. (5) Surgeons now know that massive intravenous fluid re-placement is necessary to prevent the renal problems which were common 15 years ago. (6) The development of sophisticated techniques of pulmonary and cardiac support and the ready availability of a critical care unit during the postoperative period have significantly reduced the risks to the patient.

Although the collected recent statistics for operative mortality shown in Table 1 are variable, it is clear that the risk of elective operation is invariably much lower than that of postrupture operation. Similar evidence is found by comparing long-term survival rates of operated versus nonoperated patients

261

TABLE 1.  Recent Reported Crude Mortality Rates for Elective and
Postrupture Operations for Abdominal Aortic Aneurysms

| Author | Years | Place | Elective Operation | | Postrupture Operation | |
|---|---|---|---|---|---|---|
| | | | Number of Patients | Mortality (Per Cent) | Number of Patients | Mortality (Per Cent) |
| Couch, et al.[8] | 1964–68 | P. B. Brigham Hosp., Boston | 55 | 15 | 15 | 60 |
| Gardner, et al.[14] | 1966–68 | W. Virginia Univ., Morgantown | 39 | 8 | | |
| Darling[10] | 1961–69 | Massachusetts General Hosp., Boston | 155 | 2.6 | 60 | 40 |
| Van Heeckeren[27] | 1964–69 | Yale, New Haven | | | 26 | 60 |
| Baker and Roberts[3] | 1966–69 | Univ. Pennsylvania, Philadelphia | 150 | 2.7 | | |
| Szilagyi et al.[25] | 1966–70 | Henry Ford Hosp., Detroit | 7 | | | 42.9 |
| Yashar[30] | 1958–71 | Providence, R.I. | 105 | 5.6 | 32 | 56 |
| David et al.[11] | 1960–71 | Louisiana State Univ., New Orleans | 69 | 2.6 | 14 | 100 |
| Williams et al.[28] | 1968–71 | Ft. Lauderdale, Fla. | 66 | 7.4 | 48 | 34 |
| Ameli et al.[2] | 1970–71 | Toronto, Canada | 162 | 6.7 | | |
| Key and Sokol[18] | 1957–72 | Toronto, Canada | 146 | 0.0 | 43 | |
| Cooley[7] | 1963–73 | Texas Heart Inst., Houston | 1092 | 5.8 | | 16 |
| Hicks et al.[17] | 1966–73 | Univ. Rochester, N.Y. | 242 | 8.4 | 56 | 55 |
| Thompson et al.[26] | 1968–74 | Baylor Univ., Dallas | 108 | 5.5 | | |
| Malan et al.[21] | | Milan, Italy | 154 | 6.7 | 44 | 69.9 |
| Stokes and Butcher[23] | | Barnes Hosp. and St. Lukes Hosp., St. Louis | 87 | 3.4 | 13 | 15 |

with aneurysms. For example, Szilagyi et al.[24] compared 244 surgical and 105 nonsurgical cases followed for as long as 13 years. At 5 years, the operated patient survival rate was 49 per cent as opposed to the 17 per cent rate for nonoperated patients, and the 10-year figures were 28 per cent versus 2 per cent. It is therefore generally agreed that elective aneurysmectomy should be done prior to rupture in most instances.

It has been contended by some, however, that small aneurysms are an exception to the general rule because the risk of rupture is less.[22] Wolffe and Colcher[29] reported no ruptures among 25 aneurysms less than 4.5 cm. in diameter, and Klippel and Butcher's study[19] of 30 patients also seems to support this conclusion since the two patients who died of rupture had a 6 and a 10 cm. lesion respectively. In 1967, Bernstein et al.[6] collected data and concluded that the incidence of rupture of small aneurysms was low and that the mortality risk was less than the risk of operation.

However, later experience indicates that the risk of rupture is appreciable and that the mortality risk is greater than the low risk associated with removal of a small aneurysm. Foster et al.[13] in 1969 reported that 16 per cent of nonoperated abdominal aortic aneurysms of less than 6 cm. in diameter ruptured at some variable time after detection, and Darling[10] found that 18 per cent of aneurysms less than 5 cm. in diameter ruptured. In 1972, Szilagyi et al.[25] summarized the results of nonsurgical treatment of abdominal aortic aneurysms and stated that death was due to rupture of 31 per cent of the 22 small (< 6 cm.) abdominal aortic aneurysms versus 42 per cent of those greater than 6 cm. More recently, Baker and Munns[4] noted that while they had treated no ruptured aneurysms smaller than 5 cm. in diameter, there had been 11 ruptured aneurysms of 5 to 7.5 cm. among a total of 58 patients over 70 years of age. Such data suggest that no aneurysm is immune to rupture, although smaller ones are less likely to do so.

It is difficult to determine precisely the size of the aneurysm. Most reports do not specify whether size was determined by palpation of the abdomen, laparotomy, autopsy, plain radiographs, reflected ultrasound, or isotope aortography. All available methods should be used to complement each other since any one tends to have inherent error. However, if all aneurysms are to be corrected, then differences of 1 to 2 cm. are of little practical concern.

The outline in Table 2 shows a reasonable management program for patients with abdominal aortic aneurysms. To be stressed is the necessity for immediate operation, without delaying in the emergency room for blood replacement, for the patient with a ruptured aneurysm. Needless laboratory work will delay control of bleeding. When the referring telephone diagnosis seems reliable, we prepare the operating room and have personnel standing by for the estimated time of arrival and transfer the patient from the ambulance through the emergency room without moving him from the ambulance stretcher to a bed and without making any particular effort to remove clothing other than to expose the abdomen as rapidly as possible in the operating room.

Aneurysms that have become acutely symptomatic in terms of pain are considered as threatening perforation, and such patients should be operated upon on the day of admission to the hospital after suitable brief diagnostic study and laboratory examination are completed. If correctable heart disease, diabetes, or other problem requires several hours of examination, it is undertaken in the critical care unit and the patient is carefully observed for changes which might signal actual rupture and require a shift to immediate operation.

For patients with asymptomatic aneurysms of large size, operation is scheduled at an early elective time. The intervening period of days is used for correction of any coexisting medical problems. For patients with small asymptomatic aneurysms, operation is similarly scheduled on an elective basis unless some factor exists which indicates that the risks of operation may be increased. When cardiac disease, pulmonary disease, carcinoma, or other noncorrectable disease is present, an individual decision is made based on the best possible estimate of the risk of operation versus that of a nonoperative course.

The various factors to be considered prior to recommending removal of a small asymptomatic abdominal aortic aneurysm are summarized in Table 3. Physiologic rather than chronologic age is stressed, along with recognition of

TABLE 2.  Indications in Abdominal Aortic Aneurysms

Rupture: immediate operation
Acute symptoms: early elective operation
Asymptomatic: large → elective operation
           small − good risk → elective operation
                 contraindication → observation

TABLE 3. Factors Affecting the Decision To Operate upon
a Small Aortic Aneurysm

Patient — general physiologic age
        coexisting conditions
              cardiovascular disease
              noncardiovascular disease
              obesity
Aneurysm — size
        evidence of growth
        symptoms
        position
Surgeon — personal experience
        team experience
Environment — anesthesia capability
        consultants
        intensive care facilities

other important disease processes. The most serious of these are hypertensive cardiovascular disease, previous myocardial infarction, and congestive heart failure, all of which increase somewhat the risk of operation.

There are no known statistics on the difference in the risk of operation in obese and thin patients, yet there is a clinical impression not only that obese patients are more difficult to operate upon but also that their postoperative convalescence is often more complicated. For this reason when the aneurysm is asymptomatic and small, the surgeon may require that the patient embark on a crash program of weight loss before he will accept him for operation. Some of these patients are actually able to rid themselves of 20 to 30 pounds in a period of several months, although they often regain them in the postoperative period.

The experience of the surgeon and his team are important considerations. Each surgeon must review his own results from time to time so that he can understand his personal statistics. Delusional identification of oneself with a more successful surgeon in terms of results occurs in the field of vascular surgery as well as in other areas of operative endeavor. The importance of the supporting team for the surgeon, who occasionally works outside his usual haunts, should be obvious.

Intraoperative care from a first-rate anesthesiologist, which provides respiratory support and fluid balance maintenance, together with other supportive measures available in the well-run intensive care facility can prevent complications which otherwise would be more likely to occur. In sum, they reduce mortality as much as does a rapid, efficient, and technically correct operative procedure.

## Summary

An abdominal aortic aneurysm, whatever its size, is dangerous to life, and unless there is a clear contraindication, is its own indication for operative repair.

# References

1. Alpert, J. A., Brief, D. K., and Parsonnet, V.: Surgery for the ruptured aortic aneurysm. J.A.M.A. *212*:1355, 1970.
2. Ameli, F. M., Gunstensen, J., Jain, K., Poilly, N., Spratt, E. H., and Tutassaura, H.: Surgical treatment of abdominal aortic aneurysms in Toronto: a study of 1013 patients. Can. Med. Assoc. J. *107*:1091, 1972.
3. Baker, A. G., and Roberts, B.: Long-term survival following abdominal aortic aneurysmectomy. J.A.M.A. *212*:445, 1970.
4. Baker, W. H., and Munns, J. R.: Aneurysmectomy in the aged. Arch. Surg. *110*:513, 1975.
5. Bergan, J. J., and Yao, J. S.: Modern management of abdominal aortic aneurysms. Surg. Clin. North Am. *54*:175, 1974.
6. Bernstein, E. F., Fisher, J. C., and Varco, R. L.: Is excision the optimum treatment for all abdominal aortic aneurysms? Surgery *61*:83, 1967.
7. Cooley, D. A.: Discussion. *In* Shumacker, H. B., Jr., Barnes, D. L., and King, H.: Ruptured abdominal aneurysm. Ann. Surg. *177*:772, 1973.
8. Couch, N. P., Lane, F. C., and Crane, C.: Management and mortality in resection of abdominal aortic aneurysm. Am. J. Surg. *119*:408, 1970.
9. Crisler, C., and Bahnson, H. T.: Aneurysms of the aorta. Curr. Probl. Surg. *1*:64, 1972.
10. Darling, R. C.: Ruptured arteriosclerotic abdominal aortic aneurysms. Am. J. Surg. *119*:397, 1970.
11. David, J. P., Marks, C., and Bonneval, M.: A ten year institutional experience with abdominal aneurysms. Surg. Gynecol. Obstet. *138*:591, 1974.
12. Esselstyn, C. B., Humphries, A. W., Young, J. R., Beven, E. G., and De Wolfe, V. C.: Aneurysmectomy in the aged? Surgery *67*:34, 1970.
13. Foster, J. H., Bolasny, B. L., Gobbel, W. G., and Scott, H. W.: Comparative study of elective resection and expectant treatment of abdominal aortic aneurysm. Surg. Gynecol. Obstet. *129*:1, 1969.
14. Gardner, R. J., Lancaster, J. R., and Tarnay, J. J.: Five year history of surgically treated abdominal aortic aneurysms. Surg. Gynecol. Obstet. *130*:981, 1970.
15. Hall, A. D., Zubrin, J. R., Moore, W. S., and Thomas, A. N.: Surgical treatment of aortic aneurysm in the aged. Arch. Surg. *100*:455, 1970.
16. Hardy, J. D.: Discussion. *In* Esselstyn, C. B., Humphries, A. W., Young, J. R., Beven, E. G., and De Wolfe, V. C.: Aneurysmectomy in the aged? Surgery *67*:34, 1970.
17. Hicks, O. L., Eastland, W. M., DeWeese, J. A., May, A. G., and Rob, C. G.: Survival improvement following aortic aneurysm resection. Ann. Surg. *181*:863, 1975.
18. Key, J. A., and Sokol, D. M.: The symptomless abdominal aneurysm: a 15 year review. Can. J. Surg. *16*:297, 1973.
19. Klippel, A. P., and Butcher, H. R.: The Unoperated abdominal aortic aneurysm. Am. J. Surg. *111*:629, 1966.
20. Lord, J. W.: Discussion. *In* Esselstyn, C. B., Humphries, A. W., Young, J. R., Beven, E. G., and DeWolfe, V. C.: Aneurysmectomy in the aged? Surgery *67*:34, 1970.
21. Malan, E., Ruberti, U., Tiberio, G., DeMetz, A., and Biglioli, P.: Abdominal aortic aneurysms: results with surgical treatment in 198 cases. Cardiovasc. Surg. *13*:576, 1972.
22. Schatz, I. J., Fairbairn, J. F., and Juergens, J. L.: Abdominal aortic aneurysms: a reappraisal. Circulation *26*:200, 1962.
23. Stokes, J., and Butcher, H. R., Jr.: Abdominal aortic aneurysms. Factors influencing operative mortality and criteria of operability. Arch. Surg. *107*:297, 1973.
24. Szilagyi, D. E., Smith, R. F., DeRusso, F. J., and Elliott, J. P.: Contribution of abdominal aortic aneurysmectomy to prolongation of life. Ann. Surg. *164*:678, 1966.
25. Szilagyi, D. E., Elliott, J. P., and Smith, R. F.: Clinical fate of the patient with asymptomatic abdominal aortic aneurysm unfit for surgical treatment. Arch. Surg. *104*:600, 1972.
26. Thompson, J. E., Hollier, L. H., Patman, R. D., and Persson, A. V.: Surgical management of abdominal aortic aneurysms: factors influencing mortality and morbidity: a 20 year experience. Ann. Surg. *181*:654, 1975.
27. Van Heeckeren, D. W.: Ruptured abdominal aortic aneurysm. Am. J. Surg. *119*:402, 1970.
28. Williams, R. D., Fisher, F. W., and Dickey, J. W.: Problems in the diagnosis and treatment of abdominal aortic aneurysms. Am. J. Surg. *123*:698, 1972.
29. Wolffe, J. B., and Colcher, R. E.: Diagnosis and conservative treatment of atherosclerotic aneurysms of the abdominal aorta. Vasc. Dis. *3*:49, 1966.
30. Yashar, J. J.: Surgical resection of aneurysm of the abdominal aorta: experience with 137 consecutive cases. Elective operation improves survival expectancy significantly. R.I. Med. J. *55*:43, 1972.

# Considerations in the Management of Poor-Risk Patients with Small Asymptomatic Abdominal Aortic Aneurysms

EUGENE F. BERNSTEIN

*University of California, San Diego, School of Medicine*

"It is foolish to follow the practice of the ancient surgeons and decline to treat any aneurysms, but it is dangerous to apply surgical treatment to all types."

Antyllus (1st Century A.D., Greece)

## Statement of Position

In general, the diagnosis of an abdominal aortic aneurysm is an indication for its operative excision because of the threat of sudden rupture and death. Certainly, the aneurysm which is large (> 6 cm.), symptomatic, rapidly expanding, leaking, or ruptured must be operated upon, essentially regardless of the patient's general condition, because under these circumstances mortality from aneurysm rupture is prohibitive unless efficient operative intervention is undertaken. In asymptomatic, small aneurysms, too, elective operation is advisable in good risk patients since the aneurysm will only expand with time and present a greater risk of rupture in the future when the patient's general condition and operative risk may no longer be as good. In none of these areas is there any controversy. However, in patients with small asymptomatic abdominal aneurysms who are relatively poor operative risks, there is a place for the judicious selection of nonoperative management, which will provide this group of patients with life expectancy equal to or greater than that following routine operative therapy. More recent data will permit such choices to be based on firmer, more quantitative grounds.

## Supporting Evidence

1. Following successful operation for abdominal aortic aneurysms, long-term survival is poor, averaging about 50 per cent in 5 years, despite decreasing elective operative mortality rates (Table 1).

2. The long-term outlook for the unoperated patient is better than formerly thought, with the survival rate ranging from 10 to 36 per cent in seven recent clinical series (Table 2). However, with small asymptomatic aneurysms, the outlook for unoperated patients (Wolffe,[34] 30 per cent; Szilagyi,[29] 48 per cent) approaches the long-term survival rate following operation.

3. Aneurysm size strongly influences the likelihood of rupture, which is 20 per cent or less with aneurysms 6 cm. in diameter or less (Table 3). Much of the argument for withholding operation from the poor risk patient with the asymptomatic small aneurysm is based on such data indicating a relatively low incidence of rupture under these circumstances. These data are based almost exclusively on measurements performed at autopsy, which may produce an underestimate of aneurysm size during life since the aorta is measured without the distension due to physiologic blood pressure. Nevertheless, these autopsy data document a rupture rate of 2 per cent or less for aneurysms *under 5 cm.* in size, with the exception of the recent series of Darling,[6] which cites an 18 per cent rupture rate in this small-aneurysm

TABLE 1.  Recent Data on Elective Operative Mortality and 5-Year Survival Following Abdominal Aneurysmectomy

| Institution | Recent Mortality – Elective Operation | | | | Long-Term Survival | |
|---|---|---|---|---|---|---|
| | Number of Years Included | Number of Cases | Operative Mortality (Per Cent) | Year Reported | 5-Year Survival (Per Cent) | Year Reported |
| Baylor U.[7] | 2 | 533 | 5 | 1964 | 58 | 1964 |
| Henry Ford Hosp.[29] | 2 | 127 | 6 | 1966 | 49 | 1969 |
| Georgetown U.[12] | 1 | 100 | 4 | 1967 | – | – |
| U. Rochester[23] | 2 | 39 | 7 | 1968 | 49 | 1968 |
| Vanderbilt U.[11] | 4 | 52 | 8 | 1969 | 50° | 1969 |
| U. California, S.F., V.A. Hosp., S.F.[13] | 13 | 62 | 5 | 1969 | 47 | 1969 |
| Massachusetts General Hosp.[6] | 8 | 155 | 3 | 1970 | – | – |
| U. Pennsylvania[1] | 3 | 145 | 3 | 1970 | 54 | 1970 |
| U. W. Virginia[13] | 5 | 56 | 13 | – | – | – |
| Barnes Hosp.[28] | 6 | 87 | 4 | 1973 | 53 | 1973 |
| MEAN | | | 5.8 | | 51 | |

° Elective operations only.

TABLE 2.   Five-Year Survival in Untreated Patients with
Abdominal Aortic Aneurysms (Clinical Series)

| Author | Number of Patients | Per Cent With Rupture | 5-Year Survival (Per Cent) |
|---|---|---|---|
| Estes[9] | 102 | 63 | 19 |
| Foster[11] | 75 | 38 | 18 |
| Klippel[21] | 30 | 10 | 27 |
| Schatz[24] | 119 | 44 | 36 |
| Steinberg[27] | 96 | 20 | 35 |
| Szilagyi[29] | 156° | 28 | 10 |
| Szilagyi[30]† | 44 | 20 | 48 |
| Wolffe[34]† | 33 | 0 | 30 |
| MEAN | | | 20 |

° Rejected for operation as medically unfit.
† Aneurysms < 6 cm.

group. Further data indicate a rupture rate of 4 to 20 per cent in aneurysms *under 6 cm.* in size and provide the basis for believing that there is a sharp dividing line for risk of rupture, since all series indicate a rupture rate of greater than 70 per cent in aneurysms measuring *7 cm. or more.* For these compelling reasons, early operative intervention is indicated for essentially all aneurysms greater than 6 cm. in diameter, regardless of the presence of symptoms or other factors suggesting a high operative risk. However, in the small asymptomatic lesion, the rupture risk of up to 20 per cent must be balanced against the risk of immediate operative mortality and the likelihood of early death from other existing conditions. Accurate delineation of aneurysm size is clearly critical in weighing these risks, and the easy availability of ul-

TABLE 3.   Effect of Size on Aneurysm Rupture Rate

| Year Reported | Author | Number of Cases | Per Cent Ruptured |
|---|---|---|---|
| | SMALL ANEURYSMS (<5 cm.) | | |
| 1957 | Shapiro[25] | 16 | 0 |
| 1959 | Sommerville[26] | 117 | 1 |
| 1967 | Fomon[10] | 54 | 2 |
| 1970 | Darling[6] | 182 | 18 |
| TOTAL | | 369 | MEAN 5 |
| | SMALL ANEURYSMS (<6 cm.) | | |
| 1955 | Crane[5] | 26 | 4 |
| 1966 | Szilagyi[29] | 130 (operative) | 16 |
| | | 82 (nonop.) | 20 |
| 1969 | Foster[11] | 38 | 16 |
| TOTAL | | 276 | MEAN 16 |
| | LARGE ANEURYSMS (≥7 cm.) | | |
| 1955 | Crane[5] | 17 | 82 |
| 1957 | Shapiro[25] | 9 | 78 |
| 1957 | Gliedman[14] | 32 | 72 |
| 1959 | Sommerville[26] | 19 | 80 |
| 1967 | Fomon[10] | 10 | 70 |
| 1970 | Darling[6] | 47 | 75 |
| TOTAL | | 134 | MEAN 76 |

TABLE 4.   Cause of Late Death in Patients with Abdominal Aneurysms

|  | Progressive Arteriosclerosis (Per Cent) | Aneurysm Rupture (Per Cent) | Late Deaths Related to Operation (Per Cent) | All Other Causes (Per Cent) |
|---|---|---|---|---|
| Nonoperative (Szilagyi[29]) | 56 | 28 | – | 17 |
| Operative – UCLA[4] | 43 | – | 14 | 43 |
| U. Pennsylvania[1] | 41 | – | 29 | 29 |
| U. Kansas[19] | 48 | – | 13 | 39 |
| Columbia U.[32] | 52 | – | 30 | 17 |
| Baylor U.[7] | 64 | – | 11 | 25 |
| U. Minnesota[3] | 47 | – | 29 | 24 |

trasonic echography, with its demonstrated accuracy (within 3 mm.) in estimating aneurysm size,[22] makes this technique essential to the knowledgeable assessment of risks with either form of management in the borderline patient.

4. Most late deaths are from arteriosclerotic complications in the heart, brain, and kidney, not from aneurysm rupture, whether or not the aneurysm has been operated upon (Table 4). Both the immediate operative mortality and the late mortality due to complications of the operation or progressive disease (e.g., aortoenteric fistula, late intestinal obstruction) must be considered in calculating the price of operative treatment in the poor risk patient.

5. Aneurysm growth rates are quite slow for small aneurysms. Thirty-four patients have been identified in our clinic over the past 5 years who meet our requirements for further nonoperative observation of small asymptomatic abdominal aortic aneurysms in poor risk patients. By remeasuring these aneurysms periodically (every 3 months) with the ultrasonic A-mode and B-scan echogram, data have been obtained regarding the growth rates of these lesions over periods ranging from 6 to 60 months (Table 5; Fig. 1). Patients originally assigned to this group have been re-evaluated at the time of each examination and subjected to operation on the basis of (1) rapid growth, (2) the aneurysm reaching a diameter of 6 cm. or more, or (3) the development of symptoms or signs suggestive of expansion or rupture. To date, 12 patients have been operated upon, including one for frank rupture.

TABLE 5.   Summary of Abdominal Aortic Aneurysm Growth Rate Data Obtained in Poor Risk Patients with Small (<6 cm.) Asymptomatic Aneurysms Followed with Ultrasonic Echography Scans at 3-Month Intervals for at Least 1 Year

| Initial Aneurysm Size (cm.) | Patient Months of Observation | Mean Growth Rate (cm./yr.) |
|---|---|---|
| 3.0–3.9 | 179 | 0.15 |
| 4.0–4.9 | 248 | 0.54 |
| 5.0–5.9 | 79 | 0.15 |
|  | 506 patient months or 42.2 patient years | 0.34 |

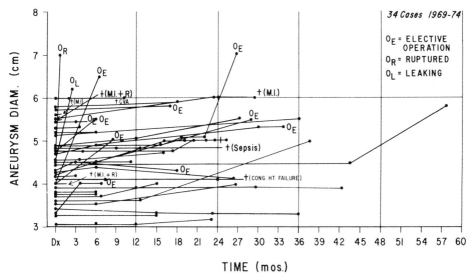

*Figure 1.* Echographic evaluation of growth rates of abdominal aortic aneurysms in poor risk patients.

Two others died with myocardial infarction and aneurysm rupture of unknown duration. Five additional patients have succumbed to other diseases, with their aneurysms remaining intact. The remainder continue in the protocol. From this experience, it is clear that even the very small aneurysm can be treacherous, become symptomatic, or expand rapidly. This unpredictable rupture rate approximates 5 per cent per year. However, most of these lesions remain quite stable for long periods of time. Based on currently available data for this group of patients who have been followed for over 42 patient-years, the average aneurysm growth rate appears to be approximately 0.34 cm. per year of observation. These two figures, the rupture rate per year and the average growth rate per year for stable lesions, offer a quantitative assessment of the risk of the lesion to the patient, against which the risk of the operation may be weighed.

## Gaps in Our Evidence

There is no truly prospective, randomized study of the outcome of the particular patient group in question, alternately treated by selective criteria and by routine operation.

## Flaws in the Opposing Point of View

1. Previously published comparative retrospective clinical studies of operated and nonoperated groups are misleading, no matter how well matched the groups, since there must have been an important reason for the

surgeons to have rejected the members of the nonoperative group as medically unfit, which clearly biased their outcome. Such studies are not randomized trials of operation but rather are a comparison of the life spans of good and poor risk patients with abdominal aneurysms, in regard to which aneurysmectomy may be a relatively unimportant factor. To settle this issue, a prospective, randomized trial of uniform versus selective operative treatment in poor risk asymptomatic patients with small (< 6 cm.) aneurysms is required.

2. Until recently, the diagnosis of an abdominal aneurysm was considered reasonably secure when based on the physical findings of a pulsatile abdominal mass, evidence of calcification on a lateral abdominal roentgenograph, and, in a few clinics, an aortogram. Data regarding the accuracy of each of these techniques is currently available (Table 6) and confirms the clinical impression that there is more than an occasional error, in both the positive and negative directions. These diagnostic errors are of particular pertinence to the present discussion, since the bulk of data relating to the unoperated patient is based upon such diagnostic criteria.

More recently, the echogram and the radionucleotide scan have become available; these offer greater accuracy than contrast aortography, without invasion or patient risk. The A-mode echogram is also capable of accurately delineating aneurysm size (±3 mm.) since it measures outer wall dimensions in contrast to the conventional and radionucleotide aortograms, which depict intraluminal diameter and are misleading in lesions commonly filled with layers of atheromatous material and thrombus.

## Additional Factors

### Influence of Hypertension

Elevated arterial blood pressure is common in patients with abdominal aneurysms, with an average incidence of 45 per cent.[15] However, whether

TABLE 6. Accuracy and Limitations of Various Diagnostic Techniques in Detecting and Evaluating Abdominal Aortic Aneurysms[*]

| Technique | Accuracy (Per Cent) | Limitations |
|---|---|---|
| 1. Physical examination | 88 | Body habitus, kyphosis, transmitted pulsations, tortuous aorta. |
| 2. Lateral abdominal X-ray | 55–85 | Two dimensional. Not all aneurysms are calcified. |
| 3. Aortography | 90 | Only demonstrates lumen—may be falsely narrow, or negative. Two dimensional. Risk of arterial puncture. |
| 4. Radionucleotide aortic scan | 90+ | Same as aortography, but no arterial puncture. |
| 5. Ultrasonic echography | 100 | Three dimensional representation, demonstrates outer walls and true size. No risk. |

[*]From Gore, I., and Hirst, A. E., Jr.: Arteriosclerotic aneurysms of the abdominal aorta: a review. Prog. Cardiovasc. Dis. 16:113–150, 1973. Reproduced by permission.

hypertension influences the likelihood of aneurysm rupture is unclear. In the autopsy reports of Gliedman[14] and Sommerville,[26] hypertension was no more frequent in those patients who died of aneurysm rupture than in patients who died of other causes. On the other hand, Szilagyi[30] found a strong correlation between those patients in whom arterial hypertension was present and rupture occurred (67 per cent) and those patients deemed medically unfit for elective operation in whom rupture did not occur, in whom the incidence of hypertension was 23 per cent. Furthermore, rupture occurred in two thirds of the patients in whom hypertension was the specific contraindication for operation. As a result, Szilagyi has suggested that the presence of hypertension should favor the surgical approach, despite its correlation with an increased operative mortality. Foster,[11] too, cites evidence that diastolic hypertension is more likely to lead to rupture, which occurred in 72 per cent of his patients who had the combination of diastolic hypertension (> 100 mm. Hg) and an untreated aneurysm. On the basis of these clinical data, hypertension should be an indication for strongly considering elective operation, even in the relatively poor risk patient.

### The Aged

Whether an arbitrary age limit should be adopted for the elective operative treatment of asymptomatic aneurysms is not uniformly accepted, although many authors, including Szilagyi[29, 30] and Bergan[2] believe that patients over 80 years of age should not be operated on without compelling indications. The reports of Esselstyn[8] and Hardy[20] indicate a substantially higher operative mortality rate (14 and 15 per cent respectively) for aneurysm operation in patients over 75 years of age, and Wilder[33] reports that patients over 80 years of age had a 33 per cent mortality rate for all types of operations and that 42 per cent were dead within 6 months of their operations. In view of these data, I would be selective in accepting patients over 75 years of age for elective aneurysm operation and would accept a patient over 80 only if he was physiologically younger and free of all other serious complicating diseases.

## Summary

In concluding, I agree completely with the following statements:

Good risk patients should have elective resection of an existing abdominal aortic aneurysm, regardless of the size of the aneurysm. Resection is recommended in poor risk patients with symptomatic aneurysms because the chance of rupture is great. For the same reason, resection is also advised in most poor risk patients with large asymptomatic aneurysms. A more conservative attitude is justified in patients with significant cardiovascular disease and small asymptomatic aneurysms, since ruptured aneurysm is much less likely to be the cause of death in such patients. These patients should be studied carefully and operation deferred until signs or symptoms of enlargement of the aneurysm are noted.[11]

Although we choose to call this a "conservative" approach, while other vascular surgeons refer to their attitudes as "aggressive," in practice, it is clear that little difference of opinion exists regarding proper treatment for the patient group in question, the poor risk patients. It is a matter of viewing the glass as half full or half empty. The availability of newer, more accurate methods for the diagnosis and measurement of abdominal aneurysms should permit a more quantitative evaluation of the costs and benefits of elective operation to these poor risk patients.

## References

1. Baker, A. G., and Robers, B.: Long-term survival following abdominal aortic aneurysmectomy. J.A.M.A. 212:445, 1970.
2. Bergan, J. J., and Yao, J. S. T.: Modern management of abdominal aortic aneurysms. Surg. Clin. North Am. 54:175, 1974.
3. Bernstein, E. F., Fisher, J. C., and Varco, R. L.: Is excision optimum treatment for all abdominal aortic aneurysms? Surgery 61:83, 1967.
4. Cannon, J. A., Van De Water, J., and Barker, W. F.: Experience with the surgical management of 100 consecutive cases of abdominal aortic aneurysms. Am. J. Surg. 106:128, 1963.
5. Crane, C.: Arteriosclerotic aneurysm of abdominal aorta. N. Engl. J. Med. 253:954, 1955.
6. Darling, R. C.: Ruptured arteriosclerotic abdominal aortic aneurysms. Am. J. Surg. 119:397, 1970.
7. DeBakey, M. E., Crawford, E. S., Cooley, D. A., Morris, G. C., Jr., Roysten, T. S., and Abbott, W. P.: Aneurysm of abdominal aorta. Analysis of results of graft replacement therapy one to eleven years after operation. Ann. Surg. 160:622, 1964.
8. Esselstyn, C. B., Jr., Humphries, A. W., Young, J. R., Beven, E., and De Wolfe, V. G.: Aneurysmectomy in the aged? Surgery 67:34, 1970.
9. Estes, J. E.: Abdominal aortic aneurysm: study of one hundred and two cases. Circulation 2:258, 1950.
10. Fomon, J. J., Kurzweg, F. T., and Broadway, R. K.: Aneurysms of aorta: review. Ann. Surg. 165:557, 1967.
11. Foster, J. H., Bolasny, B. L., Gobbel, W. G., and Scott, H. W.: Comparative study of elective resection and expectant treatment of abdominal aortic aneurysm. Surg. Gynecol. Obstet. 129:1, 1969.
12. Friedman, S. A., Hufuagel, C. A., Conrad, P. W., Simmons, E. M., and Weintraub, A.: Abdominal aortic aneurysms. J.A.M.A. 200:1147, 1969.
13. Gardner, R. J., Lancaster, J. R., Tarnay, T. J., Warden, H. E., and Curie, R. A.: Five year history of surgically treated abdominal aortic aneurysms. Surg. Gynecol. Obstet. 130:981, 1970.
14. Gliedman, M. L., Ayres, W. B., and Vestal, B. L.: Aneurysms of abdominal aorta and its branches. Ann. Surg. 146:207, 1957.
15. Gore, S., and Hirst, A. E., Jr.: Arteriosclerotic aneurysms of the abdominal aorta: a review. Progr. Cardiovasc. Dis. 16:113, 1973.
16. Gwathmey, O., Adkins, P. C., and Blades, B.: Emergency and elective surgical treatment of abdominal aortic aneurysms. Postgrad. Med. 25:677, 1959.
17. Hall, A. D., Zubrin, J. R., Moore, W. S., and Thomas, A. N.: Surgical treatment of aortic aneurysm in the aged. Arch. Surg. 100:455, 1970.
18. Halpert, B., and Willms, R. K.: Aneurysms of aorta. Arch. Pathol. 74:163, 1962.
19. Hardin, C. A.: Survival and complications after 121 surgically treated abdominal aneurysms. Surg. Gynecol. Obstet. 118:541, 1964.
20. Hardy, J. D.: Discussion. In Esselstyn, C. B., Jr., Humphries, A. W., Young, J. R., Beven, E., and DeWolfe, V. G.: Aneurysmectomy in the aged? Surgery 67:34, 1970.
21. Klippel, A. P., and Butcher, H. R.: The unoperated abdominal aortic aneurysm. Am. J. Surg. 111:629, 1966.
22. Leopold, G. R., Goldberger, L. E., and Bernstein, E. F.: Ultrasonic detection and evaluation of abdominal aortic aneurysms. Surgery 72:939, 1972.

23. May, A. G., DeWeese, J. A., Frani, I., Mahoney, E. B., and Rob, C. G.: Surgical treatment of abdominal aortic aneurysms. Surgery 63:711, 1968.
24. Schatz, I. J., Fairbairn, J. F., II, and Juergens, J. L.: Abdominal aortic aneurysms: reappraisal. Circulation 36:200, 1962.
25. Shapiro, E.: Aneurysms of the abdominal aorta: prognosis if untreated. Calif. Med. 87:155, 1957.
26. Sommerville, R. L., Allen, E. V., and Edwards, J. E.: Bland and infected arteriosclerotic abdominal aortic aneurysms. Medicine 38:207, 1959.
27. Steinberg, I., and Tobier, N.: Study of 200 consecutive patients with abdominal aneurysms diagnosed by intravenous aortography: comparative longevity with and without aneurysmectomy. Circulation 35:530, 1967.
28. Stokes, J., and Butcher, H. R.: Abdominal aortic aneurysms: factors influencing operative mortality and criteria of operability. Arch. Surg. 107:297, 1973.
29. Szilagyi, D. E., Smith, R. F., DeRusso, F. J., Elliott, J. P., and Sherrin, F. W.: Contribution of abdominal aortic aneurysmectomy to prolongation of life. Ann. Surg. 164:678, 1966.
30. Szilagyi, D. E., Elliott, J. P., and Smith, R. F.: Clinical fate of the patient with asymptomatic abdominal aortic aneurysm unfit for surgical treatment. Arch. Surg. 104:600, 1972.
31. Van Heeckeren, D. W.: Ruptured abdominal aortic aneurysms. Am. J. Surg. 119:402, 1970.
32. Voorhees, A. B., Jr., and McAllister, F. F.: Long-term results following resection of arteriosclerotic abdominal aortic aneurysms. Surg. Gynecol. Obstet. 117:355, 1963.
33. Wilder, R. J., and Fishbein, R. H.: Operative experience with patients over 80 years of age. Surg. Gynecol. Obstet. 113:205, 1961.
34. Wolffe, J. B., and Colcher, R. E.: Diagnosis and conservative management of atherosclerotic aneurysms of abdominal aorta. Vasc. Dis. 3:49, 1966.

# 13

# *Prevention of Postoperative Pulmonary Embolism*

Is Postoperative Pulmonary
Embolism a Preventable
Complication?
*by V. V. Kakkar*

Postoperative Pulmonary
Embolism is a Preventable
Complication
*by Richard E. C. Collins
and Edwin W. Salzman*

## Statement of the Problem

*The discussants address themselves to the efficacy and hazards of various methods aimed at preventing postoperative venous thrombosis and pulmonary embolism.*

*Provide data which serve to define high-risk patients in terms of such factors as age, obesity, varicose veins, pre-existing diseases, type of operation, and type of injury.*

*Discuss and judge Coumadin, heparin, "mini-heparin," dextran, Persantine, and aspirin as prophylactic agents. What are the data regarding these agents with respect to intraoperative bleeding, postoperative bleeding, wound infection, prevention of venous thrombosis, prevention of pulmonary embolus, cost, and difficulty of control?*

*Analyze existing data regarding the efficacy for preventing venous thrombosis of: (1) leg wrapping, (2) early ambulation, (3) elevation of foot of the bed, and (4) active and passive physical therapy.*

# Is Postoperative Pulmonary Embolism a Preventable Complication?

V. V. KAKKAR

*King's College Hospital Medical School*

Venous thromboembolism is a frequent complication in hospital patients. Apart from the immediate risk to life, one must also consider the late sequelae of extensive deep vein thrombosis—swelling of the legs, varicose veins, ulceration, and other trophic changes which represent an equally distressing situation. It is often asked whether postoperative pulmonary embolism is preventable, and furthermore, whether it is worth preventing, since the mortality due to this complication is extremely low and all prophylactic measures require supervision, extra work, organization, and vigilance? The data presented in this paper support the argument that not only should this complication be prevented but also that several prophylactic measures are now available which make prevention a practical proposition.

## The Need for Prophylaxis

This need can best be illustrated by consideration of the following facts: Despite advances in the management of pulmonary embolism, the mortality due to this condition is increasing; the deaths recorded in the Registrar General's report for England and Wales indicate that there has been nearly a six-fold increase in mortality due to pulmonary embolism during the last 30 years. It has been estimated that approximately 21,000 patients die each year from this cause in the United Kingdom,[1] while the figures reported for the United States vary between 47,000 and 140,000.[2,3] Several autopsy studies have shown that most cases of major embolism are not diagnosed during life and thus are not treated.[4,5,6] Two thirds of the deaths from pulmonary embolism occur within 30 minutes after the embolic event[7]—too brief a

279

period for even pulmonary embolectomy to be performed or for any benefit to be derived from thrombolytic therapy, which has been shown to be highly effective in producing rapid lysis of emboli.[8, 9, 10] Furthermore, approximately 80 per cent of pulmonary emboli occur without premonitory signs of peripheral venous thrombosis, and consequently, treatment with heparin and oral anticoagulants to prevent embolism is often not given. Thus, to say that one's policy is to treat massive pulmonary embolism or its precursor, peripheral venous thrombosis, is to expose patients to an unacceptable risk of fatal complications.

The most rational approach would therefore seem to be that of developing an effective method of prophylaxis, if the mortality due to pulmonary embolism and the misery due to the postphlebitic syndrome are to be significantly reduced. If such a method is to be adopted on a wide scale, it must fulfill the following criteria: it must be simple, safe and effective; it must be applicable to all types of patients at risk of developing deep vein thrombosis; and it must cover the period of risk, which in surgical patients has been shown to extend from the time of operation through the first 7 to 10 postoperative days.

## Available Methods

Venous thrombi are generally regarded as an expression of blood coagulation and fibrin formation in the presence of venous stasis. The main attempts to prevent deep vein thrombosis can be conveniently divided into two groups: those directed toward the elimination of stasis in the deep veins of the legs and those employed to counteract changes in blood coagulability.

### ELIMINATION OF STASIS

Despite general agreement that stasis plays a significant role in the pathogenesis of venous thrombosis and despite increasing awareness of the hazards of bed rest, there is conflicting evidence as to the efficacy of early ambulation and leg exercises in reducing the incidence of deep vein thrombosis: some workers say they are of value[11, 12, 13, 14] while others deny this.[15, 16, 17, 18] Unfortunately, these conclusions are based on physical signs alone, which are often quite inadequate to diagnose the existence of a venous thrombosis. Although elastic stockings have been shown to increase the rate of venous return,[19] recent studies using the $^{125}$I-labelled fibrinogen test (an accurate and objective method of detecting deep vein thrombosis) have failed to confirm the beneficial effects in surgical patients who wore elastic stockings throughout their hospital stay.[20] Elevation of the lower extremities has also been claimed to increase the rate of venous return,[21] but again, controlled studies have shown this to be ineffective in preventing venous thrombosis.[22]

The limitations of intensive physical prophylaxis in general surgical cases were clearly demonstrated by Flanc, Kakkar, and Clarke, using the [125]I-fibrinogen test to detect leg vein thrombi.[23] In this study, patients wore elastic stockings from admission to discharge, had frequent and vigorous leg exercises before and after operation, had the foot of the bed elevated, and were provided with a foot board to aid plantar flexion against resistance; pressure on the calves during operation was avoided by the use of a sorbo-rubber stand, and after operation, the legs were kept elevated until consciousness permitted exercise and movement. Ambulation began between the first and third postoperative day, depending on the operation. Despite all efforts, the overall results of these physical measures were disappointing: thrombosis was detected in 25 per cent of 67 patients having intensive physiotherapy and in 35 per cent of 65 concurrent controls. However, a significant reduction was seen in the elderly patients undergoing major operation, in whom the incidence of thrombosis was 24 per cent, compared with 61 per cent in the controls. However, different results have been reported by Tsapogas and co-workers, who found these methods to be highly effective.[24]

More specific attempts have now been made to prevent stasis during operation, and several methods for increasing venous return from the lower limbs have recently been investigated. One of these is electrical stimulation of the calf muscles during operation: two electrodes are applied to the calf and a low voltage current is used to contract the muscles every 2 to 4 seconds. The beneficial results of this method of preventing stasis and consequently of reducing thrombosis, first reported by Doran, Drury, and Sivyer in 1964,[17] have now been investigated by several other workers, using the radioactive fibrinogen test for assessment.

Another method, pneumatic compression of the calves,[26] involves encasing the legs in an envelope of plastic material and rhythmically altering the pressure to squeeze the calf muscles and increase venous return. In practice, an electric pump inflates each legging alternately so that compression at 40 to 45 mm. Hg for 1 minute is achieved, followed by relaxation for 1 minute. The advantage of this method is that it can be used not only during operation but also in the postoperative period. The third method which has been investigated consists of passive plantar and dorsiflexion of the foot during operation by means of motor-driven pedals, which again increases blood flow.[27] The results of some of the studies using these different methods are shown in Table 1. In each study, the radioactive fibrinogen test was used to detect the presence of deep vein thrombosis.

There is little doubt that all these methods lessen stasis and lower the incidence of venous thrombosis, except in "high risk" patients undergoing operation for malignant disease. However, such physical methods present almost insuperable difficulties as a long-term solution: they must be applied to both legs, and during certain types of operation—for example, for repair of fractured neck of femur or those in which the patient is in the lithotomy position—they are either impracticable or extremely inconvenient. These prophylactic measures must be applied not only during operation but also at regular intervals for the first 10 postoperative days and perhaps even longer. Some of the methods are uncomfortable for conscious patients, and, most importantly the logistical problem of applying such physical measures on a

TABLE 1. Prophylaxis: Effect of Elimination of Stasis on the Incidence of Postoperative Deep Vein Thrombosis as Detected by the $^{125}$I-Fibrinogen Test

| | Control Group | | Treated Group | | |
| --- | --- | --- | --- | --- | --- |
| Study | Number Studied | Deep Vein Thrombosis | Number Studied | Deep Vein Thrombosis | Statistical Significance |
| Electrical stimulation of calf muscles[63] | 110 limbs | 23(20.9%) | 110 limbs | 9(8.2%) | 0.001 < p < 0.01 |
| Pneumatic compression of the calves[26] | 16 patients | 8(50%) | 9 patients | 5(55.5%)° | |
| | 34 patients | 7(21%) | 41 patients | 1(2.4%)† | p = 0.015 |
| Passive flexion of calf muscles[27] | 47 limbs | 13(27.6%) | 47 limbs | 3(6.4%) | 5%‡ |

° Patients with malignant disease.
† Patients without malignant disease.
‡ Sequential analysis—the line of significance corresponds to a probability level of 5 per cent.

large scale would strain the resources of even the most lavishly equipped hospital. Experience with less complicated regimens of intensive prophylaxis supports this view. Thus physical methods are unlikely to be the choice for the future.

## COUNTERACTING BLOOD COAGULABILITY

Many attempts have also been made to prevent thrombosis by simpler means, such as the use of chemical agents. These agents can be broadly classified into three main groups. It has been suggested that adhesion of platelets to subendothelial connective tissue at the site of presumed-damaged venous endothelium and subsequent events leading to platelet aggregation may account for thrombus formation. If this platelet aggregation can be prevented, it is conceivable that the thrombus will not form. It is with this background that various drugs have been investigated which interfere with the different aspects of platelet function; these include dextran (usually dextran 70), dipyridamole, aspirin, and chloroquine.

The second chemical approach has involved the use of drugs which interfere with the coagulation mechanism. A vital step in the sequence of coagulation is the conversion of prothrombin to thrombin, under the influence of activated Factor X. The thrombin so formed acts on fibrinogen to convert it into fibrin, which in turn forms the essential network of a venous thrombus. To block the coagulation sequence, two different types of drugs have been used: oral anticoagulants, which act by reducing synthesis in the liver of various clotting factors such as prothrombin, Factor X, and others; and heparin, which acts primarily by increasing Factor X inhibitor activity.[28] Therefore, small doses of heparin given before Factor X is activated are effective in preventing thrombosis but do not affect the clotting time.

The third group of drugs is thought to act on venous endothelium to increase naturally occurring fibrinolytic activity in the body. Astrup[29] has suggested that thrombosis may be due in part to a local or generalized imbalance between coagulation and fibrinolysis. A shift in the balance toward fibrinolysis could prevent thrombosis or rapidly lyse recent thrombi, while impairment of fibrinolysis would encourage the growth of the thrombus. Various investigators[30, 31, 32] have shown that fibrinolytic activity in the blood and vein walls is abnormally low in the majority of patients with recent deep vein thrombosis or superficial thrombophlebitis.

A large number of papers have recently been published claiming success or otherwise with these various types of drugs: their results are summarized in Table 2. Analysis of these data clearly shows a good deal of confusion, and the reason for this is that in the majority of studies, clinical methods were used to assess the effectiveness of the agent used. This form of assessment has now been shown to be unreliable for detecting the presence or absence of thrombosis.

The evidence that drugs such as aspirin and dipyridamole (known to interfere with platelet function) effectively reduce the incidence of deep vein thrombosis is unconvincing, and these agents should probably not be used for the prophylaxis of venous thrombosis. In a recent double-blind, randomized trial, the efficacy of aspirin in preventing postoperative venous thromboembolism was assessed.[33] In this study, 303 patients over the age of 28 admitted for elective operation were included; they were randomly allocated to either a control or a treated group and received either 600 mg. of aspirin or a placebo—plain white tablets. Deep vein thrombosis was diagnosed by the [125]I-fibrinogen test. Twenty-two per cent of the patients who received the placebo developed isotopic thrombi, compared with 27.5 per cent of those receiving aspirin.

Similar disappointing results were reported by O'Brien.[34] However, different results were reported by Salzman and his colleagues,[35] who compared the protective effect of warfarin, dipyridamole, dextran 40, and aspirin in 69 patients who were admitted for hip arthroplasty. It was claimed that the results with aspirin were better than those in an untreated group reported previously. One interesting point in this study was that while the incidence

TABLE 2. Prophylaxis: Drugs which Affect Platelet Function and the Incidence of Postoperative Deep Vein Thrombosis

| Study | Diagnostic Technique | Incidence of Deep Vein Thrombosis | |
|---|---|---|---|
| | | Control Group | Treated Group |
| *Aspirin* | | | |
| Salzman, Harris, and DeSanctis (1971)[35] | Clinical | 23/67 (34%) | 4/43 (9%) |
| Medical Research Council (1972)[33] | [125]I-fibrinogen test | 32/150(22%) | 20/153(27.5%) |
| *Dextran* | | | |
| Johnson, Bygdeman, and Eliasson (1968)[69] | | 13/25 (52%) | 1/27 (4%) |
| Sawyer (1968)[64] | Clinical | 5/53 (9.4%) | 3/51 (6%) |
| Brisman, Parks, and Haller (1971)[39] | Clinical/autopsy | 14/90 (15.5%) | 11/89 (12.4%) |
| Kakkar (1972)[68] | [125]I-fibrinogen test | 23/40 (35%) | 16/43 (27%) |
| Bonnar and Walsh (1972)[65] | [125]I-fibrinogen test | 15/140(10.7%) | 1/120(0.8%) |
| *Dipyridamole* | | | |
| Browse and Hall (1969)[66] | Clinical | 7/334(2.1%) | 12/315(3.8%) |

of deep vein thrombosis (as detected by clinical criteria) was lower in the aspirin-treated patients as compared with the control group, the incidence of pulmonary embolism was not reduced. This paradoxical result raises the question of whether the administration of aspirin (1 to 2 grams daily) may have masked some of the clinical features, such as pain, tenderness, and increased temperature. The apparent success of aspirin in preventing clinically detectable venous thrombosis and its lack of success in preventing pulmonary emboli may be explained by the fact that aspirin prevents synthesis[36] and release[37] of prostaglandins from platelets; prostaglandins are known to be mediators of inflammatory response.

The role of dextran is still uncertain and its efficacy in reducing the incidence of fatal pulmonary embolism has yet to be determined. Concurrent trials by several workers, especially in Sweden, have shown that dextran (usually dextran 70) reduces the incidence of thromboembolism among general surgical patients, in patients with fractured neck of femur, and in gynecologic patients undergoing operation. Bygdeman et al.[38] listed eight surgical studies in which a total of 1321 patients were given dextran 70 prophylactically and compared them with a similar number of control patients. There was approximately a fourfold reduction in fatal emboli in the dextran-treated patients. However, in 6 of these 8 studies there was no significant difference between control and treated patients in the incidence of fatal emboli; caution is required in accepting a statistically significant difference that may be present in the aggregate but is absent in the individual trials.

A recent prospective, double-blind, randomly allocated trial at the Johns Hopkins Hospital found that the prophylactic administration of dextran 70 to "high risk" surgical patients reduced neither the incidence of pulmonary emboli nor the overall mortality rate.[39] The advantages claimed for dextran prophylaxis are the absence of bleeding complications and the lack of need for laboratory control of therapy, as compared with oral anticoagulant drugs. It has been suggested that the bleeding complications of dextran therapy approach those of oral anticoagulants;[40] other major complications include pulmonary edema in patients with limited cardiac reserve, occasional renal failure, mild allergic reactions, and anaphylactic response.

There is no doubt that drugs which are known to enhance naturally occurring fibrinolytic activity, such as phenformin and ethylestranol, are totally effective in preventing deep vein thrombosis in surgical patients.[41] However, oral anticoagulant therapy, properly employed (started well before operation), is the most effective and proven method of preventing venous thrombosis. In a controlled, randomly allocated clinical trial involving nearly 300 patients who were operated upon for fractured neck of femur, Sevitt and Gallagher[67] found clinical and postmortem evidence of venous thrombosis in 2.7 per cent of those receiving oral anticoagulants, compared with 28.7 per cent of the control patients. Pulmonary embolism was not encountered in treated patients, but in the controls, embolism occurred in 18 per cent and fatal embolism in 10 per cent. Subsequent studies have reported similar results in patients undergoing orthopedic procedures,[42, 43] those having gynecologic and other pelvic operations,[44] and "high risk" surgical patients.[45, 46] However, a major drawback of oral anticoagulant therapy is the risk of massive hemorrhage during and after operation, in spite of laboratory control of the dosage given. The incidence of severe hemorrhage in the various reported studies has varied between 2.0 and 6.97 per cent and the mortality rate has been in the range of 0.08 to 0.1 per cent.[47] The risk of hemorrhage and the need for strict laboratory control have undoubtedly contributed to the relatively low level of acceptance of this form of prophylaxis among surgeons generally—at least in the United States and the United Kingdom.

A form of therapy which is both effective and devoid of the drawbacks of oral anticoagulant therapy would therefore meet a real need. Ideally, any agent used for the prophylaxis of deep vein thrombosis should be well tolerated by the patient, have no side effects, require no special monitoring, and produce no bleeding in a clinical situation in which the patient is subjected to major tissue trauma. One promising approach is the use of low-dose heparin, given subcutaneously, which has been claimed to prevent thrombosis without increasing the risk of bleeding. Such a proposal, however, is not new; for many years there have been suggestions that small doses of heparin after operation reduce the incidence of postoperative thrombosis.[48, 49, 50] The effectiveness of this form of prophylaxis has recently been investigated by several workers[51, 52, 53, 54, 55, 56, 57, 58, 59] in patients undergoing general surgical, thoracic, orthopedic, and urologic operations. The incidence of deep vein thrombosis detected by the [125]I-labelled fibrinogen test has been reduced from approximately 30 per cent in the control group to less than 10 per cent in those receiving heparin (Table 3). However, this form of prophylaxis failed to protect patients subjected to emergency operation for fracture of the femoral neck and those undergoing total hip replacement.[60, 61] These observations tend to indicate that when the coagulation sequence has already been activated beyond the stage of thrombin generation (as happens in

TABLE 3. Prophylaxis: Effect of Low Doses of Heparin on the Incidence of Postoperative Deep Vein Thrombosis as Assessed in Controlled Clinical Trials

| Study | Control Group | | Treated Group | | Statistical Significance |
|---|---|---|---|---|---|
| | Number of Patients | Deep Vein Thrombosis | Number of Patients | Deep Vein Thrombosis | |
| Kakkar et al. (1971)[51] | 27 | 7(26%) | 26 | 1(4%) | $0.05 > p > 0.025$ |
| Williams (1971)[53] | 29 | 12(41%) | 27 | 4(15%) | $0.02 > p > 0.01$ |
| Gordon-Smith et al. (1972)[54]° | 50 | 21(42%) | 52 | 7(13.5%) | $p < 0.003$ |
| | | | 48 | 4(8.3%) | $p < 0.001$ |
| Kakkar et al. (1972)[52]† | 39 | 17(42%) | 39 | 3(8%) | $p < 0.001$ |
| | | | 133 | 13(9.7%) | |
| | | | 50 | 20(40%) | |
| Nicolaides et al. (1972)[56] | 122 | 29(24%) | 122 | 1(0.8%) | $p < 0.000003$ |
| Gallus et al. (1973)[55] | 118 | 19(16%) | 108 | 2(2%) | $p < 0.003$ |

° A trial comparing two different regimens.
† Double-blind randomly allocated trial.

patients with hip fractures before heparin prophylaxis is started) or when the stimulus to thrombin generation is overwhelming, then probably more heparin is required than is at present given.[62] However, an important question that arises is whether low-dose heparin prophylaxis is equally effective in preventing postoperative fatal pulmonary embolism. To answer this question, a multicenter trial has been organized; in this trial, patients over the age of 40 who are undergoing major elective operation are randomly allocated to a control or treated group. To date, 4050 patients have entered the trial and the early results in this limited number of patients suggest that the regimen of low-dose heparin prophylaxis being investigated is effective in preventing fatal pulmonary embolism in surgical patients.

## THE "HIGH RISK" GROUP

As already mentioned, the incidence of postoperative fatal pulmonary embolism is low and a form of prophylaxis which is effective and devoid of side effects is not available at present. It therefore seems logical that prophylactic attempts should be directed toward the patient at high risk of developing this complication. Using the $^{125}$I-labelled fibrinogen test (a sensitive and accurate method of detecting thrombi) the effects of various factors known to influence the incidence of venous thrombosis were assessed (Table 4) and it was found that those who have had pulmonary embolism or deep vein thrombosis in the past are highly likely to develop these conditions again following operation. With regard to the generally accepted danger of thromboembolism in women who are using the contraceptive pill, it is our practice whenever possible to stop the pill for at least 6 weeks prior to operation.

## Comments

The published evidence presented in this paper tends to indicate that postoperative pulmonary embolism is a complication both preventable and

TABLE 4.   "High Risk" Group: Effect of Various Factors on the Incidence of DVT

| | Number of Patients Studied | | |
| --- | --- | --- | --- |
| | DVT | No DVT | Total |
| Overall incidence | 62 (30.5%) | 141 | 203 |
| Age: | | | |
|   40–60 years | 35 (25.4%) | 108 | 143 |
|   61–80 years | 27 (45.0%) | 33 | 60 |
| Type of operation: | | | |
|   Minor | 15 (23.8%) | 49 | 64 |
|   Major | 46 (33.3%) | 93 | 139 |
| Malignancy | 24 (40.9%) | 35 | 59 |
| Varicose veins | 22 (56.5%) | 17 | 39 |
| Previous DVT | 13 (68.4%) | 6 | 19 |
| Previous pulmonary embolism | 6 (100%) | 0 | 6 |

worth preventing. A standard regimen of 5000 I.U. of heparin given 2 hours before operation, followed by the same dose every 8 to 12 hours until the patient is fully ambulant, can be recommended as a method of primary prevention for all adults undergoing major abdominal, pelvic, or thoracic—but not, as yet, orthopedic—operation. A standard regimen fulfills most of the criteria demanded of an ideal prophylactic agent: it is well tolerated by the patient, is free of side effects, requires no monitoring other than that the patient receives the drug appropriately, and finally, does not produce excessive bleeding when the patient is subjected to major tissue trauma. For patients undergoing orthopedic operations, including hip reconstruction, anticoagulation with warfarin still remains the method of choice.

## References

1. Department of Health and Social Security. Annual Report of the Chief Medical Officers of the Department of Health and Social Security for 1970. London, H.M.S.O., 1970.
2. Hume, M., Sevitt, S., and Thomas, D. P.: *Venous Thrombosis and Pulmonary Embolism*. Cambridge, Mass., Harvard University Press, 1970, p. 3.
3. Morrell, M. T., Truelove, S. C., and Barr, A.: Pulmonary embolism. Br. Med. J. *5361*:830, 1963.
4. Freiman, D. G., Suyemoto, J., and Wessler, S.: Frequency of pulmonary thromboembolism in man. N. Engl. J. Med. *272*:1278, 1965.
5. Sevitt, S.: Venous thrombosis and pulmonary embolism: their prevention by oral anticoagulants. Am. J. Med. *33*:703, 1962.
6. Coon, W. W., and Coller, F. A.: Clinicopathologic correlation in thromboembolism. Surg. Gynecol. Obstet. *109*:259, 1959.
7. Donaldson, G. A., Williams, C., Scannel, J. G., et al.: A reappraisal of the application of the Trendelenburg operation to massive fatal embolism. N. Engl. J. Med. *268*:171, 1963.
8. Hirsh, J., Hale, G. S., McDonald, I. G., et al.: Streptokinase therapy in acute major pulmonary embolism: effectiveness and problems. Br. Med. J. *41*:729, 1968.
9. Miller, G. A. H., Sutton, G. C., Kerr, I. H., et al.: Comparison of streptokinase and heparin treatment of isolated acute massive pulmonary embolism. Br. Med. J. *2*:681, 1971.
10. N.H.L.I. Urokinase Pulmonary Embolism Trial. J.A.M.A. *214*:2163, 1970.
11. Hunter, W. C., Krygier, J. J., Kennedy, J. C., and Sneeden, V. D.: Etiology and prevention of thrombosis of the deep leg veins: a study of in vivo cases. Surgery *17*:178, 1945.
12. McCann, J. C.: Thromboembolism: a comparison of the effect of early postoperative ambulation and Dicumarol on its incidence. N. Engl. J. Med. *242*:203, 1950.
13. Sharnoff, J. G., and Rosenberg, M.: Effects of age and immobilisation on the incidence of postoperative thromboembolism. Lancet *1*:845, 1964.
14. Murley, R. S.: Postoperative venous thrombosis and pulmonary embolism with particular reference to current methods of treatment. Ann. R. Coll. Surg. Engl. *6*:283, 1950.
15. Blodgett, J., and Beattie, E. J.: Early postoperative rising: a statistical study of hospital complications. Surg. Gynecol. Obstet. *82*:485, 1946.
16. Powers, J. H.: Prompt postoperative activity after hernioplasty: its influence on incidence of complications and rate of recovery. Arch. Surg. *59*:601, 1949.
17. Doran, F. S. A., Drury, M., and Sivyer, A.: A simple way to combat the venous stasis which occurs in the lower limbs during surgical operations. Br. J. Surg. *51*:486, 1964.
18. Kakkar, V. V.: The problem of thrombosis in the deep veins of the leg. Ann. R. Coll. Surg. Engl. *45*:259, 1969.
19. Mayerowitz, B. R., and Nelson, R.: Measurement of the velocity of blood in lower limb veins with and without compression. Surgery *56*:481, 1964.
20. Rosengarten, D. S., Laird, J., Jeyasingh, K., et al.: The failure of compression stockings (Tubigrip) to prevent deep venous thrombosis after operation. Br. J. Surg. *57*:296, 1970.
21. Clark, G., and Cotton, L. T.: Blood-flow in deep veins of leg: recording technique and evaluation of methods to increase flow during operation. Br. J. Surg. *55*:211, 1968.
22. Rosengarten, D. S., and Laird, J.: The effect of leg elevation on the incidence of deep vein thrombosis after operation. Br. J. Surg. *58*:182, 1971.

23. Flanc, C., Kakkar, V. V., and Clarke, M. B.: Postoperative deep vein thrombosis: effect of intensive prophylaxis. Lancet 1:477, 1969.

24. Tsapogas, M. J., Goussous, H., Peabody, R. A., et al.: Postoperative venous thrombosis and the effectiveness of prophylactic measures. Arch. Surg. 103:561, 1971.

25. Doran, F. S. A., and White, H. M.: A demonstration that the risk of postoperative deep vein thrombosis is reduced by stimulating the calf muscles electrically during the operation. Br. J. Surg. 54:686, 1967.

26. Hills, N. H., Pflug, J. J., Jeyasingh, K., et al.: Prevention of deep vein thrombosis by intermittent pneumatic compression of calf. Br. Med. J. 1:131, 1972.

27. Sabri, S., Roberts, V. C., and Cotton, L. T.: Prevention of early postoperative deep vein thrombosis by passive exercise of leg during surgery. Br. Med. J. 3:82, 1971.

28. Yin, E. T., Wessler, S., and Stoll, P. J.: Biological properties of the naturally occurring plasma inhibitor to activated Factor X. J. Biol. Chem. 246:3703, 1971.

29. Astrup, T.: Fibrinolysis in the organism. Blood 11:781, 1956.

30. Nilsson, I. M., Pandolfi, M., and Robertson, B.: Properties of fibrinolytic activators appearing after venous stasis and intravenous injection of nicotinic acid. Coagulation 3:13, 1970.

31. Pandolfi, M., Isacson, S., and Nilsson, I. M.: Low fibrinolytic activity in the walls of veins in patients with thrombosis. Acta Med. Scand. 186:1, 1969.

32. Isacson, S., and Nilsson, I. M.: Defective fibrinolysis in blood and vein walls in recurrent "idiopathic" venous thrombosis. Acta Chir. Scand. 138:313, 1972.

33. Report of the steering committee of a trial sponsored by the Medical Research Council. Effect of aspirin on postoperative venous thrombosis. Lancet 2:441, 1972.

34. O'Brien, J. R.: Two in-vivo studies comparing high and low aspirin dosage. Lancet 1:399, 1971.

35. Salzman, E. W., Harris, W. M., and DeSanctis, R. W.: Reduction in venous thrombosis by agents affecting platelet function. N. Engl. J. Med. 284:1287, 1971.

36. Vane, J. R.: Inhibition of prostaglandin synthesis as a mechanism of action for aspirin-like drugs. Nature [New Biol.] 231:235, 1971.

37. Smith, J. B., and Willis, A. L.: Aspirin selectively inhibits prostaglandin production in human platelets. Nature [New Biol.] 231:235, 1971.

38. Bygdeman, S., Svensjo, E., and Tollerz, G.: Prevention of venous thrombosis. Lancet 2:419, 1970.

39. Brisman, R., Parks, L. C., and Haller, J. A., Jr.: Dextran prophylaxis in surgery. Ann. Surg. 174:137, 1971.

40. Harris, W. H., Salzman, E. W., Desanctis, R. W., et al.: Prevention of venous thromboembolism following total hip replacement: warfarin vs. dextran 40. J.A.M.A. 220:1319, 1972.

41. Fossard, D. P., Friend, J. R., Field, E. S., Kakkar, V. V., et al.: Fibrinolytic activity and postoperative deep vein thrombosis. Lancet 1:9, 1974.

42. Tubiana, R., and Duparc, J.: Prevention of thrombo-embolic complications in orthopaedic and accident surgery. J. Bone Joint Surg. [Br.] 43:7, 1961.

43. Neu, L. T., Jr., Waterfield, J. R., and Ash, C. J.: Prophylactic anticoagulant therapy in the orthopedic patient. Ann. Intern. Med. 62:463, 1965.

44. Pyorala, T., and Lampinen, V.: Preoperative anticoagulant treatment in gynaecological surgery. Acta Obstet. Gynaecol. Scand. 49:215, 1970.

45. Storm, O.: Anticoagulant protection in surgery. Thromb. Diath. Haemorrh. 2:484, 1958.

46. Skinner, D. B., and Salzman, E. W.: Anticoagulant prophylaxis in surgical patients. Surg. Gynecol. Obstet. 125:741, 1967.

47. Hume, M., Sevitt, S., and Thomas, D. P.: Venous Thrombosis and Pulmonary Embolism. Cambridge, Mass. Harvard University Press, 1970, p. 3.

48. DeTakats, G.: Anticoagulants in surgery. J.A.M.A. 142:527, 1950.

49. Bauer, G.: Thirteen years experience with heparin therapy. In Koller, T. H., and Merz, W. R. (eds.): Proceedings of the First International Conference on Thrombosis and Embolism. Basel, Schwalis Verlag, 1954, p. 721.

50. Lenggenhager, K.: Genese und Prophylaxe der Postopertiven Fernthrombose. Helvetica Chir. Acta 24:316, 1957.

51. Kakkar, V. V., Field, E. S., Nicolaides, A. N., et al.: Low doses of heparin in the prevention of deep vein thrombosis. Lancet 2:669, 1971.

52. Kakkar, V. V., Corrigan, T. P., Spindler, J., et al.: Efficacy of low doses of heparin in prevention of deep vein thrombosis after major surgery. A double-blind randomized trial. Lancet 2:101, 1972.

53. Williams, H. T.: Prevention of postoperative deep vein thrombosis with perioperative subcutaneous heparin. Lancet 2:950, 1971.

54. Gordon-Smith, I. C., Grundy, D. J., Le Quesne, L. P., et al.: Controlled trial of two regimens of subcutaneous heparin in prevention of postoperative deep vein thrombosis. A double blind randomized trial. Lancet 1:1133, 1972.
55. Gallus, A. S., Hirsh, H., Tuttle, R. J., et al.: The use of small doses of heparin to prevent venous thrombosis in surgical and medical patients. N. Engl. J. Med. 288:545, 1973.
56. Nicolaides, A. N., Dupont, P. A., Desai, S., et al.: Small doses of subcutaneous sodium heparin in preventing deep venous thrombosis after major surgery. Lancet 2:890, 1972.
57. Van Vroonhoven, T. J., Van Zijl, J., and Muller, H.: Low-dose subcutaneous heparin versus oral anticoagulants in the prevention of postoperative deep venous thrombosis. A controlled clinical trial. Lancet 1:375, 1974.
58. Wessler, S., and Yin, E. T.: The theory and practice of mini-dose heparin in surgical patients: a status report. Circulation 47:661, 1973.
59. Ballard, R. M., Bradley-Watson, P. J., Johnstone, F. D., et al.: Low-dose subcutaneous heparin in prevention of D.V.T. in gynaecological patients. J. Obstet. Gynaecol. Br. Commonw. 80:469, 1973.
60. Corrigan, T. P., Kakkar, V. V., and Fossard, D. P.: Low-dose subcutaneous heparin—optimal dose regimen. Br. J. Surg. 61:320, 1974.
61. Hume, M., Kuriakose, T. X., Zuch, L., et al.: [125]I-fibrinogen in the prevention of venous thrombosis. Arch. Surg. 107:803, 1973.
62. Kakkar, V. V.: Low dose heparin in the prevention of venous thromboembolism. Rationale and results. Thrombo. Diath. Haemorrh. 33:87, 1975.
63. Browse, N. L., and Negus, D.: Prevention of postoperative leg vein thrombosis by electrical muscle stimulation. An evaluation with [125]I-labelled fibrinogen. Br. Med. J. 3:615, 1970.
64. Sawyer, R. B.: Clinical experiences with dextran treatment. Acta Chir. Scand. Suppl. 387:58, 1968.
65. Bonnar, J., and Walsh, J.: Prevention of thrombosis after pelvic surgery by British dextran 70. Lancet 1:614, 1972.
66. Browse, N. L., and Hall, J. H.: Effect of dipyridamole on the incidence of clinically detectable deep-vein thrombosis. Lancet 2:718, 1969.
67. Sevitt, S., and Gallagher, N. G.: Prevention of venous thrombosis and pulmonary embolism in injured patients: a trial of anticoagulant prophylaxis with phenindione in middle aged and elderly patients with fractured necks of femur. Lancet 2:981, 1959.
68. Kakkar, V. V.: Platelets, drugs and venous thrombosis. Symposium, Hamilton, Ontario, 1972. Basel, S. Karger, 1975, pp. 292–300.
69. Johnson, S. R., Bygdeman, S., and Eliasson, R.: Effect of dextran on post-operative thrombosis. Acta Chir. Scand. 80(Suppl):387, 1968.

# Postoperative Pulmonary Embolism Is a Preventable Complication*

RICHARD E. C. COLLINS

*Canterbury and Thanet Hospitals, Canterbury, England*

*and* EDWIN W. SALZMAN

*Harvard Medical School*

Venous thromboembolism can hardly be overemphasized as a major health problem. Coon and Coller[20] judged in 1959 that pulmonary embolism (PE) was the cause of 9 per cent of hospital deaths in the United States. In Britain, the Registrar-General's Report for England and Wales[74] showed nearly a tenfold increase in mortality due to pulmonary embolism over the last 35 years.

Any attack on the incidence of pulmonary embolism should concentrate on its precursor, deep vein thrombosis (DVT), for there is ample evidence that clots in the deep veins of the lower limb and pelvic veins are the origin of the great majority of pulmonary emboli.[83] Three approaches are feasible:

1. Using better methods for diagnosing DVT, in order to permit treatment before PE.

2. Developing more effective methods of treatment of established DVT.

3. Lowering the incidence of postoperative DVT by various prophylactic techniques.

By far the greatest impact on the problem can be made through the last approach, and we have elected to confine our remarks to this aspect of the general subject. To compare the efficacy of various prophylactic regimens, accurate diagnosis is essential, so a discussion of prevention must first consider the diagnostic methods currently available.

*Supported by Grants HE 13754 and HL 11414 from the National Institutes of Health.

291

## Diagnostic Methods

### Clinical Evidence

Until recently, physical examination and autopsy were the only commonly employed methods of diagnosing DVT, and the former is very insensitive. Sevitt and Gallagher[83] reported an absence of clinical signs of DVT in 50 per cent of patients dying with pulmonary embolism, and others have found up to 80 per cent of PE occurring without premonitory signs of DVT,[41] even though at least 75 per cent of PE appear to originate in the lower limbs.[38, 83] Kakkar[49] has claimed that 35 per cent of patients with physical signs suggesting DVT are found actually not to have this problem when they are examined by more objective modern diagnostic techniques. False positives may run as high as 50 per cent when the signs of tenderness, pain, and edema are confined to the limb below the knee.

### Radiographic Phlebography

Radiographic phlebography is probably the most sensitive and accurate diagnostic test for DVT and is the yardstick against which all other methods must be compared. The technique of Rabinov and Paulin[73] appears to be the most satisfactory method available at present, from the standpoint of reproducibility and dependable filling of all the veins of the lower extremity. The deep veins of the limb are opacified by the injection of 100 to 150 ml. of contrast medium into a dorsal toe vein while the patient lies on an x-ray table which is tilted 30 to 45 degrees foot down. The limb being examined hangs free and is nonweight-bearing. No tourniquets are employed. The process of filling is observed on an image intensifier, and multiple spot films are made in various positions. The femoral and iliac veins are demonstrated by making the patient flex the ankle, thus driving the dye out of the calf vein sinuses. At the end of the procedure, the venous system is flushed out with a rapid infusion of normal saline containing heparin. We have found this technique to be highly efficient in demonstrating even tiny thrombi in small calf veins.

The objections to phlebography for routine screening are obvious: the expense, the demands on the time and resources of the radiology staff and equipment, the radiation hazard, and the possibility of inducing thrombosis as a complication of the procedure. Additionally, difficulty in selecting the correct time to perform phlebography can result in failure to diagnose DVT which forms after the investigation. However, the technique is unsurpassed as a standard of comparison for other methods and as the final arbiter of the presence, localization, and extent of DVT in the living patient.

### The [125]Iodine-Labelled Fibrinogen Scan

This test, which was first used clinically in Britain and reported in 1968 by Negus et al.[67] and Flanc et al.,[31] has since gained widespread popularity. Table 1 shows the diagnostic accuracy claimed by some of its advocates, most of whom were investigating general surgical patients.

TABLE 1. Diagnosis of DVT by [125]I-Fibrinogen Test as
Compared with Radiologic Phlebography

| Study | DVT | | |
|---|---|---|---|
| | Detected by [125]I-Fibrinogen Test | Confirmed by Venography | Correlation (Per Cent) |
| Flanc et al. (1968)[31] | 18 | 17 | 94 |
| Negus et al. (1968)[67] | 28 | 26 | 93 |
| Kakkar et al. (1969)[56] | 40 | 39 | 97 |
| Lambie et al. (1970)[59] | 44 | 40 | 89 |
| Pinto (1970)[72] | 22 | 20 | 90 |
| Kakkar (1972)[51] | 36 | 32 | 88 |
| Milne et al. (1971)[63] | 18 | 18 | 100 |
| Bonnar and Walsh (1972)[8] | 15 | 15 | 100 |
| Hume and Gurewich (1972)[45] | 12 | 10 | 83 |

It is our belief, however, that the [125]I-fibrinogen test has an appreciable incidence of false negative results in certain circumstances — mainly in diagnosing thrombi in the ilio-femoral veins. This is especially so after hip operation, when wound hematoma may cause difficulty in interpreting the scan. Harris and co-workers[40] have shown that the overall accuracy of the [125]I-fibrinogen scan, as compared with phlebography, was only 76 per cent in a group of patients undergoing total hip replacement. The main source of error in this study was failure of the scan accurately to identify thrombi forming in the thigh or pelvis. Field et al.[30] and Kakkar[49] have suggested that most DVT originate in the calf veins and that propagation above the knee usually commences from these vessels. In contrast, Harris et al.[40] have shown by phlebography in patients undergoing total hip replacement that 28 per cent of DVT occurred in the proximal area of the thigh with no evidence of thrombi in calf veins.

This test relies on the incorporation of radioactive fibrinogen into a thrombus during its formation. It is essential therefore to inject the label *before* the thrombus forms, because the label will not necessarily attach itself to an already formed clot.

The method is expensive in technician time and suffers from the theoretical hazard of inducing hepatitis. Nevertheless, the technique is undoubtedly of great value as a screening procedure in high risk patients and as a diagnostic tool for clinical studies, provided its limitations are recognized. It may prove to be more useful when combined with a suitable noninvasive method for recognizing thrombosis in proximal veins.

## Plethysmography

The technique of impedance plethysmography as described by Wheeler and colleagues[94] was shown by Johnston et al.,[47] Harris et al.,[42] and Steer et al.[88] to have a poor correlation with phlebography. The method may be improved by using an inflatable thigh pressure cuff rather than a prolonged deep breath to trap venous blood before measurement of the maximum rate of venous emptying. The method is generally useful only for recognition of thrombi above the knee. Early or small DVT in the calf are often missed, and thrombi in the femoral or iliac system may also be overlooked if they are nonocclusive. However, this test is of value in that it will sometimes diagnose a large preformed thrombus which the [125]I-fibrinogen test may fail to detect.

Cranley and co-workers[23] developed a technique of mechanical plethysmography using two cuffs, and they report encouraging results. Since they reported investigation only of patients suspected of having DVT, their paper does not indicate the sensitivity of the method for detection of silent DVT. The method suffers from the same difficulty in diagnosing small calf vein thrombosis as does impedance plethysmography.

### Reflected Ultrasound

Like plethysmography, this quick and simple method depends on detection of the obstruction to blood flow produced by a thrombus. Unfortunately, the technique has not lived up to its early promise.[26, 85] Kakkar[51] could find positive correlation with phlebography in only 65 per cent of cases. His claim that the method rarely shows calf vein thrombi is an important criticism. The test is probably of greatest value in detecting large occluding clots above the knee; however, a warning about its use in this situation was given by Brown and Polak,[9] who reported producing a fatal pulmonary embolus during the test.

### Other Methods

Blood tests for intermediate products of coagulation, such as that described by Niewiarowski and Gurewich[69] eventually may be of value in detecting DVT, but at present their sensitivity and specificity are not adequate. Clagett et al.[18] found that platelet survival studies did not help to diagnose postoperative DVT. Thrombus uptake of labelled macro-aggregated albumin[25] gives less accurate results than phlebography or [125]I-fibrinogen scan. Venous flow studies with [99]technetium[46] are subject to the same criticism. [77]Bromine-labelled fibrinogen[58] and highly iodinated fibrinogen[43] are being developed but have not yet been subjected to rigorous clinical trials.

In summary, as a tool for clinical use in high risk patients, the labelled fibrinogen scan is probably the most suitable. It will be more helpful if an improved method can be developed for diagnosis of thrombi in proximal veins. The insensitivity of presently available noninvasive techniques seriously limits their value.

Radiographic phlebography is the most dependable method for confirmation of a suspected diagnosis of DVT and is the most sensitive diagnostic procedure for use in clinical tests. Data derived from studies based on less discriminating techniques must be viewed with recognition of their shortcomings.

In order to scrutinize reports that claim an influence on the incidence of PE, the difficulties in making this diagnosis should also be understood.

Acute massive PE may present the typical clinical picture of collapse, dyspnea, and right heart strain, but sometimes it is difficult to distinguish this from other major catastrophes such as myocardial infarction. In this situation, Oakley[70] favors pulmonary angiography as the special investigation of choice; ECG, lung scan, and blood gas studies may also give valuable information.

Of more consequence to our topic, however, is the diagnosis of small, often clinically silent pulmonary emboli. Browse et al.[10] have stated that 18 per cent of a series of general surgical patients had clinically silent pulmonary emboli when investigated by the technique of combined lung perfusion and ventilation imaging. Williams and co-workers[96] have claimed that this technique eliminates the false positive results associated with standard perfusion studies (as found sometimes with asthma and bronchitis). It is clear from postmortem studies, such as those of Wessler,[93] that, as with DVT, the true incidence of PE has been grossly underestimated. When considering reports of the incidence of PE, the diagnostic criteria should be analyzed with care. Clinical signs and the appearances of simple chest radiographs are not sufficiently specific for unequivocal diagnosis.

Trials of various techniques for diagnosing DVT have also identified certain patients at high risk. These include patients with a prior history of DVT or PE, those with varicose veins, those with malignancy, and those over 61 years of age having major operations.[57] Additionally, Sevitt and Gallagher[83] documented the frequent association with trauma; Harris and colleagues reported an 80 per cent incidence in patients undergoing hip operation; Mayo et al.[62] have described similar findings among men undergoing open prostatectomy; and Coon and Coller[21] have shown that the obese also are greatly at risk.

## Prophylaxis of DVT

Interpretation of the early literature on this subject is difficult because DVT was diagnosed only on clinical grounds or at postmortem examination. The use of new techniques has clarified and confirmed many but not all of the clinical impressions.

The [125]I-fibrinogen technique is, by popular acceptance, employed for comparison of one prophylactic regime with another. Correct use of the method is obviously important; thus, any studies in which patients are scanned only after the appearance of clinical signs[61] or in which the thigh has not been counted[64] are to be viewed critically. Furthermore, the possibility of thrombosis above the area of applicability of the test must be kept in mind.

Three main categories of prophylactic techniques have appeared: (1) physical methods to prevent stasis; (2) drugs interfering with blood coagulation; and (3) drugs interfering with platelet activity. Regardless of the prophylactic technique selected, it should be instituted early with respect to the predisposition to thrombosis. In surgical patients, prophylaxis is best initiated before operation. It is claimed that up to half the patients with positive fibrinogen scans after operation develop the abnormality within the first 24 hours.[51]

### Physical Methods

Virchow[92] included stasis of blood in his triad of features influencing thrombosis, along with the predisposition of the blood to clot and abnormalities in the vessel wall. The belief that immobilization in bed or on the operating table leads to a reduction in venous flow suggested that efforts to accelerate flow or to produce periodic emptying of the veins of the lower extremities might reduce the incidence of DVT. A variety of methods have been investigated, primarily with the $^{125}$I-fibrinogen scan.

Flanc and co-workers[32] showed that raising the foot of the bed did not significantly reduce the incidence of postoperative DVT except for a slight effect in the elderly. Tsagopas et al.[90] claimed that active and passive leg exercises postoperatively were beneficial, but their patient groups are very small and the results were not statistically significant. Rosengarten and Laird[76] could find no significant effect from elevating the legs during operation. Rosengarten et al.[77] have shown that elastic compression stockings have no prophylactic value.

Sabri and co-workers[78] reported that passive leg exercises in which a motorized device flexes the ankle during operation significantly lowered the incidence of postoperative DVT. The technique is cumbersome and has not been widely adopted. The authors felt that the mode of action was regular compression of the veins of the soleal plexus.

After demonstrating that intermittent pneumatic compression using specially designed boots caused rhythmic alterations in the venous blood flow of the legs of greyhounds, Calnan et al.[14] were encouraged to extend the technique to human subjects. The results from their study[44] and from that of Clark et al.[19] have shown significant protection. However, patients with malignant disease are said not to benefit, an observation that has led Allenby et al.[3] to suggest that activation of fibrinolysis is involved rather than simple mechanical compression. This straightforward, if somewhat clumsy, technique may prove to be the prophylactic method of choice for patients in whom any interference with hemostatic mechanisms by drugs cannot be accepted. Trials are currently in progress to evaluate the effectiveness of the method in neurosurgical and urologic patients.

Early ambulation may prevent some DVT and is to be encouraged, but Flanc and colleagues[32] have shown that only limited protection is obtained, especially in the high risk patient. Furthermore, "early ambulation" is often wrongly interpreted to mean sitting in a chair with the feet and legs in a dependent position, thereby negating any possible beneficial effects of being out of bed.

Active leg exercises, using an ergometer and a physiotherapist, as suggested by Gibbs in 1959,[35] have not been adequately investigated by modern techniques. Clinical observations suggest some value, but Doran et al.[24] quote Gibbs as reporting that the method has been abandoned because of dissatisfaction expressed by the nursing staff.

Finally, Browse and co-workers[12] have reported encouraging results from electrical stimulation of the leg muscles during operation. The problem of concomitant use of a diathermy current may limit the application of the method. The same physiologic response is probably obtained by the simpler technique of intermittent pneumatic compression.

## Drugs Interfering with Blood Coagulation

A substantial part of a venous thrombus is fibrin, so the use of drugs that inhibit conversion of fibrinogen to fibrin is a rational approach to reduction of the incidence of DVT. Both heparin, administered either intravenously or subcutaneously, and oral anticoagulants have been used.

HEPARIN. Prophylactic intravenous heparin was described first in a clinical report in 1938 by Murray and Best[65] and subsequently by several other groups,[5, 6, 22, 48] but its use was restricted by the high cost and tedium of its administration. While no sophisticated analyses were performed, the clinical impression was favorable. However, hemorrhagic complications were sufficiently frequent to lead most clinicians to reject intravenous heparin for prophylactic use (as distinguished from its therapeutic use for established thromboembolism).

Yin and Wessler[97] have shown that small doses of heparin can increase the activity of a natural inhibitor of the activated form of clotting Factor X before the clotting time is affected. Their work has given a rational basis to the use of small doses of subcutaneous heparin ("mini-dose heparin") before and after operation to prevent DVT and PE, as first suggested by Sharnoff.[84] This method and its modifications have gained widespread approval recently, and impressive results have emerged from several trials in surgical patients (Table 2). It appears to be established beyond any reasonable doubt that subcutaneous mini-dose heparin can prevent DVT, at least in patients at moderate risk. Further, low-dose heparin has been shown to reduce the frequency of fatal pulmonary embolism, especially in patients undergoing elective general surgical operations.[57a] The rate of bleeding complications

TABLE 2.  Prophylaxis: Effect of Low Doses of Heparin on Incidence of DVT Diagnosed by $^{125}$I-Fibrinogen Scans

| Study | Control Group | | Treated Group | |
|---|---|---|---|---|
| | Number of Patients | DVT | Number of Patients | DVT |
| Kakkar et al. (1971)[55] | 27 | 7(26%) | 26 | 1(4%) |
| Williams (1971)[95] | 29 | 12(41%) | 27 | 4(15%) |
| Gordon-Smith et al. (1972)[36] | 50 | 21(42%) | 52 | 7(13.5%) |
| | | | 48 | 4(8.3%) |
| Kakkar et al. (1972)[54] | 39 | 17(42%) | 39 | 3(8%) |
| | | | 133 | 13(9.7%) |
| Nicolaides et al. (1972)[68] | 122 | 29(24%) | 122 | 1(0.8%) |
| Gallus et al. (1973)[33] | 118 | 19(16%) | 108 | 2(2%) |
| Van Vroonhoven et al. (1974)[91] | other prophylaxis | | 50 | 1(2%) |
| Scottish Multi-Unit Trial (1974)[81] | 128 | 47(37%) | 125 | 15(12%) |

appears to be low and is substantially less than with intravenous heparin in therapeutic dosage. Most reports of the use of mini-dose heparin have remarked on the freedom from bleeding despite the apparently striking antithrombotic effect of the regimen, but a few contradictory reports have appeared. Brozovic et al.[13] have suggested that bleeding is a function of excessive plasma levels of heparin and believe it is essential to monitor plasma heparin levels when employing this form of prophylaxis, although Kakkar[53] disputes the evidence for their claim. Bonnar and Denson[7] have suggested that the hazard of bleeding from uncontrolled administration of low-dose heparin is sufficient to outweigh its advantages and advocate a monitoring scheme using a simple plasma heparin assay. In a Scottish multi-unit controlled trial of prophylactic mini-dose heparin,[81] the statement was made that among 128 patients given the drug, its use was prematurely abandoned in 7 because "at operation or in the early postoperative period the surgeon was concerned about bleeding." We have found hemorrhagic complications to be few but have encountered serious bleeding in two patients with previously unrecognized congenital Factor XI deficiency. To avoid such an accident, we advise determination of the partial thromboplastin time and one-stage prothrombin time to screen for underlying coagulation defects before initiation of a course of mini-dose heparin. We have not found the use of laboratory tests of coagulation necessary for regulation of dosage.

It is apparent from studies such as those by Williams,[95] Hampson et al.,[37] Evarts and Alfidi,[28] and Harris et al.[39] that the efficacy of mini-dose heparin is not as high in patients undergoing prostatic or hip operation. One might argue that the prostatectomy group should be excluded anyway on the grounds of bleeding hazards, but they represent a high risk population for thromboembolism.[62] Some alternative form of prophylaxis probably would be preferable in such patients. Morris and co-workers[64] recently have claimed that mini-dose heparin prevents DVT after reconstructive hip operation, but since they based their claims on evidence from [125]I-fibrinogen scans that excluded the thigh on the side of operation, their conclusions cannot be regarded as proved.

The evidence available at present suggests that patients with malignant disease respond to mini-dose heparin in a satisfactory way. Gordon-Smith et al.[36] reported that an abbreviated three-dose regimen did not protect such patients.

The ideal dosage regimen also has been debated. Most would agree that a dose of 5000 units, given 2 hours before operation and then every 8 or 12 hours thereafter, is adequate. The former schedule (every 8 hours) probably is accompanied more frequently by bleeding complications. The duration of treatment has varied in reported series; it seems prudent to continue it at least until the patient is fully ambulatory. A predisposition to thromboembolism probably persists for several weeks after operation. Cases have been reported in which DVT developed after mini-dose heparin was discontinued.[34]

ORAL ANTICOAGULANTS.    Vitamin K antagonists have been used prophylactically in Europe for many years, and it is reported that 60 per cent of Dutch surgeons routinely use this form of prophylaxis.[60] In the United States and the United Kingdom, prophylactic oral anticoagulants have been much less widely used,[86] despite overwhelming evidence of their efficacy.[1]

There is no doubt that the fear of bleeding, which has limited the use of coumarin derivatives, has been exaggerated. With careful control of dosage, operation is safe and hemorrhagic complications infrequent and seldom serious. Our practice is to insist that the prothrombin time not exceed twice the control value during operation and in the early postoperative period. One must also observe certain contraindications to anticoagulation, such as active peptic ulcer, intracranial or visceral injury, hemorrhagic diathesis, gastrointestinal bleeding, severe diastolic hypertension, and gross hematuria or hemoptysis.

Many earlier studies employing autopsy or clinical estimation of the incidence of DVT and PE suggested a beneficial effect of warfarin.[79, 83] However, Pinto,[72] using the [125]I-fibrinogen test, claimed that prophylactic warfarin was of no value in patients undergoing hip operation. We have noted earlier that Harris[40] has demonstrated a poor correlation between phlebography and the [125]I-scan in these patients, but of greater consequence in interpreting Pinto's results is the fact that over 75 per cent of the DVT noted occurred within 36 hours of operation. Since warfarin was given only a few hours before operation, it is unlikely that it would have had any effect on these small early thrombi because it takes several days for oral anticoagulants to become effective. It would seem that if warfarin is given only a short time before operation, it may not prevent the development of small thrombi forming in the calf. It does appear, however, to limit their growth and prevent the development of large occluding thrombi which are the ones most likely to produce physical signs of DVT and proceed to PE. A recent study by Harris and co-workers,[39] using phlebography in patients undergoing total hip replacement found that of 51 patients with warfarin prophylaxis, 10 developed DVT, as opposed to 12 of 15 patients receiving prophylactic mini-dose heparin. While these figures show a clear superiority in results, the warfarin group still had a DVT incidence of 18 per cent. Thus, the use of warfarin, although representing a significant advance, is still not the final answer for this difficult-to-treat group of patients.

Van Vroonhoven et al.,[91] in a controlled clinical trial with general surgical patients monitored by the [125]I-fibrinogen test, claimed that another oral anticoagulant, acenocoumarol (nicoumalone) was significantly *less* effective than mini-dose heparin, with DVT rates of 18 per cent and 2 per cent respectively in a series of 100 patients. They monitored the oral anticoagulants by regulating the daily dose in response to daily thrombotests, aiming for a value of 5 to 10 per cent of normal. Eighteen per cent of these patients were not satisfactorily kept in this therapeutic range, and it is of interest that all but one of the patients developing DVT were in this poorly controlled group. A major criticism of this study is the fact that the acenocoumarol was commenced only after operation; in view of the slow onset in action of vitamin K antagonists, the possibility of a beneficial effect was minimized. Lambie et al.[59] claimed that in a controlled study of gynecologic patients in which [125]I-fibrinogen was used, warfarin was inferior to dextran and permitted a 30 per cent incidence of DVT.

These are the only trials of oral anticoagulants as prophylactic agents evaluated by modern diagnostic tests. There is strong evidence that warfarin is far superior to mini-dose heparin in patients undergoing hip operation. Studies cited previously might suggest that the reverse is true in other surgical patients, but such a conclusion would, in our view, be inappropriate in view of the massive accumulation of evidence of the prophylactic efficacy of vitamin K antagonists from trials based on clinical diagnosis or autopsy data.

### Drugs Interfering with Platelet Activity

Patersen[17] and Sevitt[82] have demonstrated that platelet deposition behind venous valve cusps is often the first event in development of a venous thrombus. Drugs that interfere with platelet activity have therefore been investigated as agents to reduce the incidence of DVT. The drugs most widely studied in this context are low molecular weight dextran (average molecular weight, 40,000) or "clinical" dextran (average molecular weight, 70,000). Their mechanism of action is incompletely understood, but it may be related to interaction with plasma proteins necessary for platelet aggregation[2] or to rendering fibrin clots more susceptible to lysis.[66] Evarts and Feil[29] and Harris et al.[39] have shown that dextran can lower the incidence of DVT in hip surgery patients. Bonnar and Walsh[8] made similar claims in regard to pelvic and gynecologic surgery. Lambie and colleagues[59] have suggested that the protective effect of dextran 70 in gynecologic patients is significantly greater than that of warfarin. Harris et al.[39] have compared dextran with aspirin, warfarin, and mini-dose heparin and contend that the first three result in a similar and much lower incidence of DVT than does mini-dose heparin. A Scottish multi-center controlled trial[81] compared dextran with mini-dose heparin in general surgical patients and concluded that heparin was significantly more effective than dextran.

Dextrans are not without problems: fluid overload, congestive heart failure, bleeding, occasional severe allergy, and renal failure may attend their administration. In addition, they are relatively expensive.[17] It would appear that the dextrans clearly have value as prophylactic agents but in most cases probably are not the agents of first choice.

Dipyridamole, another drug which affects platelet function, has been found ineffective in preventing thromboembolic disease in two trials.[11, 80]

Aspirin also alters platelet function, and a trial based on clinical diagnosis found it of prophylactic value in hip surgery patients.[79] A British Medical Research Council trial[75] could not confirm these results in general surgical patients. Clagett et al.[18] found a significant improvement with this agent (using a higher dose than that used in the MRC trial). Using aspirin prophylaxis Zekert et al.[98] also claimed a reduction in the incidence of thromboembolic episodes (judged clinically) in patients undergoing operation for fractured neck of femur and an eight-times lower incidence of fatal PE diagnosed at autopsy. Harris and co-workers[39] have also found aspirin to be of value in hip surgery patients. Operative bleeding can occur with the use of aspirin, and there may be damage to the gastric mucosal barrier in the postoperative state. The ultimate place of aspirin in prophylaxis against venous thromboembolism is not established, but it seems likely that the agent will prove of some value.

Carter and Eban[16] have confirmed an earlier claim[15] that hydroxychloroquine has a significant prophylactic action in general surgical patients, based on its effect on platelet function. Of particular interest is the apparent value of this drug in prostatic surgery.

Steele and colleagues[87] and Evans and Gent[27] have shown that the incidence of clinically demonstrable idiopathic recurrent venous thrombosis can be reduced with sulfinpyrazone. This suggests that the drug may be of value as a prophylactic agent in surgical patients, but no data are yet available to support this idea.

### Fibrinolytic Agents

Lysis of already formed venous thrombi by agents such as streptokinase, urokinase, and ancrod (which also reduces plasma fibrinogen levels) is an established form of therapy.[52, 89] Recently Barrie et al.[4] have presented evidence suggesting a possible beneficial effect of prophylactic ancrod in hip surgery patients. Further data on this approach are awaited.

## Conclusions

It is clear that the incidence of postoperative DVT and PE can be reduced by employing a suitable prophylactic regimen. Because the highly effective preventive measures now available have shortcomings, recommendations must be regarded as tentative and subject to change. Present evidence suggests that all adults undergoing operation should be given the benefit of some form of prophylaxis against venous thromboembolic disease. In terms of safety and effectiveness, mini-dose heparin appears to be the best regimen for general purposes, but there are two categories of patients in whom it is not appropriate. Patients in whom the risk of bleeding is high, from either coexisting disease or the nature of the operation, should probably not receive mini-dose heparin or any other antithrombotic drug. Such patients might include those undergoing neurosurgical or ophthalmologic procedures and possibly prostatectomies. For these patients, one of the physical methods is probably more suitable, and of these, external pneumatic compression of the legs seems the best currently available. The other group in whom mini-dose heparin is not appropriate includes patients in whom the risk of thromboembolism is so high that mini-dose heparin cannot be relied upon to give adequate protection: for example, patients undergoing hip operation, those with fracture of the hip, and general surgical patients with a past history of venous thromboembolism. These patients should be given oral anticoagulants in full therapeutic doses. The roles of hydroxychloroquine, aspirin, and dextran are not yet certain, but they may prove to be valuable.

Advances of the last 10 years permit one optimistically to forecast a continued decrease in the incidence of postoperative thromboembolic disease. Although all regimens available at present have some drawbacks, the therapeutic benefit-to-risk ratio is acceptable, and their use is to be encouraged. Postoperative venous thromboembolism is now a preventable complication; surgeons are obliged to consider the use of prophylactic measures in all patients undergoing operation.

# References

1. Aggeler, P. M., and Kosmin, M.: Anticoagulant prophylaxis and treatment of venous thromboembolic disease. In Sherry, S., Brinkhous, K. M., Genton, E., and Stengle, J. M. (eds.): Thrombosis. Washington, D.C., National Academy of Sciences, 1969, p. 639.
2. Alexander, B.: Recent studies on plasma colloid substitutes: their effects on coagulation and hemostasis. In Fox, C. L., and Nahas, G. G. (eds.): Body Fluid Replacement. New York, Grune & Stratton, Inc., 1970, p. 157.
3. Allenby, F., Boardman, L., Pflug, J. J., and Calnan, J. S.: Effects of external pneumatic intermittent compression on fibrinolysis in man. Lancet 2:1412, 1973.
4. Barrie, W. W., Wood, E. H., Crumlish, P., Forbes, C. D., and Prentice, C. R. M.: Low-dosage ancrod for prevention of thrombotic complications after surgery for fractured neck of femur. Br. Med. J. 4:130, 1974.
5. Bauer, G.: Early diagnosis of venous thrombosis by means of venography and abortive treatment with heparin. Acta Med. Scand. 107:136, 1941.
6. Bauer, G.: Heparin therapy in acute deep venous thrombosis. J.A.M.A., 131:196, 1946.
7. Bonnar, J., and Denson, K. W.: Letter to the Editor. Lancet 2:956, 1974.
8. Bonnar, J., and Walsh, J.: Prevention of thrombosis after pelvic surgery by British dextran 70. Lancet 1:614, 1972.
9. Brown, J. N., and Polak, A.: Letter to the Editor. Br. Med. J. 1:108, 1973.
10. Browse, N. L., Clemenson, G., and Croft, D. N.: Fibrinogen-detectable thrombosis in the legs and pulmonary embolism. Br. Med. J. 1:603, 1974.
11. Browse, N. L., and Hall, J. H.: Effect of dipyridamole on the incidence of clinically detectable deep vein thrombosis. Lancet 2:718, 1969.
12. Browse, N. L., and Negus, D.: Prevention of post-operative leg vein thrombosis by electrical muscle stimulation. An evaluation with $^{125}$I-labelled fibrinogen. Br. Med. J. 3:615, 1970.
13. Brozovic, M., Stirling, Y., Klenerman, L., and Lowe, L.: Letter to the Editor. Lancet 2:99, 1974.
14. Calnan, J. S., Pflug, J. J., and Mills, C. J.: Pneumatic intermittent compression legging simulating calf-muscle pump. Lancet 2:502, 1970.
15. Carter, A. E., Eban, R., and Perrett, R. D.: Prevention of post-operative deep venous thrombosis and pulmonary embolism. Br. Med. J. 1:312, 1971.
16. Carter, A. E., and Eban, R.: Prevention of post-operative deep venous thrombosis in legs by orally administered hydroxychloroquine sulphate. Br. Med. J. 3:94, 1974.
17. Clagett, G. P., and Salzman, E. W.: Prevention of venous thromboembolism in surgical patients. N. Engl. J. Med. 290:93, 1974.
18. Claggett, G. P., Schneider, P., Rosoff, C. B., and Salzman, E. W.: The influence of aspirin on post-operative platelet kinetics and venous thrombosis. Surgery 77:61, 1975.
19. Clark, W. B., Macgregor, A. B., Prescott, R. J., and Ruckley, C. V.: Pneumatic compression of the calf and postoperative deep vein thrombosis. Lancet 2:5, 1974.
20. Coon, W. W., and Coller, F. A.: Clinico-pathologic correlation in thromboembolism. Surgery 109:259, 1959.
21. Coon, W. W., and Coller, F. A.: Some epidemiologic considerations of thromboembolism. Surgery 109:487, 1959.
22. Crafoord, C., and Jorpes, E.: Heparin as a prophylactic against thrombosis. J.A.M.A. 116:2831, 1941.
23. Cranley, J. J., Gay, A. Y., Grass, A. M., and Simeone, F. A.: A plethysmographic technique for the diagnosis of deep venous thrombosis of the lower extremities. Surg. Gynecol. Obstet. 136:385, 1973.

24. Doran, F. S. A., White, M., and Drury, M.: A clinical trial designed to test the relative value of two simple methods of reducing the risk of venous stasis in the lower limbs during surgical operations: the danger of thrombosis and a subsequent pulmonary embolus, with a survey of the problem. Br. J. Surg. 57:20, 1970.

25. Duffy, G. J., D'Auria, D., Brien, T. G., Ormond, D., and Mehigan, J. A.: New radioisotope test for detection of deep vein thrombosis in the legs. Br. Med. J. 1:712, 1973.

26. Evans, D. S.: The early diagnosis of deep vein thrombosis by ultrasound. Br. J. Surg. 57:726, 1970.

27. Evans, G., and Gent, M.: The effect of platelet suppressive drugs on arterial and venous thromboembolism. In Cade, J. F., et al. (eds.): Platelets, Drugs, and Thrombosis: Proceedings. Symposium, Hamilton, Ontario, Canada, October, 1972. White Plains, N. Y., Phiebig, 1974, p. 258.

28. Evarts, C. M., and Alfidi, R. J.: Thromboembolism after total hip reconstruction. Failure of low doses of heparin in prevention. J.A.M.A. 225:515, 1973.

29. Evarts, C. M., and Feil, E. J.: Prevention of thromboembolic disease after elective surgery of the hip. J. Bone Joint Surg. 53:1271, 1971.

30. Field, E. S., Nicolaides, A. N., Kakkar, V. V., and Crellin, R. Q.: Deep-vein thrombosis in patients with fractures of the femoral neck. Br. J. Surg. 59:377, 1972.

31. Flanc, C., Kakkar, V. V., and Clarke, M. B.: The detection of venous thrombosis of the legs using $^{125}$I-labelled fibrinogen. Br. J. Surg. 55:742, 1968.

32. Flanc, C., Kakkar, V. V., and Clarke, M. B.: Post-operative deep vein thrombosis: effect of intense prophylaxis. Lancet 1:477, 1969.

33. Gallus, A. S., Hirsh, J., Tutle, R. J., Trebilcock, R., O'Brien, S. E., Carroll, J. J., Minden, J. H., and Hudecki, S. M.: Small subcutaneous doses of heparin in prevention of venous thrombosis. N. Engl. J. Med. 288:545, 1973.

34. Gallus, A. S., and Hirsh, J.: Low-dose heparin prophylaxis in elective surgery—a randomized study. Circulation 49 and 50 (Suppl. III):298, 1974.

35. Gibbs, N. M.: The prophylaxis of pulmonary embolism. Br. J. Surg. 47:282, 1959.

36. Gordon-Smith, I. C., Grundy, D. J., Lequesne, L. P., Newcombe, J. F., and Bramble, F. J.: Controlled trial of two regimens of subcutaneous heparin in prevention of post-operative deep vein thrombosis Lancet 1:1133, 1972.

37. Hampson, W. G. J., Harris, F. C., Lucas, H. K., Roberts, P. H., McCall, I. W., Jackson, P. C., Powell, N. L., and Staddon, G. E.: Failure of low-dose heparin to prevent deep-vein thrombosis after hip-replacement arthroplasty. Lancet 2:795, 1974.

38. Hampton, A. O., and Castleman, B.: Correlation of post-mortem chest teleroentgenograms and autopsy findings with special reference to pulmonary embolism and infarction. Am. J. Roentgenol. Radium Ther. 43:305, 1940.

39. Harris, W. H., Salzman, E. W., Athanasoulis, C., Waltman, A. C., Baum, S., and DeSanctis, R. W.: Comparison of warfarin, low molecular weight dextran, aspirin and subcutaneous heparin in prevention of venous thromboembolism following total hip replacement. J. Bone Joint Surg. [Am.] 56:1552, 1974.

40. Harris, W. H., Salzman, E. W., Athanasoulis, C., Waltman, A. C., Baum, S., DeSanctis, R. W., Potsaid, M., and Sise, H.: Comparison of $^{125}$I-fibrinogen count scanning with phlebography for detection of venous thrombi following elective hip surgery. N. Engl. J. Med. 292:665, 1975.

41. Harris, W. H., Salzman, E. W., and DeSanctis, R. W.: The prevention of thromboembolic disease by prophylactic anticoagulation. J. Bone Joint Surg. 49:81, 1967.

42. Harris, W. H., Sara, S. M., Salzman, E. W., DeSanctis, R. W., Waltman, A. C., and Athanasoulis, C.: Impedance phlebography: a correlation with lower limb venography in the diagnosis of deep vein thrombosis. Surgery 74:385, 1973.

43. Harwig, J. F., Coleman, R. E., Harwig, S. S. L., Welch, M. J., Sherman, L. A., and Siegel, B. A.: Highly iodinated fibrinogen; a new thrombus localizing agent. Circulation 50 (Suppl. III):285, 1974.

44. Hills, N. H., Pflug, J. J., Jeyasingh, K., Boardman, L., and Calnan, J. S.: Prevention of deep vein thrombosis by intermittent pneumatic compression of the calf. Br. Med. J. 1:131, 1972.

45. Hume, M., and Gurewich, V.: Letter to the Editor. Lancet 1:845, 1972.

46. Johnson, W. C.: Evaluation of newer techniques for the diagnosis of venous thrombosis. J. Surg. Res. 16:473, 1974.

47. Johnston, K. W., and Kakkar, V. V.: Plethysmographic diagnosis of deep vein thrombosis. Surg. Gynecol. Obstet. 139:41, 1974.

48. Jorpes, E.: Pure heparin for the prevention and treatment of thrombosis. Acta Med. Scand. 107:107, 1941

49. Kakkar, V. V.: Medical treatment of deep vein thrombosis. Br. J. Hosp. Med. 6:741, 1971.
50. Kakkar, V. V.: Proceedings of the 2nd Congress of the International Society of Thrombosis and Hemostasis. Stuttgart, Schattaner, 1972, p. 253.
51. Kakkar, V. V.: The diagnosis of deep vein thrombosis using the $^{125}$I-fibrinogen test. Arch. Surg. 104:152, 1972.
52. Kakkar, V. V.: Results of streptokinase therapy in deep venous thrombosis. Postgrad. Med. J. August Suppl., 1973, p. 60.
53. Kakkar, V. V.: Letter to the Editor. Lancet 2:784, 1974.
54. Kakkar, V. V., Corrigan, T., Spindler, J., Fossard, D. P., Flute, P. T., and Crellin, R. Q.: Efficacy of low doses of heparin in prevention of deep vein thrombosis after major surgery. Lancet 2:101, 1972.
55. Kakkar, V. V., Field, E. S., Nicolaides, A. N., Flute, P. T., Wessler, S., and Yin, E. T.: Low doses of heparin in prevention of deep vein thrombosis. Lancet 2:669, 1971.
56. Kakkar, V. V., Howe, C. T., Flanc, C., and Clarke, M. B.: Natural history of post-operative deep vein thrombosis. Lancet 2:230, 1969.
57. Kakkar, V. V., Howe, C. T., Nicolaides, A. N., Renney, J. T. G., and Clarke, M. B.: Deep vein thrombosis of the leg: is there a high risk group? Am. J. Surg. 120:527, 1970.
57a. Kakkar, V. V.: Prevention of fatal postoperative pulmonary embolism by low doses of heparin; an international multicentre trial. Lancet 2:45, 1975.
58. Knight, L. C., Harwug, S. S. L., and Welch, M. J.: The preparation of bromine-77 labelled fibrinogen. Circulation 49 and 50 (Suppl. III):285, 1974.
59. Lambie, J. M., Mahaffy, R. G., Barber, D. C., Karmody, A. M., Scott, M. M., and Matheson, N. A.: Diagnostic accuracy in venous thrombosis. Br. Med. J. 2:142, 1970.
60. Leading Article: Subcutaneous heparin. Lancet 2:502, 1974.
61. Mavor, G. E., Mahaffy, R. G., Walker, M. G., Duthie, J. S., Dhall, D. P., Gaddie, J., and Reid, J. F.: Peripheral venous scanning with $^{125}$I-tagged fibrinogen. Lancet 1:661, 1972.
62. Mayo, M. E., Halil, T., and Browse, N. L.: The incidence of deep vein thrombosis after prostatectomy. Br. J. Urol. 43:738, 1971.
63. Milne, R. M., Griffiths, J. M. T., Gunn, A. A., and Ruckley, C. V.: Post-operative deep vein thrombosis: a comparison of diagnostic techniques. Lancet 2:445, 1971.
64. Morris, G. K., Henry, A. P. J., and Preston, B. J.: Prevention of deep vein thrombosis by low dose heparin in patients undergoing total hip replacement. Lancet 2:797, 1974.
65. Murray, D. G., and Best, C. H.: The use of heparin in thrombosis. Ann. Surg. 108:163, 1938.
66. Muzaffar, T. Z., Stalker, A. L., Bryce, W. A. J., and Dhall, D. P.: Dextrans and fibrin morphology. Nature 238:288, 1972.
67. Negus, D., Pinto, D. J., Lequesne, L. P., Brown, N., and Chapman, M.: $^{125}$I-labelled fibrinogen in the diagnosis of deep vein thrombosis and its correlation with phlebography. Br. J. Surg. 55:835, 1968.
68. Nicolaides, A. N., DuPont, P. A., Desai, S., Lewis, J. D., Douglas, J. N., Dodsworth, H., Fourides, G., Luck, R. J., and Jamieson, C. W.: Small doses of subcutaneous sodium heparin in preventing deep venous thrombosis after major surgery. Lancet 2:890, 1972.
69. Niewiarowski, S., and Gurewich, V.: Laboratory identification of intravascular coagulation. J. Lab. Clin. Med. 77:665, 1971.
70. Oakley, C. M.: Diagnosis of pulmonary embolism. Br. Med. J. 2:773, 1970.
71. Patersen, J. C.: The pathology of venous thrombi. In Sherry, S., Brinkhous, K. M., Genton, E., and Stengle, J. M. (eds.): Thrombosis. Washington, D. C., National Academy of Sciences, 1969, p. 321.
72. Pinto, D. J.: Controlled trial of an anticoagulant (warfarin sodium) in the prevention of venous thrombosis following hip surgery. Br. J. Surg. 57:349, 1970.
73. Rabinov, K., and Paulin, S.: Roentgen diagnosis of venous thrombosis in the leg. Arch. Surg. 104:134, 1972.
74. Registrar-General. Statistical Reviews of England and Wales. Part 1, Medical. London, H.M.S.O., 1970.
75. Report of the Steering Committee of a Trial Sponsored by the Medical Research Council: Effect of aspirin on post-operative venous thrombosis. Lancet 2:441, 1972.
76. Rosengarten, D. S., and Laird, J.: The effect of leg-elevation on the incidence of deep vein thrombosis after operation. Br. J. Surg. 58:182, 1971.
77. Rosengarten, D. S., Laird, J., Jeyasingh, K., and Martin, P.: The failure of compression stockings (Tubigrip) to prevent deep venous thrombosis after operation. Br. J. Surg. 57:296, 1970.
78. Sabri, S., Roberts, V. C., and Cotton, L. T.: The effects of intermittently applied external pressure on the haemodynamics of the hind-limb in greyhound dogs. Br. J. Surg. 59:219, 1972.

79. Salzman, E. W., Harris, W. H., and DeSanctis, R. W.: Anticoagulation for prevention of thrombo-embolism following fractures of the hip. N. Engl. J. Med. 275:122, 1966.
80. Salzman, E. W., Harris, W. H., and DeSanctis, R. W.: Reduction in venous thromboembolism by agents affecting platelet function. N. Engl. J. Med. 284:1287, 1971.
81. Scottish Multi-Unit Trial. Heparin versus dextran in the prevention of deep vein thrombosis. Lancet 2:118, 1974.
82. Sevitt, S.: The structure and growth of valve pocket thrombi in femoral veins. J. Clin. Pathol. In press.
83. Sevitt, S., and Gallagher, N. G.: Prevention of venous thrombosis and pulmonary embolism in injured patients—a trial of anticoagulant prophylaxis with phenindione in middle-aged and elderly patients with fractured necks of femur. Lancet 2:981, 1959.
84. Sharnoff, J. G.: Results in the prophylaxis of post-operative thrombo-embolism. Surg. Gynecol. Obstet. 123:303, 1966.
85. Sigel, B., Popky, L., Wagner, D. K., Boland, J. P., Mapp, E., and Feigel, P.: A Doppler ultrasound method for diagnosing lower extremity venous disease. Surg. Gynecol. Obstet. 127:339, 1968.
86. Simon, T. L., and Stengle, J. M.: Antithrombotic practice in orthopaedic surgery—results of a survey. Clin. Orthop. 102:181, 1974.
87. Steele, P. P., Weily, H. S., and Genton, E.: Platelet survival and adhesiveness in recurrent venous thrombosis. N. Engl. J. Med. 288:1148, 1973.
88. Steer, M. L., Spotnitz, A. J., Cohen, S. I., Paulin, S., and Salzman, E. W.: Limitations of impedance phlebography for diagnosis of venous thrombosis. Arch. Surg. 106:44, 1973.
89. Tibbutt, D. A., Williams, E. W., Walker, M. W., Chesterman, C. N., Holt, J. M., and Sharp, A. A.: Controlled trial of ancrod and streptokinase in the treatment of deep vein thrombosis of lower limb. Br. J. Haematol. 27:407, 1974.
90. Tsagopas, M. J., Goussous, H., Peabody, R. A., Karmody, A. M., and Eckert, C.: Post-operative venous thrombosis and the effectiveness of prophylactic measures. Arch. Surg. 103:561, 1971.
91. Van Vroonhoven, T. J., Van Zijl, J., and Muller, H.: Low-dose subcutaneous heparin versus oral anticoagulants in the prevention of post-operative deep-venous thrombosis—a controlled clinical trial. Lancet 1:375, 1974.
92. Virchow, R.: Cellular Pathology as Based upon Physiological and Pathological Histology. London, Churchill, 1860, p. 197.
93. Wessler, S.: Thrombosis in the presence of vascular stasis. Am. J. Med. 33:648, 1962.
94. Wheeler, H. B., and Mullick, S. C.: Detection of venous obstruction in the leg by measurement of electrical impedance. Ann. N. Y. Acad. Sci. 170:804, 1970.
95. Williams, H. T.: Prevention of post-operative deep vein thrombosis with perioperative subcutaneous heparin. Lancet 2:950, 1971.
96. Williams, O., Lyall, J., Vernon, M., and Croft, D. N.: Ventilation-perfusion lung scanning for pulmonary emboli. Br. Med. J. 1:600, 1974.
97. Yin, E. T., and Wessler, S.: Evidence for a naturally occurring plasma inhibitor of activated Factor X: its isolation and partial purification. Throm. Diath. Haemorrh. 21:398, 1969.
98. Zekert, F., Kohn, I., Vormittag, E., and Poigenfurst, J.: Prophylaxis of thromboembolic diseases in traumatologic patients. Proceedings of the IV Congress of the International Society of Thrombosis and Haemostasis. Vienna, 1973, p. 246.

# 14

# Treatment of Pulmonary Embolism

OPERATIVE INTERVENTION FOR
MASSIVE PULMONARY EMBOLUS
*by George J. Reul, Jr.,
and Denton A. Cooley*

THE USE OF THE "UMBRELLA"
IN THE TREATMENT OF
THROMBOEMBOLISM
*by Kazi Mobin-Uddin*

THE TREATMENT OF LIFE-
THREATENING MASSIVE
PULMONARY EMBOLISM
*by Richard D. Sautter*

TREATMENT OF POSTOPERATIVE
PULMONARY EMBOLUS
*by W. Clayton Davis*

## Statement of the Problem

*The discussants address themselves to the problem of a noninfected post-operative pulmonary embolus clearly established by clinical means plus lung scan or angiogram. The issues are the choice of pharmacologic agents, the timing and method of caval interruption, and the factors that guide these decisions. The aggressive operative approach for removing emboli is also debated.*

*For the patient with clinical deep vein thrombosis, what are the data on the effectiveness of (1) heparin, (2) fibrinolytic agents, and (3) platelet inhibitors in preventing fatal pulmonary emboli?*

*What is the accuracy of a lung scan compared to that of angiography for diagnosing a pulmonary embolus?*

*In what circumstances should caval interruption be the treatment of choice? What are the contraindications to caval ligation?*

*Give early and late data supporting the technique you prefer: umbrella, ligation, or plication. What are the late follow-up data regarding patency after caval plication or umbrella placement? Does residual caval patency serve a useful purpose in minimizing early leg swelling?*

*Should anticoagulants be used following management by umbrella? Ligation? Plication? If so, how soon after the procedure should they be started? What agents should be used, and how long should they be continued?*

*Assuming clinically effective prevention of subsequent pulmonary emboli, cite evidence, if any, that anticoagulant treatment favorably alters clot propagation and canalization in the pulmonary arteries. Does anticoagulation influence ultimate pulmonary hypertension?*

*If you favor embolectomy, do you require angiographic proof of a pulmonary embolus prior to the operation? By what other means is the diagnosis of pulmonary embolus established—clinical signs, symptoms, scan, operative exploration? Are serum enzyme measurements of value?*

*Identify these institutional requirements most importantly contributive to successful embolectomy—experienced cardiovascular team, standby pump team, emergency angiography, and necessary equipment. Outline the supportive measures to be used preceding operation.*

*Provide data on the outcome of pulmonary embolectomy from both personal and literature review. Contrast these data with those on nonoperative heparin and/or lytic agent therapy in comparable groups of patients.*

# Operative Intervention for Massive Pulmonary Embolus

GEORGE J. REUL, JR.,
and DENTON A. COOLEY

*Texas Heart Institute, St. Luke's Episcopal and Texas Children's Hospitals, Houston, Texas*

Although the clinical importance of pulmonary embolism is well known, optimum methods of treatment remain debatable. The major area of contention has been the role of operation in the management of massive pulmonary embolus. Some have claimed that operative extraction of the pulmonary clots is unnecessary because of the inherent ability of thrombolysis, the recent addition of substances which theoretically accelerate clot lysis, the improvement in medical monitoring and management, and the high operative mortality reported in some series. Those who propose medical management for all clinically evident pulmonary emboli have used heparin and/or urokinase or streptokinase infusions added to the usual standard medical therapy. The medical regimen is one which allows slow improvement under careful observation, with the hope of preventing further emboli or sudden cardiovascular deterioration. Proponents of operative management have used the same standard medical therapy plus pulmonary embolectomy under cardiopulmonary bypass and inferior vena cava ligation or postoperative heparin therapy. Most have agreed that cardiac arrest from massive pulmonary embolus is an indication for operative treatment. The major disagreement has been over the need for operative intervention in the patient who has massive pulmonary embolism with or without hypotension, shock, and hypoxemia. Many factors have been responsible for the controversy. The following discussion will attempt to analyze these factors and to present our current plan of therapy, together with the rationale behind an operative approach to the treatment of massive pulmonary embolus.

## Definition

Pulmonary embolism may range in severity from an asymptomatic, rather insignificant pulmonary infiltrate demonstrated on chest x-ray films to

309

the rare occurrence of sudden death. The extent of pulmonary embolus has been described as nonmassive, submassive, or massive (MPE). In the urokinase cooperative study, MPE was defined as "the presence of obstructions or significant filling defects involving two or more lobar pulmonary arteries or an equivalent amount of emboli in other vessels."[5] Various subjective and objective subcategories have been added. On the other hand, in most operative reports, MPE has been defined as one which involves more than 50 per cent of the major pulmonary arterial distribution and results in cardiopulmonary deterioration, usually in the form of systemic hypotension and shock.[6-9] The difference in the medical and surgical definitions of MPE may have evolved because of the inherent limitations of the proposed medical treatment and the type of patients the medical consultant treats, in contrast to the status of the patients that the surgeon usually is asked to see in consultation. For the purpose of this discussion, MPE will be used to denote a pulmonary embolus involving 50 per cent or more of the pulmonary arteries, accompanied by systemic hypotension, shock, and hypoxemia (arterial systolic pressure < 90 mm. Hg; urine output < 20 ml./hr.; arterial oxygen tension [$PaO_2$] < 60 mm. Hg).

## Pathophysiology

The catastrophic events of MPE are initiated by mechanical obstruction of the main or branch pulmonary arteries, usually in excess of 50 per cent of the pulmonary arterial distribution. The end result is right ventricular outflow obstruction, right ventricular and pulmonary artery hypertension, and elevation in the right ventricular end diastolic pressure, right atrial pressure, and central venous pressure with arterial hypoxemia.[10] There is a marked decrease in pulmonary blood volume and pulmonary vascular compliance.[11] Because of the accompanying cardiovascular reflexes, decrease in myocardial blood flow has also been proposed;[12] however, most data indicate that a coronary vasodilatation in response to pulmonary embolus occurs.[13-18] Increased hemodynamic load on the right ventricle causes a proportional increase in right ventricular myocardial blood flow. Further increase in the right ventricular afterload causes increased demands for oxygen and eventually may terminate in right ventricular failure. Right ventricular failure may occur earlier with relatively smaller emboli in patients who have preexisting coronary artery disease, because coronary vasodilatation may not be possible. Many patients who have a pulmonary embolus may also have coronary artery occlusive disease.[19] Furthermore, many have had previous myocardial infarctions, either remote or recent. Experimentally, previous myocardial damage has been shown to be a major factor in determining tolerance to a pulmonary embolus.[10] While some patients may tolerate fairly large emboli well, others with underlying cardiac or pulmonary disease tolerate MPE poorly. In these patients, the amount of embolic obstruction is not necessarily related to the clinical results, and the final outcome is determined not only by the size of the mechanical obstruction but also by the amount of preexisting cardiopulmonary disease. Therefore, important considerations in evaluating patients for potential therapy or in interpreting the results of clinical studies are not only the extent of the mechanical obstruction but also the cardiopulmonary status of the patients prior to MPE.

## Evolution of Operative and Medical Treatment

Some confusion as to the proper management of MPE has been produced by the conflicting results in many clinical reports. We reported the first successful pulmonary embolectomy using temporary cardiopulmonary bypass for an acute massive embolism.[20] Sharp later reported on a more chronic case of MPE treated with successful embolectomy.[21] Subsequent development of pulmonary embolectomy has been described in more detail.[22, 23] The operative approach has been based on the simple premise that mechanical obstruction causes the tenuous clinical state. Therefore, prompt removal of this obstruction should result in an excellent clinical response. Unfortunately, without the use of cardiopulmonary bypass, early operative results were poor.[23] Once the adaptation of cardiopulmonary bypass for the removal of pulmonary emboli was initiated, a dramatic and successful form of treatment for MPE was made available.[20-26] Results then became more dependent on the preoperative condition of the patient rather than on the technique itself. Most patients were originally treated on medical services, and some responded successfully to heparin and supportive therapy. Those who did not improve were referred for operative treatment, usually after prolonged low perfusion states, and were in moribund condition or actually in the process of resuscitation following cardiac arrest. As mortality for pulmonary embolectomy became higher, early embolectomy became even less attractive, and the indications for embolectomy were restricted further by some to only moribund patients or those who had cardiac arrest. The cause of death in most of these patients was the underlying preoperative condition of the patient and was not inherent to the procedure itself.

To further complicate analysis of the data, in 1967 Cross and Mowlem[27] accumulated a series of 157 patients from 28 different institutions treated by embolectomy with a survival rate of only 43 per cent (Table 1). Unfortunately, this summarized series of patients is still used as the basis of reference for operative survival in MPE. Taken in context, the survival rate of 43 per cent was excellent for the group of patients operated upon. Most patients in Cross's series had MPE with shock, hypotension, or cardiac arrest.[27] Patient selection differed from that in most medical reports in that the reports of medical treatment included large numbers of patients without hypotension or other signs of cardiac collapse. It also differed from the report of Coon and Coller,[28] which showed a survival rate of only 38 per cent in the first hour following massive pulmonary embolus without any treatment.

Not only was the patient population different, but also the operative techniques utilized varied from institution to institution. Some type of mechanical circulatory assist prior to operation was utilized in only 35 per cent of Cross's series.[27] Cardiopulmonary bypass was not utilized for extraction of the clots in all patients. Thus, as in any review of results from dif-

TABLE 1.   Survival Rates Following Pulmonary Embolectomy in
Accumulated Series Prior to and after 1967

| Year | Author | Total Number | Survivors | Survival Rate (%) |
|------|--------|--------------|-----------|-------------------|
| 1967 | Cross and Mowlem[27] | 157° | 67 | 43 |
| 1973 | Turnier et al.[23] | 104 | 74 | 71.2 |

°Only 35 per cent had preoperative mechanical circulatory support.

ferent institutions, the survival rate of 43 per cent should not be utilized as an absolute survival rate. However, the report was important in establishing the role of early initiation of mechanical circulatory support in MPE.

As operative treatment advanced, medical treatment likewise improved. The medical treatment consisted of the usual supportive care similar to the preoperative, intraoperative, and postoperative care given in operative treatment, along with heparin and/or the experimental thrombolytic agents. The well-known effects of heparin were to prevent further embolization. Experimental and clinical evidence has shown that pulmonary emboli actually undergo reduction in size by intrinsic thrombolytic mechanism.[29-31] However, this process takes days to weeks, and some emboli never really resolve completely. Nevertheless, most patients treated by a strict medical regimen were found to improve clinically following a rather hectic period of treatment.

Although usually satisfactory, inherent thrombolysis, even with heparin therapy, did not resolve all emboli at a fast enough rate, particularly in patients with MPE. In an attempt to develop a substance which would accelerate the thrombolytic process, urokinase, a plasminogen activator derived from human urine, was studied extensively. In 1967, the National Heart and Lung Institute organized a controlled clinical trial comparing the effects of the thrombolytic agent urokinase with the well-known effects of heparin in "MPE" as defined by the urokinase cooperative study.[5] At a number of institutions between 1968 and 1970, 160 patients were included for study; 78 received heparin, 82 urokinase (Table 2). Excellent clinical results were reported in both groups. The urokinase study group, however, was not comparable to patients reported in most operative series. In the urokinase cooperative study, the mortality rate was only reported to 14 days, and only 11 of the 160 original patients had "shock" prior to treatment. None of the patients had cardiac arrest. Nevertheless, 6 of 82 (7.4 per cent) urokinase patients died, and 7 of 78 (9 per cent) heparin patients died. Two of the 11 patients (18.1 per cent) with shock died. Almost half of the patients in the urokinase group developed bleeding during urokinase treatment, and almost a third in the heparin group bled. Pulmonary embolism recurred in 17 per cent of the patients in the urokinase group and in 23 per cent of the patients in the heparin group. Inferior vena cava ligation was required in 4 per cent of the urokinase group and in 9 per cent of the heparin group. Radiologic filling defects were still present in 25 per cent of the patients on one year follow-up angiograms. The results of urokinase treatment compared well with those of heparin treatment, except that more patients had bleeding problems in the

TABLE 2.  Survival Rates with Medical Therapy

| | Total Patients | | | With "Shock" | | |
|---|---|---|---|---|---|---|
| | Number | Survivors | Survival Rate (%) | Number | Survivors | Survival Rate (%) |
| Cooperative study, 1973 | 160 | 147 | 91.9 | 11 | 9 | 81.1 |
| Sautter et al., 1972[32] | 10° | 10 | 100 | 3 | 3 | 100 |
| Heimbecker et al., 1973[36] | 7 | 6 | 85.7 | 5† | 3 | 100 |

° Seven cases of "submassive emboli."
† Two cases with cardiac arrest.

urokinase group. Other isolated reports of urokinase therapy appeared and were favorable or unfavorable, depending on the type of patients involved and the complication from the treatment itself.[32]

It is obvious that, despite randomization, the patients studied in the urokinase cooperative clinical trial were different from those undergoing operative embolectomy. Frequent comparisons of the survival rates have been made between the urokinase group and the group of embolectomy patients summarized by Cross.[27] As previously stated, in Cross's[27] report the indications for operation for most of the patients who had pulmonary embolectomy were systemic hypotension, refractory shock, or cardiac arrest. In the urokinase study group, only 7 per cent of the patients had hypotension, and none had previous cardiac arrest. The two groups, then, are dissimilar with regard to patient population, and the survival rates of the two groups cannot be compared.

Furthermore, the overall survival rates of Cross's summarized report have been improved upon in more recent operative series. Despite the use of hypotension and/or cardiac arrest as indications for pulmonary embolectomy, reports have appeared subsequent to 1967 showing a rather consistent survival rate of over 70 per cent (Table 3).[7-9, 33-36] The small numbers of patients from each center would seem to indicate that the patients were highly selected—that is, were only the most critically ill following MPE. Survival rate following preoperative cardiac arrest was approximately two out of every three patients (Table 3).

TABLE 3.  Survival Rates in Recent Series of Pulmonary Embolectomies

| Author        Year | Total Number | Survivors | Survival Rate (%) | With Cardiac Arrest | Survivors | Rate (%) |
|---|---|---|---|---|---|---|
| Stansel et al., 1967[8] | 10 | 7 | 70 | 2 | 1 | 50 |
| Gentsch et al., 1969[7] | 10 | 7 | 70 | 3 | 2 | 66.7 |
| Paneth, 1969[33] | 34 | 26 | 76 | — | — | — |
| Taber and Arciniegas, 1973[34] | 18 | 13 | 72 | (1)° | — | — |
| Berger, 1973[35] | 17 | 13 | 76.4 | (3) | — | — |
| Heimbecker et al., 1973[36] | 11 | 10 | 90.9 | 4 | 4 | 100 |
| Reul and Beall, 1974[9] | 17 | 11 | 64.7 | 9 | 5 | 55.6 |
| Overall | 117 | 87 | 74.3 | 18 | 12 | 66.7 |

° Parentheses indicate that survival in patients with cardiac arrest was not stated.

In the patient with MPE and shock, the most important determining factor for survival is establishment of tissue perfusion to prevent irreversible changes. Rapid initiation of cardiopulmonary bypass has achieved this goal more satisfactorily than have vasopressors, cardiotonic agents, and thrombolytic substances. Extraction of the clots from the pulmonary artery naturally follows the initiation of cardiopulmonary bypass and can rapidly reverse the clinical state, depending on the underlying cardiopulmonary status of the patient and the perfusion state prior to resuscitation. To initiate cardiopulmonary bypass and wait for natural or accelerated thrombolysis to occur would be foolhardy, when embolectomy can be so easily accomplished.

The most frequent cause of death was poor perfusion and hypoxemia, which had occurred from the time of MPE until the initiation of cardiopulmonary bypass.[6-9, 33-36] Many moribund patients underwent pulmonary embolectomy in desperate attempts and died of neurologic or cardiac injury incurred prior to resuscitation. On the other hand, many dramatic results were achieved when cardiopulmonary bypass could be rapidly initiated and perfusion established. Most of the patients in the operative group would not have survived without the operation, since extracorporeal circulation was the sole method of cardiopulmonary support. Most patients were operated on because initial medical therapy had failed; that is, shock was not reversed by the standard medical therapy, including use of vasopressors.

The reasons for the recently improved results following embolectomy in MPE have been (1) initiation of cardiopulmonary bypass under local anesthesia prior to induction of general anesthesia by the use of femoral vein to femoral artery extracorporeal circulation; (2) accurate diagnosis of pulmonary embolus by preoperative angiography; (3) pump standby for inferior vena cava ligation; (4) rapid diagnosis and initiation of resuscitation; and (5) rapidly available pulmonary arteriography and cardiopulmonary bypass.

Recently Heimbecker et al.[36] have reported excellent results with both conservative and operative therapy and have stressed the early institution of cardiopulmonary bypass under local anesthesia in patients who have refractory shock. They have proposed that vigorous manual external cardiac massage fractionates the blood clots into the peripheral pulmonary arteries and results in relief of obstruction with increase in arterial oxygen saturation. As with other reports, early initiation of cardiopulmonary bypass played the most important role in the good results. All patients who had cardiac arrest in our series had vigorous manual massage prior to initiation of cardiopulmonary bypass.[9] None with MPE had clots lodged only in the nonmajor pulmonary arteries. Once cardiac arrest occurred, resuscitation was virtually impossible without cardiopulmonary bypass. When cardiopulmonary bypass has been initiated, it is a simple step to perform pulmonary embolectomy in these critically ill patients.

## Current Method of Treatment

Utilizing this information and experience as a basis for logical management of massive pulmonary embolus, we use an operative approach for the patient who has MPE accompanied by electrocardiographic changes, decreased cardiac output, lowered blood pressure, tachycardia, and acidosis. Presumptive evidence of MPE is present whenever a patient suffers sudden cardiac arrest or sudden deterioration with arterial hypoxemia, electrocardiographic changes of right ventricular strain, and evidence of pulmonary hypertension by increased pulmonary second sound on auscultation. Elevation of the central venous pressure or pulmonary artery pressure is usually present when measured. Although pulmonary scanning has been helpful in postoperative assessment and in the assessment of nonmassive or submassive pulmonary embolism or infarction, in the acute MPE accompanied by hypotension and cardiac arrest, lung scanning is not practical. Serum enzyme elevations are of no benefit in the acute situation. The final clinical diagnosis of pulmonary embolism is never determined until a pulmonary angiogram is completed.

Angiography should be done by injection of contrast media directly into the pulmonary artery. Serial x-ray films are necessary to make the diagnosis and to demonstrate the amount of arterial involvement. A single film by injection into a central venous catheter or indwelling pulmonary artery catheter is more misleading than diagnostic. Measurement of the pulmonary artery pressure, right ventricular pressure, and right and left ventricular end diastolic pressures is desirable.

In most instances, angiographic proof of pulmonary embolus should be present prior to pulmonary embolectomy. The only way this may be obtained in patients who have cardiac arrest is by initiating portable cardiopulmonary bypass or by the use of portable angiography equipment. If there is any question as to the patient's cardiac stability, cardiopulmonary bypass by femoral vein to femoral artery cannulation should be done immediately under local anesthesia. In the instance of cardiac arrest or refractory shock, the patient must be taken to an x-ray facility or x-ray taken to him while he is supported by cardiopulmonary bypass.

In the rare instance in which cardiac arrest has occurred and cardiopulmonary bypass is initiated for resuscitation but pulmonary angiography is not available, operative exploration may be indicated. If pulmonary embolus is not found, usually cardiopulmonary bypass is necessary to resuscitate the patient in the first place, and appropriate coronary arteriography or transfer to another mechanical circulatory assist device may be undertaken. We have utilized portable or operating room cardiopulmonary bypass to resuscitate many patients, and there have been several long-term survivors, even when pulmonary embolus was not found.

An appropriate plan of attack in MPE has evolved (Figure 1). Any patient with sudden cardiac arrest or refractory hypotension is rapidly evaluated. Noncardiopulmonary causes can usually be excluded by interpretation of the electrocardiogram and arterial blood gases. Supportive therapy should be given to this group. Patients with cardiopulmonary causes of cardiac arrest or refractory hypotension are treated with the usual resuscitative medications and techniques. If resuscitation is successful and MPE is suspected on clinical grounds, heparin is given and an immediate pulmonary angiogram is done with cardiopulmonary bypass standby in the x-ray room. If the angio-

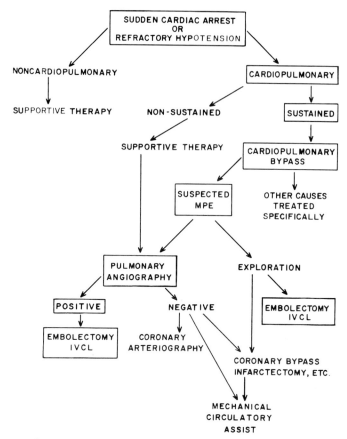

*Figure 1.* The general procedure for sudden cardiac arrest or refractory hypotension in potentially salvageable patients is shown. After resuscitative measures, noncardiopulmonary causes receive supportive therapy as indicated. Cardiopulmonary causes are treated according to the duration of the cardiac arrest or refractory hypotension. If there is recovery, then supportive therapy with pulmonary angiography and subsequent embolectomy with inferior vena cava ligation may be done. If cardiac arrest or refractory hypotension is sustained, cardiopulmonary bypass is immediately instituted and the patient treated according to the lesion causing the cardiopulmonary arrest. If these techniques fail, the patient may be placed on whichever mechanical circulatory assist device is indicated. This technique can be utilized for treating all patients with refractory hypotension or sudden cardiac arrest. (MPE = massive pulmonary embolus; IVCL = inferior vena cava ligation.)

gram is positive, cannulation of the femoral artery and vein under local anesthesia is done prior to induction of general anesthesia, and pulmonary embolectomy under total cardiopulmonary bypass is accomplished, as previously described.[9, 20, 24-26] Inferior vena cava ligation is done at the end of the procedure (Figure 2).

In patients who have refractory hypotension or cardiac arrest, cardiopulmonary bypass is initiated under local anesthesia at the bedside, and if there is suspected MPE, pulmonary angiography may be done with portable cardiopulmonary bypass support. Immediate operative exploration may be done

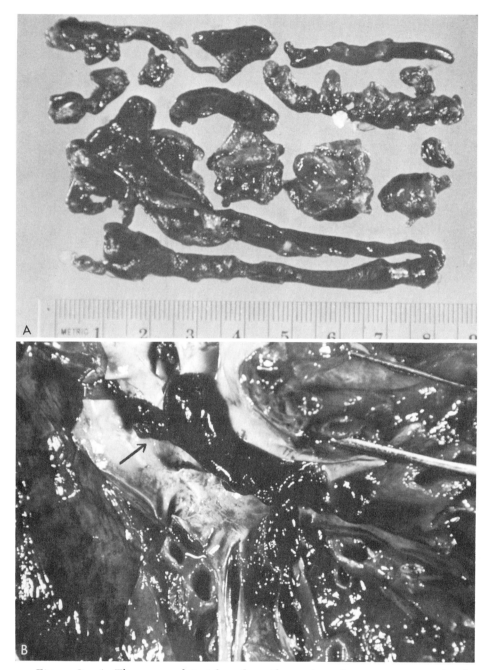

*Figure 2.* A, The many clots taken from the main pulmonary artery and right and left branches are shown. The patient was satisfactorily resuscitated following a massive pulmonary embolus by portable cardiopulmonary bypass. Inferior vena cava ligation was not done following pulmonary embolectomy. Her postoperative course was benign until the sixth postoperative day, at which time another massive pulmonary embolus occurred, resulting in death. *B,* There is fresh embolus lodged in the major pulmonary artery (arrow). This and similar cases in our experience have shown the importance of inferior vena cava ligation following embolectomy.

if pulmonary angiography is not available. If pulmonary embolism is present, pulmonary embolectomy is done, followed by inferior vena cava ligation. If pulmonary embolus is not present, further evaluation of the cause of the cardiac arrest can be done at the operating table by palpation of the coronary arteries or coronary arteriography, examination for acute myocardial infarction, and direct measurement of intracardiac and arterial pressure. Possible coronary artery bypass, infarctectomy, aneurysmectomy, valve replacement, repair of ventricular septal defect, or insertion of an epicardial pacemaker may follow. If none of these procedures is indicated and further cardiopulmonary bypass support is necessary, then the patient may be transferred to one of the other types of mechanical circulatory assist, including intra-aortic balloon counterpulsation, left atrial to femoral artery bypass, and extracorporeal bypass utilizing the membrane oxygenator or mechanical heart when available. This plan for management of cardiac arrest and refractory hypotension includes all patients who are potentially salvageable — that is, according to underlying condition, age, neurologic status, etc. In the more common instance when pulmonary embolus occurs and there is no evidence of shock or cardiac decompensation, intravenous heparin therapy is begun, with careful observation. If hypotension occurs, pulmonary arteriography should be done with cardiopulmonary bypass standby. In the case in which refractory hypotension suddenly occurs, the above plan is followed. This technique screens out the patients who do not require operation for MPE yet has the advantage of immediate applicability if sudden clinical deterioration occurs.

Obviously, specially trained personnel and equipment are necessary for this type of approach, but we believe that any medical unit specializing in cardiopulmonary disease should have this capacity. Portable cardiopulmonary bypass equipment, such as the Travenol EPO unit,* is ideal for transporting patients to pulmonary angiography and bringing cardiopulmonary bypass to the patient's bedside. The portable unit may be set up with sterile connections to the oxygenator and tubing in place ready for cardiopulmonary bypass, except for priming. Priming by hemodilution technique takes a matter of minutes, and the house staff should be familiar with the techniques of priming the pump. Once the groin is cannulated with a set of portable instruments at the bedside, cardiopulmonary bypass may be initiated. If the patient is close to the operating room and the portable pump is not available, then immediate transport to the operating room for resuscitation and placement on standard cardiopulmonary bypass may be done, and operative exploration may take place. In any event, some type of cardiopulmonary bypass should be available within minutes for immediate resuscitation to avoid cerebral hypoxemia or irreversible damage to other systems.

Pulmonary angiography likewise should be immediately available. Emergency coronary arteriography and/or cardiac catheterization is also essential to total patient management.

Not much controversy exists regarding definitive treatment of the pa-

---

*Travenol Laboratories, Morton Grove, Illinois.

tient with MPE causing cardiac arrest. Immediate resuscitation and embolectomy are indicated in this group of patients. Prolonged cardiopulmonary bypass while attempting to resuscitate the patient or prolonged membrane oxygenation during the few days that clot lysis will occur carries a much higher mortality, and is a drain on personnel time, than simple pulmonary embolectomy. In the patient with hypotension refractory to medical therapy including vasopressors, medical management alone will fail. In the patient who becomes hypotensive and requires vasopressors or is unstable, pulmonary embolectomy should be done because of the low mortality involved in this group. In the patient with one episode of hypotension followed by good recovery, medical therapy will have equally good results, provided pulmonary embolization does not recur, the patient does not have severe underlying cardiac disease, and less than 50 per cent of the pulmonary arterial distribution is involved.

In summary, MPE is a catastrophic occurrence which results from mechanical obstruction of the right ventricular outflow tract. The overall effect is related to the size of the embolus and the underlying cardiopulmonary status of the patient. Immediate relief of obstruction results in reversal to preembolic conditions. The limiting factor to success in pulmonary embolectomy is the duration of the low perfusion state and accompanying system failure caused by MPE prior to initiation of cardiopulmonary bypass support and institution of adequate perfusion. Therefore, immediate initiation of cardiopulmonary bypass by femoral vein to femoral artery cannulation has resulted in a markedly decreased mortality rate in pulmonary embolectomy, except in patients with missed diagnosis, in those with severe underlying cardiopulmonary disease, or in those in whom the operation is undertaken after prolonged perfusion deficits. In the latter group of patients, the critical moment of potential salvage has passed, and, regardless of the treatment, the situation is usually irreversible. We therefore strongly urge pulmonary embolectomy in patients who have MPE with systemic hypotension, shock, or cardiac arrest. Rapid relief of the pulmonary artery obstruction and hypoxemia by a simple operation is essential for survival.

# References

1. Kakkar, V. V., Howe, C. T., Nicolaides, A. N., Renny, J. T. G., and Clarke, M. B.: Deep vein thrombosis of the leg: Is there a "high risk" group? Am. J. Surg. 120:527, 1970.
2. Jeffcoate, T. N. A., Miller, J., Ross, R. F., and Tindall, V. R.: Puerperal thromboembolism in relation to the inhibition of lactation by oestrogen therapy. Br. Med. J. 3:19, 1968.
3. Belt, T. H.: Thrombosis and pulmonary embolism, Am. J. Pathol. 10:129, 1934.
4. Hampton, A. O., and Castleman, B.: Correlation of postmortem chest teleroentgenograms with autopsy findings; with special reference to pulmonary embolism and infarction. Am. J. Roentgenol. 43:305, 1940.
5. Urokinase-Pulmonary Embolism Trial. Circulation (Suppl. II) 47:5, 1973.
6. Berger, R. L., Gibson, H., and Ferris, E. J.: A reappraisal of the indications of pulmonary embolectomy. Am. J. Surg. 116:403, 1968.
7. Gentsch, T. O., Larsen, P. B., Daughtry, D. C., Chesney, J. G., and Spea, H. C.: Community-wide availability of pulmonary embolectomy with cardiopulmonary bypass. Ann. Thorac. Surg. 7:97, 1969.

8. Stansel, H. C., Jr., Hume, M., and Glenn, W. W. L.: Pulmonary embolectomy: Results in ten patients. New Engl. J. Med. 276:717, 1967.
9. Reul, G. J., Jr., and Beall, A. C., Jr.: Emergency pulmonary embolectomy for massive pulmonary embolism, Circulation 50:II–236, 1974.
10. McIntyre, K. M., and Sasahara, A. A.: Determinants of right ventricular function and hemodynamics after pulmonary embolism. Chest 65:534, 1974.
11. Alpert, J. S., Haynes, F. W., Dalen, J. E., and Dexter, L.: Experimental pulmonary embolism: Effect on pulmonary blood volume and vascular compliance. Circulation 49:152, 1974.
12. Dack, S., Master, A. M., Horn, H., Grishman, A., and Field, L. E.: Acute coronary insufficiency due to pulmonary embolism. Am. J. Med. 7:464, 1949.
13. Oldham, H. N., Jr., Cox, J. L., Pass, H. I., Wechsler, A. S., and Sabiston, D. C., Jr.: Effects of pulmonary embolism on regional myocardial blood flow. Surgery 76:160, 1974.
14. Sharma, G. V. R. K., Wrenn, C. E., Godin, P. F., O'Neil, D. M., and Sasahara, A. A.: Regional and transmural myocardial blood flow distribution in experimental pulmonary embolism. Circulation (Suppl. II)45–46:57, 1972.
15. Spotnitz, H. M., Berman, M. A., and Epstein, S. E.: Pathophysiology and experimental treatment of acute pulmonary embolism. Am. Heart J. 82:511, 1971.
16. Stein, P. D., Alshabkhoun, S., Hawkins, H. F., Hyland, J. W., and Jarrett, C. E.: Right coronary blood flow in acute pulmonary embolism. Am. Heart J. 77:356, 1969.
17. Symbas, P. N., and Bonanno, J. A.: Coronary blood flow in acute experimental pulmonary embolization. J. Surg. Res. 10:377, 1970.
18. Vatner, S. F., and Van Citters, R. L.: Effects of acute pulmonary embolism on coronary dynamics in the conscious dog. Am. Heart J. 83:50, 1972.
19. Sasahara, A. A., CAnilla, J. E., Morse, R. L., et al.: Clinical and physiologic studies in pulmonary thromboembolism. Am. J. Cardiol. 20:10, 1967.
20. Cooley, D. A., Beall, A. C., Jr., and Alexander, J. K.: Acute massive pulmonary embolism. Successful surgical treatment using temporary cardiopulmonary bypass. J.A.M.A. 177:283, 1961.
21. Sharp, E. H.: Pulmonary embolectomy: Successful removal of a massive pulmonary embolus with the support of cardiopulmonary bypass: Case report. Ann. Surg. 156:1, 1962.
22. Beall, A. C., Jr., Fred, H. L., and Cooley, D. A.: Pulmonary Embolism. In Current Problems in Surgery. Philadelphia, W. B. Saunders Co., 1964, pp. 31–39.
23. Turnier, E., Hill, J. D., Kerth, W. J., and Gerbode, F.: Massive pulmonary embolism. Surgery 125:611, 1973.
24. Cooley, D. A., and Beall, A. C., Jr.: A technique of pulmonary embolectomy using temporary cardiopulmonary bypass. J. Cardiovasc. Surg. 2:469, 1961.
25. Cooley, D. A., and Beall, A. C., Jr.: Surgical treatment of acute massive pulmonary embolism using temporary cardiopulmonary bypass. Dis. Chest 41:102, 1962.
26. Cooley, D. A., Beall, A. C., Jr., and Alexander, J. K.: Acute massive pulmonary embolism: successful surgical treatment using temporary cardiopulmonary bypass. J.A.M.A. 177:283, 1961.
27. Cross, F. S., and Mowlem, A.: A survey of the current status of pulmonary embolectomy for massive pulmonary embolism. Circulation (Suppl. I) 35:86, 1967.
28. Coon, W. W., and Coller, F. A.: Clinicopathologic correlation in thromboembolism. Surg. Gynecol. Obstet. 109:259, 1959.
29. Fred, H. L., Axelard, M. A., Lewis, J. M., and Alexander, J. K.: Rapid resolution of pulmonary thromboemboli in man. J.A.M.A. 196:1137, 1966.
30. Dalen, J. E., Banas, J. S., Jr., Brooks, H. L., Evans, G. L., Paraskos, J. A., and Dexter, L.: Resolution rate of acute pulmonary embolism in man. New Engl. J. Med. 280:1194, 1969.
31. McDonald, I. G., Hirsh, J., and Hale, G. S.: The rate of resolution of pulmonary embolism and its effects on early survival. Aust. Ann. Med. (Suppl.) 19:46, 1970.
32. Sautter, R. D., Myers, W. O., and Wenzel, F. J.: Implications of the urokinase study concerning the surgical treatment of pulmonary embolism. J. Thorac. Cardiovasc. Surg. 63:54, 1972.
33. Paneth, M.: Pulmonary embolism: Surgical treatment of massive pulmonary embolism. Trans. Med. Soc. London LXXXV, p. 27, 1969.
34. Taber, R. E., and Arciniegas, E.: An aggressive approach to thromboembolic disease. J. Cardiovasc. Surg. (Torino) 14:306, 1973.
35. Berger, R. L.: Pulmonary embolectomy with preoperative circulatory support. Ann. Thorac. Surg. 16:217, 1973.
36. Heimbecker, R. O., Keon, W. J., and Richards, K. U.: Massive pulmonary embolism. Arch. Surg. 107:740, 1973.

# The Use of the "Umbrella" in the Treatment of Thromboembolism

KAZI MOBIN-UDDIN

*The Frederick C. Smith Clinic, Marion, Ohio*

With the advent of new methods for the diagnosis of venous thrombosis and the prevention of pulmonary embolism, there has been a widespread renewal of interest in thromboembolic disease. Following a literature review, one gets the distinct impression that nothing about pulmonary embolism is clearly established. The reported autopsy incidence varies from 6 to 64 per cent. The estimated mortality in the United States varies from 47,000 to 200,000 per year. Diagnosis is elusive in 70 per cent of patients, and many aspects of management remain controversial. No general agreement exists as to indications for venous interruption, and opinions vary considerably as to the role of pulmonary embolectomy in massive pulmonary embolism. The use of thrombolytic agents in the management of thromboembolic disease remains investigational.

This article is intended to review the clinical data for effectiveness of therapy in thromboembolic disease, with special reference to the use of the inferior vena cava umbrella filter (IVC-UF).

## Deep Venous Thrombosis

Nearly all emboli arise from thrombi in the lower extremity or pelvic veins. Seventy-three per cent of major or fatal emboli come from the large veins of the pelvis or thigh.[1] Lower limb thrombi can be significant when they extend into the popliteal vein or proximally. Approximately one-half of those who die of pulmonary embolism have no premonitory signs, and one-half to two-thirds of those with deep venous thrombosis (DVT) in the lower extremities discovered at autopsy had no clinical manifestations.[2] In 30 per

321

cent of patients with a clinical diagnosis of DVT, phlebography is normal.[3] The treatment of DVT cannot be assessed on clinical grounds alone, because the physical signs may give little indication of the extent or progression of the disease. Considerable controversy exists concerning the optimal therapy of acute DVT. Anticoagulants, thrombolytic agents, and platelet inhibiting drugs have been used clinically in the treatment of established DVT.

## ANTICOAGULANT THERAPY

Heparin and coumarin compounds, alone or in combination, have been used in the treatment of acute DVT. Heparin[4] in adequate doses blocks the coagulation mechanism and thus prevents further thrombus formation. Its use is prophylactic, and it has no effect on preformed thrombi, except to prevent distal propagation. The fate of venous thrombi is primarily dependent on the endogenous mechanisms — thrombolysis, thrombus fragmentation, organization, and recanalization — rather than on the direct action of heparin. Thrombolysis may result in complete dissolution of thrombi. Thrombus fragmentation and detachment result in embolization to the lungs. When thrombosed veins recanalize, the valves either are destroyed[5] or become incompetent.[6] Subsequently, pain in the legs, swelling, varicose veins, eczema, ulceration, and other trophic changes — the postphlebitic syndrome — may develop.

Clinical improvement following heparin therapy in DVT is not due to anatomical lysis of thrombi, as repeat radiographic findings are practically unchanged.[7] Heparin therapy does not prevent scarring of the venous valve when recanalization occurs. Fifty to 75 per cent of patients with DVT suffer persistent symptoms in the affected extremity and stand one chance in four of developing postphlebitic syndrome.[8] The severity of the postphlebitic syndrome depends on the extent of phlebitis rather than on treatment. Butcher,[9] after a study of 272 patients with DVT, concluded that the results in 163 patients initially treated with heparin followed by coumarin compound did not differ significantly from those in the 109 patients treated only by bed rest, limb elevation, and elastic support.

Pulmonary embolism is a dreaded complication of DVT. Byrne[10] reported the results of anticoagulant therapy in 118 patients with DVT. Fifty-four patients were treated with bishydroxycoumarin; 13 deaths occurred, giving a mortality rate of 24 per cent. Sixty-four patients were treated with heparin alone; nine deaths, occurred, giving a mortality rate of 14 per cent. Thus the overall anticoagulant mortality rate was 18.6 per cent.

Bleeding complications are a constant threat to patients on anticoagulant therapy. Salzman and associates,[11] in a group of 100 consecutive patients receiving heparin in therapeutic dosage, reported major bleeding in 11 of 56 medical patients, 5 of 28 surgical patients, 1 of 6 orthopedic patients, and 4 of 10 obstetric and gynecologic patients. Two patients died from bleeding.

In the Urokinase Pulmonary Embolism Trial Phase I cooperative study,[12] moderate to severe bleeding complications were reported in 27 per cent of patients on heparin therapy.

## Defibrinating Agents

Anticoagulant therapy by defibrination with Arvin has been used clinically in the treatment of established DVT. Small clinical trials[7, 13-17] suggest that Arvin effectively produces a state of anticoagulation which prevents thrombus formation and has no direct thrombolytic effects. More extensive clinical trials are needed before firm conclusions can be drawn as to the superiority of Arvin over heparin and oral anticoagulation.

## PLATELET INHIBITORS

Bernard et al.,[18] in a prospective study of the use of clinical dextran in established DVT, found no beneficial effect over that obtained by saline.

## THROMBOLYTIC THERAPY

Since anticoagulants are prophylactic and have no direct effect on the preformed thrombi, much attention is being given to acceleration of thrombus dissolution by thrombolytic agents. Rapid thrombolysis not only may decrease the risk of pulmonary embolism but also may prevent postphlebitic syndrome by preservation of venous valve function.

There have been several controlled studies comparing the effects of streptokinase with those of heparin on the resolution of thrombi as judged by phlebography. It has been shown that there is accelerated resolution of thrombi after streptokinase therapy as compared with that occurring after heparin therapy. Combining the results of these five studies,[19] of 47 patients, 22 (47 per cent) achieved complete lysis after 24 to 48 hours of streptokinase therapy, while only 5 of 40 (12.5 per cent) patients achieved similar lysis after heparin therapy. On the other hand, Silver[20] reported on the results of urokinase therapy in seven patients with thrombi in the iliofemoral or leg veins; only two improved, and in no instance was there complete lysis of the thrombi.

Venous thrombi detected by the fibrinogen uptake method, when they are limited to the legs, usually resolve spontaneously without any therapy. Thrombi extending into the proximal veins are associated with greater risk of pulmonary embolism.[21] Early treatment with thrombolytic enzymes is more likely to dissolve thrombi and to preserve the function of venous valves.[16] Patients with extensive DVT are less likely to have accelerated resolution because of limited access of the fibrinolytic enzymes to the affected areas.

In the Urokinase Pulmonary Embolism Trial Phase I[12] cooperative study, treatment with thrombolytic enzymes was of little value in preventing recurrent pulmonary embolism. During the 2-week observation period, possible recurrent embolism (defined by the presence of clinical and/or lung scan evidence) was described with nearly equal frequency in the two treatment groups. It occurred in 15 per cent of the group given urokinase and in 18 per cent of the heparin group. Six of the urokinase-treated patients (7 per cent) and seven heparin-treated patients (9 per cent) died of pulmonary embolism during the observation period. Neither streptokinase nor urokinase is available except for investigational purposes.

## OPERATIVE TREATMENT

### Indications for Inferior Vena Cava–Umbrella Filter Insertion in Patients with DVT

1. When anticoagulant therapy is contraindicated.

2. When recurrent thrombophlebitis requires repeated hospitalization, especially if long-term adequate anticoagulant therapy is difficult to maintain.

3. Hip fractures. Sevitt and Gallagher[2] demonstrated an 83 per cent incidence of venous thrombosis in autopsy studies of patients who died following fractures of the hip. Freeark and Fardin[22] reported that 36 per cent of a series of 50 patients with hip fractures had deep leg vein thrombosis shown by venography. The study of Fitts and associates[23] showed that 38 per cent of 161 patients dying with hip fractures and undergoing autopsy had pulmonary emboli as the cause of death. In several comparative studies, prophylactic anticoagulation[24-27] reduced the incidence of thromboembolic complications in hip operations, particularly in elective cases. However, it did not appreciably affect the mortality rates in elderly patients with hip fractures.[2, 26] Sevitt and Gallagher reduced thromboembolic incidence from 37 per cent in controls to 3 per cent in the treated group. The mortality rate in the treated group was 17 per cent, and in the control group 28 per cent. Salzman and associates reduced thromboembolism from a 26 per cent incidence to a 7 per cent incidence with warfarin, but reduced the mortality rate only from 27 per cent to 24 per cent.

Fullen and associates[28] reported the prophylactic use of the IVC-UF in hip fracture patients, with a controlled study group. Fifty-nine patients were in the control group. Of 70 patients offered the IVC-UF, 22 refused the procedure, and in 7 patients the IVC-UF could not be inserted because of technical reasons. The two groups were similar in regard to age, associated disease, type of fractures, and the time delay between admission and fracture fixation. They reported no clinically detectable pulmonary emboli in the treated group versus a 20 per cent incidence in the controls. The mortality rate in the treated group was 10 per cent, as compared to 24 per cent in the control group. No patient in the treated group died from pulmonary embolism. In the control group, pulmonary embolism was considered to be the cause of death in 8 (13.5 per cent).

4. Prophylactic IVC-UF insertion was performed at the University of Kentucky Medical Center in five patients who had developed DVT, confirmed by venography, while awaiting hip operation. These patients were considered to be at great risk of developing fatal pulmonary embolism following hip operation. All patients recovered without clinical evidence of pulmonary embolism.

## *Pulmonary Embolism*

Pulmonary thromboembolic disease continues to be a major cause of morbidity and mortality in hospitalized patients on surgical as well as medical services.

### ANTICOAGULANT THERAPY

Based on the work of Murray and Best,[29] anticoagulant therapy with heparin has become the standard treatment for patients with pulmonary embolism. An often quoted prospective controlled study whose results favored anticoagulant therapy is the report by Barritt and Jordan.[30] After 35 patients were admitted into the trial, 2 of 19 not receiving anticoagulants died of recurrent pulmonary embolism, and 5 others had nonfatal recurrences. There was no death from recurrent pulmonary emboli in the treated group. The treated group received 10,000 units of heparin intravenously every 6 hours for six doses without laboratory control. Nicoumalone was begun concurrently and continued for 14 days. Clinical methods were used for diagnosis and evaluation of therapy.

The reported results of anticoagulant therapy vary widely. Currently positions range from, "Recurrent pulmonary embolism rarely occurs following anticoagulant therapy," to "Anticoagulants can give patients a false sense of security and can provide little or no protection against further thrombotic disease or recurrent pulmonary emboli, and they produce an added hazard from bleeding."[31] The results of uncontrolled studies[32] report fatal recurrent embolization rates ranging from 0 to 18.6 per cent. Failure of anticoagulant therapy in preventing recurrent pulmonary embolism indicates that heparin in adequate doses can prevent thrombus formation or propagation but cannot prevent fragmentation and detachment of a nonadherent thrombus.

### OPERATIVE TREATMENT

Crane[33] reported the results in 341 patients with thromboembolism treated by femoral vein ligation and in 104 treated by inferior vena cava ligation. Subsequent embolism occurred in 10 per cent of femoral vein ligations and in 1 per cent of the IVC ligations; fatal embolism occurred in 5 per cent of femoral and in 1 per cent of the caval ligations. Crane concluded that "ligation of the IVC is a most effective procedure for preventing pulmonary embolism." However, operative ligation of IVC under general anesthesia is accompanied by an operative mortality rate that varies from 5[34] to 40[35] per cent, depending upon the severity of the underlying disease and the extent of obstruction to pulmonary blood flow.

Transvenous insertion of the IVC umbrella filter[36-41] is performed under local anesthesia, avoids a major operation, does not decrease the cardiac output, and at the same time protects the patient from potentially lethal pulmonary embolism. The present report includes the author's experience with the IVC-UF, as well as experiences reported by other physicians.

## SELECTION OF PATIENTS FOR UMBRELLA INSERTION

### Contraindications to Anticoagulants

Contraindications to heparin therapy may be absolute or relative; treatment for each patient should be individualized and the need for therapy verified against the probable risk of hemorrhage. Usually heparin is not given to patients with recent cerebral vascular accident, operation, or severe trauma, or to those patients with actively bleeding lesions. Women over 60 years of age have a 50 per cent risk of bleeding complications.[42]

### Failure of Anticoagulants

The main indication for the IVC-UF insertion has been in those patients in whom adequate heparinization (Lee-White clotting time > 20 minutes) has failed to prevent recurrent embolic episodes. Recurrent pulmonary embolism is common in patients who have a basic predisposing cause for continued thromboembolism, such as chronic congestive heart failure and recurrent thrombophlebitis. In some patients, the source of recurrent emboli may be thrombi formed in the IVC in the cul-de-sac just above the ligation site but below the renal veins. The IVC-UF should be implanted above the thrombus just below the renal veins.

### Presence of Potentially Fatal Thrombi in
### Iliofemoral Veins or IVC

Potentially fatal thromboemboli frequently arise in iliofemoral veins[43] and can be readily demonstrated by phlebography.[41, 44] A fresh, nonadherent thrombus appears as a radiolucent defect within the vein, with a thin white line representing contrast medium between the thrombus and the vein wall on each side.[44] We perform phlebograms in all patients with pulmonary embolism to determine the location, extent, and nature of residual venous thrombi. IVC-UF insertion is recommended if large, nonadherent thrombi are demonstrated in iliofemoral veins or IVC.

## CONTRAINDICATIONS TO IVC-UF INSERTION

IVC-UF insertion is not recommended in patients with septic emboli or in those with septicemia. We have advised removal of the IVC-UF and ligation of IVC in one patient with postoperative septicemia. The organisms cultured from the blood and from the clot on the proximal surface of the filter were identical.

## MANAGEMENT — POST-UMBRELLA INSERTION

Following IVC-UF implantation, systemic anticoagulant therapy is withheld for 12 hours to minimize the possibility of bleeding in the neck incision or into the retroperitoneal space. Thereafter, intravenous heparin is resumed, if there is no contraindication to its use, for 7 to 10 days, preferably by continuous infusion, to maintain partial thromboplastin time or the Lee-White clotting time at two times the control value. Oral anticoagulation with warfarin sodium is started on the third postoperative day and continued for three months. Postoperative systemic anticoagulation plays an important part in the prevention of formation or propagation of peripheral thrombi. In patients with a continuing predisposition for recurrent emboli, long-term anticoagulant therapy is advised.

In an attempt to resist or prevent thrombus formation on the proximal surface of the IVC-UF, preoperative heparin impregnation[45] of the filter with TDMAC/heparin complex* is recommended. There is considerable experimental evidence to suggest that the filters preoperatively impregnated with heparin are less thrombogenic.[37] Local along with systemic anticoagulation can prevent or resist thrombus formation and allow for endothelium to grow in between the fenestrations of the IVC-UF. How long the heparin bonding is effective is not known. Once the IVC-UF is endothelialized, a process usually complete within 3 months, local or systemic anticoagulation is no longer necessary to maintain patency of the IVC. Our objective is to maintain patency of the ostia of the IVC-UF, except when they entrap emboli.

# *Results*

### AUTHOR'S EXPERIENCE

IVC-UF insertion was performed in 163 patients between July, 1968, and June, 1975. One hundred filter implants (July, 1968, to June, 1970) were done at the University of Miami Hospitals; 51 filter implants (July, 1970, to June, 1974) were done at the University of Kentucky Medical Center at Lexington, Kentucky; and 12 filter implants (July, 1974, to June, 1975) were done at the Community Med-Center Hospital in Marion, Ohio.

The results are summarized in Table 1.

### *Mortality and Recurrent Embolism*

Significant retroperitoneal bleeding following IVC-UF insertion may have contributed to the death of a 75-year-old man with chronic congestive heart failure who died on the fifth postoperative day. The bleeding was not recognized clinically. A 25-year-old markedly obese woman had sudden cardiac arrest 12 hours after IVC-UF insertion and could not be resuscitated. At

---

*Polysciences Inc., Paul Valley Industrial Park, Warrington, Pennsylvania 18976.

TABLE 1.    Inferior Vena Cava Umbrella Filter:
Author's Experience
(July, 1968–June, 1975)

| Complication | Number of Patients (Total of 163) |
| --- | --- |
| Filter migration | 0 |
| Retroperitoneal bleeding | 1 |
| Recurrent emboli | 3 |
| Recurrent phlebitis | 10 |

autopsy, recent thrombosis of the right and left main pulmonary arteries was found, and there was also an old resolving thrombus in the right main pulmonary artery. The IVC-UF was securely fixed in the IVC and had no evidence of thrombus formation. No source of emboli could be found. This may well have been a case of hypercoagulable state with primary thrombosis of the pulmonary arteries. Fatal recurrent pulmonary embolism occurred in a markedly obese patient 8 months after IVC-UF insertion. The filter was inadvertently placed at the junction of the left common iliac vein with the IVC. Thrombosis in the opposite iliac vein appeared to be the source of the pulmonary embolus. Recurrent pulmonary embolism with areas of infarction in lower lobe segments was documented at autopsy in two patients who died of heart disease 2 months after IVC-UF insertion. The embolization probably occurred via collateral veins.

### Filter Migration

Filter migration has not occurred in our own experience. In one patient, tilting of the device was noted immediately after insertion. Another IVC-UF was implanted just above the dislodged filter to prevent migration.

### IVC Patency

Of the first 50 patients in whom the IVC-UF impregnated with the TDMAC/heparin complex was used, 16 had IVC angiograms performed within 6 weeks after the filter insertion. Patency of the filter was demonstrated in 5 patients and occlusion of the IVC in the remaining 11 patients. Repeat angiograms in two of the five patients in whom the filter was patent, done at 6 months after the filter insertion in one and at 1 year and 3 months in the other, demonstrated free flow of blood through the IVC. IVC angiograms done in patients in whom unheparinized IVC-UF were used demonstrated occlusion of IVC within 1 to 2 weeks.

### PHYSICIANS' EXPERIENCES

The IVC-UF was released for general clinical use in January, 1970. According to the estimates made by the Edwards Laboratories,* 10,000 filters

---

*Santa Anna, California.

TABLE 2. Inferior Vena Cava Umbrella Filter:
Physicians' Experiences
(January, 1970 – October, 1975)

| Complication | Number of Patients (Total of 3415) |
|---|---|
| Filter migration | 1.0% |
| Misplacements | 1.0% |
| Recurrent embolism | 2.2% |
| Clinical edema | 5.1% |
| Phlebitis | 1.5% |

were implanted in the United States between January, 1970, and October, 1975. However, complete data, as reported by the evaluating physician, have been accumulated for only 3415 filter implants during the first 5 years of their use; these form the basis of this report.

The results are summarized in Table 2.

## Mortality and Recurrent Embolism

Recurrent pulmonary embolism has occurred in 2.2 per cent of patients (fatal, 0.5 per cent). For three patients, blood clots from the proximal surface of the IVC-UF were implicated as the source of recurrent embolus.

## Filter Migration

The clinical data for patients in whom filters migrated are given in Table 3. The IVC-UF has migrated in 1 per cent of patients. The original caval umbrella was 23 mm. in diameter, but episodes of migration led to the development of the 28-mm. device. With the introduction of the 28-mm. filter, the incidence of migration has been reduced to 0.6 per cent. The main causes of filter migration have neen (1) inadequate seating of the filter in the IVC; (2) exceptionally large IVC; and (3) sudden embolic obstruction of the filter by a large thrombus, resulting in dilation of IVC and permitting dislodgment and migration of the filter along with the embolus.

Partial dislodgment of the IVC-UF without migration has occurred in 20

TABLE 3. Inferior Vena Cava Umbrella Filter:
Physicians' Experiences
(January, 1970–October, 1975)

| Filter Migrated To | Number of Patients |
|---|---|
| Pulmonary artery | 17 |
| Right ventricle | 3 |
| Right atrium | 4 |
| Suprarenal IVC | 4 |
| Right iliac vein* | 6 |

*Following closed cardiac massage.

patients. To prevent migration, the larger 28-mm. filter was implanted just above the dislodged filter in six patients. In the remaining patients, either nothing was done or the IVC was ligated operatively with or without removal of the filter.

### Misplacement of the Filter

The IVC-UF was misplaced in the suprarenal IVC in three patients. The filters were pushed down by the applicator capsule into the infrarenal IVC. The IVC-UF was misplaced in the right renal vein in seven patients. In three of these, the filter was removed by a direct operative approach. The IVC-UF was mistakenly placed in the iliac vein in 20 patients. These patients have been treated either by implanting another filter in the IVC or by ligation of IVC with or without removal of the filter.

### Miscellaneous Complications

Significant retroperitoneal bleeding has occurred in five patients, right recurrent laryngeal nerve injury in two, air embolism in two, perforation of duodenum in one, and perforation of ureter in one. Postoperative septicemia led to removal of the filter in two patients.

### Stasis Sequelae

Significant edema developed in 115 patients (5.1 per cent), and phlebitis of the lower extremities, not previously present, developed in 35 (1.5 per cent). The majority of these patients improved with standard medical treatment.

Gradual occlusion of the IVC-UF allows for the progressive development of the collateral circulation, thereby avoiding acute venous pooling of blood in the lower extremities. Edema of the lower extremities following IVC-UF insertion is less of a problem. The majority of patients with severe venous stasis problems had a history of preexisting venous disease. Occlusion of the cava with peripheral edema can result from sudden thromboembolic obstruction of the IVC-UF.

As physicians have gained experience with the use of the IVC-UF, the complication rate has significantly decreased. To prevent dislodgment of the filter, tiny barbs have been placed at the distal tips of the spokes of the umbrella. The initial experimental results from implanting the barbed 28-mm. filter in calves have been satisfactory, and a clinical trial is in progress. It is hoped that the use of the barbed filters will eliminate filter migration as a problem.

## Massive Pulmonary Embolism

In any discussion of acute massive pulmonary embolism (AMPE), it is appropriate to begin with a definition of this entity. AMPE is a clinical syndrome characterized by severe respiratory distress with sustained hypotension or profound shock. Pulmonary arteriography in these patients usually shows thrombotic obstruction of more than one-half of the pulmonary circulation. Pulmonary embolism not accompanied by unyielding circulatory collapse is not considered life-threatening and is not germane to a discussion of pulmonary embolectomy.

It is estimated that pulmonary embolism causes approximately 200,000 deaths per year in the United States. Pulmonary embolism is the sole cause of death in 100,000 and is a major contributing cause in another 100,000.[46] Death in AMPE is directly related to the severity of obstruction to the pulmonary circulation and to that patient's cardiopulmonary reserve. Patients with preexisting cardiopulmonary disease tolerate much less additional obstruction than do those without preexisting disease.

The time elapsed between the onset of symptoms and death in patients with AMPE is of major clinical importance. In the autopsy series of 100 patients with proved fatal massive pulmonary embolism reported by Gorham,[47] 44 per cent died within 15 minutes, an additional 22 per cent lived up to 2 hours, and the remaining patients lived up to several days. Another autopsy review by Flemma and associates[48] involving 52 patients with fatal pulmonary embolism separated them into two groups: previously healthy patients and others with obvious terminal illnesses. In the former group, 55 per cent lived longer than 2 hours, and 48 per cent survived longer than 8 hours. Only 32 per cent of the terminally ill patients survived longer than 2 hours. Thus more than 50 per cent of patients with AMPE without terminal illnesses survived long enough to confirm the diagnosis and perform pulmonary embolectomy under cardiopulmonary bypass.

Spontaneous lysis of massive pulmonary emboli by intrinsic fibrinolytic system within several days to several weeks has been reported by several investigators.[49, 50] The rate of lysis varies, depending upon the age of thromboemboli and the fibrinolytic system.

Closed cardiac massage in patients with AMPE with cardiac arrest has been reported to produce effective fragmentation.[51, 52] In our own recent experience with three patients with massive pulmonary embolism and cardiac arrest, we were unable to resuscitate all by means of cardiac massage.

## OPERATIVE TREATMENT

### Inferior Vena Cava Interruption

Patients with massive pulmonary embolism who have survived the acute insult can die from (1) arrhythmias, (2) low cardiac output, and (3) recurrent pulmonary embolism. IVC ligation is usually recommended in these patients, as reliance on anticoagulant therapy alone is not justified since any additional embolization can be fatal. In acute massive pulmonary embolism, a direct operative approach for IVC ligation under general anesthesia carries a prohibitive risk. Berger[53] reported seven patients with massive embolism, five of whom developed circulatory collapse during operative ligation of IVC. Two patients died, and three were salvaged by pulmonary embolectomy. Six of Sautter's[54] pulmonary embolectomies were precipitated by rapid deterioration of the patient's condition during or just after the induction of anesthesia for caval ligation.

Transvenous insertion of the IVC-UF is the method of choice in these acutely ill patients, as the procedure is done under local anesthesia and avoids a major operation. Bloomfield[55] reported IVC-UF insertion in patients who had survived massive pulmonary embolism by 1 to 2 hours. Of the 12 patients, 8 made uncomplicated complete recovery. Bloomfield noted marked improvement within 2 to 12 hours after the IVC-UF insertion, as documented by symptomatic relief, objective increase in arterial oxygen partial pressure, and systemic blood pressure maintenance without vasopressor agents. Similar improvement was also noted previously by us.[38]

### Experiences with Pulmonary Embolectomy

Trendelenburg[56] in 1908 first proposed pulmonary embolectomy, but none of the patients survived. Kirschner,[57] a student of Trendelenburg, performed the first successful pulmonary embolectomy in 1924. The mortality of the Trendelenburg operation was high, as the procedure was attempted only on dying patients. Sharp[58] in 1961 introduced the use of cardiopulmonary bypass during the performance of pulmonary embolectomy. Those patients who deteriorated and developed irreversible cardiovascular collapse during induction of anesthesia benefited by the establishment of peripheral circulatory support with femorofemoral cannulation and the pump oxygenator prior to the induction of anesthesia. This technique provides a better chance for a successful outcome.

The criteria for selection of patients for pulmonary embolectomy have been the subject of considerable debate and remain controversial. The following views on pulmonary embolectomy exemplify the extreme divergence of opinion held on this subject: (1) There is no indication for pulmonary embolectomy.[59] (2) All but minor emboli should now be removed by pulmonary embolectomy.[60] (3) The successful completion of emergency angiography virtually precludes the need for pulmonary embolectomy.[61] (4) Ideally, in some patients, pulmonary embolectomy should be done before the onset of systemic arterial hypotension.[62]

Those who admit no indication for pulmonary embolectomy suggest that patients dying of massive pulmonary embolism can be kept on cardiopulmonary bypass until sufficient fragmentation and/or lysis occurs to allow recovery. The authors[59] report two patients treated by this modality: one requiring intermittent 6-hour perfusions survived; the other, on 27-hour perfusion, died. Prolonged extracorporeal support has limited application because of the expertise and facilities required.

From hemodynamic data obtained during right heart catheterization and prior to pulmonary arteriography, certain investigators suggest the following guide lines for recommending pulmonary embolectomy: (1) right ventricular mean pressure greater than 22 mg. Hg in the absence of other causes of pulmonary hypertension;[63] (2) mean pulmonary artery pressure greater than 30 per cent of mean systolic arterial pressure.[64] However, patients with increased right ventricular end diastolic pressures have survived without embolectomy.[65] In making the decision for subsequent management, I believe the degree of elevation of right ventricular end diastolic pressure, as suggested by Del Guercio, is the most sensitive and reliable index and should be considered in combination with the response to treatment and the severity of obstruction to pulmonary circulation, as determined by angiography.

If the peripheral signs of shock recede and urinary output is greater than 20 ml./hr. with the arterial pH returning toward normal, one can conclude that cardiac output is improving. A lack of improvement within 1 to 2 hours in association with arteriographic evidence of severe obstruction to pulmonary blood flow should lead to a prompt decision for embolectomy.

The results of pulmonary embolectomy depend on a variety of factors. The mortality rate is extremely high in patients who have been in shock for several hours and have developed metabolic and myocardial failure. It is 100 per cent after cardiac arrest not responding to resuscitative measures. The mortality of pulmonary embolectomy with cardiopulmonary bypass remains high. Cross and Mowlem[66] surveyed pulmonary embolectomies performed in 28 institutions. The mortality in 115 patients was 57 per cent. In 44 of 115 patients, preoperative circulatory support was utilized. The results in this group of patients were not reported separately. Pulmonary embolectomy in patients in whom preoperative mechanical circulatory support with pump oxygenator is established under local anesthesia prior to the induction of general anesthesia can carry a lower mortality. Berger[67] had survivals in seven of ten patients who underwent pulmonary embolectomy after preoperative peripheral circulatory support. The three deaths in this series were due to (1) an error in diagnosis, (2) irreversible cerebral ischemia during cardiac arrest prior to embolectomy, and (3) exsanguination during IVC ligation following pulmonary embolectomy. Heimbecker et al.,[52] using similar indications and embolectomy techniques, reported survival in nine of ten patients.

The causes of death following pulmonary embolectomy are (1) irreversible metabolic deterioration with myocardial failure; (2) irreversible ischemic brain injury during cardiopulmonary resuscitation; (3) hemorrhage into the lung following embolectomy; this usually occurs in subacute cases; (4) recurrent massive embolism, if caval interruption is not performed; (5) failure to clear the emboli; and (6) associated disease.

## EXPERIENCE WITH THROMBOLYTIC THERAPY

Under the sponsorship of The National Heart and Lung Institute, a controlled multicenter study, the Urokinase Pulmonary Embolism Trial Phase I[12] compared urokinase followed by anticoagulation therapy with anticoagulant therapy alone. The study design evaluated differences in the resolution rate of thromboemboli in the two groups. Of the 160 patients entered in the trial, 78 received heparin and 82 urokinase.

Those given urokinase had a loading dose of 2000 CTH units per pound and 200 units/hr. thereafter for 12 hours. Patients given heparin had a loading dose of 75 units per pound, followed by a constant infusion of 10 units per pound for a 12-hour period. After the completion of both 12-hour infusions, both groups received intravenous heparin for 5 days, followed by oral anticoagulant therapy.

Follow-up right heart catheterization, pulmonary arteriograms, and lung scans were performed within 24 hours after completion of the heparin and urokinase infusions. Lung scans were repeated frequently in the follow-up.

This study demonstrated only a modestly enhanced resolution rate for pulmonary emboli at 24 hours, as estimated by angiography, lung scanning, and hemodynamic measurements, in patients treated with urokinase followed by heparin. This modest increase in thrombolysis did not result in cardiopulmonary improvement sufficient to influence favorably the subsequent course in patients with massive pulmonary embolism. The resolution rate for pulmonary emboli within two treatment groups was indistinguishable after 5 days. Patients critically ill with pulmonary embolism or those in whom an operation (venous interruption or pulmonary embolectomy) was contemplated were not admitted into the trial. Of the 14 patients who developed clinical shock—five in the heparin and nine in the urokinase group—five died (one in the heparin and four in the urokinase group).

In my opinion, since thrombolytic agents are not immediately effective in relieving obstruction to pulmonary circulation, patients with massive pulmonary embolism and right ventricular decompensation unresponsive to intensive medical therapy are best treated by pulmonary embolectomy after preoperative circulatory support.

## References

1. McLachlin, J., and Paterson, J. C.: Some basic observations on venous thrombosis and pulmonary embolism. Surg. Gynecol. Obstet. 93:1, 1951.
2. Sevitt, S., and Gallagher, N. G.: Prevention of venous thrombosis and pulmonary embolism in injured patients. A trial of anticoagulant prophylaxis with phenindione in middle aged and elderly patients with fractured necks of femur. Lancet 2:981, 1959.
3. Kakkar, V. V.: The $^{125}$I-labelled fibrinogen test and phlebography in the diagnosis of deep vein thrombosis. Milbank Memorial Fund Quarterly (Suppl. 2) 50:206, 1972.
4. Deykin, D.: The use of heparin. New Engl. J. Med. 280:937, 1969.
5. Edwards, E. A., and Edwards, J. E.: Effect of thrombophlebitis on venous valve. Surg. Gynecol. Obstet. 65:310, 1937.
6. Linton, R. R., and Hardy, I. B., Jr.: Postthrombotic syndrome of lower extremity; treatment by interruption of superficial femoral vein and ligation and stripping of long and short saphenous veins. Surgery 24:452, 1948.
7. Kakkar, V. V., Flanc, C., Howe, C. T., O'Shea, M., and Flute, P. T.: Treatment of deep vein thrombosis: A trial of heparin, streptokinase and Arvin. Br. Med. J. 1:806, 1969.
8. Dodd, H., and Cockett, F. B.: Pathology and Surgery of the Veins of the Lower Limb. Edinburgh, E. & S. Livingstone, Ltd., 1956.
9. Butcher, H. R.: Anticoagulant drug therapy for thrombophlebitis in the lower extremities. Arch. Surg. 80:864, 1960.
10. Byrne, J. J.: Phlebitis: A study of 979 cases at the Boston City Hospital. J.A.M.A. 174:113, 1960.

11. Salzman, E. W., Deykin, D., Shapiro, R. M., and Rosenberg, R.: Management of heparin therapy. New Engl. J. Med. 292:1046, 1975.
12. Urokinase Pulmonary Embolism Trial Phase I Results (A Cooperative Study). J.A.M.A. 214:2163, 1970.
13. Bell, W. R., Pitney, W. R., and Goodwin, J. F.: Therapeutic defibrination in the treatment of thrombotic disease. Lancet 1:490, 1968.
14. Sharp, A. A., Warren, B. A., Paxton, A. M., and Allington, M. J.: Anticoagulant therapy with a purified fraction of Malayan pit viper venom. Lancet 1:493, 1968.
15. Pitney, W. R.: Clinical experience with "Arvin." Thromb. Diath. Haemorrh. Suppl. 38:81, 1969.
16. Kakkar, V. V., Howe, C. T., Laws, J. W., and Flanc, C.: Late results of treatment of deep vein thrombosis. Br. Med. J. 1:810, 1969.
17. Davies, J. A., Merrick, M. V., Sharp, A. A., and Holt, J. M.: Controlled trial of ancrod and heparin in the treatment of deep vein thrombosis of lower limb. Lancet 1:113, 1972.
18. Bernard, H. R., Powers, S. R., Leather, R. P., and Clark, W. R., Jr.: A prospective double blind study of clinical dextran in thrombophlebitis. Surgery 65:191, 1969.
19. Hirsh, J., Jr., Gallus, A. S., and Cade, J. F.: Streptokinase therapy in pulmonary embolism. In Mobin-Uddin, K. (ed.): Pulmonary Thromboembolism. Illinois, Charles C Thomas, Publisher, 1975.
20. Silver, D.: Urokinase in the management of acute arterial and venous thrombosis. Arch. Surg. 97:910, 1968.
21. Kakkar, V. V., Howe, C. T., Flanc, C., and Clarke, M. B.: Natural history of deep vein thrombosis. Lancet 2:230, 1969.
22. Freeark, R. J., and Fardin, R.: Venographic study of the lower extremity in patients with fracture of the hip. Surg. Forum 17:444, 1966.
23. Fitts, W. T., Jr., Lehr, H. B., Bitner, R. L., and Spelman, J. W.: An analysis of 950 fatal injuries. Surgery 56:663, 1964.
24. Harris, W. H., Salzman, E. W., and Desanctis, R. W.: The prevention of thromboembolic disease by prophylactic anticoagulation. J. Bone Joint Surg. 49–A:81, 1967.
25. Neu, L. T., Jr., Waterfield, J. R., and Ash, C. J.: Prophylactic anticoagulant therapy in the orthopedic patient. Ann. Intern. Med. 62:463, 1965.
26. Salzman, E. W., Harris, W. H., and Desanctis, R. W.: Anticoagulation for prevention of thromboembolism following fractures of the hip. New Engl. J. Med. 275:122, 1966.
27. Salzman, E. W., Harris, W. H., and Desanctis, R. W.: Reduction in venous thromboembolism by agents affecting platelet function. New Engl. J. Med. 284:1287, 1971.
28. Fullen, W. D., Miller, E. H., Steele, W. F., and McDonough, J. J.: Prophylactic vena cava interruption in hip fractures. J. Trauma 13:403, 1973.
29. Murray, G. D. W., and Best, C. H.: Use of heparin in thrombosis. Ann. Surg. 108:163, 1938.
30. Barritt, D. W., and Jordan, S. C.: Anticoagulant drugs in treatment of pulmonary embolism: Controlled trial. Lancet 1:1309, 1960.
31. Eberlein, T. J., and Carey, L. C.: Comparison of surgical managements for pulmonary emboli. Ann. Surg. 179:836, 1974.
32. Aggeler, P. M., and Kosmin, M.: Anticoagulant prophylaxis and treatment of venous thromboembolic disease. In Sherry, S., Brinkhous, K. M., Genton, E., and Stengle, J. E. (eds.): Conference on Thrombosis. Wasington, D.C., National Academy of Sciences, 1969.
33. Crane, C.: Femoral vs. caval interruption for venous thromboembolism. New Engl. J. Med. 270:819, 1964.
34. Krause, R. J., Cranley, J. J., Hallaba, M. A. S., Strasser, E. S., and Hafner, C. D.: Caval ligation in thromboemboli disease. Arch. Surg. 87:184, 1963.
35. Amador, E., Li, T. K., and Crane, C.: Ligation of inferior vena cava for thromboembolism. J.A.M.A. 206:1758, 1968.
36. Mobin-Uddin, K., McLean, R., and Jude, J. R.: A new catheter technique of interruption of inferior vena cava for prevention of pulmonary embolism. Am. Surg. 35:889, 1969.
37. Mobin-Uddin, K., McLean, R., Bolooki, H., and Jude, J. R.: Caval interruption for prevention of pulmonary embolism. Arch. Surg. 99:711, 1969.
38. Mobin-Uddin, K., Trinkle, J. K., and Bryant, L. R.: Present status of the inferior vena cava umbrella filter. Surgery 70:914, 1971.
39. Mobin-Uddin, K., Callard, G. M., Bolooki, H., Rubinson, R., Michie, D., and Jude, J. R.: Transvenous caval interruption with umbrella filter. New Engl. J. Med. 286:55, 1972.
40. Mobin-Uddin, K., Utley, J. R., and Bryant, L. R.: The inferior vena cava umbrella filter. Progr. Cardiovasc. Dis. 17:391, 1975.
41. Mobin-Uddin, K., Bolooki, J., and Jude, J. R.: Intravenous caval interruption for pulmonary embolism in cardiac disease. Circulation (Suppl. 2) 41:152, 1970.

42. Jick, H., Slone, D., Bold, I. T., and Shapiro, S.: Efficacy and toxicity of heparin in relation to age and sex. New Engl. J. Med. *279*:284, 1968.

43. Browse, N. L., Thomas, M. L., and Solan, M. J.: Management of source of pulmonary emboli: Value of phlebography. Br. Med. J. *4*:596, 1967.

44. Thomas, M. L., Andress, M. R., Browse, N. L., Fletcher, E. W. L., Phillips, J. D., Pim, H. P., McAllister, N., Stephenson, R. H., and Tonge, K.: Phlebography in the prevention of recurrent pulmonary embolism—Technique and value. Am. J. Roentgenol. Radium Ther. Nucl. Med. *110*:725, 1970.

45. Grode, G. A., Falb, R. D., and Crowley, J. P.: Bio-compatible materials for use in vascular systems. J. Biomed. Mater. Res. *6*:77, 1972.

46. Dalen, J. E., and Alpert, J. S.: Natural history of pulmonary embolism. Prog. Cardiovasc. Dis. *17*:257, 1975.

47. Gorham, L. W.: A study of pulmonary embolism. Arch. Intern. Med. *108*:8–22, 189–207, 418–426, 1961.

48. Flemma, R. J., Young, W. G., Wallace, A., Whalen, R. E., and Freese, J.: Feasibility of pulmonary embolectomy: A case report. Circulation *30*:234, 1964.

49. Sautter, R. D., Fletcher, F. W., Emanuel, D. A., Lawton, B. R., and Olsen, T. G.: Complete resolution of massive pulmonary thromboembolism. J.A.M.A. *189*:948, 1964.

50. Fred, H. L., Axelrad, M. A., Lewis, J. M., and Alexander, J. K.: Rapid resolution of pulmonary thromboemboli in man: Angiographic study. J.A.M.A. *196*:1137, 1966.

51. Oakley, C. M.: Conservative management of pulmonary embolism. Br. J. Surg. *55*:801, 1968.

52. Heimbecker, R. O., Keon, W. J., and Richards, K. U.: Massive pulmonary embolism: A new look at surgical management. Arch. Surg. *107*:740, 1973.

53. Berger, R. L.: Pulmonary embolectomy for massive embolization. Am. J. Surg. *121*:437, 1971.

54. Sautter, R. D., Myers, W. O., and Wenzel, F. J.: Implications of the urokinase study concerning the surgical treatment of pulmonary embolism. J. Thorac. Cardiovasc. Surg. *63*:54, 1972.

55. Bloomfield, D. A.: The use of intracaval umbrella filters in massive pulmonary embolism. *In* Mobin-Uddin, K. (ed.): *Pulmonary Thromboembolism*. Illinois, Charles C Thomas, Publisher, 1975.

56. Trendelenburg, F.: Ueber die operative Behandlung der Embolie der Lungenarterie. Arch. Klin. Chir. *86*:686, 1908.

57. Kirschner, M.: Ein Durch die Trendelenburgsche operation geheilter Fall von Embolie der Art. pulmonalis. Arch. Klin. Chir. *133*:312, 1924.

58. Sharp, E. H.: Pulmonary embolectomy: Successful removal of a massive pulmonary embolus with support of cardiopulmonary bypass: Case report. Ann. Surg. *156*:1, 1962.

59. Sautter, R. D., Myers, W. O., Ray, J. F., III, and Wenzel, F. J.: Pulmonary embolectomy: Review and current status. Progr. Cardiovasc. Dis. *17*:371, 1975.

60. Pisko-Dubienski, Z. A.: A new approach to pulmonary embolism. Br. J. Surg. *55*:138, 1968.

61. Crane, C., Hartsuck, J., Birtch, A., Couch, N. P., Zollinger, R., Jr., Matloff, T., Dalen, J., and Dexter, L.: The management of major pulmonary embolism. Surg. Gynecol. Obstet. *128*:27, 1969.

62. Fred, H. L., and Natelson, E. A.: Selection of patients for pulmonary embolectomy. Dis. Chest *56*:139, 1969.

63. Del Guercio, L. R. M., Cohn, J. D., Feins, N. R., Coo-maraswamy, R. P., and Mantle, L.: Screening for pulmonary embolism shock. Physiologic basis of a bedside screening test. J.A.M.A. *196*:751, 1966.

64. Diacoff, G. R., Rams, J. J., and Moulder, P. V.: Pulmonary embolectomy. Surg. Clin. North Am. *46*:27, 1966.

65. Wechsler, B. M., Karlson, K. E., Summers, D. N., Krasnow, N., Garzon, A. A., and Chart, A.: Pulmonary embolism: Influence of cardiac hemodynamics and natural history on selection of patients for embolectomy and inferior vena cava ligation. Surgery *65*:182, 1969.

66. Cross, F. S., and Mowlem, A.: A survey of the current status of pulmonary embolectomy for massive pulmonary embolism. Circulation (Suppl. 1) *35*:86, 1967.

67. Berger, R. L.: Treatment of massive pulmonary embolism. The advantages of pulmonary embolectomy. *In* Ingelfinger, J., Ebert, R. V., Finland, M., and Relman, A. S. (eds.): *Controversy in Internal Medicine II*. Philadelphia, W. B. Saunders Co., 1974.

# The Treatment of Life-Threatening Massive Pulmonary Embolism

RICHARD D. SAUTTER

*Marshfield Clinic and Marshfield Medical Foundation,*
*Marshfield, Wisconsin*

It goes without saying that my opinions are worth no more than your appraisal of their rationality. One of the most attractive features of medicine for many of you who cerebrate upon a liberal pattern is the fact that no one confronted by a medical problem is ever wholly right.

Cecil K. Drinker (*Pulmonary Edema and Inflammation*. Cambridge, Harvard
University Press, 1945, p. 64.)

## Introduction

Massive pulmonary embolism is defined as 50 per cent or greater angiographic obstruction of the pulmonary artery. It is important and crucial to point out that the majority of patients with massive pulmonary emboli are not in immediate danger of death, as they manifest no signs of cardiopulmonary collapse. There should be little debate that such patients are properly managed by supportive therapy, the cornerstone of which is sodium heparin infusion, complemented when indicated by venous interruption.

The controversy over therapy for massive pulmonary embolism centers around the patient who has a severely compromised cardiorespiratory system (cyanosis, shock, cardiovascular collapse) and who *seems* to be in imme-

337

diate danger of death. The question of *when* pulmonary embolectomy is indicated is the focal point of that controversy. At present and for the foreseeable future, there will be insufficient data to provide a definitive answer to the question. The course the physician will follow in treating such a patient will depend upon the abilities and the facilities available to him.

The multiple interrelated factors which must be considered in order to provide optimum therapy for such a patient are:

1. Angiographic diagnosis of massive pulmonary embolism.
2. Fate of pulmonary emboli.
3. Time from onset of cardiovascular collapse to death.
4. Preoperative cardiopulmonary status of the patient.
5. Role of lytic agents in the treatment of massive embolism.
6. Closed cardiac massage.
7. Pulmonary embolectomy.
8. Venous interruption.

The physician should critically evaluate these factors to determine what action is *most likely* to prevent the patient's death. Embolectomy should be considered *only* on a highly individualized basis. Routine or planned embolectomy for those patients who *appear* to be in imminent danger of death (i.e., hypotension, oliguria, cyanosis, dyspnea) is not rational. A far more logical approach is to provide intensive supportive measures, buying time to allow stabilization of the compromised cardiovascular system. Either by fragmentation or by lysis of the emboli, the obstruction within the pulmonary artery will ultimately decrease to restore homeostasis.

## Diagnosis of Life-Threatening Massive Pulmonary Embolism

A positive diagnosis is essential for the specific treatment of any disease. When one is confronted with possible catastrophic massive pulmonary embolism, speed and accuracy of diagnosis are essential and can *only* be provided by pulmonary arteriography. No patient is too ill to undergo this procedure if a massive embolus is suspected. Pulmonary arteriography has been done safely in many critically ill patients and should be performed regardless of the type of treatment anticipated.[1] Pulmonary embolectomy should never be considered until the diagnosis is confirmed by arteriography. Embolectomies undertaken with a mistaken diagnosis are uniformly fatal. It may be necessary to do the pulmonary arteriogram while the patient is supported by femorofemoral cardiopulmonary bypass either in the operating suite with portable x-ray equipment[2] or in the department of radiology with portable bypass equipment.[3]

Pulmonary scintillation scanning and perfusion or ventilation techniques are now highly refined and, when combined, can provide a highly accurate diagnosis in most institutions. These techniques, however, are time-consuming. More importantly, most departments of nuclear medicine are not geared or psychologically prepared for urgent, much less emergent, situations. These are excellent screening procedures, but in the case of an immediate life-threatening pulmonary embolus, the pulmonary arteriogram is the most direct and accurate approach to diagnosis.

The movement of such critically ill patients to more than one area for diagnosis and therapy is hazardous and should be avoided. Pulmonary arteriography should be done in an area where the equipment is available for lower-extremity venography and, if indicated, the insertion of a caval umbrella.

## Ultimate Fate of Pulmonary Emboli

If given enough time, massive pulmonary emboli lyse spontaneously. Several studies[4-9] using serial pulmonary arteriography have shown the disappearance of such emboli. Further, chronic obstruction of a lobar or larger pulmonary artery is an extremely rare autopsy finding. The prosector does find fibrous bands and webs as the *only* residua of pulmonary emboli.[10] Prevention of recurrent emboli is essential if complete lysis is to be seen uniformly. Although it is not completely proved, it is likely that recurrent showers of emboli impede resolution by overwhelming the intrinsic fibrinolytic system.

In the absence of recurrent embolism, chronic cor pulmonale as a result of a single massive embolic episode is not satisfactorily documented. In an anecdotal report in 1960, Phear[11] suggested that one-third of the patients suffering a massive pulmonary embolus develop chronic cor pulmonale. In a recent report[12] of 43 patients who had suffered a massive embolus, only one developed chronic cor pulmonale, a patient who had recurrent episodes of massive embolization. Chronic cor pulmonale is a rare condition which, when it results from embolization, is almost always the result of recurrent showers of microemboli.

There is no clinical evidence of chronic pulmonary insufficiency in those patients who survive a massive embolus. We studied 14 such patients by means of conventional tests of pulmonary function. Six had no deficit; the other eight had minimal deficit, which was adequately explained by preembolic cardiorespiratory disease.

The major clinical implications of this information are that (1) pulmonary embolectomy for the preservation of pulmonary function is *never* indicated, and (2) the prevention of recurrent embolization is mandatory.

## Time from Onset of Cardiovascular Collapse to Death

Fifteen minutes following cardiovascular collapse, one-half (50 per cent) of the patients *who will succumb as a result of a massive pulmonary embolus* will be dead. Only one-third (33 per cent) survive 1 hour, and only one-fourth (25 per cent) are alive 2 hours following the onset of symptoms.

Three large autopsy series[13-15] provide the evidence supporting these statements.

Because the majority of patients who suffer a massive pulmonary embolus do not succumb, some care must be exercised in extrapolating this information obtained from cadavers to human patients. First, the information is not current, the reports having appeared in 1959,[13] 1963,[14] and 1967.[15] Second, there is no information regarding supportive therapy, which has greatly improved, even since the 1967 report. Third, nothing is known about recurrent embolization or other severe diseases that may have been present. Additional information such as this may help explain the late deaths.

Still, it is clear that those patients who die from massive pulmonary embolism do so early. The patient who has survived 2 hours has already demonstrated a greater cardiopulmonary reserve than the patient who dies after 15 minutes. It then seems logical that the longer a patient survives the initial insult, the greater that patient's cardiopulmonary reserve and the more likely that such a patient will respond to prompt, intensive, supportive measures.

This contention is supported by the Urokinase Pulmonary Embolism Trial (UPET),[16] in which 11 patients in shock were treated with either lytic agents or heparin. None of them died of the embolic event.

To the clinician, the most important information is the *critical time frame* provided into which specific forms of therapy must be integrated. For instance, unless a pulmonary arteriogram can be done, a heart surgery team assembled, and an operation begun in 2 hours or less, 75 per cent of the patients most likely to benefit from this procedure are dead. Obviously, to be really effective, embolectomy should be performed within 1 hour. If the mortality of pulmonary embolectomy done within 1 hour from the onset of symptoms were 20 per cent, I would be compelled to reevaluate my position regarding this procedure.

## Pre-Embolic Cardiopulmonary Status of the Patient

Whether or not a patient will die following a massive pulmonary embolus depends upon that patient's pre-embolic cardiopulmonary status and the degree of his pulmonary obstruction. We have observed elderly patients with chronic obstructive lung disease or cardiac failure who suffered severe cardiopulmonary collapse with only 50 per cent obstruction of the pulmonary arterial tree. We have also observed young patients with no preexisting cardiopulmonary disease tolerate 75 per cent obstruction of the pulmonary arterial tree without shock or cardiopulmonary collapse. It is rare to see cardiovascular collapse or death from 50 per cent or less obstruction of the pulmonary arterial tree. Conversely, seldom does a patient survive 80 per cent obstruction of the pulmonary arterial tree. The individual patient's cardiopulmonary reserve accounts for these differences. The clinical implication is that therapy should be based on the response of the patient's cardiovascular system to the embolus rather than on the percentage obstruction demonstrated by pulmonary arteriography.[17]

## Role of Lytic Agents

The lytic agents urokinase and streptokinase accelerate the lysis of pulmonary emboli, a fact well documented by rigidly controlled, double-blind, randomized trials.[16, 19] These studies also demonstrated that *massive* emboli are especially prone to lysis by these agents. The lytic process, however, does not occur early enough to help significantly the patient in extremis, nor does lysis occur in every instance. Both agents carry the hazard of bleeding and are contraindicated in a significant group of patients. The most specific contraindication for their use is major surgery within the previous 10 days. Such patients are prone to develop massive pulmonary embolism.

There is no convincing evidence to suggest that emboli are more completely resolved by these agents than by the natural lytic process. Although they provide little benefit to the patient in extremis, these agents may benefit the patient who survives the initial insult of a massive embolus by more rapid restoration of cardiopulmonary reserve in the subsequent 24 to 72 hours.

These agents have not yet earned a definitive place in the treatment regimen for massive pulmonary embolism.

## Cardiac Massage and the Fragmentation of Pulmonary Emboli

Heimbecker et al.[20] demonstrated unequivocally that closed chest massage can fragment pulmonary emboli and propel them distally, with immediate improvement in blood gases, arterial and venous pulmonary and aortic pressures, and cardiac output. This same author reported three patients who, after suffering cardiac arrests following massive pulmonary emboli, were treated with closed cardiac massage and who survived without the additional hazard of embolectomy. Oakley[21] reported a similar experience with one patient. We have utilized closed chest massage in the treatment of two very elderly patients with massive pulmonary emboli, but both attempts were unsuccessful. In one patient, a second pulmonary arteriogram after 1 hour of closed chest massage showed the pulmonary emboli unchanged.

Fragmentation depends upon many factors, most important of which is the degree of organization of the thrombus. That is, a highly organized or old thrombus will not fragment as easily as a loose, gelatinous, poorly organized thrombus.

Because this maneuver requires no special skills or equipment, it can be almost universally applied. Therefore, it deserves further clinical investigation.

## *Pulmonary Embolectomy*

If pulmonary embolectomy is to be performed, it is best to support the patient's circulation with cardiopulmonary bypass before, during, and perhaps even following the procedure. When so performed, it represents a simple cardiac procedure with optimal operating conditions.

After a longitudinal arteriotomy in the pulmonary artery, the emboli can be removed by gallstone forceps, right-angle clamps, sponge forceps, suction catheter, etc. Massage of the lung toward the hilum should be discouraged because hemorrhagic atelectasis has been observed and undoubtedly is related to the fact the patient is totally heparinized. Prevention of recurrent embolism is best assured by insertion of a caval umbrella via the right atrial appendage, thus avoiding an abdominal or cervical incision.[17]

When so performed, pulmonary embolectomy has resulted in a mortality rate ranging from 80 per cent to 20 per cent. In our series of 22 patients, the mortality rate was 80+ per cent. A similar-size series reported by Berger[22] indicated a 20 per cent mortality. This discrepancy undoubtedly is explained by patient selection. The time from onset of symptoms to embolectomy in our series averaged 1 hour. In Berger's series, this interval was slightly more than 7 hours. As pointed out earlier, a delay of even 2 hours allows 75 per cent of those who are to die of massive embolization to do so. Comparison of mortality rates in these two groups of patients is impossible because of the overpowering bias introduced by patient selection.

A possible flaw in my argument is that, since 1970, we have not proceeded with pulmonary embolectomy after several hours of intensive support, even if the patient was deteriorating. The reason for this is that, of all of the suggested indications or criteria for embolectomy, *none* is infallible. There is no way to be certain that a patient will die unless he is submitted to embolectomy, even though the patient is deteriorating during intensive support. Sasahara's indications for embolectomy are, to most observers, conservative (see Table 1). We, however, have encountered four patients fulfilling all of his criteria for embolectomy, and two of them survived without embolectomy. Surely it would be foolish to avoid embolectomy if one were certain the patient would not survive without it. The absolutely critical information to support an unchallenged position regarding embolectomy is lacking.

In addition to Sasahara's suggested indications, shock or cardiovascular collapse has been presented as a critical indication for pulmonary embolectomy. I will reemphasize that shock does not preclude survival without

**TABLE 1.   Sasahara's Indications for Embolectomy**

If after 1 hour of maximum medical management:
- the systolic blood pressure is less than 90 mm. Hg
- urine output is less than 20 cc. per hour
- arterial $pO_2$ is less than 60 mm. Hg

embolectomy. Three patients admitted to our pilot study of urokinase were in shock; all survived. The 11 patients accessed to the UPET who were in shock survived. Even cardiac arrest does not preclude survival, as demonstrated in reports by Heimbecker et al.[20] and Oakley,[21] in which the only procedure used was closed chest massage.

There have been many methods described for pulmonary embolectomy without support of the patient with cardiopulmonary bypass.[17] The majority of these methods are modifications of the original Trendelenburg procedure. Some are quite ingenious, and their obvious advantage is that embolectomy can be quickly undertaken without special equipment. They do require a daring and very skilled surgeon and most likely a great deal of luck to be successful. These techniques, without the positive diagnosis provided by a pulmonary arteriogram, are grossly deficient. Attempted embolectomy with a mistaken diagnosis is uniformly fatal. Surely, if these techniques were widely employed, more patients would die because of mistaken diagnosis than would be saved from the effects of massive emboli.

Removal of pulmonary emboli by suction apparatus introduced via the iliac vein has been described.[24, 25] This is an innovative concept which must still be regarded as experimental. If refined, the procedure might become an important tool in the treatment of patients with massive pulmonary emboli.

The decision to proceed with embolectomy, or for that matter to avoid the procedure, cannot be based on fact but remains one of judgment.

## Venous Interruption

It is beyond the scope of this discussion to review all the indications for venous interruption. However, once the diagnosis of massive pulmonary embolism is confirmed by arteriography, it is mandatory that bilateral venograms be done. If a life-threatening thrombus is identified in the caval drainage, venous interruption is indicated.[26]

Because the patient with a massive pulmonary embolus has a compromised cardiopulmonary status, general anesthesia must be avoided. The insertion of a Mobin-Uddin caval umbrella requires only local anesthesia and a short cervical incision and can be done in 30 minutes or less. At present, it is the only method acceptable for the patient who has sustained a massive embolus.

Venous interruption is essential to prevent recurrent and likely fatal emboli.

## Comment

To summarize the factors influencing therapy for the patient with massive pulmonary embolism:

1. The diagnosis of massive pulmonary embolism must be confirmed by pulmonary arteriography.

2. Spontaneous resolution of massive emboli is the rule.

3. The majority of patients (75 per cent) who will die of a massive pulmonary embolus do so in the first 2 hours.

4. The patient's pre-embolic cardiopulmonary status and the amount of pulmonary arterial obstruction determine whether the patient will survive a massive pulmonary embolus.

5. Lytic agents (streptokinase, urokinase), while accelerating the lysis of massive pulmonary emboli, do not act quickly enough to benefit the patient in extremis. Precise indications for the use of these agents are not yet identified.

6. Closed cardiac massage has been shown to fragment massive pulmonary emboli, resulting in immediate improvement of the patient's cardiopulmonary status.

7. Pulmonary embolectomy, if employed, should be done using cardiopulmonary bypass support; indications are based on judgment, not fact.

8. Venous interruption to prevent recurrent emboli is mandatory if life-threatening thrombi are demonstrated by venography.

## Discussion

The preceding discussion is essential in order to address the following question raised by the editors: "Given a patient with a massive pulmonary embolus which is life-threatening, with electrocardiographic changes, decreased cardiac output, lower blood pressure, tachycardia, and acidosis, is survival more likely with direct operative embolectomy or nonoperative measures?"

The vast majority of patients who receive intensive medical therapy will survive without pulmonary embolectomy. In order to clarify what is meant by intensive medical therapy, I will describe how such a patient would be treated at our institution.

While we prepare to confirm the diagnosis by pulmonary arteriography, the patient immediately receives 10,000 to 15,000 units of sodium heparin intravenously, unless there are *very* strong contraindications. Acidosis is corrected by appropriate amounts of sodium bicarbonate given intravenously. Hypotension is corrected by the intravenous infusion of either isoproterenol or epinephrine. Oxygen is administered by mask or, in critical circumstances, by endotracheal intubation and positive-pressure breathing apparatus.

Following the confirmation of the diagnosis by pulmonary arteriography, bilateral venography is performed. The demonstration of a large, residual, life-threatening thrombus in the inferior caval circulation demands immediate caval interruption utilizing the Mobin-Uddin vena caval umbrella. The cardiac catheter is left in the pulmonary artery and an arterial needle inserted. Pulmonary artery and arterial pressures are continuously monitored. Mixed central venous and arterial blood gases are monitored often enough to provide optimal management of the patient's compromised cardiovascular system. An indwelling urethral catheter is inserted and urinary output recorded hourly. Such a patient is managed identically to the patient who has undergone open-heart surgery. If the agents were available to me and there were no overwhelming contraindications, I would administer urokinase or streptokinase in an attempt to restore cardiopulmonary reserve more rapidly.

If the patient has an additional severe illness (incurable cancer, end-stage renal or cardiac disease), the question of embolectomy is moot.

For the elderly patient with only moderately severe concurrent illnesses, we have on three occasions used prolonged partial cardiopulmonary bypass, which in one instance was successful. Prolonged bypass, however, is not a panacea because of the many technical difficulties which arise the longer one utilizes this modality. Except in very experienced hands, prolonged bypass support can be utilized for no more than 24 hours.

The rationale for using prolonged cardiopulmonary bypass is sound. First, it provides excellent support for the vital organ systems. Secondly, fragmentation or lysis of the emboli to reduce pulmonary artery obstruction will ultimately occur. The expertise and equipment necessary do limit broad application.

If the patient is young, has no other illnesses, and is deteriorating under intensive medical management, I would consider embolectomy. This, however, is a circumstance I have not experienced.

Between these extremes are a great variety of circumstances in which the problems of judgment become even more difficult. Ultimately, however, the decision to perform embolectomy still rests precariously on judgment rather than fact. These decisions are difficult and agonizing. The arguments presented here are advanced as much to rationalize my positions as to convince the reader. Divine guidance aside, I will continue to search for convincing evidence.

ACKNOWLEDGMENT: The author wishes to thank Dr. Jefferson F. Ray, III, Dr. William O. Myers, Mr. Frederick J. Wenzel, Mr. Al Zimmermann, and Mrs. Ardell Specht for their assistance in the preparation of this article.

# References

1. Dalen, J. E., Brooks, H. L., Johnson, L. W., et al.: Pulmonary angiography in acute pulmonary embolism. Indications, technique and results in 367 patients. Am. Heart J. 81:175, 1971.
2. Sautter, R. D., Fletcher, F. W., Emanuel, D. A., and Wenzel, F. J.: Pulmonary arteriography in the operating room. Chest 57:423, 1970.
3. Beall, A. C., and Cooley, D. A.: Experience with pulmonary embolectomy using temporary cardiopulmonary bypass. J. Cardiovasc. Surg. (Suppl.)48:201, 1965.
4. Sautter, R. D., Fletcher, F. W., Emanuel, D. A., Lawton, B. R., and Olsen, T. G.: Complete resolution of massive pulmonary thromboembolism. J.A.M.A. 189:948, 1964.
5. Fred, H. L., Axelrad, M. A., Lewis, J. M., and Alexander, J. K.: Rapid resolution of pulmonary thromboemboli in man: Angiographic study. J.A.M.A. 196:1137, 1966.
6. Murphy, M. L., and Bulloch, R. T.: Resolution of pulmonary emboli as determined by angiography and scanning. Clin. Res. 15:348, 1967.

7. Mounts, R. J., Molnar, W., Marable, S. A., and Wooley, C. F.: Angiography in recent pulmonary embolism with follow-up studies: Preliminary report. Radiology 87:713, 1966.
8. Sautter, R. D., Fletcher, F. W., Ousley, J. L., and Wenzel, F. J.: Extremely rapid resolution of a pulmonary embolus: Report of a case. Dis. Chest 52:825, 1967.
9. Dalen, J. E., Banas, J. S., Brooks, H. L., Evans, G. L., et al.: Resolution rate of acute pulmonary embolism in man. New Engl. J. Med. 280:1194, 1969.
10. Edwards, J. E.: Personal communication, 1973.
11. Phear, D.: Pulmonary embolism. A study of late prognosis. Lancet 2:832, 1960.
12. Paraskos, J. A., Adelstein, S. J., Smith, R. E., et al.: Late prognosis of acute pulmonary embolism. New Engl. J. Med. 289:55, 1973.
13. Coon, W. W., and Coller, F. A.: Some epidemiologic considerations of thromboembolism. Surg. Gynecol. Obstet. 109:487, 1959.
14. Donaldson, G. A., Williams, C., Scannel, J. G., and Shaw, R. S.: A reappraisal of the application of the Trendelenburg operation to massive fatal embolism. New Engl. J. Med. 268:171, 1963.
15. Soloff, L. A., and Rodman, T.: Acute pulmonary embolism. II. Clinical. Am. Heart J. 74:829, 1967.
16. The Urokinase-Pulmonary Embolism Trial, A National Cooperative Study. Circulation 47 and 48 (Suppl. II): 1, 1973.
17. Sautter, R. D., Myers, W. O., Ray, J. F., III, and Wenzel, F. J. Pulmonary embolectomy: review and current status. Prog. Cardiovasc. Dis. 17:371, 1975.
18. Urokinase-Streptokinase Embolism Trial, Phase 2 Results. A Cooperative Study. J.A.M.A. 229:1606, 1974.
19. Sautter, R. D., Ray, J. F., III, and Myers, W. O.: Massive pulmonary thromboembolism— fibrinolytic therapy. In Mobin-Uddin, K. (ed.): Pulmonary Thromboembolism. Springfield, Ill., Charles C Thomas, 1975, pp. 354–363.
20. Heimbecker, R. O., Keon, W. J., and Richards, K. U.: Massive pulmonary embolism: A new look at surgical management. Arch. Surg. 107:740, 1973.
21. Oakley, C. M.: Conservative management of pulmonary embolism. Br. J. Surg. 55:801, 1968.
22. Berger, R. L.: Pulmonary embolectomy with preoperative circulatory support. Ann. Thorac. Surg. 16:217, 1973.
23. Sasahara, A. A., and Barsamian, E. M.: Another look at pulmonary embolectomy. Ann. Thorac. Surg. 16:317, 1973.
24. Greenfield, L. J., Bruce, T. A., and Nichols, N. B.: Transvenous pulmonary embolectomy by catheter device. Ann. Surg. 174:881, 1971.
25. Greenfield, L. J., Reif, M. E., and Guenter, C. E.: Hemodynamic and respiratory responses to transvenous pulmonary embolectomy. J. Thorac. Cardiovasc. Surg. 62:890, 1971.
26. Ray, J. F., III, Myers, W. O., Lawton, B. R., and Sautter, R. D. Vena cava umbrella placement—its place in the overall management of thromboembolic disease. Am. J. Surg. 127:545, 1974.

# Treatment of Postoperative Pulmonary Embolus

W. CLAYTON DAVIS

*York Hospital, York, Pennsylvania*

It is fortunate for the large number of patients who in the future may or will have pulmonary emboli that most of the decisions on treatment will not be made by the enthusiasts proposing the broad variety of procedures noted during the last several years. Each proposed method of operative and nonoperative prevention and treatment of pulmonary embolus has important complications and incidences of failures.

The diagnosis of pulmonary embolus should be suspected in every patient with sudden tachypnea, dyspnea, or sense of impending doom. Chest pain and hemoptysis are not often reported by the patient, since these are seen only in infarction, and pulmonary infarction is demonstrated in only about 5 per cent of patients with proven pulmonary emboli.[1] Failure to consider pulmonary embolus is the most common cause for misdiagnosis and delay in treatment of this catastrophe. Repeated examinations of the lower extremities in postoperative patients not only will afford the opportunities to prevent the formation of venous thrombosis but also will increase the index of suspicion when emboli do occur. On a surgical service, over 95 per cent of pulmonary emboli arise in pelvic or lower extremity veins, and any cardiac sources have almost always become evident during the preoperative studies.

Pulmonary arteriography is the most definitive of the currently available methods of diagnosing pulmonary emboli. It should be performed by the selective catheter technique. It is the only method which permits visualization and accurate localization of embolic occlusions. Information of this type becomes indispensable as increasing efforts are directed toward earlier diagnosis and more aggressive management of the disease. Current techniques permit satisfactory visualization of vessels larger than 2 mm. in diameter. Hence, arteriography cannot provide definitive information in patients who suffer from recurrent small or miliary pulmonary emboli.

Radioisotope lung scanning for pulmonary embolism has gained considerable interest during the past few years. Its simplicity and safety have made it available to many hospitals which are unable to maintain facilities for selective pulmonary arteriography. The information obtained by scanning relates only to distribution of pulmonary blood flow without regard to etiologic factors. Hence, diseases such as pneumonia, emphysema, or carcinoma of the lung must be excluded by routine roentgenography before a perfusion defect can be ascribed to pulmonary embolism. It has become evident that a single-plane scan of the lungs cannot adequately define the total pulmonary vasculature. Multiple views such as anterior, posterior, and right and left laterals are necessary. When multiple views are obtained, the lung scan is a sensitive indicator of abnormal distribution of pulmonary blood flow. Despite its lack of etiologic specificity, scanning provides flow dimensions which, when combined with anatomic information obtained by arteriography, become a positive means of diagnosing pulmonary embolic disease.[2, 3]

Nonoperative treatment has included the use of poor anticoagulants, given in inadequate doses and delivered through questionable routes. The administration of anticoagulants is not synonymous with anticoagulation. For approximately 20 years I have utilized a loading dose of intravenous heparin, followed by continuous intravenous heparin, to maintain the Lee-White coagulation time at over 30 minutes or comparable tests at comparable levels for anticoagulation.[4] This has been successful and uncomplicated, except in the postoperative period following procedures which required major extraperitoneal dissection or prosthetic vascular replacements. This method of treatment would certainly be contraindicated following intracranial hemorrhages or operations. We have not seen proven pulmonary emboli during this method of therapy but have seen it with all other techniques of so-called anticoagulation. The treatment is continued for 3 weeks after the disappearance of all signs and symptoms of pulmonary emboli.

It is mandatory that, when there is any evaluation of treatment, all the instances of pulmonary emboli are proved. We believe that the only adequate method of diagnosing a pulmonary embolus is selective pulmonary arteriography. I would give the loading dose of heparin on the suspicion of a pulmonary embolus and support the diagnosis with a pulmonary arteriogram.[5] Our aim is to prevent the propagation of the thrombus distal to the embolus. If a patient survives a major pulmonary embolus, the cause of death following this should be the propagation of the thrombus.[6]

In recent years there has been a rebirth of application of the Trendelenburg operation of pulmonary embolectomy. Certainly this procedure is not indicated if the diagnosis is not established. Mortality rates for this procedure remain high in the best of hands. I personally believe that no treatment would yield a better survival.[3, 6] Greenfield's[7] suggestion of a transvenous extraction of emboli is exciting but still should be listed as an experimental procedure.

The various operative methods[8, 9, 10] for preventing future pulmonary emboli following episodes of proven pulmonary emboli range from the outmoded ligation of the femoral veins[11] to the insertion of filters[12] in the vena cava and, on occasion, in many other veins unwittingly. It is most disappointing to see an extremely large series of these procedures reported when one realizes that the incidence of pulmonary embolus could not possibly match the figures of the application of the operation. Even if this procedure were absolutely safe and uncomplicated, there seems to be no indication to perform such an operation when the diagnosis is not established. Each of these operations, be it plication, filter, clip, etc., has been followed by proven pulmonary emboli.[13]

Several years ago we proposed ligation and division of the inferior vena cava just below the level of the renal veins.[14] The division was performed to afford retraction of the stump of the proximal vena cava, thus avoiding any cul-de-sac which automatically appears with ligation alone. All patients were on continuous intravenous heparin before, during, and after the operation. Four years ago we reported 15 cases,[15] which now have been followed for 6 to 13 years. All of the procedures were performed for pulmonary emboli which had been at least recurrent and proven. All but one of these patients is free of intermittent recurrent thrombophlebitis and peripheral edema. We believe that the absence of edema as contrasted with the case in other reported series of caval interruption, is due to the use of adequate anticoagulation before, during, and after the procedure. This prevents early thrombosis of collaterals. Five of these 15 patients had had previous partial or complete occlusion of their vena cava performed to prevent pulmonary emboli. These five patients all had proven recurrences of pulmonary emboli after the other procedures. Our series of patients shows no proven pulmonary emboli after high ligation and division of the vena cava. The series is small, since the indications for the operation were strict. We suggest this operation for patients with proven recurrent pulmonary emboli occurring after heparin has been stopped or for those in whom adequate anticoagulation is contraindicated. We suggest that complete occlusion and division of the vena cava is definitely indicated when septic pelvic thrombophlebitis is the source of the pulmonary emboli. In three of our patients, we evaluated proximal and distal vena caval pressures before and after the ligation, as well as studied the cardiac output. Immediately after the ligation, there was either minimal or no change in cardiac output when these operations were performed under continuous intravenous heparin therapy. We carried out a series of animal experiments which supported these clinical observations. All patients studied showed a return to normal cardiac output within 15 minutes of ligation and division of the inferior vena cava under adequate anticoagulation. In our animal experimentation, these findings were supported only in animals with high ligation and division with adequate continuous intravenous heparin. Low ligation, and high ligation without heparin both caused major alterations in cardiac output and showed increased distal venous pressure.

Once we have survived the pleasures of learning the gymnastics of pulmonary embolectomy and the other operations suggested for the prevention or treatment of pulmonary emboli, it will be simpler to decide on the indications for each of the suggested procedures.

I propose that the application of the filters will be indicated in the extremely poor-risk patients. I would also propose that pulmonary embolus may be the kindest cause of death in patients with terminal carcinoma and far advanced cardiac disease. If any of these procedures are proposed for terminal conditions, I suggest that our philosophy of indications for operations and treatment should be reexamined.

The following is from J. Barzun's article, So Long as Doctors Have to Think. Bulletin of the New York Academy of Medicine 47:234, 1971:

Granted that speeches and articles should not always deal with local particulars, they should always deal with *some* particulars, if only by way of illustration. Otherwise, writer and audience waste their time in sterile agreement over absolute unknowns. In this world, at any rate, no art or science can long afford to invite assent of this kind to what is unproductive, to what will make no difference in action—including the action of thinking.

# References

1. Freiman, D. G.: Pathologic observations on experimental and human thromboembolism. *In* Sasahara, A. A., and Stein, M. (eds.): *Pulmonary Embolic Disease*. New York, Grune & Stratton, 1965, pp. 81–85.
2. Sasahara, A. A., Belko, J. S., and Simpson, R. G.: Blended scintiscans of lungs with a dual detector system. Radiology 88:363, 1967.
3. Davis, W. C., and Sasahara, A. A.: Management of pulmonary embolus in the postoperative patient. Surg. Clin. North Am. 48:869, 1968.
4. Baden, J. P., Sonnenfield, M., Ferlic, R. M., and Seller, R. D.: The bason test: A rapid bedside test for control of heparin therapy. Surg. Forum 22:172, 1971.
5. Sasahara, A. A., Potchen, E. J., Thomas, D. P., Wagner, H. N., and Davis, W. C.: Diagnostic requirements and therapeutic decisions in pulmonary embolus. J.A.M.A. 202:553, 1967.
6. Davis, W. C.: (Discussion of pulmonary embolectomy by Heimbecker, R. O., Keon, W. J., and Elliott, G.). Arch. Surg. 96:582, 1967.
7. Greenfield, L. J., Peyton, M. D., Brown, P. P., and Elkins, R. C.: Transvenous management of pulmonary embolic disease. Ann. Surg. 180:461, 1974.
8. DeWeese, M. S., and Hunter, D. C., Jr.: A vena cava filter for the prevention of pulmonary embolism. Arch. Surg. 86:852, 1963.
9. Moretz, W. H., Rhode, C. M., and Shepherd, M. H.: Prevention of pulmonary emboli by partial occlusion of the inferior vena cava. Am. Surg. 25:617, 1959.
10. Spencer, F. C., Quattlebaum, J. K., Quattlebaum, J. K., Jr., Sharp, E. H., and Jude, J. R.: Plication of the inferior vena cava for pulmonary embolism: A report of 20 cases. Ann. Surg. 155:827, 1962.
11. Anlyan, W. G., Campbell, F. H., Shingleton, W. W., and Gardner, C. R., Jr.: Pulmonary embolism following venous ligation. Arch. Surg. 64:200, 1952.
12. Mobin-Uddin, K., Trinkle, J. K., and Bryant, L. R.: Present status of the inferior vena cava umbrella filter. Surgery 70:914, 1971.
13. DeMeester, T. R., Rutherford, R. B., Blaizek, J. V., and Zuidema, J. D.: Plication of the inferior vena cava for thromboembolism. J. Surg. 62:56, 1967.
14. Davis, W. C., Davie, F. M., and Maxwell, J. W., Jr.: Evaluation of inferior vena caval ligation for pulmonary embolus. Am. Surg. 31:234, 1965.
15. Davis, W. C., McManus, W. F., Freeman, D. E., and LeVeen, R. F.: Evaluation of inferior vena caval occlusion to prevent pulmonary emboli. Am. Surg. 38:268, 1972.

# 15

# *Venous Thrombectomy*

## Statement of the Problem

*The alternatives of anticoagulation alone versus management which includes operative thrombectomy, with particular emphasis on late results, constitute the controversy.*

*Analyze variables which determine patient selection for iliofemoral thrombectomy.*

*During venous thrombectomy, should direct proximal caval control be secured for prevention of embolization? Will indirect control with balloon catheters assure adequate protection?*

*What anticoagulants are used intraoperatively? Postoperatively? What laboratory values are used to control anticoagulant levels? How long should anticoagulation be maintained? Do you recommend other ancillary measures?*

*Compare data on early and late results after heparin administration alone and after mechanical removal of the thrombus. To what degree does the age of the thrombotic process determine the success of thrombectomy?*

*Cite evidence regarding the state of venous valvar function after thrombectomy.*

*Analyze data comparing incidence of late venous patency and post-thrombophlebitic sequelae after heparin treatment alone and after thrombectomy for iliofemoral thrombosis.*

# Thrombectomy for Iliofemoral Venous Thrombosis: A Position Against

**VALLEE L. WILLMAN**

*St. Louis University School of Medicine*

Clot removal has a considerable history as a method of treating the symptoms and sequelae of acute iliofemoral venous thrombosis. Leriche and Geisendorf[27] advocated removal of the clot along with the involved vein (phlebectomy), intending to reduce the pain and the presumed arteriospasm. Läwen[26] advocated clot removal with vein preservation, while Allen[1] and Homans extracted the clot and ligated the vein. These procedures were proposed as measures to relieve the pain of thrombophlebitis and to lessen the threat of pulmonary embolus. Mahorner[29] became a leading advocate of clot extraction and vein reconstruction, proposing that not only was there relief of pain and swelling along with lessening of the risk of embolus, but also there was an improved long-term outlook for the leg. Many favorable clinical reports followed his,[3, 12, 15-18, 22, 32, 34] all advocating clot extraction and vein reconstruction, together with heparin anticoagulation begun preoperatively and continued into the postoperative period.

It is of considerable importance to note that heparin, which became available at about the same time that thrombectomy was adopted, has been established as a valuable agent for the lessening of the probability of pulmonary embolus and for facilitating the reduction of pain and swelling.[4, 7, 33] Not only does heparin have several effects upon the coagulation mechanism,[35] but also it has been reported to have fibrinolytic[13] and anti-inflammatory[11] effects, as well as several other biologic activities.[21, 33] Heparin not only alters coagulation and ameliorates the immediate manifestations of the disease but also might influence the long-term outcome of iliofemoral thrombophlebitis. An assessment of its effect on this aspect of the entity has never been made; therefore, the long-term results of heparin therapy are at this time undetermined.

Although the procedure of iliofemoral venous thrombectomy has been extensively employed during the past 20 years, it has not been possible to

353

evaluate it critically as compared with heparin therapy alone. This is in part the result of the very poor clinical characterization of the entity, as well as the failure to establish commonly agreed upon, reproducibly measurable end points. Thus, conclusions from comparisons of retrospective treatments are tenuous. The desideratum, which is for thrombectomy with anticoagulant (heparin) therapy to be evaluated against anticoagulant therapy alone in a concurrent, prospective study, is not available. A comparison of the operative and the nonoperative procedures must be made, therefore, on a descriptive and post hoc basis, discussing the advantages of the two approaches and drawing inferences, rather than deducing firm conclusions from factual data. Appropriate areas for consideration might be (1) relief of pain and swelling, (2) threat of pulmonary embolus, (3) limb loss, and (4) prevention of long-term sequelae (postphlebitic syndrome).

## Pain Relief and Reduction of Swelling

Thrombectomy can be expected to relieve pain promptly and generally results in dramatic reduction in limb size.[12] Failure of these results to occur indicates inadequate removal of the major obstructing clots. Such failure usually occurs in those operations undertaken a considerable time after clot deposition.[12, 18, 26] The ability to obtain a good immediate result is lessened if the clot is judged to be older than 10 days.[18] Controversy exists as to the natural sequential history of the disease. The classic teaching advanced by Bauer[5] is that the process begins in the vessels of the calf, and the presentation in the groin is an extension centrally. This implies a process of some duration prior to the appearance of symptoms of acute iliofemoral thrombophlebitis and limits the ability to extract the soleus vessel clots. This concept has been challenged by Mavor and Galloway,[30] who believe that the process is usually initiated at the groin or in the major veins of the pelvis and that total clot extraction is therefore often possible. Unfortunately, there have not been adequate efforts to obtain pretreatment diagnostic venography to determine the extent of the vascular involvement.

Heparin therapy is clearly less dramatic than thrombectomy in relieving pain and reducing swelling, but it is certainly effective in most instances.[9, 33] The occasional progression of symptoms during heparin anticoagulation and the inability to attain adequate heparinization in several clinical circumstances make this approach somewhat less certain than thrombectomy. Countering this disadvantage, however, is the risk of operation.

The operative insult in our hands has been substantial. In the first 49 patients we operated upon, the average volume of blood replacement was 650 ml., with 19 of the 49 patients losing more than a liter and only 12 receiving no transfusion.[22] This blood loss is not unusual.[25] Although the procedure is conducted with local anesthesia, there can be little doubt that some risk is incurred by these patients, who are often severely ill. Wounds in the edematous groins of heparinized patients fail to heal primarily in nearly a fourth of the instances, and lymph drainage for as long as a week is not unusual.[22] The presence of an open wound in the groin is of concern in the heparinized, bed-ridden patient.

The hospitalization time of patients treated nonoperatively for acute iliofemoral venous thrombosis has not been well documented but is probably little different from that of those undergoing thrombectomy—a mean of 30 days.[25]

For the management of pain and swelling, it would seem reasonable to attempt to utilize selectively the advantages of both methods in the treatment of any patient. We therefore choose to initiate heparin therapy promptly and to observe for complications of anticoagulation or failure to improve. Evidence of failure of this regimen shifts attention to consideration of the risks and benefits of thrombectomy. Employing such a plan in the past 3 years, we have found it prudent to perform thrombectomy in only one instance in the management of over 30 patients. We clearly favor heparin therapy alone as the first attempt in managing pain and swelling in acute iliofemoral thrombophlebitis.

## Pulmonary Embolus

The dramatic and awesome complication of thrombophlebitis is pulmonary embolus. Advocates of thrombectomy have indicated both an anticipation of decreasing incidence and a concern for actual induction of clot dislodgment.[16, 32] Most large series of operations report at least one acute fatal episode. In our own experience, we have observed two fatal emboli—both in patients being prepared for operation—one during transport to the operating room, and one during preoperative preparation of the leg. It is uncertain whether these are operative or nonoperative casualties. Reported incidences of pulmonary embolism in patients operated upon vary from 1 per cent to 6.6 per cent. The fear of intraoperative embolism has prompted some to occlude the vena cava.[14, 24] The incidence of fatal pulmonary embolism with heparin therapy alone is not readily available from the literature. There is some evidence to suggest that it is no higher than that of thrombectomy.[7, 8, 9] Thus at present, there is no evidence to favor thrombectomy as a means of lessening the risk of pulmonary embolism.

## Limb Loss

The progression of venous thrombosis to the point of capillary stasis and infarction, be this simply by dynamic back pressure[6] or complicated by autonomic vascular activity, is an infrequent although real threat. DeBakey's review[10] in 1949 included 56 instances—only three in the United States. These occurred prior to the extensive use of heparin and the enthusiasm for thrombectomy.

As the indications for thrombectomy have developed during the past 20 years, threatened loss of tissue has been generally accepted as an indication, and it is not now possible to obtain information on the incidence of limb loss in the absence of operation. Although threatened loss as an indication for thrombectomy has been reported by some[6, 9, 32] to be frequent, we in over 100 instances have not seen a circumstance in which threatened loss of the part prompted clot removal. It must be quite rare. Fear of progression of the process sufficient to threaten limb loss would not seem to justify thrombectomy as a prophylactic measure. If progression does occur to the point of pulse obliteration, we would certainly undertake operation.

## Prevention of Late Sequelae

If an advantage of thrombectomy over anticoagulant therapy is to be realized, it must be in the long-term results of preventing the pain, swelling, and ulceration that occur after recanalization, which sometimes present as long as 15 to 20 years after the acute episode.[5, 20]

Clearly, this extent of follow-up observation is not available and will indeed be difficult to obtain in numbers sufficient for meaningful analysis. We are unaware of any prospective studies underway that will permit comparison of concurrent nonoperative treatment with that which adds thrombectomy. It is reasonable, however, to assume a relationship between the resultant venous anatomy and the expected long-term result, anticipating that recanalized or occluded deep veins eventually lead to stasis, edema, and ulceration.[31]

McLachlin's animal experiment,[28] in which induced femoral venous thrombosis was untreated, treated with heparin, or treated with heparin and thrombectomy, failed to provide data favoring thrombectomy, as documented by vein patency or competent valves at 6 weeks.

Although a few clinical venographic studies performed early after operation have been interpreted as favorable,[18, 19] several late studies substantiate the very high incidence of venous occlusion or recanalization.[23, 25]

Lansing and Davis[25] reported upon 17 patients who were a part of the 45 constituting the earlier report of Haller in 1963.[18] These were the traceable patients 5 years later, all of whom had been operated upon within 10 days of the onset of symptoms. With a single exception, all had edema and wore elastic support; one had a stasis ulcer. Venograms performed on 15 patients were interpreted as indicating incompetency in all cases and absence of functioning valves. Even in the instance of the patient without symptoms, striking venous abnormalities were present.

Barner et al.[2] have reviewed the course of 29 of the 70 patients undergoing thrombectomy at our institution in the 10 years between 1958 and 1968. These patients had had postoperative venograms. The radiographic studies were compared to the clinical results, graded as excellent, good, fair, and poor. No edema without elastic support was considered an excellent result. There was only one patient with this result. Freedom from symptoms (and swelling) if elastic support was employed was considered a good result; 21 patients were in this category. Swelling without ulceration was considered a fair result; six patients were in this category. Of great concern was the extent of venous abnormalities in these postoperative venograms. In only one instance did the veins look normal. This was in a 50-year-old man studied 72 months postoperatively. The extent of abnormality in the other instances caused great concern as to the likelihood that function was normal. The post-treatment venograms of those receiving heparin alone could hardly be more abnormal.

## Summary

If there is an advantage to thrombectomy, it is not so impressive as to overshadow these inferences:

1. The current evidence suggests that the disadvantages of thrombectomy may outweigh the advantage of more prompt relief of pain and swelling.

2. Thrombectomy does not have a clear advantage in lessening pulmonary embolus.

3. Limb loss is rare in patients treated with heparin, and thrombectomy can be employed therapeutically when that threat is manifest.

4. The long-term fate of limbs in patients currently treated with heparin alone, as well as in those cases managed by heparin and thrombectomy, remains uncertain.

The case for thrombectomy would seem to rest, therefore, on tenuous logic. If it is to be established as a valuable procedure, it must meet the sterner test of prospective, randomized comparison with current nonoperative treatment. This study would involve:

1. Establishment of diagnostic measures, which must include venography.

2. A prospective study, including immediate post-treatment evaluation by venography.

3. Repeat venography at an intermediate period (2 to 5 years).

4. Long-term (10 to 15 years) clinical follow-up.

## References

1. Allen, A. W.: The present evaluation of the prophylaxis and treatment of venous thrombosis and pulmonary embolism. Surgery 26:1, 1949.
2. Barner, H. B., Willman, V. L., Kaiser, G. C., et al.: Thrombectomy for iliofemoral venous thrombosis. J.A.M.A. 208:2442, 1969.
3. Bradham, R. R., and Buxton, J. T.: Thrombectomy for acute iliofemoral venous thrombosis. Surg. Gynecol. Obstet. 119:1271, 1964.
4. Bauer, G.: Nine years' experience with heparin in acute venous thrombosis. Angiology 1:161, 1950.
5. Bauer, G.: A roentgenologic and clinical study of the sequels of thrombosis. Acta Chir. Scand. (Suppl. 74) 86:5, 1942.
6. Brockman, S. K., and Vasko, J. S.: Phlegmasia cerulea dolens. Surg. Gynecol. Obstet. 121:1347, 1965.

7. Coon, W. W., Willis, P. W., and Symons, M. J.: Assessment of anticoagulant treatment of venous thromboembolism. Ann. Surg. 170:559, 1969.
8. Crane, C.: Deep venous thrombosis and pulmonary embolism: Experience with 391 patients treated with heparin and 126 patients treated by venous division with a review of the literature. New Engl. J. Med. 257:147, 1957.
9. Dale, W. A., and Lewis, M. R.: Heparin control of venous thromboembolism. Arch. Surg. 101:744, 1970.
10. DeBakey, M., and Ochsner, A.: Phlegmasia cerulea dolens and gangrene associated with thrombophlebitis. Surgery 26:16, 1949.
11. DeTakats, G.: Vascular Surgery. Philadelphia, W. B. Saunders Co., 1959, p. 281.
12. DeWeese, J. A., Jones, T. I., Lyon, J., et al.: Evaluation of thrombectomy in the management of iliofemoral venous thrombosis. Surgery 47:140, 1960.
13. Ehrlich, J., and Stivala, S. S.: Chemistry and pharmacology of heparin. J. Pharm. Sci. 62:517, 1973.
14. Fogarty, T. J., and Hallin, R. W.: Temporary caval occlusion during thrombectomy. Surg. Gynecol. Obstet. 122:1269, 1966.
15. Fogarty, T. J., Cranley, J. J., Krause, R. J., et al.: Surgical management of phlegmasia cerulea dolens. Arch. Surg. 86:256, 1963.
16. Fontaine, R., and Tuckmann, L.: Role of thrombectomy in deep venous thromboses: Indications and results. J. Cardiovasc. Surg. 5:298, 1964.
17. Haller, J. A.: Thrombectomy for acute iliofemoral venous thrombosis. Arch. Surg. 83:448, 1961.
18. Haller, J. A., and Abrams, B. L.: Use of thrombectomy in the treatment of acute iliofemoral venous thrombosis in forty-five patients. Ann. Surg. 158:561, 1963.
19. Harris, E. J., and Brown, W. H.: Patency after thrombectomy for iliofemoral thrombosis. Ann. Surg. 167:91, 1968.
20. Höjensgård, I. C.: Sequelae of deep thrombosis in the lower limbs: Follow-up study of patients initially treated by conservative measures. Angiology 3:42, 1952.
21. Hunt, P. S., Reeve, T. S., and Hollings, R. M.: A "standard" experimental thrombus: Observations on its production, pathology, response to heparin, and thrombectomy. Surgery 59:812, 1966.
22. Kaiser, G. C., Murray, R. C., Willman, V. L., et al.: Iliofemoral thrombectomy for venous occlusion. Arch. Surg. 90:574, 1965.
23. Karp, R. B., and Wylie, E. J.: Recurrent thrombosis after iliofemoral venous thrombectomy. Surg. Forum 17:147, 1966.
24. Kitainik, E., and Quirós, R. S.: Thrombectomy and caval interruption: Indications and results. J. Cardiovasc. Surg. 13:440, 1972.
25. Lansing, A. M., and Davis, W. M.: Five-year follow-up study of iliofemoral venous thrombectomy. Ann. Surg. 168:620, 1968.
26. Läwen, A.: Uber Thrombektomie bei Venenthrombose und Arterio-spasmus. Zentralbl. Chir. 64:961, 1937.
27. Leriche, R., and Geisendorf, W.: Résultats d'un thrombectomie precoce avec résection veineuse dans une phlebite grave des deux membris inferieurs. Presse Med. 47:1301, 1939.
28. McLachlin, A. D., Carrol, S. E., Clark, R. L., et al.: Experimental venous thrombectomy. Ann. Surg. 171:956, 1970.
29. Mahorner, H., Castleberry, J. W., and Coleman, W. O.: Attempts to restore function in major veins which are the site of massive thrombosis. Ann. Surg. 146:510, 1957.
30. Mavor, G. E., and Galloway, J. D. M.: Iliofemoral venous thrombosis: Pathological considerations and surgical management. Br. J. Surg. 56:45, 1969.
31. Phillips, R. S.: Prognosis in deep venous thrombosis. Arch. Surg. 87:732, 1963.
32. Rossi, N., Lawrence, M. S., and Ehrenhaft, J. L.: Surgical treatment of massive iliofemoral venous thrombosis. Am. J. Surg., 113:533, 1967.
33. Sawyer, P. N., Schaefer, H. C., Domingo, R. T., et al.: Comparative therapy of thrombophlebitis. Surgery 55:113, 1963.
34. Smith, G. W.: Therapy for iliofemoral venous thrombosis. Surg. Gynecol. Obstet. 121:1298, 1965.
35. Wessler, S., and Morris, L. E.: Studies in intravascular coagulation: IV. The effect of heparin and dicumarol on serum-induced venous thrombosis. Circulation 12:553, 1955.

# Venous Thrombectomy for Acute Iliofemoral Thrombosis

WALLY S. BUCH
and THOMAS J. FOGARTY

*Stanford University Hospital*

The clinical presentation of iliofemoral venous thrombosis is nearly always acute. However, the underlying pathologic process responsible for the clinical picture is often of a chronic nature. It is this apparent paradox which makes the treatment of iliofemoral venous thrombosis difficult and controversial and to a large extent explains the variable results reported with thrombectomy.

Only by careful historical analysis and clinical observation can a particular episode of venous thrombosis be located upon the spectrum of pathologic processes presenting as an "acute" thrombosis. Only by determining the extent to which a chronic component exists concomitantly with an acute clinical presentation can a rational approach to therapy be designed. In this setting, the results of medical or operative therapy can be intelligently analyzed.

## Diagnosis

Acute iliofemoral venous thrombosis occurs in two distinct clinical patterns, usually referred to as phlegmasia alba dolens and phlegmasia cerulea dolens. Since the therapeutic implications differ in the two forms, they are best discussed separately.

### PHLEGMASIA ALBA DOLENS

This is the more benign form of iliofemoral venous thrombosis. The patient presents acutely with pain in the involved leg, soon followed by diffuse

359

edema and a peculiar pale coloration ("milk leg"). On physical examination the superficial veins are dilated, and tenderness can often be elicited over the femoral canal. Arterial pulsations are usually normal.

Although the clinical picture is that of an acute process, in only 30 per cent of cases is the occlusion pathologically as well as nosologically acute. Most commonly, the acute form is due to extension of clot into the iliofemoral system from the calf veins or the saphenous vein. Less frequently, iatrogenic interventions (e.g., femoral vein cannulation), inguinal infection, or hematoma will be responsible.[1]

However, in 70 per cent of cases the pathologic process is chronic, and the acute episode is precipitated by occlusion of a previously patent collateral pathway in a chronically occluded deep venous system, or by total occlusion of a major venous tributary previously only partially obstructed by malignancy, retroperitoneal inflammatory disease, or intramural thrombus.[1]

## PHLEGMASIA CERULEA DOLENS

From a pathophysiologic standpoint, this clinical form represents the most severe form of iliofemoral venous thrombosis. There is virtually complete venous obstruction, with severe edema, impeded arterial inflow, and tissue necrosis. Massive pooling in the extremity and profound edema may cause hypovolemic shock. The typical violaceous discoloration in the early phase of the process progresses to bullae formation and frank gangrene and ultimately requires amputation.

Despite the more malignant clinical picture, cerulea dolens is quite likely to represent an acute pathologic process. Indeed, the major component of the obstruction is usually acute thrombus. Over half of the patients have a recent history of trauma or operative complications, or are pregnant or in a postpartum state. One-third of the patients exhibit an advanced retroperitoneal or abdominal malignancy with extrinsic venous compression. The remainder have no other obvious clinical abnormality.

## *Sequelae of Venous Thrombosis*

In either clinical form, iliofemoral venous thrombosis can lead to massive pulmonary embolism and/or a disabling postphlebitis syndrome.[2, 3, 4] In phlegmasia cerulea dolens, there is the added threat of gangrene.

If thrombectomy is to be a viable adjunct to medical therapy in the management of these disorders, it must be shown that operative intervention (1) reduces the likelihood of pulmonary embolism; (2) reduces the incidence of serious postphlebitic changes; (3) results in patency of venous channels and valvar competency; and (4) in the case of phlegmasia cerulea, reduces the incidence of gangrene and amputation. With proper patient selection and operative technique, these goals can be realized.

## *Selection of Patients for Thrombectomy*

As noted previously, candidates for thrombectomy should be selected after a careful assessment of the nature of the pathologic process responsible for the acute clinical presentation. It is intuitively obvious that patients with pathologically acute thrombosis represent the more favorable candidates. Patients with thrombosis on a chronic basis are unlikely to achieve a satisfactory postoperative clinical result because of organization and adherence of the thrombus to the endothelium and chronic propagation of thrombus into venous collaterals.

Even with pathologically acute thrombosis, time is an important element. Venous thrombosis present more than 9 to 10 days cannot be completely alleviated because of propagation and organization of the thrombus and intimal inflammation.[4-9]

Our policy regarding operability is based on the etiology of the thrombosis, the chronicity of the pathologic process, and the degree of embarrassment to venous outflow.

### Phlegmasia Alba Dolens

Indications for operability are iliofemoral venous occlusion of less than 10 days' duration without (1) chronic venous insufficiency, (2) bilateral involvement, or (3) pelvic pathology. When these criteria are applied, about 30 per cent of patients with "white phlebitis" are candidates for thrombectomy. Operative technique and postoperative management are described below.

Thrombectomy has been performed on 50 patients with phlegmasia alba dolens (Table 1). Follow-up is available on 44 patients ranging from 1 to 6 years. There were no operative deaths, and no amputation was required. Clinically, 32 patients (73 per cent) are free of any edema. Only two patients (5 per cent) have edema which interferes with their lifestyles.

Forty-nine venograms have been performed on 37 patients 6 to 25 months postoperatively. Sixteen reveal normal venous anatomy from the popliteal vein to the inferior vena cava. Four of these patients have small filling defects in veins below the popliteal segment. All have competent valves. Seven patients have patent iliofemoral venous segments with persistent nonocclusive intraluminal defects. Five patients in this subgroup have competent venous valves. Ten patients have a total occlusion of a femoral or

TABLE 1.   Phlegmasia Alba Dolens: Late Results of Primary Venous
Thrombectomy (44 Cases)

| | |
|---|---|
| Follow-up | 1 to 6 years |
| Edema-free | 32 |
| Venograms (37 pts.) | Normal anatomy — 16 |

iliac segment with extensive collaterals. There is an excellent correlation between venographic appearance and clinical findings.

### PHLEGMASIA CERULEA DOLENS

The indication for operability is iliofemoral venous occlusion in the absence of terminal illness. A combined approach is utilized, employing pre- and postoperative heparin therapy, inferior vena caval interruption, thrombectomy, and, when indicated, fasciotomy. Caval interruption is employed, because many of these patients have already sustained a pulmonary embolus, and, in the remainder, the rate of embolization is high. Interruption is also beneficial because of the high incidence of late, recurrent phlebitis in this group.

Table 2 summarizes 40 cases of phlegmasia cerulea dolens. Nine patients had a terminal malignancy and were not treated with thrombectomy. Early in our experience, eight patients were treated with heparin, elastic support, and steep elevation. Clotting times (Lee-White) were maintained at two to three times control. Four patients (50 per cent) died—two of massive pulmonary emboli, one of a diffuse coagulopathy—and in one the cause of death was obscure. Two of the four survivors required amputation. Of the remaining two patients, one has a disabling postphlebitic syndrome, while the other has minimal edema.

Twenty-three patients were treated operatively. There were two deaths, one from a pulmonary embolus (no caval interruption) 4 weeks postoperatively, and the other from an acute myocardial infarction 6 weeks after operation.

Of the 21 survivors, all are available for follow-up ranging from 1 to 5 years. Eleven (52 per cent) have no peripheral edema, seven have mild edema, and three have a severe postphlebitic syndrome. Venography has been performed on nine patients in the late postoperative period. Two patients have totally patent venous systems up to the level of the caval interruption. The remaining seven show varying degrees of chronic superficial femoral obstruction and recanalization.

## Operative and Postoperative Techniques

Prior to operation, all patients are systemically heparinized. We prefer to use intravenous heparin, approximately 5000 units every 4 to 6 hours. The degree of anticoagulation is monitored with either Lee-White whole blood

**TABLE 2.  Phlegmasia Cerulea Dolens (40 Cases)**

| Type of Management | Number of Cases | Deaths | Amputations | Pulmonary Emboli |
|---|---|---|---|---|
| Terminal | 9 | 9 | 0 | 5 |
| Medical | 8 | 4 | 2 | 4 |
| Surgical | 23 | 2 | 0 | 1 |

clotting times or partial thromboplastin time determinations. With either method, values of two to three times control are ideal.

Operation is carried out under local anesthesia with general anesthesia standby. Following preparation of both lower extremities and the abdomen, a vertical incision is made in the groin. In cerulea, the vena cava is plicated prior to exploration of the vein.

If caval plication is not to be done, the opposite vein is exposed and an 8 to 10 French venous thrombectomy catheter introduced into the inferior cava to prevent inadvertent embolization from the involved side during the operation. There have been no pulmonary emboli with this technique. Following exposure of the involved venous system, all major branches of the vein are encircled with Silastic loops. A transverse venotomy is made in the common femoral vein just above its bifurcation. Clot will often extrude from the vein. A 6 French venous thrombectomy catheter is passed proximally, and, with great care to avoid rupture of the valves, clot is extracted. Distally, the leg is compressed with rubberized bandages. Concomitantly, calf and thigh compression and vigorous extension and flexion of the foot and leg are performed. Following extrusion of clot, venous catheters are carefully manipulated into the major venous tributaries and withdrawn to remove any residual clots. Heparinized saline is then flushed into the distal circulation.

An operative venogram is usually performed, and if residual thrombus is noted, attempts are made to extract it. If it becomes obvious that chronic adherent thrombus is present, attempts to extract the material are abandoned. The venotomy is closed with fine polypropylene suture, and a vacuum drain is placed in the wound.

Heparin therapy is continued for about 7 days. Warfarin is begun on the third postoperative day. The foot of the bed is elevated on 6-inch blocks, and elastic tensor support is applied. Ambulation is encouraged, and standing or sitting are prohibited. When the edema resolves, the patient is fitted with a full-length Jobst leotard. Oral anticoagulants are continued for 4 to 6 weeks.

## Discussion

The controversy over the treatment of acute iliofemoral venous thrombosis lies only with the therapy of the less malignant form, phlegmasia alba dolens. There is general agreement, even by strong advocates of medical therapy, that phlegmasia cerulea dolens is best treated by heparinization and thrombectomy.[4, 6-8, 10, 11] This is, in itself, curious. If the clinical results after thrombectomy in phlegmasia cerulea dolens are satisfactory, should it not offer an advantage in some cases of phlegmasia alba dolens?

The advantage can only be realized if the nature of the underlying pathology and its chronicity are firmly understood. Phlegmasia cerulea dolens is usually an acute pathologic process; thus, the results of thrombectomy are excellent. The same excellent results can be obtained in phlegmasia alba dolens when proper case selection to rule out chronic pathology is joined with operative venography and the use of the thrombectomy balloon catheter.

Any discussion advocating thrombectomy would not be complete without alluding to the report of Lansing and Davis.[11] They observed late clinical and phlebographic results in a group of patients operated upon by Haller and Abrams.[4] This excellent report showed edema, valvar incompetence, and reocclusion in the vast majority of patients. Unfortunately, there is little or no information on the pathologic substrate. Operative venograms were not performed to assess the immediate result, and the thrombectomy catheter was not employed. The results might have been better if these techniques and criteria had been employed.

Our series of phlegmasia alba dolens is flawed by lack of a suitable control group. Inasmuch as no reports in the literature compare operated and nonoperated patients with respect to pathologic findings, we cannot predict what a randomized study would reveal. However, Fontaine and Tuchmann reported a large series of patients treated in a somewhat randomized fashion, with better results in the group operated upon.[6]

This series of patients with phlegmasia cerulea and alba dolens shows excellent results with thrombectomy in properly selected patients. Although very late venograms are not available, the clinical picture in the majority of patients indicates adequate venous flow. We continue to be enthusiastic about venous thrombectomy in appropriately selected patients.

## *References*

1. Fogarty, T. J.: Venous thrombectomy. *In* Delaney, J. P. (ed.): *Surgery of the Vascular System.* Minneapolis, University of Minnesota, Department of Surgery, 1973.
2. Fogarty, T. J.: Arterial embolectomy and venous thrombectomy. *In* Irvine, W. T. (ed.): *Modern Trends in Surgery.* London, Butterworths, 1971.
3. Mahorner, H., Castleberry, J. W., and Coleman, W. O.: Attempts to restore function in major veins which are the site of massive thrombosis. Ann. Surg. *146*:510, 1957.
4. Haller, J. A., Jr., and Abrams, B. L.: Use of thrombectomy in the treatment of acute iliofemoral venous thrombosis in forty-five patients. Ann. Surg. *158*:561, 1963.
5. Kakkar, V. V., Flanc, C., Howe, C. T., and Clarke, M. B.: Natural history of postoperative deep vein thrombosis. Lancet, *2*:230, 1969.
6. Fontaine, R., and Tuchmann, L.: The role of thrombectomy in deep venous thrombosis. J. Cardiovasc. Surg. *5*:298, 1964.
7. Haller, J. A.: Thrombectomy for deep thrombophlebitis of the leg. New Engl. J. Med. *267*:65, 1962.
8. Edwards, W. H., Sawyers, J. L., and Foster, J. H.: Iliofemoral venous thrombosis: Reappraisal of thrombectomy. Ann. Surg. *171*:961, 1970.
9. Kakkar, V. V., Howe, C. T., Laws, J. W., and Flanc, C.: Late results of treatment of deep vein thrombosis. Br. Med. J. *1*:810, 1969.
10. Cockett, F. B.: Surgery of ilio-femoral thrombosis. *In* Gillespie, J. A. (ed.): *Modern Trends in Vascular Surgery.* London, Butterworths, 1970.
11. Lansing, A. M., and Davis, W. M.: Five-year follow-up study of iliofemoral venous thrombectomy. Ann. Surg. *168*:620, 1968.
12. Dale, W. A.: *The Swollen Leg. Current Problems in Surgery.* Chicago, Year Book Medical Publishers, 1973.
    *An excellent monograph dealing with the entire spectrum of the acute and chronic problems associated with venous disease. Dr. Dale has referenced the monograph with numerous articles which, if pursued, will allow for an understanding of the pathophysiology of venous thrombosis.*

13. Cockett, F. B.: Surgery of Ilio-femoral thrombosis. *In* Gillespie, J. A. (ed.): *Modern Trends in Vascular Surgery.* London, Butterworths, 1970.
    *The various mechanisms by which an episode of iliofemoral venous thrombosis may be precipitated are discussed. The natural history of iliofemoral venous obstruction is clearly presented.*

# 16

# *Inguinal Hernia Repair*

COOPER'S LIGAMENT HERNIOPLASTY
  *by Chester B. McVay*

THE SHOULDICE REPAIR OF
INGUINAL HERNIA
  *by Frank Glassow*

HALSTED-FERGUSON OPERATION FOR
INGUINAL HERNIA
  *by Mark M. Ravitch*

## Statement of the Problem

*To avoid a variety of peripheral issues, the authors are asked to discuss their selection of operative management for a symptomatic groin hernia (not a small indirect hernia) in a healthy 40-year-old laborer.*

*Compare data for recurrence after the operation you prefer versus alternative operations for indirect inguinal hernia, for direct inguinal hernia, and for femoral hernia. Exclude congenital hernias in the young.*

*Include in your analysis differences in operative morbidity, patient age, type of hernia, and completeness of follow-up.*

*Justify any importance you ascribe to the position of the cord in the repair, to the use of a relaxing incision, and to the size or composition of suture material employed. Give data indicating the circumstances for use of synthetic mesh–type materials in hernia repair. When, if ever, do you advocate cord division as an aid to achieving a more secure repair?*

# Cooper's Ligament Hernioplasty

CHESTER B. McVAY

*The University of South Dakota School of Medicine*

The nature of this assignment—to discuss the validity of the use of Cooper's ligament in the repair of inguinal and femoral hernias—automatically excludes the most common of all groin hernias, the small to medium-sized indirect inguinal hernia. This group of hernias will constitute between 50 to 60 per cent of the hernias in most series. It is important, however, to be sure that there is no concomitant direct or femoral hernia. In our series there have been multiple hernias, when only one was anticipated, in 6.8 per cent of 1211 cases.[5] After the indirect hernial sac is dissected out and ligated within the preperitoneal space, the margins of the dilated abdominal inguinal ring are sharply delineated by excising all attenuated transversalis fascia. At this point, dissecting in the preperitoneal space, we inspect the femoral ring to be sure that there is no coexistent femoral hernia. We then carefully inspect the posterior inguinal wall to evaluate its strength and to be sure it is strong enough to prevent a subsequent recurrence as a direct inguinal hernia. A mistake in this regard accounted for a number of our recurrences. It should be understood that transversalis fascia alone is not strong enough to prevent direct inguinal herniation. The strength of the posterior inguinal wall is dependent upon the number of transversus abdominis aponeurotic fibers that it contains.[2] A patient who develops a direct inguinal hernia has a congenitally deficient number of aponeurotic fibers. Conversely, transversalis fascia alone is not strong enough to be used in the repair of a direct inguinal hernia.

After excision and ligation of the hernial sac and careful evaluation of the posterior inguinal wall and the femoral ring, the dilated abdominal inguinal ring is closed medial to the cord structures by suturing the transversalis fascia to the anterior femoral sheath. It would involve an unnecessary operation to incise a normal posterior inguinal wall and resuture it. The closure about the cord structures must be tight enough to prevent preperitoneal fat from protruding but loose enough to avoid a vascular compromise of the testis. Our criterion for proper size is a ring that admits the cord structures and the tip of the surgeon's fifth finger. The cord should be stripped to its main elements, the vas deferens and the internal spermatic blood vessels. Protrusions of preperitoneal fat among the cord structures are common and should always be excised. The spermatic cord should be returned to its bed and the external oblique aponeurosis closed over it to reestablish the obliquity of the inguinal canal. In our follow-up of patients for from 11 to 22 years,[5] we had a recurrence rate in the small to medium-sized indirect inguinal hernias of 3.2 per cent. The most common cause of recurrence was either a mistake in judgment as to the strength of the posterior inguinal wall or failure to close the abdominal inguinal ring tightly enough.[5]

The direct inguinal hernia and the large indirect inguinal hernia present a different problem in that the posterior inguinal wall has been destroyed. In the case of the direct inguinal hernia, there is a congenital deficiency in the number of transversus abdominis aponeurotic fibers in the transversalis fascia, and this weak wall gradually stretches to become a direct inguinal hernia. In the case of the large indirect inguinal hernia, it has been present many years, and as the abdominal inguinal ring enlarges, it attenuates the intact posterior inguinal wall, so that when it is very large, the posterior inguinal wall is completely destroyed.

My opinion that Cooper's ligament should be the anchoring structure for the new posterior inguinal wall antedated any experience in the operating room by several years and was based upon anatomic studies while I was an instructor in the Anatomy Department at Northwestern University Medical School in the mid-1930's. A portion of this work appeared in the *Anatomical Record* in 1940.[8] Another observation in this original anatomic study was that the medial margin of the femoral ring was not the lacunar ligament but the lateralmost attachment of the transversus abdominis aponeurosis into Cooper's ligament. When a femoral hernia is present, the transversus abdominis aponeurosis attachment to Cooper's ligament is pushed medially until it eventually abuts the more superficial retinaculum, the inguinal lacunar ligament system. The latter structure is in no way etiologic in the causation of a femoral hernia, and it certainly should not be used in the repair of a femoral hernia. The anatomy of the femoral hernia problem was restudied in 1960.[9] Rather than repeat the rather extensive bibliography in the field of inguinal anatomy and inguinal and femoral hernioplasty, the reader is referred to pages 486 to 532 in the Anson-McVay *Surgical Anatomy*.[2] In this source, one will also find drawings and descriptions of the operative techniques for inguinal and femoral hernioplasty.

The Cooper's ligament hernioplasty is based upon detailed studies of the normal and pathologic anatomy of the inguinofemoral region. Very simply stated, we use Cooper's ligament to anchor the new posterior inguinal wall, because Cooper's ligament is the normal insertion of the transversus abdominis aponeurosis and transversalis fascia which is the posterior inguinal wall. In a direct inguinal hernia or a large indirect inguinal hernia, the posterior wall is destroyed, and the problem then resolves into what to do about it. There are a number of methods in use today to repair the absent posterior inguinal wall. Classically, since the time of Bassini and Halsted, the "conjoined tendon" was sutured to the inguinal ligament. The "conjoined tendon" is a combination of the lower fibers of the internal oblique and the transversus abdominis aponeuroses, but these fibers do not become conjoined or fused until they form the rectus sheath. Variations in and modifications of this original technique are legion, and in careful follow-up studies, the recurrence rate in direct inguinal hernias is unacceptable.[1] The reasons are obvious to an anatomist. The closure is under tension unless a relaxing incision is used, and the inguinal ligament is a free margin which can easily be displaced in a cephalad direction; moreover, the parallel fibers are easily fragmented.

Fundamentally, the inguinal ligament is not the insertion of the transversus abdominis layer, and it is not a suitable substitute. The inguinal ligament is a free margin, except where its attachment medially is broadened by the lacunar ligament for 1.5 cm., and in its lateral one-fourth, where some of the external oblique aponeurosis fibers insert into the iliopsoas fascia. In between, it lies in a fascial bed at the line along which the innominate fascia becomes the fascia lata. This can be demonstrated easily at the operating table by sliding the handle of a knife under the inguinal ligament and moving it back and forth. Furthermore, the inguinal ligament is not a condensation of aponeurotic fibers to form a true ligament. It is simply the lowermost parallel fibers of the external oblique aponeurosis and is only 1-fiber thick at any one point. The illusion that it is a ligament is due to the fact that, at its medial end, the fibers turn approximately 90 degrees to form the attachment to the pubic tubercle and the medial extent of Cooper's ligament, and this portion is labeled the lacunar ligament. At the operating table, by untwisting this 90-degree turn, one will see that the inguinal ligament is nothing more than the single parallel fibers of the caudalmost external oblique aponeurosis.[8]

In the past 20 years, other alternative methods have been advocated, which in my opinion are either anatomically incorrect or technically unsound. The procedure that incises the bulging posterior inguinal wall in a direct inguinal hernia and then imbricates it is advocated by some.[4] While this obviously suffices for a short-term follow-up, I would question the long-term results, because imbrication of two weak layers of transversalis fascia, containing only scattered aponeurotic fibers, cannot form a layer strong enough to withstand the repeated surges of increased intra-abdominal pressure that accompany everyday occurrences. If a relaxing incision were added to this technique, a stronger upper margin could be utilized without tension, but the lower, or inferior, margin is still too weak to anchor the repair. In any event, why not attach the upper margin of the defect in the transversus to its normal insertion, Cooper's ligament? It is unfortunate that there is not a long-term follow-up (10 to 20 years) of, say, 90 to 95 per cent of the cases repaired by this technique.

Another technique excises the bulge of the attenuated transversus abdominis layer and then sutures the fresh-cut margins together.[7] A relaxing incision is not used, and in my opinion the approximated layers are not strong enough to withstand the surges of increased intra-abdominal pressure over many years. Again, a resolution of this question can only be accomplished by a long-term follow-up upon 90 to 95 per cent of the cases operated upon.

Among the more controversial techniques in recent years has been the preperitoneal approach to inguinal and femoral hernias. While I would agree that the small indirect inguinal and the femoral hernias can be just as effectively repaired by this approach, it is an unnecessarily complicated approach to simple, anatomic problems that are easily repaired by the more conventional anterior approach. We have used the preperitoneal approach through the years when we have performed a lower abdominal celiotomy for other reasons and an indirect or a femoral hernioplasty is the secondary operation. I think it is appropriate to point out that the surgeon who does an occasional preperitoneal hernioplasty may not understand the anatomy of the region as it presents in the posterior approach. For a number of reasons, we do not believe that the preperitoneal approach should be used for direct inguinal hernias, and the reported results show a formidable recurrence rate on short-term follow-up.[3]

First, the margins that one approximates are essentially the same as in the anterior technique that excises the bulge and sutures the cut margins together.[7] In other words, it is a closure with weak layers, and tension on the suture line is not appreciated because of the more cephalad incision that is used for the preperitoneal approach. A relaxing incision is not used, so excessive tension on the suture line is a certainty. In a recent publication, Dr. Raymond Read[10] has added a proximal transverse relaxing incision to the preperitoneal repair of direct inguinal hernias, but it is only through the anterior rectus sheath above the main incision, so it cannot possibly reduce tension in the transversus layer. He reports an 8.2 per cent recurrence rate in 523 cases of direct inguinal hernia after 1 to 6 years of follow-up. One must realize that Dr. Read has had extensive experience with preperitoneal hernioplasty. However, if one projects the recurrence rate (8.2 per cent) to 25 years, as we have done, then the eventual recurrence rate will be between 16 and 20 per cent, which is not acceptable.

Second, the preperitoneal hernioplasty anchors the repair into the so-called iliopubic tract. As an anatomist, I have repeatedly called attention to the fact that no such structure exists in normal anatomy. If one carefully removes all of the preperitoneal connective tissue from the transversalis fascia in a posterior approach to the inguinal region, no such structure can be identified in an inguinal region without a hernia. Similarly, the interfoveolar ligament of Hesselbach fails to materialize. That portion of the "iliopubic tract" over the vascular lacuna is simply the line along which the transversalis fascia turns forward to pass into the thigh as the anterior layer of the femoral sheath. The medial portion of the "iliopubic tract" is an illusion that appears in the patient with a direct inguinal hernia. Such a lip of tissue attached to Cooper's ligament is apparent in both anterior and posterior dissections in the patient with a direct inguinal hernia. As the posterior inguinal wall attenuates with the development of a direct inguinal hernia, the inferior, or caudal, 4 or 5 mm. of the posterior inguinal wall above the attachment to Cooper's ligament is prevented from bulging by the more superficial support of the inguinal-lacunar ligament system. After the attenuated posterior inguinal wall is excised, this ledge of fascia remains, and rather than use this weakened layer, we excise it and place our sutures into Cooper's ligament, because it is strong. Furthermore, why not use the normal attachment rather than the remnant of the posterior inguinal wall attachment? Hopefully, I have again explained the myth of the iliopubic tract of Thomson.

Some recent reports have suggested the prophylactic use of prosthetic materials in all direct inguinal hernioplasties.[6] I cannot accept this dictum and, as in the past, use a prosthesis only when there is no other way to close the defect. The last detailed analysis of our series was a report on 1211 hernioplasties, in which the study period ended in 1968.[5] We used a prosthesis 22 times, or in 1.8 per cent of our cases, and this includes all of the single and multiple recurrent hernias. We have now done almost 2000 hernioplasties and have used a prosthesis in 30 cases, or 1.5 per cent of the total series.

The foregoing is a critique of popular methods of hernioplasty that we do not endorse. Why, then, do we continue to use the "Cooper's ligament hernioplasty" for large indirect and direct inguinal hernias? First of all, we believe in anchoring the medial part of the repair to Cooper's ligament because it is the normal insertion of the transversus abdominis aponeurosis and transversalis fascia, and it is strong. We close the lateral part of the defect (over the vascular lacuna) by suturing the transversalis fascia to the anterior femoral sheath, because this reestablishes normal fascial continuity. The most simple and most effective way to repair the aponeuroticofascial defect in a large direct inguinal hernia is to make the relaxing incision and shift or slide the aponeurotic rectus sheath into the position of a new posterior inguinal wall. This is accomplished without tension, and the rectus abdominis muscle and the rectus fascia prevent herniation through the defect created by the relaxing incision.

The repair of a femoral hernia is an exercise in precise, anatomic restoration. It cannot be done correctly through the femoral approach, and plugging the defect with wads of fascia or prosthetic material is anatomically unsound. An attempt to suture the inguinal ligament to Cooper's ligament via the femoral approach in order to close the femoral ring is doomed to failure for two reasons. First, this is the wrong layer to close, and it leaves the femoral ring open; second, the closure is under extreme tension, and one will get pressure necrosis of the inguinal ligament. If one understands that the defect in a femoral hernia is a narrowing of the insertion of the transversus abdominis aponeurosis onto Cooper's ligament, then the repair is simple, because all one has to do is to broaden this attachment so that the femoral ring is closed.[9] The anterior or inguinal approach is a beautiful dissection of normal anatomic layers. The preperitoneal approach is also a nice demonstration of the anatomic defect that permits a femoral hernia to develop; likewise, the broadening of the transversus attachment is easy and accurate.

The following numbered paragraphs are in answer to specific questions by the editors.

1. We believe that the spermatic cord should always be replaced against the posterior inguinal wall and the external oblique aponeurosis closed over it. This restores the obliquity of the inguinal canal and avoids placing the subcutaneous inguinal ring directly over the abdominal inguinal ring closure, as in the Halsted I operation. Dr. Halsted rather promptly recognized

this error and shortly began closing the external oblique aponeurosis over the cord—the Halsted II operation.

2. We believe that the relaxing incision is mandatory in all direct and large indirect inguinal hernias for reasons stated before.

3. Most present-day surgeons use nonabsorbable sutures, since several studies many years ago showed a much higher recurrence rate when the repair was done with catgut. The type of nonabsorbable suture material is relatively unimportant and will depend upon the preference of the individual surgeon. In general, there is no point in using a suture material that is stronger than the tissues to be approximated.

4. We never divide the spermatic cord for the purpose of a more secure repair. However, in the scar of multiple recurrent hernias, one frequently finds the cord so fragmented that there is no alternative. It may be excised either deliberately or accidentally. In our experience, if one does not dissect the cord beyond the pubic tubercle, sufficient collateral circulation develops to prevent testicular slough. The testis may or may not atrophy following severance of the cord structures, and the result is certainly dependent upon the effectiveness of the collateral blood supply in the scrotum.

5. Morbidity is closely related to age, but we do not deny an aged person a hernia operation when it is indicated, because we prefer an elective procedure under local anesthesia to an emergency operation because of strangulation. There is rarely morbidity as regards the hernia operation, but it frequently aggravates other conditions, such as obstructive uropathy.

The evaluation of a given technique for hernia repair is dependent upon the number of long-term cures. It is almost impossible to compare one series with another, because of variations in the length and completeness of follow-up. Also, some surgeons do not consider a different type of groin hernia as a recurrence—e.g., the patient who develops a direct inguinal hernia 15 or 20 years following the repair of a small indirect inguinal hernia. We consider this a recurrence, because at the original operation the surgeon should have detected the weakness of the posterior inguinal wall. In our published data, we record this type of recurrence as an error in judgment of the surgeon performing the original operation. Also, in recording recurrences, the type of the original hernia should be recorded and the various categories analyzed separately; if they are all lumped together, a formidable recurrence rate for direct inguinal hernias may be obscured by the favorable recurrence rate for the very common small indirect inguinal hernia.

I have earlier given a reference for our techniques of inguinal and femoral hernioplasty. The results of a 22-year study on our series of hernioplasties is readily available,[5] and there would seem to be no point in repeating this extensive data here. From our studies and those of others, it is apparent that hernias may recur many years after the original operation; therefore, to compare a long-term series with a shorter one, we developed a formula to predict one's recurrence rate to 25 years.[5] For example, if a series of cases have all been followed for 1 year, the predicted recurrence rate at 25 years would be five times the 1-year recurrence rate. Other factors are presented in a table in this follow-up study.

Finally, I believe that the Cooper's ligament repair for the difficult groin hernias is based upon firm anatomic principles. Our recorded overall recurrence rate of 3.5 per cent, with a predicted recurrence rate to 25 years of 4.2 per cent, is not perfect, but it does reflect an acceptable recurrence rate, with the candid acknowledgment of our errors in judgment and operative technique. Perhaps with this detailed type of analysis, a younger generation of surgeons can improve upon our results.

## References

1. Andrews, E., and Bissel, A. D.: Direct hernia: A record of surgical failures. Surg. Gynecol. Obstet. 58:753, 1934.
2. Anson, B. J., and McVay, C. B.: *Surgical Anatomy.* 5th ed. Philadelphia, W. B. Saunders Co., 1971.
3. Gaspar, M. R., and Casberg, M. A.: An appraisal of preperitoneal repair of inguinal hernia. Surg. Gynecol. Obstet. *132*:207, 1971.
4. Glassow, F.: Recurrent inguinal and femoral hernia: 3000 cases. Can. J. Surg. 7:284, 1964.
5. Halverson, K., and McVay, C. B.: Inguinal and femoral hernioplasty. Arch. Surg. *101*:127, 1970.
6. Lichtenstein, I. L.: Lichtenstein's single-day herniorrhaphy. Hosp. Physician, September, 1972, p. 38.
7. Madden, J. L., Hakim, S., and Agorogiannis, A. B.: The anatomy and repair of inguinal hernias. Surg. Clin. North Am. *51*:1269, 1971.
8. McVay, C. B., and Anson, B. J.: Aponeurotic and fascial continuities in the abdomen, pelvis and thigh. Anat. Rec. 76:213, 1940.
9. McVay, C. B., and Savage, L. E.: Etiology of femoral hernia. Ann. Surg. (Suppl.) *154*:25, 1961.
10. Read, R. C.: Recurrence after preperitoneal herniorrhaphy in the adult. Arch. Surg. *110*:666, 1975.

# The Shouldice Repair of Inguinal Hernia

**FRANK GLASSOW**

*Shouldice Hospital, Toronto, Ontario, Canada*

In a 29-year period from January 1, 1945, to December 31, 1973, 84,000 inguinal hernia repairs were performed at Shouldice Hospital, Toronto, Canada. In the first 5 or 6 years of this period, the technique of repair, which has now become standardized, was being devised and developed by the late Dr. E. E. Shouldice. Since about 1951, therefore, in a series of 78,000 inguinal repairs, a relatively routine procedure has been used. Of the entire series, 9000 repairs were for recurrent inguinal hernia, the original repair(s) having been performed elsewhere. The author, in a 20-year period, has performed 15,000 of the inguinal repairs, 1761 of which were for recurrent hernia. Figure 1 shows that the overall recurrence rate for the series has fallen from 17 per cent in 1945 to approximately 1 per cent in 1952,[1] calculated on an annual basis, and has remained in that region ever since. The total recurrence rate for the entire period is 0.8 per cent.

The essence of the Shouldice repair is an overlap of the divided transversalis layer. Its most characteristic feature is the detailed technique used in this division and in the subsequent overlapping type of repair. The division commences laterally at the internal ring and is carried medially through part or all of the posterior inguinal wall to the pubic bone. This produces a lower (or lateral) leaf of transversalis approximately 1 to 2 cm. wide and an upper (or medial) transversalis flap. These two flaps are overlapped, bringing the upper one anterior to the lower to attach its free edge to Poupart's ligament. This layer is further strengthened by another double layer immediately superficial to it, which attaches medial structures, namely the conjoined tendon and internal oblique muscle, to the surface of the external oblique aponeurosis. Two continuous, monofilament, stainless steel, 34-gauge wire sutures are used, one for the first two lines of the repair and a second for the remaining two.

All but the most difficult repairs are performed using local anesthesia. This applies to 95 per cent of cases.

At the internal ring, the cord is carefully and completely freed by sharp

375

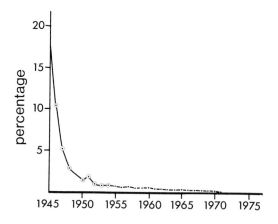

*Figure 1.* Recurrence rate following hernia repairs from 1945 to 1973.

dissection from the transversalis fascia, adherent around its entire circumference. Then the indirect hernial sac is freed from the cord to its neck. In the absence of an indirect hernia, a peritoneal protrusion here is routinely identified and similarly dealt with. After dealing with its contents, the indirect sac is usually, but not always, excised. If the freeing is well performed, the level of division and ligation of the sac is of lesser importance, for the ligated stump retracts out of sight, even when the ligation is low.[2] This technique is particularly suited to the treatment of sliding hernias, which are almost invariably indirect. After the freeing, the sliding hernia can be completely reduced within the abdomen without even opening the sac, even when it is large. If it has been opened to establish the diagnosis, it is closed again without excision. This technique simplifies the treatment of these otherwise troublesome hernias. Recurrent indirect inguinal hernia following inguinal repair here is extremely uncommon, suggesting that the technique used at the internal ring is adequate.[3, 4] Careful examination at the internal ring will detect the occasional unsuspected interstitial hernia.

Similarly, the importance of excision of the cremaster muscle is emphasized. This routine maneuver illuminates the entire anatomy of the posterior inguinal wall.

The femoral area is also examined routinely, both from below the inguinal ligament, at the commencement of the operation, and from above, later, when the posterior inguinal wall is opened, so that the occasional unsuspected femoral hernia will be revealed.

## Routine Management of an Uncomplicated Hernia in a Healthy 40-Year-Old Laborer

### Preoperative Management

The patient is encouraged to lose excess weight before operation. He is given a diet sheet and instructed to lose the weight gradually at about two pounds per week.

## Anesthesia

Adequate preoperative sedation precedes the local anesthesia. In this patient, 300 mg. of sodium pentobarbital would be given orally 90 minutes preoperatively. Then, 20 minutes preoperatively, 50 mg. of meperidine hydrochloride would be given intramuscularly. At operation, approximately 150 ml. of procaine hydrochloride, 2 per cent, without epinephrine is used, of which 100 ml. is injected at the initial subcutaneous regional infiltration. A further 10 to 20 ml. is used beneath the external oblique aponeurosis and a third injection of a similar amount around the internal ring.

## Stages of Operation

The skin incision is made in the line of the inguinal canal, and similarly in the external oblique aponeurosis in the line of its fibers, to the external ring, avoiding damage to the ilioinguinal nerve while the aponeurotic flaps are being mobilized. The cremaster muscle is divided longitudinally over the cord and each flap freed and excised. The internal ring region is now freed from all transversalis attachments as described. Routine identification of the peritoneal protrusion in cases of direct inguinal hernia will ensure that no indirect hernia is overlooked. In our series of 9000 recurrent inguinal herniorrhaphies, more than 4000 were recurrent indirect. Any indirect hernia is dealt with as described.

The assessment of the strength of the posterior wall is fundamental to the Shouldice repair. This is accomplished first by inspection and then by testing with a finger deep to the transversalis but in an extraperitoneal plane. A direct hernia is obvious protruding through part or all of the posterior inguinal wall. In some cases, only a weakness is present. In these, a prophylactic repair is performed, so that in either circumstance the Shouldice repair is applicable. The division of the posterior inguinal wall is commenced laterally where the transversalis layer has already been entered during the freeing at the internal ring (Figure 2). The division is continued medially toward the pubic bone (Figure 3). When a direct hernia is present, the transversalis layer is stretched over it and often adherent to it and has to be freed during the division. This is usually carried to the pubic bone, but if the transversalis layer is strong medially, this part may be left undisturbed. Excess attenuated transversalis may require excision. Nevertheless, firm transversalis of good quality is usually found, even in the presence of a large direct hernia. The direct hernia, usually diffuse, is freed and reduced, usually without opening. A funicular sac is excised. The bladder is rarely seen.

The basic features of the repair have been stressed. The first suture starts medially at the pubic bone (Figure 4). It attaches the free edge of the lateral transversalis flap to the back of the edge of the rectus fascia, identified as a firm white line inserting onto the pubic bone. The entire free edge is now brought upward and medially under the medial flap which overlaps it, so that a line of attachment extends to the internal ring. It is sutured medially to the edge of the rectus fascia and more laterally to the undersur-

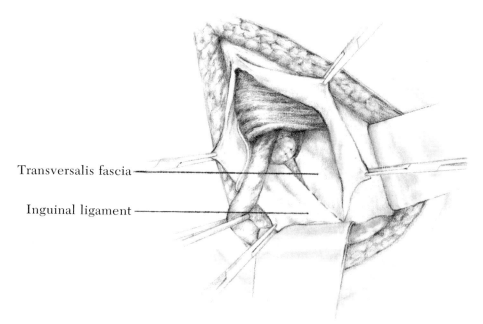

Transversalis fascia ——————

Inguinal ligament ——————

*Figure 2.* Anterior aspect of posterior wall of right inguinal canal, showing site and direction of division of transversalis fascia commencing laterally at internal ring. (Redrawn from Shearburn, E. W., and Myers, R. N.: Shouldice repair for inguinal hernia. Surgery 66:450, 1969. Redrawn by Miss Lee Goodchild, A.O.C.A., B.Sc., A.A.M., and Miss Lynn Goodchild, A.O.C.A., B.Sc., A.A.M.)

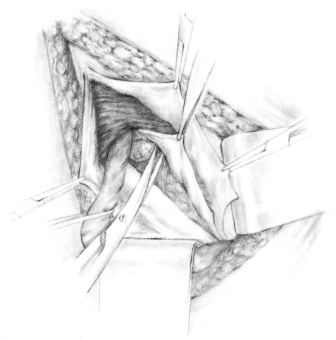

*Figure 3.* Anterior aspect of posterior wall of right inguinal canal, showing division of transversalis fascia completed from internal ring to pubic bone, with medial flap mobilized. (Redrawn from Shearburn, E. W., and Myers, R. N.: Shouldice repair for inguinal hernia. Surgery 66:450, 1969. Redrawn by Miss Lee Goodchild, A.O.C.A., B.Sc., A.A.M., and Miss Lynn Goodchild, A.O.C.A., B.Sc., A.A.M.)

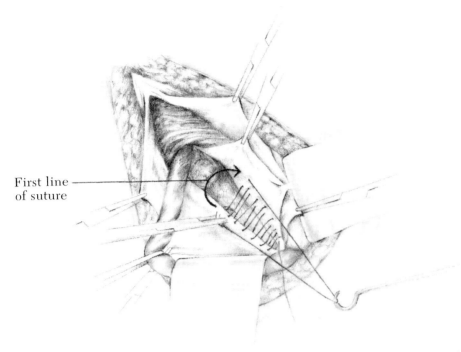

First line
of suture

**Figure 4.** Anterior aspect of posterior wall of right inguinal canal, showing first suture line approaching internal ring after commencing at pubic bone. (Redrawn from Shearburn, E. W., and Myers, R. N.: Shouldice repair for inguinal hernia. Surgery 66: 450, 1969. Redrawn by Miss Lee Goodchild, A.O.C.A., B.Sc., A.A.M., and Miss Lynn Goodchild, A.O.C.A., B.Sc., A.A.M.)

face of the internal oblique fascia. The suture line is continuous. It is inserted without tension, using small bites. At the internal ring this first suture is reversed, and it then returns to the pubic bone as the second line of the repair, where it is tied (Figure 5). This second line attaches the free edge of the medial flap of transversalis to Poupart's ligament, accurately following the contours of the femoral vessels. This first suture is basic to a successful repair. The second suture commences immediately medial to the internal ring. It attaches the internal oblique and conjoined tendon to the surface of the external oblique as the third line of the repair just superficial to both Poupart's ligament and to the original suture, thus obliterating all space beneath. It returns from the pubic bone laterally to the internal ring as the fourth line of the repair, where it is tied.

The repair should be performed without tension. A relaxing incision is practically never used. The cord is replaced and the external oblique closed over it. Neither the internal nor the external ring should be tight. Michel's skin clamps are used.

The patient is discharged on the third postoperative day after unilateral herniorrhaphy. Bilateral repairs are performed 48 hours apart.

The management of an uncomplicated case of inguinal hernia has intentionally been described in detail. It ensures that other surgeons using the Shouldice repair will do so with precision. Shearburn and Myers[5, 6] have accurately followed these principles. In their 13-year series of 953 consecutive inguinal herniorrhaphies, their recurrence rate was 0.7 per cent, the same as

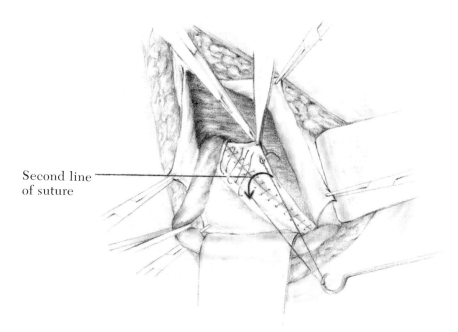

Second line
of suture

*Figure 5.*   Anterior aspect of posterior wall of right inguinal canal, showing second suture line returning to pubic bone after reversing at the internal ring, overlapping medial flap anterior to lateral flap. (Redrawn from Shearburn, E. W., and Myers, R. N.: Shouldice repair for inguinal hernia. Surgery 66:450, 1969. Redrawn by Miss Lee Goodchild, A.O.C.A., B.Sc., A.A.M., and Miss Lynn Goodchild, A.O.C.A., B.Sc., A.A.M.)

ours, while their recurrence rate for 76 recurrent inguinal herniorrhaphies in this period was 2.6 per cent.

Monofilament stainless steel is the suture material preferred. Other surgeons use different nonabsorbable sutures with excellent results, but absorbable sutures are unsatisfactory and should be abandoned. Palumbo and Sharpe[7] and McVay and Anson[8] use silk; Shearburn and Myers use Teflon-impregnated Dacron; Maingot[9] uses floss silk and Moloney[10] nylon yarn. All report low recurrence rates. The continuous nature of the suture is considered important. It distributes stresses evenly. Many direct recurrences have been repaired by the author, who found individual nonabsorbable sutures visible on either side of the neck of the hernia. Nevertheless, in a large series, Palumbo, using interrupted silk sutures, has achieved a recurrence rate of 1 per cent (Table 1).

Mesh, although very popular with many surgeons, is never used here, even for the largest hernias. Indeed, mesh has many times been removed during the repair of recurrences. I have never used it in a personal series of more than 15,000 repairs. Nevertheless, some surgeons use it with excellent results. In particular, Bellis,[11] in an impressive series of more than 9000 repairs in 3000 of which a polyester fiber mesh was inserted, achieved a very low recurrence rate of less than 0.5 per cent (Table 1), but he gives no information about his follow-up. Preston and Richards[12] have used wire mesh in a series of more than 2000 repairs but do not quote their recurrence rates.

**Table 1.** *

| Author | Period | Number of Years | Number of Operations | Type of Original Hernia | | | | | All Types | Number of Recurrences | Recurrence Rate |
|---|---|---|---|---|---|---|---|---|---|---|---|
| | | | | Inguinal | | | | Femoral | | | |
| | | | | Indirect | Direct | Recurrent | All Types | All Types | | | |
| Palumbo | 1940–1970 | 30 | 3572 | 3572 (primary) | | | | | | 30 | 1.0 |
| Maingot | 1935–1965 | 30 | 1000 (floss silk) | | | | 1000 | | | 20 | 2.0 |
| Bellis | 1944–1964 | 20 | 4432 | | | | 4432 | | | 23 | 0.5 |
| | 1960–1969 | 9 | 3083 (mesh) | | | | 3083 | | | 5 | 0.2 |
| McVay | 1946–1967 | 22 | 1211 | 646 | | | | | | 21 | 3.2 |
| | | | | | 442 | | | | | 16 | 3.6 |
| | | | | | | 135 | | | | 4 | 3.0 |
| Marsden[33] | 3-year review | | 1602 | | | | | 96 | | 3 | 3.1 |
| | | | | 1100 | | | | | | 57 | 5.2 |
| | | | | | 367 | | | | | 27 | 7.4 |
| | | | | | | 121 | | | | 23 | 19.0 |
| | | | | | | | 1602 | | | 109 | 6.8 |
| Nyhus[34] | 1955–1963 | 8 | 777 (preperitoneal) | 442 | | | | | | 12 | 2.7 |
| | | | | | 222 | | | | | 11 | 5.0 |
| | | | | | | | 664 | | | 23 | 3.5 |
| | | | | | | | | 113 | | 1 | 0.8 |
| | | | | | | | | | 123 recurrences | 8 | 6.5 |
| Margoles and Braun[35] | 1963–1966 | 3 | 150 (preperitoneal) | 61 | | | | | | 10 | 16.4 |
| | | | | | 63 | | | | | 20 | 31.7 |
| | | | | | | 35 | | | | 12 | 34.3 |
| | | | | | | | | 10 | | 0 | 0.0 |
| | | | | | | | | | 150 | 38 | 25.3 |
| | | | 625 (classical) | 215 | | | | | | 4 | 1.8 |
| | | | | | 225 | | | | | 13 | 5.7 |
| | | | | | | 109 | | | | 11 | 10.1 |
| | | | | | | | | 14 | | 2 | 14.3 |
| | | | | | | | | | 625 | 32 | 5.1 |

*This is a comparative table of recurrence rates for some other large, well-documented series. It represents only a cross section of such surveys and is in no way complete.

Lichtenstein[13] uses plastic mesh for repair of direct and recurrent hernias. Usher[14] has used Marlex mesh with considerable success.

The subcutaneous positioning of the cord is never used and is not recommended. However, the cord was encountered in this subcutaneous plane in approximately 2000 of the recurrent herniorrhaphies performed here. Of these, the recurrent hernia was indirect in half and direct in the rest. Such a technique therefore has no great merit. In almost every instance, the cord was replaced in its true anatomic plane at the end of the operation. The subsequent recurrence rate in this group was approximately 1 per cent.

Relaxing incisions[15] are very rarely used and are not recommended except in unusual circumstances of great tension. I have used a relaxing incision only two or three times in my entire series in 20 years. Tension can be avoided by other means, such as adequate weight loss preoperatively and careful operative technique. Since tension can hardly be avoided in the Cooper ligament repair,[16] a relaxing incision is almost mandatory and is accordingly recommended by Koontz,[17] McVay,[18, 19] Tanner,[20] Ponka, and others. However, the experience gained from the large series surveyed here, as well as from other large series—in particular, those published by Palumbo and Bellis, with excellent results—suggests that this maneuver has a very limited place in inguinal herniorrhaphy. Ponka says that "... it [the relaxing incision] is the most noteworthy contribution in the present century to the successful repair of hernias in which the weakness lies in Hesselbach's triangle, or the so-called floor of the inguinal canal." I do not agree with this opinion.

Orchiectomy is very rarely necessary. Cord division is almost never practiced. I have personally performed it only two or three times in my entire series. It is almost always possible to preserve the cord structures by gentle and careful dissection, even in the difficult recurrence and in the elderly. Section may have a very limited place in the patient who has had three or more recurrences. In Heifetz's[21] series of 112 cord resections, 38 patients had once recurrent hernias, 21 had twice recurrent hernias, and 1 had a hernia which recurred three times. I might have considered cord section in this last case, and I think most of the other resections were probably unnecessary.

Since immediate ambulation is practiced here, early postoperative complications are minimal. Bellis and Palumbo, as well as ourselves, are firm believers in the importance of this phase of management. Indeed, Palumbo's figures are an impressive justification of this practice. In a carefully controlled program, he demonstrated dramatically that those patients who were ambulatory on the day of operation or on the first postoperative day developed significantly fewer immediate complications and had a lower recurrence rate than those who were ambulatory from the third to the ninth postoperative days, while a third group ambulatory after the tenth postoperative day had even poorer results in this regard. In our large series, catheterization was virtually eliminated. The wound infection rate is now less than 1 per cent. A subsidiary study by the author some years ago demonstrated that postoperative wound infection plays a relatively minor etiologic role in the subsequent development of a recurrence.[22]

Return to normal activity is rapid. A patient may return to heavy physi-

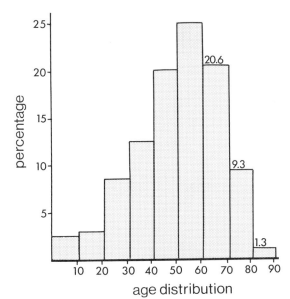

*Figure 6.* Age distribution of patients undergoing hernia repair.

cal work after 4 weeks, and he may return to a less strenuous occupation much earlier. The economic gain to both the patient and the community can easily be shown to be immense in terms of dollars. The elderly are treated no differently. They recover equally rapidly, and the recurrence rate in this group is just the same. Approximately 10 per cent of the patients, representing 8000 repairs, were more than 70 years old.[23] Figure 6[24] shows the age distribution of all patients operated upon in this series.

All authors have the same difficulty in documenting a long, continued follow-up of a large series. In this series of more than 80,000 cases, an immense statistical effort was required. A 1- to 25-year follow-up was obtained in more than 95 per cent of patients. More than 88 per cent were followed for 3 or more years. The data assembled were from a combined survey, consisting of an annual examination at this hospital, an examination by a local physician, or a questionnaire. To test the efficacy of this follow-up plan, the year 1955 was arbitrarily chosen for analysis. Table 2[25] sets forth the results obtained. The argument that the patient who is lost to the follow-up may be the one with the recurrence is unanswerable. It applies to all surgeons and all series. Nevertheless, the figures compiled and quoted throughout this article will speak for themselves. It is genuinely felt that, in view of the conscientious efforts made, the recurrence rates quoted are reasonably accurate. Hagan and Rhoads,[26] Halverson and McVay,[27] and the author have all investigated the importance of the length of the follow-up period required to exclude the probability of recurrence. Each investigation revealed that a minimum 10-year period was desirable. Figure 7 indicates the experience here. After 5 years, approximately 50 per cent of recurrences had developed and after 10 years 75 per cent. Halverson and McVay's results correspond very closely. This graph, like Halverson and McVay's table, can be used to

TABLE 2.   Follow-up of 2748 Operations Performed Upon
2270 Patients in 1955

| Year | Surviving Patients | Patients Followed-up | Percentage Followed-up | Recurrences Discovered |
|------|------|------|------|------|
| 1955 | 2270 | | | 3 |
| 1956 | 2258 | 2159 | 95.6 | 4 |
| 1957 | 2255 | 2056 | 92.4 | 1 |
| | | | | (8 in 2 years) |
| 1958 | 2190 | 1948 | 88.9 | 3 |
| 1959 | 2150 | 1823 | 84.8 | 3 |
| 1960 | 2095 | 1696 | 81.0 | 2 |
| | | | | (16 in 5 years) |
| 1961 | 2044 | 1540 | 75.3 | 2 |
| 1962 | 2007 | 1109 | 55.3 | 1 |
| 1963 | | | | 1 |
| 1964 | | | | 3 |
| | | | | (23 in 9 years°) |

°Recurrence rate after 9 years = 0.84 per cent.

predict the eventual long-term recurrence rate of any series if shorter term figures are available.

## *Recurrence Rates*

The recurrence rates for some of the different herniorrhaphy types performed at this hospital are summarized in Table 3.

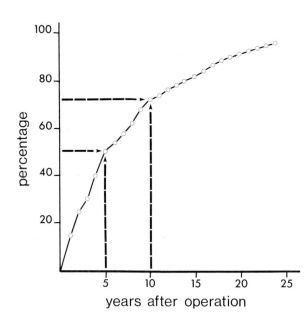

*Figure* 7. Interval between repair and evidence of recurrence. Vertical scale indicates percentage of 650 recurrences.

TABLE 3.  Recurrence Rates in Different Hernia Types

| Type of Hernia | Period | Number of Years | Number of Repairs | Number of Recurrences | Recurrence Rate as a Percentage |
|---|---|---|---|---|---|
| Inguinal (primary and recurrent) | 1945–1973 | 29 | 84,000 | 650 | 0.8 |
| Primary inguinal | 1945–1973 | 29 | 75,500 | 553 | 0.7 |
| Primary indirect | 1945–1973 | 29 | 50,500 | 335 | 0.7 |
| Primary direct | 1945–1973 | 29 | 25,000 | 218 | 0.9 |
| Recurrent inguinal (all types) | 1945–1973 | 29 | 9000 | 102 | 1.1 |
| Recurrent indirect | 1945–1973 | 29 | 4300 | 32 | 0.8 |
| Recurrent direct | 1945–1973 | 29 | 4700 | 70 | 1.5 |
| Primary indirect in women[28] | 1945–1970 | 26 | 1550 | 10 | 0.6 |
| Primary direct in women[29] | 1945–1970 | 26 | 124 | 2 | 1.6 |
| Primary femoral in women[30] | 1945–1970 | 26 | 434 | 9 | 2.1 |
| Primary femoral in men[31] | 1945–1969 | 25 | 687 | 15 | 2.2 |
| Sliding inguinal[32] | 1945–1967 | 23 | 3000 | 16 | 0.5 |

The Harkins and Nyhus preperitoneal repair, a relative newcomer in the field, has not yet established its rightful place in the surgeon's armamentarium. Gaspar and Casberg,[36] firm supporters of the technique, nevertheless quote a recurrence rate of 21 per cent for direct hernias. Margoles and Braun, discussing preperitoneal versus classic hernioplasty, concluded that the preperitoneal technique was generally unsatisfactory for inguinal hernias while reasonably good for femoral hernias. The operation is technically more difficult, involves greater morbidity, has a higher risk of more serious complications, and is followed by a higher incidence of recurrence. The same criticisms can be directed toward the Cooper ligament repair. It is deeply placed and involves tension and undue risk of damage to the femoral vein.

It is salutary to end on a note of self-criticism. Although a recurrence rate of 0.7 per cent was achieved for repair of primary inguinal hernia in the Shouldice series, representing 553 recurrences, 237 or 43 per cent of these "recurrences" were femoral in type.[37, 38] The true significance of this finding is not yet clearly understood. It may represent some missed hernias, some new hernias, or the use of too much tension at the original repair. However, it is certainly associated with bilateral direct inguinal repairs in the middle-aged male. Recurrences were significantly more frequent statistically in bilateral repairs, a point which both Palumbo and McVay corroborate. Finally, although preference in this hospital is given to the use of stainless steel wire sutures for the repair, this material requires some technical skill and an operating team familiar with its use in order to obtain the best results. When these conditions are not obtainable, several of the other nonabsorbable sutures mentioned also appear to give excellent results.

## *Summary*

The massive experience quoted herein, using the Shouldice technique of division and imbrication of the transversalis layer for repair of inguinal hernias performed under local anesthesia, gives excellent immediate and long-term results, with a recurrence rate of 0.8 per cent. It justifies a more general adoption, since the technique lends itself equally well to the treatment of all types of inguinal hernia.

Some of the popular fashions and notions can be discarded as unnecessary or irrelevant. In particular, there are only very limited indications for the Cooper ligament repair, for the use of the relaxing incision, for section of the spermatic cord, for the subcutaneous placement of the spermatic cord, and for the use of the preperitoneal approach in dealing with inguinal hernias, whether primary or recurrent. Meshes—in particular, the polyester fiber type—appear to give very good results, but is their use really necessary?

To Professor L. M. Zimmerman[39] of Chicago must belong the last word: "... the larger the series, the more valuable are the figures offered; and the percentage of patients returning for follow-up is also of great significance. . . ." Moreover, "Hernial surgery demands meticulous technique, gentle handling of tissues, free anatomical exposure, accurate approximation of sutured structures, avoidance of tension and utilization of fine, atraumatic needles and suture materials. The disregard of any of these attributes of good surgery will be reflected in a high recurrence rate. With the same method, the results will vary with the skill employed by the surgeon. . . ."

## *References*

1. Glassow, F.: The surgical repair of inguinal and femoral hernias. Can. Med. Assoc. J. *108*:308, 1973.
2. Glassow, F.: High ligation of the sac in indirect inguinal hernia. Am. J. Surg. *109*:460, 1965.
3. Glassow, F.: Recurrent inguinal and femoral hernia. Br. Med. J. *109*:1, 215, 1970.
4. Glassow, F.: Recurrent inguinal and femoral hernia: 3000 cases. Can. J. Surg. 7:284, 1964.
5. Shearburn, E. W., and Myers, R. N.: Shouldice repair of inguinal hernia. Surgery 66:450, 1969.
6. Shearburn, E. W., and Myers, R. N.: The problem of the recurrent inguinal hernia. Surg. Clin. North Am. 53:555, 1973.
7. Palumbo, L. T., and Sharpe, W. S.: Primary inguinal hernioplasty in the adult. Surg. Clin. North Am. *51*:1293, 1971.
8. McVay, C. B., and Anson, B. J.: Inguinal and femoral hernioplasty. Surg. Gynecol. Obstet. 88:473, 1949.
9. Maingot, R.: The choice of operation for inguinal hernia with special reference to the slide and lattice or darn procedures. Br. J. Clin. Pract. 27:237, 1973.
10. Moloney, G. E.: Results of nylon darn repairs of herniae. Lancet *1*:273, 1958.
11. Bellis, C. J.: Immediate unrestricted activity after inguinal herniorrhaphy—9727 personal cases with specific reference to local anesthesia and polyester fiber mesh. Int. Surg. 52:107, 1969.
12. Preston, D. J., and Richards, C. F.: Use of wire mesh prostheses in the treatment of hernia—24 years' experience. Surg. Clin. North Am. 53:549, 1973.
13. Lichtenstein, I. L.: *Hernia Repair Without Disability.* St. Louis, Mo., C. V. Mosby Co., 1970, p. 100.

14. Usher, F. C.: Hernia repair with Marlex mesh. Arch. Surg. 84:325, 1962.
15. Ponka, J. L.: The relaxing incision in hernia repair. Am. J. Surg. 115:552, 1968.
16. Harkins, H. N.: The Cooper's ligament repair of direct inguinal hernia. In Nyhus, L. M., and Harkins, H. N. (eds.): Hernia. Philadelphia, J. B. Lippincott Co., 1964, pp. 179–185.
17. Koontz, A. R.: Personal technique and results in inguinal hernia repair. J.A.M.A. 164:29. 1957.
18. McVay, C. B., and Chapp, J. D.: Inguinal and femoral hernioplasty, the evaluation of a basic concept. Ann. Surg. 148:499, 1958.
19. McVay, C. B.: The anatomy of the relaxing incision in inguinal hernioplasty. Quart. Bull. Northwestern Univ. Med. School, 36:245, 1962.
20. Tanner, N. C.: A slide operation for inguinal and femoral hernia. Br. J. Surg. 29:285, 1942.
21. Heifetz, C. J.: Resection of the spermatic cord in selected inguinal hernias. Arch. Surg. 102:36, 1971.
22. Glassow, F.: Is postoperative wound infection following simple inguinal herniorrhaphy a predisposing cause of recurrent hernia? Can. Med. Assoc. J. 91:870, 1964.
23. Welsh, D. R. J.: Hernia surgery—over seventy age group. J. Abdom. Surg. 5:29, 1963.
24. Iles, J. D. H.: Mortality from elective hernia repair. J. Abdom. Surg. 11:87, 1969.
25. Iles, J. D. H.: Specialisation in elective herniorrhaphy. Lancet 1:751, 1965.
26. Hagan, W. H., and Rhoads, J. E.: Inguinal and femoral hernias; a follow-up study. Surg. Gynecol. Obstet. 96:226, 1953.
27. Halverson, K., and McVay, C. B.: Inguinal and femoral hernioplasty: A 22-year study of the authors' methods. Arch. Surg. 101:127, 1970.
28. Glassow, F.: Inguinal hernia in the female. Surg. Gynecol. Obstet. 116:701, 1963.
29. Glassow, F.: An evaluation of the strength of the posterior wall of the inguinal canal in women. Br. J. Surg. 60:342, 1973.
30. Glassow, F.: Femoral hernia in the female. Can. Med. Assoc. J. 93:1346, 1965.
31. Glassow, F.: Femoral hernia in men. Am. J. Surg. 121:637, 1971.
32. Welsh, D. R. J.: Repair of the indirect sliding inguinal hernias. J. Abdom. Surg. 11:204, 1969.
33. Marsden, A. J.: Inguinal hernia—A three-year review of 2000 cases. Br. J. Surg. 49:384, 1961.
34. Nyhus, L. M.: The preperitoneal approach and iliopubic tract repair of all groin hernias. In Nyhus, L. M., and Harkins, H. N. (eds.): Hernia. Philadelphia, J. B. Lippincott Co., 1964, pp. 271–294.
35. Margoles, J. S., and Braun, R. A.: Preperitoneal versus classical hernioplasty. Am. J. Surg. 121:641, 1971.
36. Gaspar, M. R., and Casberg, M. A.: An appraisal of preperitoneal repair of inguinal hernia. Surg. Gynecol. Obstet. 132:207, 1971.
37. Glassow, F.: Femoral hernia: Review of 1,143 consecutive repairs. Ann. Surg. 163:227, 1966.
38. Glassow, F.: Femoral hernia following inguinal herniorrhaphy. Can. J. Surg. 13:27, 1970.
39. Zimmerman, L. M.: Recurrent inguinal hernia. Surg. Clin. North Am. 51:1317, 1321, 1971.

# Halsted-Ferguson Operation for Inguinal Hernia

MARK M. RAVITCH

*The University of Pittsburgh School of Medicine*

The operations for inguinal hernia introduced almost simultaneously by Bassini[2] and Halsted[4] some 85 years ago were immediately and widely recognized as logical and successful solutions to the problem of the radical cure of inguinal hernia. They have been widely used ever since, and numerous smaller or larger modifications have been grafted upon them. To what degree does the continued popularity of these operations and their widespread use reflect tradition and the advantage given to any operation which is the first successful attack upon the problem it is designed to treat? And to what extent does the continued use of the basic principles of these operations represent a recognition of the fact that they do, in fact, solve the problem as well as, or better than, any other operative procedure?

Both Halsted and Bassini recognized that the most important element in their repair, after the appropriate treatment of the sac, was the approximation of strong medial structures—the conjoined tendon of the internal oblique and the transversalis (and, as both of them noted, frequently the lateral border of the rectus sheath)—to Poupart's ligament. Bassini very clearly and specifically mentions the transversalis fascia as part of his medial bite. Halsted, in his first operation with the cord transplanted subcutaneously, again very clearly states that the medial bite engages the transversalis fascia and the lateral bite engages the transversalis fascia as well as the inguinal ligament. The "Hopkins hernia"[7, 9, 11] handed down from father to son from the time of the development of Halsted's second operation (without transplantation of the cord)[5] very clearly ensures that the deep bite through the conjoined tendon, and sometimes the rectus sheath medially, also includes the transversalis fascia itself in the lower portion of the repair. Bassini, and originally Halsted, carried the incision through the transversalis fascia to or above the internal ring. This is still a basic part of the Shouldice repair. After 10 years or more of experimentation with the various modifications of his repair, Halsted, like Ferguson,[3] came to the conclusion that transplantation of the cord was unnecessary and probably harmful. He gave up the long incision through the transversalis and the continuation of this incision through the internal oblique, which led to the recreation of a new internal ring above and lateral to the original one. This second operation, the Halsted-Ferguson herniorrhaphy, without transplantation of the cord, is essentially the one which we perform for all indirect inguinal hernias and for most direct inguinal hernias.[10] (In an occasional patient with an enormous defect, with multiple recurrences, or with fragile structures, we suture the medial structures to Cooper's ligament and transplant the cord subcutaneously.) The same operation is performed on both adults and children, except that in infants we do not perform the vertical paramedian rectus relaxation incision of Halsted and of Berger,[6] nor do we imbricate the aponeurosis of the external oblique. In infants, sutures between the conjoined tendon and Poupart's ligament are taken when there is a palpable gap between these medial structures and the inguinal ligament. We employ interrupted sutures of nonabsorbable material; and, except in children or in unusually complicated cases, we perform the operation under local anesthesia, with minimal sedation, and discharge the patients 1, 2, or 3 days later.

The vertical paramedian relaxation incision in the rectus sheath is made at the time when the medial flap of the aponeurosis has been reflected as close to the midline as it can be separated. At that point, the anterior rectus sheath is incised from beneath the aponeurosis and immediately lateral to its junction with the aponeurosis. The incision should be 2 or 3 cm. long; superiorly it should show the belly of the rectus muscle, and inferiorly, down to the pubis, it should show the belly of the pyramidalis muscle.

Operations bearing the same name performed in different hospitals and by different surgeons may vary widely. As illustrated in the accompanying drawings, the "Johns Hopkins" herniorrhaphy, the operation which Halsted adopted after a decade of experimentation with various combinations and permutations, is in all essential respects similar to that described by Ferguson and may be quite appropriately called the Halsted-Ferguson operation.[10] So that we may all be agreed on the elements of the operation under discussion, the illustrations (Figures 1 to 4) are accompanied by detailed legends.

This operation is, I submit, the simplest and least traumatic effective procedure. "So far as we know, no surgical clinic has undertaken a controlled series of hernia repairs by several techniques which, after several thousand operations and follow-up of all patients for a period of years, would accurately evaluate the merits of the several operations. We venture to believe that such a study would show that, if the sac is ligated high, if the repair is so performed as to produce good apposition of strong tissues, without tension, the details of the various techniques might be found to be of small importance."[9] In the absence of such controlled studies, I am inclined to think that, where disparities in cure rates occur, they may reflect the relative skill of the surgeons reporting rather than the relative merits of the operations performed. In the discussion of the relative merits of several types of hernia repair, of which this presentation is a part, I would wish simply to emphasize the rationale of the Halsted-Ferguson procedure.

*Text continued on page 395*

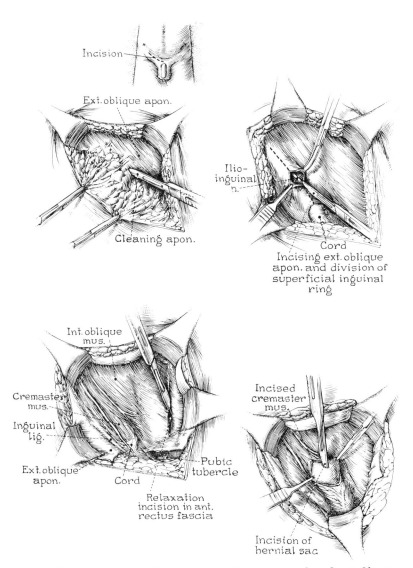

Figure 1. The operation is almost invariably performed under infiltration anesthesia. The incision should be low and extend to the midline, essentially over the pubis. It is this lower portion of the repair which may offer difficulties and in which exposure is most important. The aponeurosis is split in the line of its fibers so as to bisect the external ring. The lateral flap is dissected back to the shelving edge of Poupart's ligament and the medial flap to the point of fusion with the rectus sheath near the midline, at which point the vertical paramedian rectus relaxation incision is made. In the lower portion, this will expose the pyramidalis muscle. (From Ravitch, M. M.: *Repair of Hernias—A Handbook of Operative Surgery.* Chicago, Year Book Medical Publishers, 1969.)

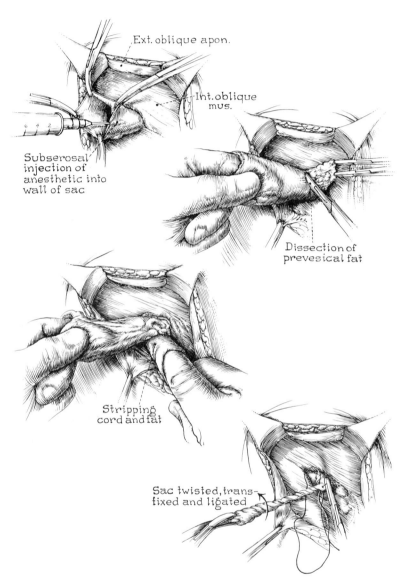

*Figure 2.* The sac may be treated in any of the usual ways, provided that a secure, high ligation is achieved. The only local anesthetic administered after the operation has been begun is injected subserosally into the opened sac. (From Ravitch, M. M.: *Repair of Hernias—A Handbook of Operative Surgery.* Chicago, Year Book Medical Publishers, 1969.)

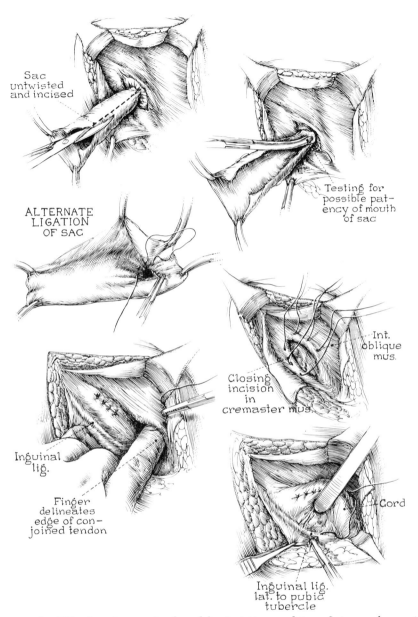

Sac untwisted and incised

ALTERNATE LIGATION OF SAC

Testing for possible patency of mouth of sac

Int. oblique mus.

Closing incision in cremaster mus.

Inguinal lig.

Finger delineates edge of conjoined tendon

Cord

Inguinal lig. lat. to pubic tubercle

*Figure 3.* Whether the sac is closed by twisting and transfixion or by an internally placed purse-string, the security of the closure must be tested before the excess of the sac is cut away. The incision in the cremaster is closed with a few fine silk sutures as a matter of neatness and because covering over the fatty layers about the cord simplifies the placement of the sutures in the next layer.

With the left index finger under the conjoined tendon, a heavy bite is taken of conjoined tendon medially and of the shelving edge of Poupart's ligament laterally. (From Ravitch, M. M.: *Repair of Hernias—A Handbook of Operative Surgery.* Chicago, Year Book Medical Publishers, 1969.)

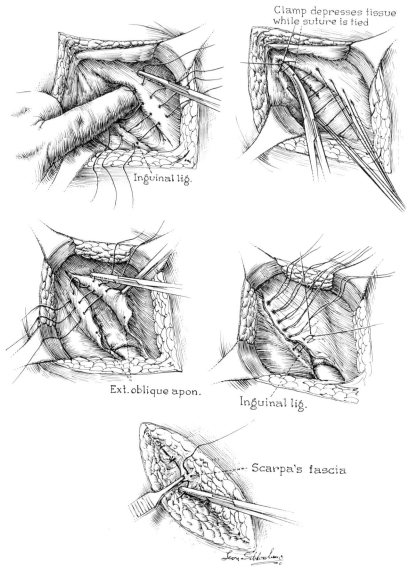

*Figure 4.* The medial bites may very well, and frequently do, include rectus sheath, at least the lower two or three sutures. The superior sutures take fairly large bites of muscle, but they are not under tension and these hold well. These sutures having been tied, the cord now emerges more or less in its normal position, and the internal oblique now attaches almost the entire length of the inguinal ligament, as is the normal situation in individuals without hernias, as Ferguson pointed out. The imbrication of the aponeurosis takes up slack, transfers tension from the deep layer, which is all important, to this layer, and provides for a broad fascia-to-fascia union. (From Ravitch, M. M.: *Repair of Hernias—A Handbook of Operative Surgery.* Chicago, Year Book Medical Publishers, 1969.)

1. The cord is left essentially undisturbed, being allowed to emerge from under the internal oblique. Ferguson[3] demonstrated 75 years ago that a principal factor in the occurrence of indirect inguinal hernia is the deficiency of the lower portion of the attachment of the internal oblique to the inguinal ligament. The Halsted-Ferguson operation corrects this, and transplantation of the cord in no way increases the effectiveness of the reconstruction.

2. The relaxation incision allows the strong medial structures to come over to Poupart's ligament with substantially less tension than would otherwise be the case. One can demonstrate the effect of the vertical paramedian rectus relaxation incision by completing the conjoined tendon–to–Poupart's ligament portion of the repair, then performing the relaxation incision; there is a sudden decrease in tension upon the suture line as the relaxing incision gapes open.

3. Since the medial suture bites not only engage the conjoined tendon but also, going deeply, pick up some of the transversalis fascia lateral to this, a very strong tissue is secured medially for approximation to the inguinal ligament laterally. In the repair of direct hernias particularly, in which the basic problem has been a deterioration in the quality of the transversalis fascia, it has never seemed to me necessary or profitable to run a separate suture line in this attenuated membrane.

4. Lotheissen,[8] to whom we owe the Cooper's ligament repair, pointed out the substantial depth in the wound at which the conjoined tendon–Cooper's ligament sutures were placed, the rigidity of Cooper's ligament, the problem of dealing with the femoral vein, and the frequency with which fluid had accumulated in the depression made by sewing the abdominal wall down so deeply. The point has been frequently made that Cooper's ligament is a good, tough, unyielding structure and that the inguinal ligament, on the other hand, is a somewhat loosely anchored, highly mobile structure. It would seem to us that healing might be at least as satisfactory between two structures that could each yield with strain as between one fixed and one mobile structure.

Fundamentally, I am willing to grant that equally good results can be obtained by any of half a dozen acceptable methods of hernia repair properly performed. Halsted's final deathbed remark in 1922 was to the effect that he had had no recurrences in 20 years. In any case, it is fruitless to compare results of methods of one operation reported by its advocates against those of another operation claimed by advocates of that operation. It is my conviction that each of the standard operations is capable of giving as good results as those of any of the other operations and that comparative statistics of this kind in uncontrolled series are more likely to reflect the skill of the individual operators or possibly their choice of clinical material than the virtues of the individual operations. It is not likely that a controlled clinical experiment of several hundred herniorrhaphies by each of the several methods carried out by the same group of surgeons and followed for 10 or 20 years will ever be performed. We are too far along in the treatment of hernia for this to be undertaken now. It is a truism that controlled clinical trials are valuable only when there is no conviction about the relative virtues of various methods of treatment and that, once a considerable measure of success has been achieved, it is difficult or impossible to undertake clinical trials. I see no virtue in routine transplantation of the cord—either interstitial, as in the Bassini operation, or subcutaneous, as in the initial Halsted operation—and therefore do not ordinarily transplant the cord.

The exposure of Cooper's ligament requires a little additional dissection, invites a little more tension on the suture line, makes for perhaps marginally more technical difficulty, and, in any event, is possible only from the lowest point of the repair to the border of the femoral vein, after which the conjoined tendon must be brought in a step-up around the femoral vein and thereafter must be sutured to the inguinal ligament. In femoral hernias, as Lotheissen pointed out, Cooper's ligament offers the best anchor for the conjoined tendon, thus excluding the femoral ring from the peritoneal boundaries. In inguinal hernias, when repeated repairs, age, or other causes result in a large defect with attenuated structures, Cooper's ligament always remains as a tough, dependable lateral anchor of the repair, but such cases are few.

The preperitoneal herniorrhaphies have a certain attractiveness, particularly if a bilateral repair is to be performed. I suspect they cannot readily be performed under local infiltration anesthesia. Even if we grant that the cure rate of the original hernia could be as high as with any of the other repairs, there is the risk that, if a wound infection results, the patient will acquire not merely a recurrence of his original hernia but also a ventral hernia. Parenthetically, the same may be said for the LaRocque maneuver (simultaneous and separate laparotomy incision for intra-abdominal traction upon and reduction of the incarcerated bowel), which probably needs to be resorted to only rarely, if at all. An exception to this might be a hernia with gangrenous bowel, if one considers a laparotomy for division and anastomosis of the bowel, with subsequent inguinal or femoral resection of the sac en masse, to be a sort of LaRocque maneuver.

5. Imbrication of the aponeurosis of the external oblique, introduced by Andrews[1] and described as part of his operation by Halsted, with the statement that he had been employing this technique before Andrews' publication, is, we think, a significant portion of the repair. Imbrication accomplishes two things. First, the 2-cm. or more overlap transfers the tension from the deep layer, which is the critical layer in the repair, to this tough aponeurotic layer, allowing the deep layer to heal without having to be concerned about holding, while its apposition is maintained by the tension on the aponeurosis. Second, the broad overlap allows for a much stronger fascia-to-fascia union than a mere edge-to-edge closure.

While we employ interrupted sutures of nonabsorbable material, still silk for the most part, the experience with wire goes back to Halsted and before, and the use of a running suture of monofilament nonabsorbable material, whether metal or synthetic, has a certain attractiveness. The use of interrupted sutures allows for a more careful adjustment of tension from one suture to the next, a smaller likelihood of catastrophic breakdown of the repair if a suture should break or come undone, and a smaller problem if infection should result.

# References

1. Andrews, E. W.: Imbrication or lap joint method: A plastic operation for hernia. Chicago Med. Rec. 9:67, 1895.
2. Bassini, E.: Sopra 100 Casi di Cura Radicale dell-Ernia Inguinale Operata col Metodo dell-autore. Archiv. Ed. Atti. Soc. Ital. Chir. 5:315, 1888.
3. Ferguson, A. H.: Oblique inguinal hernia. Typic operation for its radical cure. J.A.M.A. 33:6, 1899.
4. Halsted, W. S.: The radical cure of hernia. Johns Hopkins Hosp. Bull. 1:112, 1890.
5. Halsted, W. S.: The cure of the more difficult as well as the simpler inguinal ruptures. Johns Hopkins Hosp. Bull. 14:208, 1903.
6. Halsted, W. S.: An Additional Note on the Operation for Inguinal Hernia. Surgical papers by William Stewart Halsted. Baltimore, The Johns Hopkins Press, 1924, pp. 306–308.
7. Lewis, D.: Bassini's contribution to the radical cure of hernia. In Fasiana, G. M., and Catterina, A. (eds.): Scritti di Chirurgia Erniaria — per Commemorare il Cinquantenario della Operazione di Bassini. Vol. 1. University of Padua Press, 1937, p. 548.
8. Lotheissen, G.: Zur Radikaloperation der Schenkelhernien. Centralbl. Chir. 25:548, 1898.
9. Ravitch, M. M., and Hitzrot, J. M.: The Operations for Inguinal Hernia. St. Louis, Mo., C. V. Mosby Co., 1960.
10. Ravitch, M. M.: Repair of hernias — A Handbook of Operative Surgery. Chicago, Year Book Medical Publishers, 1969.
11. Rienhoff, W. F., Jr.: The use of the rectus fascia for closure of the lower or critical angle of the wound in the repair of inguinal hernia. Surgery 8:326, 1940.

# 17

# *Local Treatment for Carcinoma of the Rectum*

## Statement of the Problem

Abdominal perineal resection of the rectum for cancer is the standard approach. The authors compare this standard against local excision or destruction of rectal cancers by fulguration with regard to morbidity, mortality, and 5-year survival.

Give data on cure rate of rectal carcinoma by abdominal perineal resection in the presence of lymph node metastases. Cite any information that local measures might "cure" such patients.

What are the limitations of local fulguration with respect to size and location of the lesion; distance from the anus? Which cases are suitable for cure by local destruction? To what degree can a nearly circumferential carcinoma be locally destroyed without local complications or subsequent stricture? What duration of palliation can be expected in such a case?

Compare long-term survival following abdominal perineal resection or low anastomosis with that following local fulguration. Analyze factors of case selection in each clinical series.

Compare complication rates (early and late) and mortality for the two procedures.

# Limitations of Local Treatment of Carcinoma of the Rectum

MAUS W. STEARNS, JR.

*Memorial Sloan-Kettering Cancer Center*

Abdominoperineal resection (APR) is the standard approach for treatment of patients with cancer of the rectum. This statement has to be placed in context and modified before comparing the results of such treatment with those of local excision or destruction by fulguration. To do this I will cite the experience of the Rectal and Colon Service at Memorial Hospital from 1957 to 1967 with clinically infiltrating cancer of the distal 10 cm. of the large bowel.[6]

We performed an abdominoperineal type of resection in less than half of all the resections we did for infiltrating cancer of the distal 10 cm. of the bowel. When the cancer was located within 6 cm. of the anal verge, 90 per cent of patients had abdominoperineal resection, and for this portion of the rectum that was the standard treatment. When the cancer was between 6 and 11 cm., less than a quarter had abdominoperineal resection (Table 1). Very

TABLE 1.  Cancer of the Rectum 1957–1967; Operation and Level of Tumor

| Operation | Level of Tumor | |
|---|---|---|
| | *Below 6 cm.* | *6 to 10 cm.* |
| Total resections | 173 | 322 |
| APR | 155 | 72 |
| AR | 8 | 217 |
| PT | 10 | 33 |
| Utilization | | |
| APR | 90% | 22.4% |
| AR | 4.2 | 67.2 |
| PT | 5.8 | 9.4 |

401

TABLE 2.   Cancer of the Rectum 1957–1967; Operative Mortality Associated with APR

| | Age | |
| --- | --- | --- |
| | *Under 70* | *Over 70* |
| Total resections | 158 | 71 |
| Postoperative deaths | 2 | 6 |
| Postoperative mortality | 1.3% | 8.5% |

few patients with cancer in the upper rectum were electively treated by abdominoperineal resection. In almost all instances when it was done, the AP amputation was for anatomic or pathologic findings which precluded either anterior resection (AR) or pull-through (PT).

High operative mortality rates associated with abdominoperineal resection are cited as serving to negate possible advantages of that procedure over local methods. Our overall postoperative mortality in 229 patients having abdominoperineal resection was 3.5 per cent (8 patients). When we analyzed the causes of death in this group, it was apparent that age was the most important factor (Table 2); postoperative mortality was 1.3 per cent in patients under 70 and 8.5 per cent in those 70 and older. Both Crile and Turnbull[2] and Madden and Kandalaft[4] report no operative mortality associated with fulguration. This has not been our experience, as we have already had one postoperative death following fulguration in an 82-year-old male.

Undoubtedly, the postoperative complications following abdominoperineal resection are more frequent and more severe than those following fulguration. However, the complications following fulguration, as reported by Madden and Kandalaft,[4] are not insignificant. Of the 77 patients in their series, 7 required operative control of bleeding, 2 had perforation into the peritoneal cavity, and 2 developed rectovaginal fistulas.

Poor survival rates following resection in patients with cancer of the rectum having positive nodes (regional nodal metastases) are cited[4] and are apparently the basis for abandoning attempts to salvage these patients by resection. No better alternative way of treating these metastases has been offered.

The survival in our series following curative resections for cancer in the lower and upper rectum with and without regional nodal metastases is shown in Table 3. It is apparent that the prognosis is poorer for the lower-lying than for the higher lesions. This is most marked when regional nodal metastases are present. Particularly relevant to this controversy is the observation that the absolute 5-year survival without recurrent cancer at any time (N.E.C.) during the follow-up period for patients who had cancer of the upper rectum (6 to 11 cm.) and regional nodal metastases was 37 per cent—43 cured of 117 resected. It should be emphasized that more than 75 per cent of these were treated by sphincter-preserving procedures without a permanent colostomy. Less than a quarter had permanent colostomies. Many of those having abdominoperineal resections had lesions that were annular or that extensively infiltrated the vaginal wall, in which local treatment would have been precluded, as stated by Madden and Kandalaft.[4]

In view of these results as applied to the upper rectum, we believe the frequency of "cures" for patients with regional metastases is sufficient to warrant continuation of resection, even though a small number of patients will require abdominoperineal resection to effect this salvage.

The results following resection in those patients with regional nodal metastases and in those whose tumors were in the lower rectum (below 6 cm.) (90 per cent of whom had abdominoperineal resection) are less favorable — 26.5 per cent N.E.C., as indicated in Table 3. Crile and Turnbull,[2] in support of fulguration as opposed to abdominoperineal resection, stated that "the permanent cure for the patient with nodes involved and who were treated by abdomino-perineal resection was only 20%. Since only a third of the patients treated by resection had carcinoma in the nodes, the survival of 20% of them failed to compensate for the 5% immediate and delayed postoperative mortality rate of combined abdomino-perineal resections applied to the entire group." Our data pertinent to this aspect of the discussion are shown in Table 4. These data refer only to abdominoperineal resection. "Cured" refers to the 5-year survivors who did not develop cancer at any time in their subsequent course. Thus, in 158 patients under 70 years of age 2 died postresection; 16 of 60 with regional nodal metastases were "cures" — a positive balance of 14 patients. This appears to be a significant salvage and worth continuing efforts to attain. However, in those patients 70 and over, 6 of 71 died after resection, and only 4 of 27 with regional nodal metastases were "cures" — a net loss of 2 patients. While these data seem to justify continuance of resection for cancer of the lower rectum in patients

TABLE 3.   Survival in Terms of Location of Primary Tumor and Status of Regional Nodes — 1957–1967

|  | Nodes Negative | | Nodes Positive | |
|---|---|---|---|---|
|  | Below 6 cm. | 6 to 11 cm. | Below 6 cm. | 6 to 11 cm. |
| Number resections | 112 | 193 | 61 | 129 |
| Indeterminate | 20 | 30 | 12 | 12 |
| Five-year survivors | 67 | 130 | 17 | 51 |
| Cancer after 5 years | 8 | 12 | 4 | 8 |
| Five-year survival (%) |  |  |  |  |
| Overall* | 60 | 67 | 28 | 40 |
| Determinate† | 73 | 80 | 35 | 44 |
| N.E.C.‡ | 64 | 72 | 26.5 | 37 |

*Overall — 5-year survivors/total resections.
†Determinate — 5-year survivors/determinate patients (total resected excluding postoperative deaths, those dying of other disease without evidence of cancer in less than 5 years).
‡N.E.C. — 5-year survivors excluding those with recurrence after 5 years/determinate.

TABLE 4.   Mortality and "Cures" in Terms of Age of Patient

|  | Under 70 Years | 70 Years and Over |
| --- | --- | --- |
| Total resections | 158 | 71 |
| Postoperative deaths | 2 (1.3%) | 6 (8.5%) |
| With nodal metastases | 60 (38%) | 27 (38%) |
| "Cured" | 16 (29%) | 4 (24%) |

under 70 as an effective means of salvaging those with regional nodal metastases, they do not support its effectiveness in the older patients.

The foregoing data are related to patients with regional nodal metastases. Those who advocate local treatment—which offers no treatment of metastases—have apparently given up on these patients, who represent 35 to 40 per cent of all patients with rectal cancer, as being beyond reasonable expectation of cure.

When we consider the effectiveness of local control of the tumor by fulguration or resection, comparisons based on published data are quite difficult since the series of those treated by fulguration are small and overall comparisons are not particularly meaningful. There are some areas in which we can evaluate the data available in the reports by Crile and Turnbull[2] and Madden and Kandalaft.[4] First, in both reviews, survival has been reported according to configuration of the primary lesion. In the data of Crile and Turnbull, 25 of 27 patients (95 per cent) with polypoid lesions treated by fulguration survived 5 years, although 3 developed carcinoma later and 1 required abdominoperineal resection. Thus, 21 of 27 (78 per cent) were "cures" following fulguration as the sole treatment. In Madden and Kandalaft's series, there were 34 patients with polypoid cancer, of whom 21 (61.7 per cent) were alive and well after fulguration, with an average survival of 50.8 months. (It is impossible to determine from this paper how many of the group had been treated 5 or more years previously.) The overall 5-year survival for patients with polypoid cancer of the rectum following resection at Memorial Hospital, as reported by Berg, was 82 per cent.[1]

Crile and Turnbull reported on 35 patients with ulcerative lesions; 18 lived 5 years, but 2 died subsequently of carcinoma and 7 required resection. Thus, only 9 of the 35 (26 per cent) were "cures" following fulguration as the sole method of treatment. Madden and Kandalaft reported 26 patients with ulcerative and 6 with encircling lesions, of whom 13 patients were alive, although 1 had required abdominoperineal resection. Thus, 12 of 32 patients (38 per cent) with ulcerative or encircling lesions were alive following fulguration as the sole method of treatment. (Again the follow-up period is not identifiable from the report.) Berg reported a 57 per cent 5-year survival following resection in patients with similar lesions.[1] This type of lesion constitutes the majority of rectal cancers.

It would appear that, although a very satisfactory survival rate can be obtained by the local treatment of polypoid carcinoma, it is still not as high as that following resection. When the primary lesion is ulcerative or encircling, the results following resection appear to be 20 to 30 per cent better than those following fulguration alone.

## Discussion and Conclusions

Local methods of treatment—local excision, cautery snare removal, fulguration—have been shown to be quite satisfactory for villous adenomas, even though histologically infiltrating adenocarcinoma may be reported.[3, 5] The important clinical distinction is whether or not clinical infiltration of the cancer into the true muscle of the bowel wall is present.

Local methods of treatment of bulky polypoid cancer give good long-term results. They are somewhat poorer than the results following resection, probably because a number of lesions with deep infiltration into the bowel wall are included. If these were excluded, the results probably would be the same.

Attempts at local control without resection by local excision, fulguration, or high-dose, low-voltage radiation of favorable but clinically infiltrating rectal cancer are probably justified in patients with significant distant metastases, in those who are senile or otherwise incapable of caring for a colostomy, and in those who absolutely refuse a colostomy. However, with annular lesions, those invading the rectovaginal septum, or those deeply infiltrating, local methods are usually not very successful. Palliation in these patients is generally more effectively achieved by resection.

In the large majority of patients with clinically infiltrating cancer of the rectum, resection is indicated. Those having resection for ulcerative or encircling lesions have a substantially better (20 to 30 per cent) survival rate than those having fulguration alone.

Local methods of treatment offer no hope for those with regional metastases (35 to 40 per cent of all patients with clinically infiltrating cancer of the bowel), whereas resection does. In the upper rectum, resection was followed by 37 per cent "cure." To effect this, somewhat less than a quarter of patients required abdominoperineal resection; the remainder had a sphincter-preserving procedure. Among patients under 70 with cancer in the lower rectum, a substantial number in excess of the operative deaths were "cured." These would not have been salvaged by local measures. However, in the group aged 70 and over, resection could not be justified solely on the basis of its effectiveness in curing patients with regional nodal metastases. Other considerations relating to the mental and physical abilities of the patient, the clinical presentation and extent of the tumor, and the informed wishes of the patient become determining factors.

## References

1. Berg, J. W., Schottenfeld, D., Hutter, R. V. P., and Foote, F. W.: *Histology, Epidemiology and End Results.* The Memorial Hospital Cancer Registry, 1969, pp. 26–27.

2. Crile, G. J., and Turnbull, R. B., Jr.: The role of electrocoagulation in the treatment of carcinoma of the rectum. Surg. Gynecol. Obstet. *135*:391, 1972.
3. Jackman, R. J.: Conservative management of selected patients with carcinoma of the rectum. Dis. Colon Rectum *4*:429, 1961.
4. Madden, J. L., and Kandalaft, S.: Clinical evaluation of electrocoagulation in the treatment of cancer of the rectum. Am. J. Surg. *122*:347, 1971.
5. Quan, S. H. Q., and Castro, E. B.: Papillary adenoma (villous tumors): a review of 215 cases. Dis. Colon Rectum *14*:267, 1971.
6. Stearns, M. W., Jr.: The choice among anterior resection, the pull-through, and abdomino-perineal resection of the rectum. Cancer (Suppl.) *34*:969, 1974.

# Conservative Management of Certain Selected Cancers of the Lower Rectum

CLYDE E. CULP

*Mayo Clinic and Mayo Foundation*

Although abdominoperineal resection has become the standard procedure in the management of a low-lying rectal cancer, there are occasions—patient refusal or his declining general physical state—when a conservative approach must be considered. Cancer that involves the upper or the middle portion of the rectum often allows a sphincter-saving procedure to be performed. With a low-lying cancer, a colostomy is necessitated because a restorative resection usually cannot be accomplished.

To embark upon the conservative course with a "cure" in mind, the surgeon must follow rigid guidelines in patient selection; otherwise, the treatment is "palliative." A surgeon who considers these guidelines but does not apply them rigidly in his patient selection is providing less than the best management, just as is the surgeon who fails to recognize that a conservative approach is possible for selected patients. To justify routine deviation from the standard management of the low-lying rectal cancer, comparable or improved rates of morbidity and mortality with the conservative approach must be demonstrated.

In selected cases, there is justification for a conservative approach. In 1961, Jackman[5] reported the results of conservative management in 252 selected patients with carcinoma of the rectum who were seen at the Mayo Clinic. Madden and Kandalaft[6–8] and more recently Crile and Turnbull[2] have reported on the survival of patients with "low-lying" rectal carcinomas who were treated by electrocoagulation.

The low-lying neoplasm is difficult to define in its relationship to the anal verge or dentate margin. Crile and Turnbull[2] estimated that such lesions were not more than 10 cm. from the anus and at or below the level of the peritoneal reflection. Madden and Kandalaft[7,8] stated that 90 per cent of

407

their patients had lesions that were between 2 and 10 cm. from the anal orifice. The report by Culp and Jackman[3] considered the distal 8 cm. of the rectum, but a restorative resection often can be carried out for malignant lesions that are located between 6 and 8 cm. from the dentate line. Cancer presenting in the distal 6 cm. of the rectum most often necessitates a Miles procedure. Of all rectal carcinomas, lesions arising in the distal 6 cm. have the least favorable prognosis.

## Selection of Patients

Because the length of the anal canal varies from 1.5 to 5 cm.,[1, 4, 9] in the present report the dentate margin (line) or mucocutaneous junction will be considered the point of reference for the location of the rectal lesions. Therefore, only those cancers located in the distal 6 cm. of the rectum were considered low-lying lesions.

Conservative management encompasses those modalities considered to be local therapy. Many of the lesions in the present series were treated by fulguration, whereas others were excised in toto, including the muscular wall of the rectum. Radium plaque(s) was used as an adjunct for most patients.

To confirm the invasive malignancy of each lesion, all biopsy specimens were reassessed by a surgical pathologist. Similarly, when an operative specimen was available, the histopathologic findings were reviewed, and the lesion was classified by the Dukes method. Excluded from the study were patients whose rectal cancers arose in adenomas or villous tumors.

Most patients were selected for conservative management because of their refusal to undergo the abdominoperineal procedure. Others were selected because physical or mental impairments increased the operative risk of a radical operative procedure. The patients were divided into two groups: operable and inoperable.

Patients who had resectable cancers but who declined radical operation were placed in the operable group. This group also included several patients treated before 1950 whose physical disability or age was a contraindication to the Miles procedure. Patients who had malignant tumors that were limited and who thus were considered treatable by local measures were also in the operable group.

Patients with physical or mental difficulties that increased the risk of the Miles procedure or affected the care of the resultant colostomy were placed in the inoperable group. The main physical difficulties were cardiac or respiratory problems, but there were some patients with coexisting malignant disease, usually of another organ system. Senility, syphilitic paresis, cerebral insufficiency, pemphigus, and pregnancy, as well as extreme obesity with or without diabetes, were additional reasons for placement in the inoperable group.

There were 67 patients (37 men and 30 women) in the present series. This included 34 patients from Jackman's original series[5] in whom reevaluation confirmed invasive malignancy. The other 33 patients have been treated since 1961 by various members of the Section of Proctologic Surgery. The average age was 63.6 years, the youngest patient being a 31-year-old pregnant woman and the oldest an 89-year-old woman. The operable group comprised 48 patients (24 men and 24 women) whose average age was 61.8 years. The inoperable group consisted of 19 patients (13 men and 6 women) whose average age was 68.1 years.

# Evaluation of Lesions

### Size and Gross Characteristics

As determined at proctoscopy, the lesions ranged in size from one that was 0.6 cm. in diameter to one that was almost annular. The diameters of 56 lesions ranged between 1 and 4 cm.; 3 had diameters less than 1 cm., and 5 had diameters greater than 5 cm.; for 3 lesions, the size was not stated.

The lesions were described by the proctoscopist as being one or more of the following: flat, ulcerated, eroded, carcinomatous, sessile, polypoid (no true pedicle), indurated, or infiltrated. From this gross description the tumors were categorized into two types: ulcerative[2, 7] and polypoid carcinomas. Thirty-nine patients had ulcerative lesions and 28 had polypoid lesions. Of the 67 lesions, 36 (53.7 per cent), whether polypoid or ulcerative, were mobile or movable to the examining finger or the edge of the proctosigmoidoscope.

### Pathologic Features

Of the 67 lesions, 2 were Grade 4 by Broders' classification, 4 were Grade 3, and 12 were invasive Grade 1 tumors. The remaining 49 lesions were Grade 2 adenocarcinomas.

Twenty operative specimens resulting from local extirpation of the lesion were categorized according to the Kirklin modification of Dukes' classification of rectal cancer. Of these 20 specimens, 1 lesion was Dukes A (mucosal involvement), 1 was Dukes C (nodal involvement), and 18 were Dukes B, with 13 being $B_1$ (into muscularis propria) and 5, $B_2$ (through muscularis propria).

# Treatment

In this series, conservative treatment of rectal cancer was defined as local therapy involving fulguration, local excision, or cautery snare, often supplemented by the use of radium.

Fulguration is a form of electrocoagulation in which the active electrode is held a few millimeters from the surface of the lesion. With activation, a shower of sparks emanates from the blunt tip of the electrode, causing destruction of the lesion by electrodesiccation. Madden and Kandalaft,[7, 8] in describing their technique, used a needlepoint electrode inserted into the tissue and applied the coagulation current of a Bovie type of unit. Crile and Turnbull[2] utilized a brass wire loop electrode of about 1 cm. in diameter and a low-intensity cutting current to remove the malignant tissue. Whatever type of electrocautery is selected, thorough application to the lesion is most important.

Mobile polypoid but sessile cancers may be removed by excision with the electrocautery snare. Fulguration of the exposed muscle may be supplemental treatment.

In local excision of a small rectal carcinoma, either most or all of the underlying rectal wall should be included.

All of these procedures are conducted with the patient under caudal anesthesia. Adequate relaxation of the anorectal sphincters is provided to allow exposure of the lesions with the use of a bivalved anal speculum or retractors. A proctosigmoidoscope with a vent for removal of smoke is used for most of the fulguration procedures.

Radium plaque(s) can be applied by the therapeutic radiologist to the treated area. Although the radium can be placed during the original treatment, placement should be delayed until the fulguration slough has begun to separate. Inspection of the resultant ulcer may reveal additional neoplastic tissue that needs to be treated.

Fulguration was used to treat 36 patients in the operable group, with radium as an added modality in 18 patients. The growth was excised in 12 patients either by scalpel or by electrocautery snare; radium was applied in 6 of these (Table 1).

Similar methods were employed to treat patients in the inoperable group. Fulguration alone was not used, but 11 patients had combined fulguration and radium. The cancer was excised in 8 patients, and radium was applied in 3 of these (Table 1).

TABLE 1.   Results of Conservative Treatment for Carcinoma of the Lower Rectum*

| Method | Operable Group (48 Patients) | | | | Inoperable Group (19 Patients) | | | | Overall Total |
|---|---|---|---|---|---|---|---|---|---|
| | Alive and Well | Unrelated Death | Treatment Failed | Total | Alive and Well | Unrelated Death | Treatment Failed | Total | |
| Fulguration | | | | | | | | | |
| Alone | 7 (7)† | 6 (5) | 5 (4)‡ | 18 (16) | 0 | 0 | 0 | 0 | 18 |
| With radium | 10 (10) | 5 (5) | 3 (1) | 18 (16) | 1 (0) | 5 (1) | 5 (0) | 11 (1) | 29 |
| Excision | | | | | | | | | |
| Alone | 3 (1) | 2 (2) | 1 (1) | 6 (4) | 1 (1) | 3 (3) | 1 (0) | 5 (4) | 11 |
| With radium | 2 (2) | 1 (1) | 2 (0) | 5 (3) | 2 (2) | 1 (0) | 0 | 3 (2) | 8 |
| Cautery snare with radium | 1 (0) | 0 | 0 | 1 (0) | 0 | 0 | 0 | 0 | 1 |
| Total | 23 (20) | 14 (13) | 11 (6) | 48 (39) | 4 (3) | 9 (4) | 6 (0) | 19 (7) | 67 |

*Distal 6 cm. of rectum.
†Numbers within parentheses represent status at 5-year follow-up.
‡One patient died of cancer, survived more than 5 years.

Only 1 of the 67 patients suffered a complication after conservative therapy; difficulties have been reported by others.[7, 8] The one complication involved a patient who was placed in the inoperable group because of macroglobulinemia. This patient had postfulguration bleeding of sufficient degree to require blood replacement.

## Results

The patients either returned to the clinic for examination or answered letters sent periodically by the Department of Statistics. Forty-six of the 67 patients were followed for 5 years or more. In the operable group, 39 of the 48 patients were followed for 5 years or more, with 14 reporting their progress for 15 years or more. The inoperable group, as might be expected, had a shorter follow-up. However, of the 19 patients in this group, 13 survived 5 years or more and 4 died of unrelated causes; of these 7, 3 were followed for 10 years or more.

Fulguration alone or combined with radium was used in 47 patients (Table 1). The remaining 20 patients underwent local excision of the tumor. For 9 of these patients radium was added, and in 1 patient electrocautery snare was utilized. Of the 20 patients whose lesion was excised locally, 9 were alive and well and 7 were dead of unrelated causes.

A patient was considered to be a treatment failure if recurrent malignant tissue was present at any time during the follow-up period, even though additional local treatment was successful. Four patients treated by fulguration alone were treatment failures; however, one of these patients lived more than 5 years before dying of cancer.

Of the 67 patients, 17 (25 per cent) were treatment failures. Secondary treatment, either radical resection (8 patients) or further local therapy (9 patients), was done in these 17 patients (Table 2). Of the 17 patients, 11 died of rectal cancer, and 1 patient died during the immediate postoperative period after a Miles procedure. Of the other 5 patients, 2 were alive and apparently free of rectal cancer 6 years or more from the time of their original conservative treatment, and 3 patients died of unrelated causes. These 5 patients had undergone secondary treatment that included additional local therapy in 4 and radical operation in 1.

Of the 48 patients in the operable group, 11 were treatment failures. Two were dead of rectal cancer: one woman with a Grade 4 lesion died at 4 months, and a man died at 2 years. Four patients lived 4 years or more before they died of rectal cancer. The remaining 5 patients who were treatment failures have survived 5 years or more. Of these 11 patients, 5 had fulguration, 3 had fulguration and radium, and 3 had local excision. Radium was used as supplemental treatment in 2 of the 3 patients managed by local excision of the neoplasm. Five of the 11 patients underwent abdominoperineal resection: 1 died after operation necessitated by recurrent cancer 4 years after the original local therapy; a second patient died of a heart attack 13 years after the operation; and a third patient was alive and well 6½ years

TABLE 2.    Fate of 17 Patients in Whom Conservative Management for Carcinoma
of the Lower Rectum* Failed

| Method | Operable Group (11 Patients) | | | | Inoperable Group (6 Patients) | | | | Overall Total |
|---|---|---|---|---|---|---|---|---|---|
| | Died, Cancer | Alive and Well | Unrelated Death | Total | Died, Cancer | Alive and Well | Unrelated Death | Total | |
| Fulguration | | | | | | | | | |
| Alone | 2† | 0 | 3 | 5/18 | 0 | 0 | 0 | 0 | 5/18 |
| With radium | 2‡ | 1 | 0 | 3/18 | 5 | 0 | 0 | 5/11 | 8/29 |
| Excision | | | | | | | | | |
| Alone | 0 | 1 | 0 | 1/6 | 1 | 0 | 0 | 1/5 | 2/11 |
| With radium | 2 | 0 | 0 | 2/5 | 0 | 0 | 0 | 0/3 | 2/8 |
| Total | 6 | 2 | 3 | 11/47 | 6 | 0 | 0 | 6/19 | 17/66§ |

*Distal 6 cm. of rectum.
†One patient lived more than 5 years.
‡One patient died after Miles procedure.
§One patient excluded from series (patient with cautery snare without failure).

later. The remaining 2 patients had recurrent tumors 1 and 2 years after resection. Additional local therapy seemed to be sufficient, because 2 of 3 patients died of unrelated causes 17 and 18 years later. The third patient developed a second recurrence 8½ years after the initial treatment and was treated by fulguration and radium at the age of 91 years; when she was reexamined 18 months later, the treated area in the rectum was negative.

Of the 19 patients in the inoperable group, 6 were treatment failures. Although 15 patients died, only 6 of the deaths were directly attributed to rectal carcinoma. Of these 6 patients whose treatment failed, 5 had fulguration and radium, and the other patient had excision of a Dukes B₂ lesion. These 6 patients in the inoperable group who died of their disease did not tolerate the recurrence as well as did those in the operable group. Only 1 patient lived 4 years, but 4 others lived more than 2 years.

A tumor of Broders' Grade 2 may be considered to represent an average degree of malignancy. Forty-nine of the 67 low-lying rectal cancers were Grade 2. Thirty-two patients in the operable group had Grade 2 lesions, and 27 of these survived 5 or more years (Table 3). Seventeen patients in the inoperable group had Grade 2 lesions. Of these 17 patients, 11 did not survive 5 years, but none of the deaths could be attributed to rectal cancer. Of the 49 patients with Grade 2 cancers, 32 were treated by fulguration. The 10 patients in whom fulguration was used alone survived 5 years, whereas only 12 of the 22 to whom supplemental radium was applied were alive at 5 years (Table 3). Local excision was done in 9 patients, and 6 survived 5 years. Radium as an adjunct to local excision was used in 7 other patients, and 5 of these were alive and well at 5 years.

Of the 67 patients, 23 have died from causes unrelated to rectal malignancy. Fourteen of the 23 were in the operable group. The autopsy was negative for carcinoma in one case, and in 9 others the survivor informants specifically noted that the rectal condition had not recurred. Nine of the patients in the inoperable group died from conditions unrelated to rectal carcinoma. Autopsy studies were carried out in 3 cases, with negative findings for rectal cancer. In 3 other cases, the rectal condition was reported by their relatives to be negative for cancer at the time of the patient's death.

The prognosis in low-lying rectal cancer is guarded, even when there is no nodal involvement. The overall 5-year survival rate has not been substantially improved over the years, although resectability rates have gradually increased. A comparison of several studies was made to determine the 5-year survival in reference to the level of the rectal carcinoma. Waugh and Kirklin[11] reported a 5-year survival of 43 of 93 patients (46 per cent) when the tumor was located from 0 to 5 cm. above the "anal margin." Stearns and Binkley[10] found that when the rectal lesion was between 0 and 6 cm. from the "anal margin," 64 of 121 patients (53 per cent) survived 5 years. Of the 67 patients in the present series, 46 (69 per cent) survived 5 years. When patients with Grade 2 lesions were studied for 5-year survival, Waugh and Kriklin[11] found that 30 of 66 patients were alive, Stearns and Binkley[10] reported that 37 of 62 patients survived, and 33 of 49 patients in the present series were alive.

## Discussion

Among patients with rectal carcinoma, the most suitable candidates for conservative management are those with small lesions (less than 4 cm. in diameter), mobile lesions, and protuberant or polypoid (rather than flat, ulcerated) growths.

When fulguration is used to destroy the tumor, the charred tissue should be wiped away with a gauzed finger or picked free with forceps. The process should be continued until neoplastic tissue is no longer evident. Fulguration should include a border of normal-appearing tissue. Frozen-section studies of suspect tissue should be done. After the tumor has been removed completely, the defect is charred further to reduce the chance of troublesome

TABLE 3.   Results of Conservative Treatment for Carcinoma of Grade 2 of the Lower Rectum*

| Method | Operable Group (32 Patients) | | | | Inoperable Group (17 Patients) | | | | Overall Total |
|---|---|---|---|---|---|---|---|---|---|
| | Alive and Well | Unrelated Death | Treatment Failed | Total | Alive and Well | Unrelated Death | Treatment Failed | Total | |
| Fulguration | | | | | | | | | |
| Alone | 4 (4)† | 4 (4) | 2 (2)‡ | 10 (10) | 0 | 0 | 0 | 0 | 10 (10) |
| With radium | 8 (8) | 3 (3) | 2 (1) | 13 (12) | 0 | 4 (0) | 5 (0) | 9 (0) | 22 (12) |
| Excision | | | | | | | | | |
| Alone | 2 (0) | 1 (1) | 1 (1) | 4 (2) | 1 (1) | 3 (3) | 1 (0) | 5 (4) | 9 (6) |
| With radium | 2 (2) | 1 (1) | 1 (0) | 4 (3) | 2 (2) | 1 (0) | 0 | 3 (2) | 7 (5) |
| Cautery snare with radium | 1 (0) | 0 | 0 | 1 (0) | 0 | 0 | 0 | 0 | 1 (0) |
| Total | 17 (14) | 9 (9) | 6 (4) | 32 (27) | 3 (3) | 8 (3) | 6 (0) | 17 (6) | 49 (33) |

*Distal 6 cm. of rectum.
†Numbers within parentheses represent status at 5-year follow-up.
‡One patient died of cancer, survived more than 5 years.

oozing of blood. The fulgurated area sloughs away from the underlying tissue in 3 to 5 days. The wound should be inspected and further treatment done if necessary. Frequent follow-up examinations should be carried out to ascertain the state of the treated site in the rectum.

## Summary

At times, the surgeon is confronted by problems that make it necessary for him to deviate from standard practices. When a patient with a low-lying rectal cancer has steadfastly refused to accept radical operation or is in poor physical condition, a conservative method should be considered. Evaluation of 67 selected patients with low-lying rectal cancer who were treated by conservative means (fulguration, excision, or cautery snare, with or without application of radium) revealed that the patients could be placed into two groups, depending on the indication for conservative treatment. The operable group was composed of 48 patients, most of whom did not wish to undergo a radical operative procedure, whereas the inoperable group of 19 patients had physical or mental disturbances that contraindicated radical operation. Of the 67 patients, 46 were alive at 5 years (overall survival rate of 69 per cent). Conservative treatment failed in 17 (25 per cent). Twelve of the 17 patients died from rectal cancer, including 1 patient who died during the immediate postoperative period; 3 died of causes unrelated to rectal tumor, and 2 have survived 5 years or more.

ACKNOWLEDGMENTS: Dr. Louis H. Weiland of the Department of Surgical Pathology, Mayo Clinic, reviewed many of the histopathologic specimens.

## References

1. Bacon, H. E., and Recio, P. M.: *Surgical Anatomy of the Colon, Rectum and Anal Canal.* Philadelphia, J. B. Lippincott Co., 1962, p. 57.
2. Crile, G., Jr., and Turnbull, R. B.: The role of electrocoagulation in the treatment of carcinoma of the rectum. Surg. Gynecol. Obstet. *135*:391, 1972.
3. Culp, C. E., and Jackman, R. J.: Reappraisal of conservative management of certain selected cancers of the rectum. *In* Najarian, J. S., and Delaney, J.P.: *Surgery of the Gastrointestinal Tract.* New York, Intercontinental Medical Book Corp., 1974, pp. 511–519.
4. Gorsch, R. V.: *Proctologic Anatomy.* 2nd ed. Baltimore, The Williams & Wilkins Co., 1955, p. 5.
5. Jackman, R. J.: Conservative management of selected patients with carcinoma of the rectum. Dis. Colon Rectum *4*:429, 1961.
6. Madden, J. L., and Kandalaft, S.: Electrocoagulation: a primary and preferred method of treatment for cancer of the rectum. Ann. Surg. *166*:413, 1967.
7. Madden, J. L., and Kandalaft, S.: Clinical evaluation of electrocoagulation in the treatment of cancer of the rectum. Am. J. Surg. *122*:347, 1971.
8. Madden, J. L., and Kandalaft, S.: Electrocoagulation in the treatment of cancer of the rectum: a continuing study. Ann. Surg. *174*:530, 1971.
9. Nesselrod, J. P.: *Clinical Proctology.* 3rd ed. Philadelphia, W. B. Saunders Co., 1964, p. 2.
10. Stearns, M. W., Jr., and Binkley, G. E.: The influence of location on prognosis in operable rectal cancer. Surg. Gynecol. Obstet. *96*:368, 1953.
11. Waugh, J. M., and Kirklin, J. W.: The importance of the level of the lesion in the prognosis and treatment of carcinoma of the rectum and low sigmoid colon. Ann. Surg. *129*:22, 1949.

# 18

# *Preoperative Radiation in the Therapy of Rectal Carcinoma*

PREOPERATIVE RADIATION
FOR RECTAL CANCER
*by Theodor B. Grage*

## Statement of the Problem

One author discusses monetary costs, morbidity, and long-term results after preoperative radiation for carcinoma of the rectum.

Analyze relevant data indicating that preliminary x-ray treatment alters the cure rate of operation for carcinoma of the rectum.

Cite data regarding cures obtained in rectal carcinoma treated by radiation alone. After preoperative radiation, what is the frequency of finding no residual tumor on pathologic examination of the resected specimen.

Discuss timing, dosage, and ports used for preoperative irradiation, particularly with respect to morbidity.

Discuss information on adverse effects of preoperative radiation on the healing of low anastomoses. Does it alter perineal healing after proctectomy? Does radiation unfavorably influence healing of the abdominal incision?

Examine data which support the proposition that delay for preoperative radiation may adversely influence the outcome.

# Preoperative Radiation for Rectal Cancer*

**THEODOR B. GRAGE**

*University of Minnesota Health Sciences Center*

## Introduction

Operative resection continues to be the primary form of treatment for the patient with carcinoma of the rectum. In recent years, it has become increasingly clear that the salvage rates for carcinoma of the rectum have reached a plateau, and it is unlikely that further significant improvement will be forthcoming using operative resection alone. Despite all educational efforts to make the diagnosis of rectal cancer earlier, there has been no significant change in the incidence of the different stages of rectal cancer over the past 25 years.

The concept of radiation therapy as an adjuvant in the treatment of rectal cancer dates back to 1914, when treatment with radium resulted in complete disappearance of a gross tumor.[1] Subsequent use of radiation therapy in the treatment of rectal cancer has been characterized by periods of enthusiastic acceptance followed by disillusionment with this technique.[2, 3] Yet there are compelling reasons for reevaluating the use of preoperative radiation in the operative treatment of rectal carcinomas. In recent years, substantial progress has been made in our understanding of cellular responses to radiation therapy. The development and refinement of modern megavoltage radiation equipment and its greater availability are important considerations; moreover, there is an increasing recognition that local recurrence rates remain distressingly high after radical operations. They may be a major cause of treatment failure in rectal carcinoma. These aspects compel us to reexamine the use of preoperative radiation therapy.

Let us examine the evidence for this combined-modality treatment approach. Despite a wealth of clinical information on the use of radiation therapy in the treatment of rectal cancer, there have been very few well-con-

*Supported by U.S.P.H.S. No. CA 12282.

417

trolled prospective clinical trials clearly defining the benefits and the potential disadvantages of preoperative radiation therapy in the treatment of rectal cancer. However, well-designed, prospectively randomized clinical trials are now in progress.

## Magnitude of the Problem

The American Cancer Society estimates an incidence of about 100,000 new cases of cancer of the colon and rectum in this country for 1975, with 49,000 deaths predicted from this disease, of which 38,600 will be from colon cancer and 10,400 from rectal cancer.[4] Progressive improvement in supportive measures and operative skills during the past 30 years has materially increased the operability or resectability rates of rectal cancers, while the operative mortality rate has declined.[5] The experience of the University of Minnesota Hospitals in the treatment of rectal cancer from 1940 to 1959 revealed an overall 5-year survival rate of 27 per cent for the first decade and 30 per cent for the second decade.[6] The resectability rate rose from 76 per cent for the first period to 85 per cent in the second period.

A review of 830 cases of adenocarcinoma of the rectum treated at the Yale-New Haven Medical Center for three decades, from 1931 through 1960, revealed an increase in operability rates from 69 per cent to 73 per cent to 87 per cent, respectively.[7] The corresponding figures for the operative mortality were 21 per cent in the first decade, then 5 per cent and 8 per cent in the most recent two decades. Although improved, the overall 5-year survival rate remained discouragingly low. It was 17 per cent for all patients seen in the first decade, 21 per cent in the second decade, and 34 per cent in the last decade. Of those patients operated upon for cure, the respective survival rates were 30 per cent, 34 per cent, and 46 per cent.

Data from the End Results Group show that there has been virtually no improvement in the 3-year and 5-year survival rates for carcinoma of the rectum since 1950.[8] (Table 1). Furthermore, the stage distribution for cancer of the rectum has remained rather static throughout the three decades (Table 2).

## Radiation Therapy in the Treatment of Rectal Cancer

Operative resection continues to remain the primary form of curative therapy for rectal carcinoma, since the operation for this disease removes in continuity the primary tumor and the lymphatic drainage area, which is involved in 30 to 50 per cent of the resected specimens. For radiation therapy to be successful, the neoplasm must be substantially more radiosensitive than the surrounding normal tissue. In general, rectal cancers are not

TABLE 1. Relative Survival Rates of Carcinoma of the Rectum 1940–1959*

| | All Stages | | | | Localized | | | | Regional | | | |
|---|---|---|---|---|---|---|---|---|---|---|---|---|
| | 1940–49 | 1950–59 | 1960–64 | 1965–69 | 1940–49 | 1950–59 | 1960–64 | 1965–69 | 1940–49 | 1950–59 | 1960–64 | 1965–69 |
| Number of Cases | 6979 | 10,901 | 5819 | 5512 | 2890 | 4850 | 2688 | 2522 | 1715 | 2892 | 1758 | 1494 |
| Survival | | | | | | | | | | | | |
| 3-Year (Per Cent) | 35 | 47 | 47 | 49 | 55 | 71 | 71 | 74 | 32 | 42 | 41 | 48 |
| 5-Year (Per Cent) | 29 | 40 | 39 | | 48 | 65 | 63 | | 25 | 32 | 30 | |

*Modified from End Results of Cancer. Report No. 4, U.S. Department of Health, Education and Welfare, Public Health Service, National Institutes of Health.

TABLE 2.    Stage Distribution—Cancer of the Rectum*

| Stage at Diagnosis | Year of Diagnosis | | | |
|---|---|---|---|---|
| | 1940–49 | 1950–59 | 1960–64 | 1965–69 |
| Per cent classified as: | | | | |
| Localized | 41 | 44 | 46 | 46 |
| Regional | 25 | 27 | 30 | 27 |
| Distant | 22 | 22 | 20 | 22 |
| Unknown | 12 | 7 | 4 | 5 |

*Modified from End Results in Cancer. Report No. 4, U.S. Department of Health, Education and Welfare, Public Health Service, National Institutes of Health.

radiosensitive, and the surrounding connective and vascular tissue is almost equally radiosensitive; this makes for a very low therapeutic ratio. Even with high doses of radiation, rectal cancers are rarely curable. Williams reported a 5.5 per cent 5-year survival rate in 220 patients treated primarily by radiation therapy using the 1-MeV. machine.[9] Wang reported 6 long-term survivors among 58 patients treated with radiation therapy.[10] Two of these survivors had unresectable lesions due to extension into the pelvis; 2 had palliative resections with definite residual disease, and the other 2 patients had biopsy-proven local recurrences after combined abdominoperineal resections. All but 1 of the patients were males, and all but 1 were under 40 years of age; 4 of the 6 tumors were poorly differentiated. Treatment consisted of supravoltage radiation therapy at the rate of 1000 rads per week to a total dose of about 3500 to 5000 rads.

Earlier, patients with rectal cancer not operated upon were reported by Malbin and Stenstrom to have a 5 per cent 5-year survival rate; they reported 104 patients who were treated, using the 200- to 400-kv. machine with up to 3000 rads followed by radium tubes, radon gold, or both implanted in the rectum.[11]

Binkley, the first chief of the Colon and Rectum Service at Memorial Hospital for Cancer and Allied Diseases (New York), used external irradiation by radium pack, or the 200- to 250-kv machine and/or the insertion of radium tampon or irradiated gold seeds in 65 potentially operable patients with rectal cancers.[12] Thirty-four of these patients had been treated more than 5 years before his report, and 17 of these 34 survived the 5-year period. Most of the survivors had small (1 to 4 cm. in diameter), freely movable tumors.

Since 1948, Papillon, using a contact x-ray unit with a special Phillips-Vanderplats tube, has been treating a carefully selected group of patients.[13, 14] He reports a 5-year survival rate of 78 per cent in 133 patients thus treated. As Papillon points out, this form of therapy is limited to patients with small, well-differentiated, polypoid, noninfiltrating, freely movable tumors, particularly if the patients are poor risks for a major operative procedure.

In summary, available evidence suggests that, despite modern megavoltage techniques, radiation as a primary form of treatment has very limited usefulness in the majority of patients with rectal carcinoma.

## RADIATION THERAPY AS A PALLIATIVE FORM OF TREATMENT

For palliation, radiation has found its widest use in locally recurrent carcinoma to provide relief from pelvic pain or bleeding or in the patient with nonresectable disease.[10, 15] Generally, the amount of radiation therapy delivered defines the duration of response.

Whitely et al. treated 103 patients with local recurrence in the pelvis by 2000 to 2500 rads total midplane dose delivered in 8 to 12 consecutive treatment days, from a tele–cobalt-60 source.[16] Over 80 per cent of the patients received significant pain relief. Five per cent were treatment failures. Relief of pain and cessation of bleeding can usually be achieved with relatively modest doses of radiation; reduction in the tumor mass often requires a higher dose.

Urdaneta-LaFee et al. treated 102 patients with unresectable carcinoma of the rectum with 4000 to 4500 rads to the whole pelvis and an additional 1000 to 1500 rads concentrated to the region of the tumor, at a rate of 900 to 1000 rads per week, using supravoltage radiotherapy.[17] Eighty per cent of the patients experienced symptomatic relief. Of 35 patients who did not have a pretreatment colostomy or who did not come to operative resection later on, 25 never did require a colostomy, although all eventually died from their disease. Thirteen of 16 patients with advanced primary disease were converted from a nonresectable to a resectable status; three were alive and well over 5 years.

Williams and Horwitz gave radiation to 139 patients with unresectable primary carcinoma, including 24 patients with known distant metastases. They point out that, with modern supravoltage radiotherapy, one can expect some partial relief of symptoms due to the primary carcinoma, a reasonable chance of avoiding a colostomy, and a small 5-year survival rate.[18]

As was well stated by Wang, the use of palliative radiation therapy for the relief of symptoms in patients with locally recurrent disease often calls more for common sense than for science.[10] It should be done without too much additional discomfort to the patient, and significant relief can usually be obtained with a smaller dose and a shorter treatment course than is needed for curative radiation therapy.

## PREOPERATIVE RADIATION THERAPY: AN ADJUVANT TO OPERATIVE RESECTION OF RECTAL CANCER

Insignificant progress in the operative treatment of rectal cancer during the past two decades, high local recurrence rates which may be a major contributing factor to ultimate failure, and general progress in radiation therapy for cancer are compelling reasons for combining radiation therapy and operative treatment in rectal malignancy.

### Local Recurrence Rate of Rectal Cancer and Influence on Survival

A review of rectal cancers treated at St. Mark's Hospital for Diseases of the Rectum and Colon by Morson and co-workers revealed an overall 9.7 per cent pelvic recurrence rate.[19] The rate for the lower-third lesions of the rectum was almost three times that for upper-third rectal cancer, 14.5 per cent vs. 5.2 per cent. For high-grade malignancies it was higher than for low-grade lesions. The presence of lymphatic metastases was associated with a higher local recurrence rate. Those patients undergoing a palliative operation had a local recurrence rate of 25 per cent.

Gilbertsen reviewed the experience of the University of Minnesota Hospitals with rectal cancers and analyzed the course of failure in 125 patients who had a curative resection and follow-up to death.[6] Three-fourths died from the tumor, and half of these had known local recurrences in the pelvic area within a few centimeters of the operative field.

Floyd et al. found a local recurrence rate of 36 per cent in a select group of patients in whom the suture line or site of the previous tumor could be reexamined either at the time of reoperation or at autopsy. They noted that after local recurrence the salvage rate is low.[20, 21]

Gunderson and Sosin examined areas of failure after reoperation(s) following curative resections for adenocarcinoma of the rectum in 75 patients. Forty-eight had reoperation within 6 to 12 months after the primary resection, were asymptomatic, and had no clinical evidence of recurrent disease at the time of the "second look."[22] Twenty-six patients were symptomatic with evidence of disease prior to reoperation. Recurrent tumor was found in 52 patients, and 4 were converted to a disease-free status. Analysis of data revealed that distant metastases were an uncommon cause of failure, as was peritoneal seeding. Local recurrence and/or regional lymph node metastases were the reasons for failure in nearly 50 per cent of the patients and were a component in 92 per cent. Failure was related to the extent of the initial disease. Four of 17, or 23.3 per cent, with lymph nodes involved and the primary tumor confined to the bowel wall had local recurrence, in contrast to 33 of 40 patients, or 82.5 per cent, who had extension of tumor completely through the bowel wall and involved lymph nodes.

An analysis of 524 cases[23] of cancer of the rectum and rectosigmoid treated by anterior resection or abdominoperineal resection at Presbyterian Hospital in New York revealed that approximately one-third of the patients with Dukes C lesions and one-fourth of those with Dukes B lesions had recurrence in the pelvis. Of those with Dukes A lesions, approximately 5 per cent had local recurrence.

The precise mechanism of local recurrence is not clear.[24–28] Occult cancer can be present in the perirectal tissue or lymphatics, outside of the usual extirpation. However, local tumor implantation could be a factor. In the Presbyterian Hospital study, inadvertent bowel perforation occurred in 61 patients during the dissection, with 21 perforations at the site of the carcinoma.[23] The local recurrence rate was 60 per cent.

### Biologic Basis for Preoperative Irradiation

Since failure to cure rectal cancer by operative resection is due either to inadequate removal of tumor, to its implantation in the wound, or to its dissemination before or at the operation, the concept of preoperative irradiation therapy which renders a large percentage of tumor cells incapable of growth is attractive.[29-32]

The radiobiologic basis for preoperative irradiation rests on the demonstration of an approximate exponential relationship between the dose of radiation administered and the fraction of mammalian cells surviving.[33, 34] In vivo and in vitro studies on the response of mammalian cells to radiation have shown that the $D_{10}$, the dose that reduces the cell population to 10 per cent of the pretreatment value, lies between 500 and 2000 rads, single dose for aerobic cells. Therefore, relatively small doses will inactivate the majority of the population of cells. However, the exponential relationship between the dose of radiation and the percentage of cells killed also explains why with each given increment in dose an equal fraction of cells are inactivated and why at higher doses for each increment in dose the actual number of cells killed becomes progressively smaller. To achieve sterilization of a tumor by reducing the viable cell population to such an extent that the probability of cure is high may require doses of radiation therapy in the neighborhood of 5000 to 7000 rads or more, a dose sufficiently high to cause serious injury to the normal surrounding tissue.

It is generally accepted that the radiosensitivity of a tumor is determined by the degree of cellular differentiation and its reproductive capacity.[35, 36] The response to radiation therapy is more intense in a cell population composed of rapidly proliferating, less well-differentiated cells than in mature, non-proliferating, well-differentiated tissue.

Of great importance to the concept of preoperative radiation therapy is the fact that oxygenation in normal and malignant tissue influences its radiosensitivity.[37] The peripheral, well-vascularized tumor lying outside the operative excision is more radiosensitive than the central, less oxygenated core. Furthermore, peripheral tumor tissue is composed of a larger fraction of proliferating cells. The central bulk of the tumor consists largely of nonproliferating, hypoxic, radioresistant cells. These considerations are fundamental to combining operative extirpation of the main tumor mass and radiation therapy to the peripheral, actively growing extension of the tumor not encompassed by the standard resection.

Moreover, the manipulation of a tumor at operation forces tumor cells into the circulation. It may be reasonable to assume that adequate radiation therapy would interfere with the reproductive capacity of these dislodged tumor cells. Hoye and Smith have demonstrated that giving sublethal doses of radiation therapy to five different mice tumor systems in vivo reduced by 90 per cent the ability of intravascularly injected tumor cells to form distant metastases.[38]

Preoperative radiation therapy also may be of benefit in that it may decrease the ability of normal tissue to support tumor growth from cells implanted at the time of operation.[39, 40, 41]

Numerous studies from the experimental laboratory have supported the concept that preoperative radiation at *noncurative* doses reduces the incidence of local recurrences and enhances the cure rates of a variety of tumors in experimental animals (usually mice) over those seen when the tumors are treated surgically without prior irradiation therapy (Table 3). The studies by

TABLE 3.    Preoperative Irradiation: Experimental Studies in Animal
Tumor Systems*

| Author | Tumor | Approximate Curative Dose | Cure With Operation Alone (Per Cent) | Preoperative Irradiation Dose | Cure With Preoperative Irradiation and Operation (Per Cent) |
|---|---|---|---|---|---|
| Inch and McCredie, 1963 | Rat Walker 256 carcinocarcinoma | 6000 rads | 51 | 2000 rads | 88 |
| | C₃H mouse mammary carcinoma | 6000 rads | 57 | 2000 rads | 66 |
| Inch and McCredie, 1964 | C₃H mammary carcinoma | 6000 rads | 39 | 2000 rads | 59 |
| Powers, 1964 | B-16 melanoma | 5000 rads | 62 | 1000 rads | 82 |
| | KHAA | 5000 rads | 30 | 1000 rads | 66 |
| | KHDD | 5000 rads | 46 | 1000 rads | 67 |
| Powers and Tolmach, 1964 | 6C3HED lymphosarcoma | 3000 rads | 53 | 500 rads | 85 |
| DasGupta and Whitely, 1969 | Rabbit Vx-2 carcinoma | 5000 rads | 0 | 1000 rads | 90 |

*Modified from Perez, C. A.: Preoperative irradiation in the treatment of cancer. In *Frontiers of Radiation Therapy and Oncology*. Vol. 5. Basel, S. Karger, 1970, p. 1.

Powers, which have been instrumental in advancing this concept, suggest that the beneficial effect of preoperative radiation probably lies in the direct killing of the tumor cells by ionizing radiation rather than in alteration in the tumor bed, reducing the capacity of the tissue to support proliferation of implanted tumor cells.

We should not ignore the possibility that radiation enhances the development of metastases. Kaplan and Murphy, using transplantable mouse carcinoma, noted an increased frequency of pulmonary metastases after local irradiation of the primary tumor.[42] Yamamoto found that radiation increased the number of pulmonary metastases from experimental malignant bone tumors.[43] No evidence to date suggests that this effect occurs in man.

## Low-Dose Preoperative Radiation Therapy for Rectal Cancer

Stearns, Deddish, and Quan[44] analyzed 1276 cancers of the rectum and rectosigmoid in patients treated at the Memorial Center between 1939 and 1951.[44] Preoperative radiation at dose levels between 1500 and 2000 rads, via two anterior and two posterior pelvic ports, using the 250-kv machine, was administered to 727 patients. For tumors within 10 cm. of the anal verge, an additional perineal port was included. The remaining 549 patients received no radiation. Whether or not to administer radiation was not a random decision. The resectability rates for those who did not have preoperative irradiation therapy was 86 per cent and for those who did, 69 per cent. This could be due to the presence of more borderline resectable tumors in the irradiated group. The 5-year and 10-year survival figures were comparable for the irradiated and nonirradiated patients without lymph node metastases. However, the 5- and 10-year survival rates for patients with lymph node metastases were 37 per cent and 27 per cent, respectively, in those who received radiation therapy. In the nonirradiated group, 23 per cent survived 5 years and 10 per cent, 10 years.

Thereafter, a prospective randomized study was begun in 1957. Patients born on odd dates underwent operative resection; those born on even dates were given radiation preoperatively.[45, 46, 47] Total dosage was the same. Radiocobalt was used through single anterior and posterior ports. This unfortunate selection of the birthdate to assign patients into one of two treatment groups had the effect that the surgeon knew whether his patients were to receive radiation therapy or not prior to entering the patient in the study. It may account for the fact that, of a total of 459 patients resected, 192 received preoperative radiation therapy and 267 patients were treated by operative resection alone. The very purpose of random assignment—to minimize bias in favor of one treatment form—was essentially circumvented. The 5-year survival rate in the preoperative radiation group was 52 per cent. A 59 per cent survival rate occurred in the nonirradiated group.

This improvement in overall survival was primarily in those who had lymph node metastases. The authors concluded that refinements in operative techniques may have accounted for this gain. A subsequent updating of the study, involving 700 patients, did not alter these conclusions.[48]

The Veterans Administration Surgical Adjuvant Group (1964) initiated a prospective randomized study to evaluate the effect of low-dose (2000 to 2500 rads) radiation therapy. Preoperatively, 700 patients with operable adenocarcinoma of the rectum and rectosigmoid were entered in the study by 1969. They have now been followed for 5 years or more.[49-53] Radiation was administered through anterior and posterior parallel, opposed pelvic portals, 200 rads being delivered daily to the midplane for 10 fractions, for a total tumor dose of 2000 rads in 2 weeks. A booster dose of 50 rads daily for 10 fractions was added through a perineal port when the tumor was within the reach of the palpating finger. Supravoltage radiation was available for only 40 per cent of the patients; the remainder were treated with orthovoltage equipment. There was no demonstrable effect upon the incidence of operative complications or mortality during the first 3 postoperative months.

Comparability of patients' characteristics exists between the irradiated and the nonirradiated group with one exception: the incidence of lymph node metastases was 24 per cent in the irradiated group and 38 per cent in the nonirradiated group. This difference in positive lymph node involvement was greater in low-lying lesions, requiring abdominoperineal resection. It was also seen in patients with higher tumors undergoing anterior resection. The total number of nodes recovered in the irradiated and the nonirradiated specimens did not differ. This suggests no discrepancy in the diligence of the pathologist. It also denies the effect of radiation therapy on uninvolved nodes. The percentage of lymph node metastases was consistently lower in patients receiving a higher tumor dose for low-lying lesions, but the difference was not statistically significant.

Other studies also confirm that the incidence of metastatic disease in the regional nodes is consistently lower in patients treated by radiation than in patients treated by operative resection alone.[47, 54, 55, 56]

The survival data indicate no improvement in 5-year survival for resection other than by abdominoperineal resection when the irradiated group (38.5 per cent) and the nonirradiated group (39.8 per cent) are compared.[53] However, a statistically significant gain in the 5-year survival rate is noted after abdominoperineal resection for those who were irradiated preoperatively—40.8 per cent versus 28.4 per cent for the nonirradiated. In Dukes A and B lesions, the 5-year rate was 51.2 per cent for the treated group and 39.8 per cent for the control group. This treatment difference continues to be apparent in Dukes C lesions, with 32.4 per cent of patients surviving 5 years after radiation versus 24 per cent of those having abdominoperineal resection alone.

Of interest are observations at autopsy of the patients who had been treated by abdominoperineal resection. Cancer was found in 70 per cent of the control group and in 50 per cent of the irradiated group. The disease had recurred locally in 40 per cent of the control group and in 29 per cent of the irradiated group. The incidence of distant metastases was lower in the treated group as compared with the controls—47 per cent versus 63 percent, respectively.

The number of patients, the period of follow-up, the careful analysis of the data, and the random assignment of patients in a controlled prospective manner to one of two treatment groups make this study the strongest argument so far in support of preoperative irradiation as an adjuvant to the operative treatment of rectal carcinoma.

The Veterans Administration Surgical Adjuvant Group has now initiated a new trial with a higher dose of radiation therapy, 3150 rads, at the rate of 175 rads per day for a total of 18 treatments in 24 days.[53] The treatment field has been extended to the level of the second lumbar vertebra in order to include para-aortic lymph nodes up to the origin of the superior hemorrhoidal vessels. All of the irradiated group will be treated with megavoltage equipment.

### Moderate Preoperative Radiation Therapy for Rectal Cancer

There have been few studies employing higher-dose techniques, in contrast to low-dose radiation therapy, as an adjuvant to operative treatment. Surgeons have been reluctant to add a modality with the potential for major increases in intraoperative difficulties and interference with wound healing to the operative procedure of combined abdominoperineal resection with its 50 per cent complication rate and a postoperative mortality that averages about 10 per cent.

Allen and Fletcher have used a dosage of 5000 rads in approximately 6 weeks, utilizing the 2-Mev. Van de Graaff or the cobalt-60 tele-therapy unit.[55] Treatment fields were small and consisted of opposing anterior and posterior portals with an average size of 10 × 10 cm. No attempt was made to irradiate the lymph drainage area outside the pelvis. The operation was carried out at 4 to 6 weeks after completion of irradiation. Of 16 patients thought to have unresectable lesions, 8 were converted to a resectable situation. Only one of these, however, was alive without disease at the time of the report. In 51 patients, after completion of radiation there was no evidence of gross tumor in the resected specimen in 10, 9 of whom were alive and well at the time of the report. Positive lymph nodes were found in 10 of the 51 cases. There has been *no* clinical evidence of local recurrence in the pelvis in these 51 patients. Thirty-two of the 51 patients were alive from 6 months to 8½ years after treatment. The authors believe that there has been no increase in survival at the 2-year level. In general, patients tolerated the radiation treatment well. Minimal diarrhea in some patients was easily controlled by medication. A perineal abscess developed in two cases. One patient developed a fatal colonic perforation after completion of radiation therapy, but the relationship of the perforation to the treatment was not clear, since an autopsy was not performed. No significant healing problem was noted in these patients with one exception, a patient who received 9000 rads to the pelvis. Anterior resection in five patients included one anastomotic leak.

Kligerman et al. reported on the administration of 4400 to 4600 rads, with a 6-Mev. linear accelerator delivered in 4½ weeks.[56, 57, 58] They encompassed the primary tumor, the adjacent tissue, and the lymph node drainage area in the true pelvis and that extending along the hemorrhoidal vessels to the level of the second lumbar vertebrae. Treatment was administered through anterior and posterior portals. The field averaged about 275 cm.², of which 60 cm.² was above the pelvis. Operation was performed 4 weeks after completing radiation.

Of 49 patients treated, 18 had combined radiation and operation in a feasibility study. Then 31 cases were randomized by the flip of a coin. Sixteen patients underwent operation, and 15 had radiation before resection. No conclusions were drawn regarding long-term survival.

The resected specimens revealed no tumor in 4 of 33 patients treated with radiation therapy. Positive lymph nodes were found in 7 of 33 specimens from patients treated by radiation and in 11 of 16 specimens from patients treated by resection alone. On the basis of these data and historical controls, the authors conclude that radiation therapy may well have been a factor in reducing the incidence of lymph node metastases by one-half the expected.

Tolerance of radiation in these 33 patients was generally good. Twenty-four of 33 complained of diarrhea. It was severe in one but could otherwise be controlled by medication or by modest reduction in the daily radiation dose. Two patients had second-degree skin reaction, and one patient had a third-degree skin injury. Other complications relating to the urinary tract, perineal fistula, wound infection, colostomy problems, and pulmonary problems were essentially the same in incidence and severity to those seen in patients primarily operated upon. In nearly all irradiated patients, the tumor was resected by combined abdominoperineal resection.

On the basis of these results from the Veterans Administration Surgical Adjuvant Study Group, a joint plan for combined therapy by the Central Oncology Group (COG) and the Radiation Therapy Oncology Group

(RTOG) has been developed. It will seek to evaluate the effect of preoperative radiation therapy in patients with rectal cancer who will undergo an abdominoperineal resection upon tumor size, incidence of metastases to regional nodes, local recurrence rate, and long-term survival, with particular attention to the operative morbidity and mortality rates.[59, 60] To provide an unbiased comparison, patients will be allocated by a central randomization procedure at the statistical headquarters into one of three treatment groups: (1) operative resection alone; (2) low-dose preoperative irradiation (2000 rads) plus operative resection; (3) moderate-dose preoperative irradiation (4000 rads) plus operative resection. If the lesion is less than 8 cm. from the mucocutaneous junction, an additional 500 rads will be given through a perineal port in 50-rad increments, measured at the level of the mucocutaneous junction.

Treatment fields in both plans include the primary tumor and adjacent tissue and the lymph node drainage area in the pelvis and that extending along the superior hemorrhoidal vessels up to the second lumbar vertebra.

In the low-dose radiation group, the operative procedure will be scheduled within 1 week after completion of radiation, and after moderate-dose radiation, the operation will be performed within 3 to 5 weeks after completion of radiation.

Clinical staging preoperatively is quite inaccurate. Therefore, to distribute patients with favorable and unfavorable lesions evenly among the three treatment groups, they are stratified prior to the randomization procedure into one of eight clinical groups, depending upon three factors: (1) degree of circumferential involvement, more (or less) than one-half of the circumference of the rectum; (2) location in the lower or upper rectum, using 8 cm. from the mucocutaneous junction as an arbitrary dividing line; (3) absence or presence of tumor fixation.[61]

The number of patients entered so far is small and the period of follow-up brief. Meaningful analysis is therefore not yet possible. Accession to the study has been slow. Unwillingness to change an established treatment plan, concern over the potential for additional intraoperative and postoperative morbidity with radiation therapy, and the inevitable postponement of the operative resection in patients selected for radiation therapy, coupled with the enormous problem of confronting the patient with the uncertainty of selecting one of three treatment plans by randomization, all contribute to the hesitancy of investigators to participate in such a trial. It is hoped, however, that perseverance in this investigation will result in a significant evaluation of this treatment technique.

The Veterans Administration study and the COG-RTOG studies should provide sound clinical, pathologic, and radiobiologic data which could help in decision making and give new insights about this combined modality.

## Discussion

If a realistic look is taken at this information about the role of radiation therapy in the treatment of carcinoma of the rectum, can a strong case be made for the use of preoperative irradiation in the treatment of rectal cancer? At the moment, an affirmative answer is tentative. All of the information available strongly argues for the need to reexamine this issue by well-controlled, prospectively randomized trials in order to define the precise role of this combined modality. The arguments in favor of such trials can be summarized briefly:

1. Operative treatment alone has probably reached its zenith, and it is unlikely that further refinements in operative technique will alter today's static survival rate.

2. Local recurrence rates are high and make a significant contribution to the ultimate failure rate.

3. The intrinsic therapeutic mechanisms of radiation therapy and operative therapy complement each other in that radiation therapy is most effective in destroying tumor cells at the periphery, beyond the scope of the operation; operative extirpation is most efficient in removing the poorly oxygenated bulk of the primary tumor and its immediate nodal drainage area.

4. The experimental laboratory has provided substantial support for the superiority of the combined use of these modalities.

5. In certain patients with locally recurrent rectal cancer, or in patients with unresectable primary cancer, radiation therapy has been shown to be effective. It can reduce the total tumor volume; in some instances, all gross tumor has been eradicated, yielding a few long-term survivors.

6. The excellent Veterans Administration Surgical Adjuvant Study has clearly demonstrated a lower local recurrence rate and a significantly higher salvage rate in patients undergoing combined abdominoperineal resection when they are pretreated with a low dose of radiation therapy. This was achieved without an increase in morbidity and mortality. It also demonstrated no increase in metastases to the lung or to other sites. Clearly, this study needs confirmation.

7. A very limited experience with a higher dose of radiation therapy, 4000 to 4500 rads, so far indicates no major increase in morbidity or mortality, and tolerable side effects, which can be controlled. Its use suggests again a greater efficiency in controlling local disease through combination therapy than through resection alone.

8. The trend in several studies suggests that patients treated with preoperative radiation have a lower incidence of lymph node involvement. This important observation obviously needs confirmation. It simply sounds too good to be true, and yet it is a consistent observation and one not easily explained by any other mechanism.

Any enthusiasm for launching further trials which study preoperative radiation should be tempered by these considerations:

1. This combined approach costs the patient more in both time and money.

2. The long-term implications of carcinogenic ionizing radiation are not known.

3. Radiation therapy will delay the time of operation. It may allow the tumor to spread. With the low-dose regimen, the operation is postponed by about 3 weeks and with a higher dose about 10 weeks. We have no firm data

which allow an estimation of this risk. The time elapsed from cancer detection to inception has been estimated to be in months or possibly years. Radiation for rectal cancer may render a tumor less likely to metastasize successfully. Thus, the benefit(s) of radiation therapy may outweigh the potential disadvantage(s).

4. Radiation therapy in doses of 4000 to 4500 rads over a large treatment field, which encompasses the lymph node draining area and adjacent tissue, is not without risk.[62] Yet, preliminary studies from the few centers that have used this approach give some reassurance. A review by Roswit et al. of some 25,000 patients treated with radiation therapy for a variety of intra-abdominal malignancies concluded that the acute mucosal response would limit cumulative dose to about 4500 rads or less. A 5 per cent risk in 5 years of developing a stricture, ulceration, and/or perforation was noted.[63] As the dose approaches 6000 rads or higher, there is a steep rise in complications, particularly when a large volume of the small bowel is irradiated. The clinical pattern of chronic injury to the small bowel may be seen anywhere from 1 to 20 years after radiation therapy if the treatment was aggressive, the daily dose fraction was high, the portals used were large, and the total amount of radiation exceeded 5000 rads.

5. In the Veterans Administration Surgical Adjuvant Study, there was no indication that, following low-dose preoperative radiation, a low anterior anastomosis could not be accomplished with safety. Information relative to larger doses in the neighborhood of 4000 to 4500 rads is absent. In the study by Fletcher and Allen, the field of radiation was quite small, and both ends of the intestine to be anastomosed were outside of the field of radiation. How safe it would be to perform a low anterior resection with anastomosis in irradiated bowel is simply not known. In general, it appears that radiation therapy to moderate dose levels, 4000 to 4500 rads over a 4- to 5-week period, can be well tolerated without increasing operative morbidity and mortality. Only when radical irradiation is given with intent to cure and at doses approaching 6000 rads or more is there a steep rise in radiation injury to the vascular tissue and to the bowel wall. These effects may seriously interfere with the healing of an anastomosis. None of the ongoing trials are examining this issue.

In conclusion, we have a growing body of evidence from the experimental laboratory and from clinical investigations which suggests that preoperative irradiation is of value in the treatment of rectal cancer. More studies are urgently needed to confirm the Veterans Administration Surgical Adjuvant Study Group experience with low-dose radiation therapy and to obtain reliable answers to the question of the ability of ionizing radiation to sterilize involved lymph nodes. We need clearer definition of the optimum field size and optimum dose with the highest therapeutic benefit and reasonably accurate estimates of its cost to the patient in terms of increased morbidity and mortality.

Convincing data can come only through the mechanism of the controlled clinical trial, since the differences in the many parameters to be evaluated — e.g., nodal involvement, distant metastases, local recurrence rates, complication rate, survival rates — may not be large between the conventionally treated patients and the irradiated patients. Support for such investigations should be given the highest priority by all interested in the problem of this common malignancy. Both treatment modalities are widely available today, and the demonstration of worthwhile therapeutic benefit could promptly be translated into large-scale application to many cancer patients.

## References

1. Symonds, C. J.: Cancer of rectum: Excision after application of radium. Proc. R. Soc. Med. 7:152, 1913–14.
2. Gordon-Watson, C.: The radium problem. III. The treatment of carcinoma of the rectum with radium. Br. J. Surg. 17:643, 1929–30.
3. Gabriel, W. B.: The end-results of perineal excision and of radium in the treatment of cancer of the rectum. Br. J. Surg. 20:234, 1932–33.
4. Silverberg, E., and Holleb, A. I.: Major trends in cancer: 25-year survey. CA 25:2, 1975.
5. Polk, H. C., Ahmad, W., and Knutson, C. O.: Carcinoma of the colon and rectum. Curr. Prob. Surg., Jan., 1973.
6. Gilbertsen, V. A.: Improving the prognosis for patients with intestinal cancer. Surg. Gynecol. Obstet. 124:1253, 1967.
7. Thomas, W. H., Larson, R. A., Wright, H. K., and Cleveland, J. C.: Analysis of 830 cases of rectal adenocarcinoma. 1. Progressively improved results of treatment. Conn. Med. 33:569, 1969.
8. Axtell. L. M., and Cutler, S. J.: End Results in Cancer. Report No. 4, U.S. Department of Health, Education and Welfare, National Cancer Institute, Bethesda, Maryland, 1972.
9. Williams, I. G.: Radiotherapy of carcinoma of the rectum. In Monographs on Neoplastic Disease. Vol. 3. Baltimore, The Williams & Wilkins Co., 1960.
10. Wang, C. C.: The use of radiation in the management of cancer of the colon and rectum. Geriatrics 23:163, 1968.
11. Malbin, M., and Stenstrom, K. W.: Results of treatment of 173 cases of carcinoma of the rectum. Radiology 42:545, 1944.
12. Binkley, G. E.: Results of radiation therapy in primary operable rectal and anal cancer. Radiology 31:724, 1938.
13. Papillon, J. : Resectable rectal cancers. Treatment by curative endocavitary irradiation. J.A.M.A. 231:1385, 1975.
14. Papillon, J.: Endocavitary irradiation in the curative treatment of early rectal cancers. Dis. Colon Rectum 17:172, 1974.
15. Wang, C. C., and Schulz, M. D.: The role of radiation therapy in the management of carcinoma of the sigmoid, rectosigmoid and rectum. Radiology 79:1, 1962.
16. Whiteley, H. W., Stearns, M. W., Leaming, R. H., and Deddish, M. R.: Palliative radiation therapy in patients with cancer of the colon and rectum. Cancer 25:343, 1970.
17. Urdaneta-Lafee, N., Knowlton, A. H., and Kligerman, M. M.: Evaluation of palliative irradiation in rectal carcinoma. Radiology 104:673, 1972.
18. Williams, I. G., and Horwitz, H.: The primary treatment of adenocarcinoma of the rectum by high voltage roentgen rays (1,000 KV). Am. J. Roentgenol. Radium Ther. Nucl. Med. 76: 919, 1956.
19. Morson, B. C., Path, M. C., and Bussey, H. J. R.: Surgical pathology of rectal cancer in relation to adjuvant radiotherapy. Br. J. Radiol. 40:161, 1967.
20. Floyd, C. E., Corley, R. G., and Cohn, I.: Local recurrence of carcinoma of the colon and rectum. Am. J. Surg. 109:153, 1965.
21. Floyd, C. E., Stirling, C. T., and Cohn, I.: Cancer of the colon, rectum and anus: Review of 1,687 cases. Ann. Surg. 163:829, 1966.
22. Gunderson, L. L., and Sosin, H.: Areas of failure found at reoperation (second or symptomatic look) following "curative surgery" for adenocarcinoma of the rectum. Cancer 34:1278, 1974.
23. Slanetz, C. A., Herter, F. P., and Grinnell, R. S.: Anterior resection versus abdominoperineal resection for cancer of the rectum and rectosigmoid. Am. J. Surg. 123:110, 1972.
24. Dukes, C. E., and Bussey, H. J. R.: The spread of rectal cancer and its effect on prognosis. Br. J. Cancer 12:309, 1958.
25. Gilchrist, R. K., and David, V. C.: A consideration of pathological factors influencing five

year survival in radical resection of the large bowel and rectum for carcinoma. Ann. Surg. *126*:421, 1947.

26. Stearns, M. W., and Binkley, G. E.: The influence of location and prognosis in operable rectal cancer. Surg. Gynecol. Obstet., 96:368, 1953.

27. Waugh, J. M., and Kirklin, J. W.: The importance of the level of the lesion in the prognosis and treatment of carcinoma of the rectum and low sigmoid colon. Ann. Surg. *129*:22, 1949.

28. Dwight, R. W., Higgins, G. A., and Keehn, R. J.: Factors influencing survival after resection in cancer of the colon and rectum. Am. J. Surg. *117*:512, 1969.

29. Powers, W. E., and Palmer, L. A.: Biologic basis of preoperative radiation treatment. Am. J. Roentgenol. *102*:176, 1968.

30. Perez, C. A.: Preoperative irradiation in the treatment of cancer. *In Frontiers of Radiation Therapy and Oncology.* Vol. 5. Basel, S. Karger, 1970, p. 1.

31. Stein, J. J.: Preoperative radiation therapy for carcinoma of the rectum and rectosigmoid. Cancer 28:190, 1971.

32. Potter, J. F.: Preoperative irradiaion and surgery for certain cancers. Cancer 35:84, 1975.

33. Puck, T. T., and Marcus, P. I.: Actions of x-rays on mammalian cells. J. Exp. Med. *103*:653, 1956.

34. Whitmore, G. F., and Till, J. E.: Quantitation of cellular radiobiological responses. Ann. Rev. Nucl. Sci. *14*:347, 1964.

35. Bergonie, J., and Tribondeau, L.: Interpretation of some results of radiotherapy and an attempt at determining a logical technique of treatment. Radiat. Res. *11*:587, 1959.

36. Rubin, P.: Predictors of response in radiation oncology. *In Frontiers of Radiation Therapy and Oncology.* Vol. 9. Basel, S. Karger, 1974, p. 299.

37. Gray, L. H.: Cellular radiobiology. Radiat. Res. Suppl. *1*:1959, p. 73.

38. Hoye, R. C., and Smith, R. R.: The effectiveness of small amounts of preoperative irradiation in preventing the growth of tumor cells disseminated at surgery. Cancer *14*:284, 1961.

39. O'Brien, P. H., Sweitzer, C., Sherman, J. O., and Moss, W. T.: Tumor bed effect of ionizing irradiation in experimental cancer of the colon. Cancer 23:451, 1969.

40. Vermund, K., Stenstrom, K. W., Mosser, D. G. and Johnson, E. A.: Effects of roentgen irradiation of the tumor bed. II. The inhibiting action of different dose levels of local pre-transplantation roentgen irradiation on the growth of the mouse mammary carcinoma. Radiat. Res. 5:354, 1956.

41. Vermund, K., Stenstrom, K. W., Mosser, D. G., and Loken, M. K.: Effects of roentgen irradiation of the tumor bed. III. The different inhibiting action on the growth of mouse mammary carcinoma resulting from the pre- or post-transplantation irradiation. Radiat. Res. 8:22, 1958.

42. Kaplan, H. S., and Murphy, E. D.: The effect of local roentgen irradiation on the biological behavior of a transplantable mouse carcinoma. I. Increased frequency of pulmonary metastases. J. Natl. Cancer Inst. 9:407, 1949.

43. Yamamoto, T.: An experimental study on the effect of x-ray on metastasis of malignant tumor, especially in bones. Jap. J. Obstet. Gynecol. 19:388, 1936.

44. Stearns, M. W., Deddish, M. R., and Quan, S. H.: Preoperative roentgen therapy for cancer of the rectum. Surg. Gynecol. Obstet. 109:225, 1959.

45. Quan, S. H., Deddish, M. R., and Stearns, M. W.: The effect of preoperative roentgen therapy upon the 10 and 5 year results of the surgical treatment of cancer of the rectum. Surg. Gynecol Obstet. *111*:507, 1960.

46. Stearns, M. W., Deddish, M. R., and Quan, S. H.: Preoperative irradiation for cancer of the rectum and rectosigmoid: Preliminary review of recent experience (1957–1962). Dis. Colon Rectum *11*:281, 1968.

47. Quan, S. H., Deddish, M. R., and Stearns, M. W.: Preoperative radiation for carcinoma of the rectum. N.Y. State J. Med. 66:2243, 1966.

48. Quan, S. H.: A surgeon looks at radiotherapy in cancer of the colon and rectum. Cancer *31*:1, 1973.

49. Dwight, R. W., Higgins, G. A., Roswit, B., LeVeen, H. H., and Keehn, R. J.: Preoperative radiation and surgery for cancer of the sigmoid colon and rectum. Am. J. Surg. *123*:93, 1972.

50. Higgins, G. A., and Dwight, R. W.: The role of preoperative irradiation in cancer of the rectum and rectosigmoid. Surg. Clin. North Am. 52:847, 1972.

51. Roswit, B., Higgins, G. A., and Keehn, R. J.: A controlled study of preoperative irradiation in cancer of the sigmoid colon and rectum. Radiology 97:133, 1970.

52. Roswit, B., Higgins, G. A., Humphrey, E. W., and Robinette, C. D.: Preoperative irradiation of operable adenocarcinoma of the rectum and rectosigmoid colon. Radiology *108*:389, 1973.

53. Roswit, B., Higgins, G. A., and Keehn, R. J.: Preoperative irradiation for carcinoma of the

rectum and rectosigmoid colon: Report of a national Veterans Administration randomized study. Cancer 35:1597, 1975.

54. Ruff, C. C., Dockerty, M. B., Fricke, R. E., and Waugh, J. M.: Preoperative radiation therapy for adenocarcinoma of the rectum and rectosigmoid. Surg. Gynecol. Obstet. *112*:715, 1961.

55. Allen, C. V., and Fletcher, W. S.: Observations on preoperative irradiation of rectosigmoid carcinoma. Am. J. Roentgenol. Radium Ther. Nucl. Med. *108*:136, 1970.

56. Kligerman, M. M., Urdaneta-Lafee, N., Knowlton, A., Vidone, R., Hartman, P. V., and Vera, R.: Preoperative irradiation of rectosigmoid carcinoma including its regional lymph nodes. Am. J. Roentgenol. Radium. Ther. Nucl. Med. *120*:624, 1974.

57. Kligerman, M. M., Urdaneta-Lafee, N., Knowlton, A., Vidone, R., Hartman, P. V., and Vera, R.: Preoperative irradiation of rectosigmoid carcinoma including its regional lymph nodes. Am. J. Roentgenol. Radium Ther. Nucl. Med. *114*:498, 1972.

58. Tepper, M. Vidone, R. A., Hayes, M. A., Lindenmuth, W. W., and Kligerman, M. M.: Preoperative irradiation in rectal cancer: Initial comparison of clinical tolerance, surgical and pathologic findings. Am. J. Roentgenol. Radium Ther. Nucl. Med. *102*:587, 1968.

59. Grage, T. B., and Kligerman, M. M.: Preoperative irradiation in potentially curable adenocarcinoma of the rectum. Protocol of the Central Oncology Group, 1972, and Radiation Therapy Oncology Group. Personal communications.

60. Brady, L. W., Antoniades, J., Prasasvinighai, S., Torpie, R. J., Asbell, S. O., and Glassburn, J. R.: Preoperative radiation therapy. A plan for combined therapy for radiation therapy oncology group and the central oncology group. Cancer 34:960, 1974.

61. Buckwalter, J. A., and Kent, T. H.: Prognosis and surgical pathology of carcinoma of the colon. Surg. Gynecol. Obstet. *136*:465, 1973.

62. Roswit, B., Malsky, S. J., and Reid, C. B.: Severe radiation injuries of the stomach, small intestine, colon and rectum. Am. J. Roentgenol. *114*:460, 1972.

63. Roswit, B., Malsky, S. J., and Reid, C. B.: Radiation tolerance of the gastrointestinal tract. *In Frontiers of Radiation Therapy and Oncology*. Vol. 6. Basel, S. Karger, 1972, p. 160.

# 19

# *Endarterectomy versus Bypass Operation for Aortoiliac Occlusive Disease*

AORTOILIAC
THROMBOENDARTERECTOMY
*by Edwin J. Wylie,*
*Cornelius Olcott, IV,*
*and S. Timothy String*

AORTOILIAC OCCLUSIVE
DISEASE: ADVANTAGES OF
BYPASS GRAFTING
*by A. W. Humphries*
*and T. P. Corrigan*

## Statement of the Problem

*This dispute relates to the early and late morbidity, the mortality, and the success of these two procedures for the alleviation of aortoiliac occlusion in a patient who might be treated by either approach.*

*Compare the two procedures with respect to operative mortality, late mortality, late morbidity, and impotence. Compare morbidity and mortality from infection in the two procedures.*

*Compare the two with respect to patency, both early and late.*

*If the extent of the occlusive disease precludes use of the external iliac artery and the graft must be brought to the common femoral artery, does this increase the incidence of infection? Occlusion? Failure? Compare the morbidity of femoral and iliac anastomoses.*

*An endarterectomy is impossible or technically too hazardous in what percentage of patients?*

*Analyze failure of endarterectomy as a function of the length of the occluded segment and the size of the occluded vessels.*

*Describe the major technical aspects of the procedure that you believe are critical to a successful result.*

# Aortoiliac Thromboendarterectomy

**EDWIN J. WYLIE**
and **CORNELIUS OLCOTT, IV**
*University of California, San Francisco, Medical Center*

**S. TIMOTHY STRING**
*University of South Alabama College of Medicine*

Thromboendarterectomy as a method for the operative treatment of atherosclerotic occlusive lesions in the aortoiliac segment of the arterial tree was first introduced in this country in 1951. This was the first revascularization technique used for atherosclerosis, and its apparent early success prompted surgeons to explore its feasibility at numerous other sites of atherosclerotic occlusive disease, including the femoropopliteal arterial segments, the renal arteries, the extracranial arteries supplying the brain, and even the coronary arteries. In succeeding years, other methods of revascularization were introduced, the most notable being bypass grafting. Clinical experiences with each of these methods have been reported by numerous surgeons, and in many of these publications, attempts were made to compare the results of endarterectomy with other revascularization methods. At the time of this writing, atherosclerosis at the carotid bifurcation is the only lesion for which endarterectomy remains as the unchallenged preferable method.

The editors in their preface to this chapter have listed a number of pertinent questions. The answers to these questions, if they can be found, should provide substantial information to resolve the controversy over the relative effectiveness of the two operations for aortoiliac occlusive atherosclerosis—thromboendarterectomy (TEA) and bypass grafting (BPG). Eleven reports have recently been published describing the results of TEA. Three of these studies provided comparative data on the use of BPG. For purposes of brevity, each series is given a letter designation, and the references are given in the bibliography. The three critical indices are mortality rate, frequency of immediate failure, and long-term durability. Although the various writers have used different methods in reporting their results, it is

TABLE 1.   Operative Morbidity in Patients Treated by Aortoiliac Endarterectomy

| Series | Number of Patients | Mortality (Per Cent) | Postoperative Occlusion (Per Cent) |
|--------|--------------------|----------------------|-------------------------------------|
| A | 331 | 4 | 3 |
| B | 96 | 7 | 0 |
| C | 104 | 2 | 5.3 |
| D | 20 | ? | ? |
| E | 94 | 6 | 4 |
| F | 69 | 1.4 | 6 |
| G | 97 | 5.1 | 1 |
| H | 64 | 4 | 6 |

possible to derive figures for these indices with reasonable accuracy. Table 1 indicates the early morbidity in the eight reports dealing only with TEA. Table 2 reports similar data from the three additional reports that also include comparative data from BPG operations. Table 3 is a report of our own early morbidity data with TEA during three successive time periods. Table 4 is a comparative report of our experience with BPG over two time periods.

Two conclusions are apparent. First, there is an enormous variation in mortality rate and frequency of early failure with both operations. Second, these data provide no solid basis for comparing operative risks and technical ease. Pooling of the data would give meaningless figures, and if one were to use selected individual reports, either procedure could be shown to be superior, depending upon which report was selected.

Table 5 reports the long-term durability of TEA in terms of the

TABLE 2.   Endarterectomy and Bypass Graft: Comparative Operative Morbidity

| Series | Number of Patients | | Mortality (Per Cent) | Postoperative Occlusion (Per Cent) |
|--------|--------------------|--|----------------------|-------------------------------------|
| I | TEA | | 2.7 | 0.6 |
| | | 342 | AI–0.8 | 0 |
| | | | AF–4.6 | 1.1 |
| | BPG | | 4.4 | 1.7 |
| | | | AI–6.6 | 2.2 |
| | | | AF–2.3 | 1.1 |
| J | TEA | 159 | 6.9 | 11.2 (0–6 mo.) |
| | | | AI–1 | 0 |
| | | | AF–17 | 1.1 |
| | BPG | 57 | 17.5 | 27.2 (0–6 mo.) |
| | | | AI–14 | |
| | | | AF–21 | |
| K | TEA | 86 | 1.2 | 1.2 |
| | BPG | 91 | 7.7 | 2.2 |

TABLE 3.   Morbidity of Thromboendarterectomy in Patients Treated at the University of California, San Francisco

| Site of Operation | Operative Period | Number of Patients | Postoperative Occlusion (Per Cent) | Mortality (Per Cent) |
|---|---|---|---|---|
| Aorta–common iliac | 1951–62 | 134 | 1 | 6 |
| | 1963–67 | 66 | 0 | 0 |
| | 1968–74 | 86 | 0 | 0 |
| Aorta-iliac-femoral | 1951–62 | 251 | 6 | 7 |
| | 1963–67 | 103 | 1.3 | 1.8 |
| | 1968–74 | 87 | 0 | 0 |

TABLE 4.   Morbidity of Bypass Graft Procedures in 318 Patients Treated at the University of California, San Francisco

| | 1960–67 (Per Cent) | 1968–74 (Per Cent) |
|---|---|---|
| Mortality | 5 | 2 |
| Early occlusion (< 30 days) | 2 | 2 |

TABLE 5.   Late Occlusion After Aortoiliac Thromboendarterectomy

| Series | 2 Years (Per Cent) | 5 Years (Per Cent) | 8–10 Years (Per Cent) |
|---|---|---|---|
| A | 19 | 38° | ? |
| B | 9.5   AI–12 AF-7 | ? | ? |
| C | 8° | 14° | ? |
| D | ? | 15° | ? |
| E | 13 | 28 | 28 |
| F | 5 | 11 | 31 |
| G | 1 | 4 | 7 |
| H | 15 | 32 | ? |

°Aorta–common iliac only.

TABLE 6.   Comparative Durability of TEA and BPG

| Series | Number of Patients | | Per Cent Late Occlusion | | |
|---|---|---|---|---|---|
| | | | 2 Years | 5 Years | 8–10 Years |
| H | TEA–64 | | 25 | 32 | ? |
| | BPG–30 | | 15 | 28 | ? |
| | | No. of limbs | | | |
| I | TEA–342 | 482 | 6.0 | 9.1 | 12.5 |
| | | | | AI– 1.1    6.7 | 6.7 |
| | | | | AF-10.8    11.5 | 18.4 |
| | BPG | 177 | 9.6 | 18 | 18 |
| | | | | AI– 3.7    3.7 | 3.7 |
| | | | | AF-15.4    32 | 32 |
| J | TEA–159 | | 19 | 37 | 47 |
| | BPG–57 | | 38 | 38 | 38 |
| K | TEA–86 | | 5 | 8 | 33 |
| | BPG–91 | | 17 | 23 | 59 |

frequency of late occlusion at various time intervals in the first eight series. Table 6 reports similar data in the three series in which the results are compared with BPG. Table 7 gives the results from our own TEA series in a study concluded 10 years ago. Since there have been no substantial changes in our selection of patients or operative method, we suspect that a current study would yield similar results. The deadline for submission of this manuscript did not allow us to complete our follow-up studies on the BPG patients, but partial data suggest that there will be no appreciable difference in the durability of the two operations in our patients.

Similar comments can be applied to the durability data that were made concerning the early results. Atherosclerosis is a progressive disease, and it is not surprising that both operations are susceptible to a certain percentage of late failure. Other information is needed to explain the huge differences in the frequency of late failure.

One explanation is the method of reporting. Four of the studies report both early and late failures in terms of "limbs at risk" rather than "patients at risk." The method is of course valid and useful in one respect, but it skews the data when one tries to use it to compare the worth to the patient of the two operations. Imagine a hypothetical series of 20 patients with claudica-

TABLE 7.   Durability of Thromboendarterectomy in Patients Treated at the University of California, San Francisco 1951–1965

| Site of Operation | Number of Patients | Per Cent Late Occlusion | |
|---|---|---|---|
| | | 5 Years | 10 Years |
| Aorta–common iliac | 108 | 5 | 10 |
| Aorta-iliac-femoral | 312 | 15 | 28 |

tion who have undergone bilateral iliac reconstructive operations, all of whom developed re-occlusion on one side 2 years later with return of their former walking limitation. Using the "limbs at risk" method, the surgeon reports a 2-year success rate of 50 per cent, but for the patient the operations were a 100 per cent failure. Since some of the reports combine unilateral and bilateral operations, it is impossible to derive the actual figure for patient failure, which would obviously be higher than the failure rate in the "limbs at risk" reports.

A more important factor for exploring the differences in results has to do with the principle of weighing the variables. Comparative evaluation in any area of surgical controversy must either eliminate the variables or identify and weigh their significance. Oftentimes the significance of specific variables is not realized until late in one's surgical experience with a particular operation, and the retrieval of newly appreciated data may be impossible and too time-consuming to accomplish.

With respect to TEA and BPG, the important variables include the pathologic variations and distribution of the atherosclerotic process, both in the area of operation and in the distal arterial tree, and the age, sex, and clinical status of the patient. Some but not all of the reports include this information. The most important variable above all is the skill and experience of the operative team. Which operations were performed by residents? What was the extent of their experience? Who, if anyone, supervised or assisted them, and what was the extent of the supervisor's experience? Which operations were done by surgeons well trained in vascular disease? None of the answers to these questions are available. In vascular surgery, perhaps more than in any area of general surgery, the skill and experience of the vascular surgeon are the determining factors in the success or failure of an arterial reconstructive operation.

The editors have asked other pertinent questions which can be only partially answered from the published data. Perigraft sepsis has been a major concern to all surgeons using the BPG operation, since its results are so frequently disastrous. Series J reports on three groin infections with BPG to the common femoral arteries in 57 operations, one of which resulted in loss of the extremity. None of the other reports describe the frequency of this complication. We have had five similar infections in 318 BPG operations. One required removal of the graft and eventually led to the death of the patient. We have had 18 patients referred to us with extensive perigraft infections. Six of these died, and four lost one or both extremities. A few of our patients with extensive TEA to the common femoral arteries have developed postoperative sepsis in the groin. All recovered without compromise of the revascularization procedure.

The effect of either operation on impotence is virtually impossible to predict. The literature appears to contain nothing of statistical significance, and the results from our own operations are unenlightening. The development of impotence coincident with arterial occlusion in or proximal to the hypogastric arteries is a well-established phenomenon. Theoretically, the restoration of normal blood flow to both hypogastric arteries should reverse the phenomenon. Aortoiliac atherosclerosis is almost always associated with variable degrees of stenosis or occlusion of the hypogastric arteries. For this reason aortoiliac TEA, when combined with hypogastric endarterectomy, should provide greater assurance than BPG that potency will be restored. Although we have never seen it occur, a similar result could be obtained with a BPG to the sides of the external iliac arteries in those rare instances when the common iliac bifurcation and hypogastric arteries are free of hemodynamically significant disease.

Slightly less than half of our patients have regained sexual potency after what was thought to be an anatomically successful TEA. The sensation of orgasm was not impaired, but almost all lost forward ejaculation, presumably as a result of the division of the autonomic fibers passing into the pelvis from the anterior surface of the aorta.

The reasons for failure to restore potency in all of our patients are obscure. Postoperative occlusion of the endarterectomized hypogastric arteries where a satisfactory end point was not developed is one possibility, but postoperative aortograms performed in a few of the patients usually demonstrated patency of the hypogastric artery. We suspect that disturbance of the poorly defined autonomic mechanism is a more likely cause. Many patients who were sexually potent preoperatively became impotent following operations for aortic aneurysm, in which the hypogastric blood flow was not at risk but where the preaortic nerve fibers were uniformly divided. We have, in fact, had patients report loss of potency following aortofemoral BPG operations in which the anterior surface of the aorta had been cleared of all periaortic tissue prior to performing the proximal anastomosis.

The literature does contain one highly significant study relating to the durability of TEA. This is the report by Szilagyi et al. (Table 5, Series C) on the incidence and development of recurrent stenosis in the sites of operation in 67 patients undergoing aorta–common iliac endarterectomy who were followed for 2 to 7 years. In this study Szilagyi et al. considered each patient in terms of three operative segments—the aorta and each common iliac artery—and reported on the basis of recurrence per operated segment. Of 151 operative sites, 32 per cent showed some degree of recurrent stenosis in the follow-up period. In 84 per cent the stenosis was mild (< 20 to 30 per cent). There was eventual occlusion in four patients. The inescapable conclusion is that some patients in time will develop atherosclerosis in an endarterectomized artery, a situation only rarely reported in a fabric BPG. Unfortunately, this report by Szilagyi et al. is subject to the same difficulty in interpretation that the "limbs at risk" data presented. Did the stenoses appear in a small group of patients with all three segments at risk who were metabolically or genetically susceptible to recurrent atherosclerosis or were they spread throughout all the patients?

In our own experience, there are varying degrees of "malignancy" in the primary disease. The one most subject to recurrence is the succulent, pale, homogeneous atheroma most commonly seen in young patients. The data of Szilagyi et al. must obviously be compared to a major factor causing late obstruction of a BPG, namely the development of obstructing atheroma at the termination of the BPG and retrograde thrombosis of that limb of the graft. They do conclude that "the late results of the two types of operation are very similar."

The editors in their preface to this book have cautioned against the acceptance of "in my experience" data. The reader by this time must have realized that the use of other available data has led us into a morass of confusion. Perhaps it is wiser to resort to "my experience," since this is the basis of most surgeons' decisions in selecting the appropriate operation and the method of its performance. Since our experience with TEA predates the reports that have been cited, there may be some value in reporting on this experience.

We have already alluded to the composition of the operative team in terms of its relation to the results of either operation. It is therefore pertinent to describe our own. There are three full-time vascular surgeons, one of whom performs or assists at every operation. One, the senior author, was self-taught (the worst kind, if one inspects his results from the first reported time period). The other two are products of a general surgical residency with a year of additional training in vascular surgery. Resident service operations are performed by residents in their sixth year of training or by postresidency fellows. So much for the experience, if not the skill, of the responsible surgeons.

In our opinion the most fruitful first approach to exploring the difference in results in both the TEA data alone and the comparative data of the two operations is to describe the various forms of the atherosclerotic process which the surgeon is attempting to overcome. Many of the early operative complications and late occlusive problems appear to be traceable either to a failure to adapt the operative procedure to the specific lesion or to the failure of either operation to halt the natural progression of the disease.

Staple[1] and Mozersky et al. (Series D) have suggested that there are genuine and basic differences with respect to both the patient and his disease when one compares atherosclerosis limited to the aorta–common iliac segments with atherosclerosis in these segments but with additional lesions in the distal arterial tree. For purposes of brevity, we will label these Type I and Type II disease.

Patients with Type I disease tend to be younger. They often may live for lengthy periods (10 to 15 years or longer) before atherosclerosis appears in the external iliac or femoropopliteal segments. Of 108 patients with Type I disease followed early in our experience, only 14 per cent developed clinical evidence of atherosclerosis in the distal arterial tree within 10 years after aortoiliac endarterectomy. In this group, outflow obstruction from the advance of distal atherosclerosis, a common cause of late failure in either operation, appeared after a long interval, if it appeared at all. Arterial occlusion in the early years is thus more often attributable to technical error in the performance of the operation or to inherent defects in the new arterial conduit.

For the aorta–common iliac portion of TEA, we open the full length of the infrarenal aorta by a longitudinal aortotomy. The common iliac segments are endarterectomized by passing an arterial stripper through transverse arteriotomies in the distal common iliac arteries. The resulting iliac lumen is larger than normal (15 to 20 per cent) and larger than if longitudinal iliac arteriotomies had been used. We suspect that, if recurrent iliac atheromas are to appear, the larger lumen postpones their adverse effect on blood flow. Particular attention is paid to removing atheromas at the orifice of the external iliac arteries (using a separate distal arteriotomy if necessary) and to extracting atheromatous intima from as much of the hypogastric arteries as possible. All operations involve both common iliac arteries, regardless of the apparent extent of disease.

The reason for routinely performing this extensive an operation is based upon our observations of the pattern of progression of atherosclerosis in the aorta and common iliac segments. Generally, the earliest lesions are in the full length of both common iliac arteries. There is a peculiar pattern of progression beyond the common iliac bifurcation. Intimal atheroma usually extends into the first 1 or 2 cm. of the external iliac arteries to an abrupt end point. In the hypogastric artery, the lesions extend deep into the pelvis beyond the first major branches. As these lesions progress, the last area to become involved is the segment of the aorta between the renal and inferior mesenteric arteries.

Since progressive stenosis at either the inflow or outflow level results in late occlusion, it is apparent that the best long-term results for Type I disease will be provided by an operation which deals with the entire infrarenal aorta, the full length of both common iliac arteries, and the first 1 or 2 cm. of the external iliac arteries.

In our own experience with patients with Type I disease who require a second operation for late occlusion, a common cause of late failure is an inadequate original operation. From a review of the literature and from personal communication with other surgeons, we know that numerous methods are currently employed which, in our view, compromise the adequacy of the operation and contribute to late failure. The following are the three most common:

1. Placing the proximal end of the graft or beginning the endarterectomy in the distal portion of the infrarenal aorta. For TEA we currently remove the aortic intima to the level of the infrarenal aortic clamp, regardless of the visible or palpable disease at that level.

2. Terminating the endarterectomy in the midportion of the common iliac artery or anastomosing the iliac limb of the graft at that level. The endarterectomy should remove all of the common iliac intima, as well as any atheromatous intima within the proximal external iliac artery. The iliac arm of a graft should be anastomosed beyond the most distal level of palpable atheroma in the external iliac artery.

3. Performing a unilateral TEA or BPG for apparent unilateral iliac disease. It is almost axiomatic that atherosclerosis at all levels below the aortic bifurcation becomes bilateral in time. A seemingly insignificant lesion in the contralateral common iliac artery can be expected to become an obstructive lesion within a few years.

The first two of these "errors" in operative method could substantially influence the durability of either operative method. The published reports rarely indicate the completeness of the operative method in these respects and accordingly provide inadequate information for comparative evaluation.

The immediate complications which may appear after aortoiliac TEA or BPG are thrombosis of the operative segment, distal occlusion, and hemorrhage. These complications now almost never occur in our patients, leading us to the conclusion that they are caused by errors in technique, which can easily be avoided. Since we have been fortunate in overcoming some of our earlier problems, it seems appropriate to outline certain technical maneuvers that seem to have contributed to our improved results.

Thrombosis distal to the operative segment occurs as a result of either embolization from the operative area or stasis in the arterial tree distal to the occluding clamps. The inner surface of the aorta is often partially filled with loosely adherent atheromatous debris and mural thrombus. Endarterectomy requires complete mobilization of the infrarenal aorta and the common iliac arteries. Forceful finger manipulation, instrumental retraction, or suspension by narrow fabric slings can easily dislodge fragments which pass into the distal circulation. A helpful practice in the early phases of operation is to observe the color of the patient's feet at frequent intervals to make certain that distal occlusion has not occurred.

The conventional technique of performing an end-to-side anastomosis for the proximal end of a BPG operation introduces an additional hazard of embolization. After proximal or distal aortic clamps are applied and the aorta has been opened, inspection of the interior of the aorta often shows the lumen to be partially filled with grumous material. Although most of the visible debris can be removed, much still remains in the distal aorta crushed beneath the distal clamp. Release of this clamp to permit flushing and backbleeding is an unsatisfactory method of removing possible embolic fragments, which may be dislodged when forward aortic flow has been reestablished. This problem can be overcome by establishing an end-to-end proximal anastomosis in the BPG, thereby isolating the distal aorta from forward flow. In so doing, one accepts the possible interference with hypogastric blood flow, either at that time or at a future date when stenotic lesions at the common iliac bifurcation progress to complete obstruction. In either operation it is advisable to develop forward flow into the hypogastric arteries before opening the legs to flow, since detached debris may have been trapped in the aorta at the site of the proximal clamp. With TEA this is accomplished by staging the release of the distal clamps so that the last to be removed are those in the external iliac arteries.

Thrombosis in the distal arterial tree as a result of stasis can largely be prevented by adequate systemic heparinization during the occlusive phase of the operation. The external iliac arteries are particularly vulnerable, since there are no avenues for collateral blood flow to these isolated segments. A simple expedient is to infuse them with dilute heparin solution once the arteriotomies have been made. This is not a substitute for systemic heparinization. The portion of the perfusate which flows into the legs is rapidly diluted and has little effect beyond the external iliac arteries. Vigorous backflow after release of the external iliac clamps at intervals during the operation and especially before final release of the proximal clamps provides assurance of patency in the distal vessels.

Inspection for return of color to the patient's feet should be made at the time of clamp release in either operation. Color returns first in the heel and progresses upward to involve all of the foot within 4 to 5 minutes. If color does not return by this time, one must assume that distal occlusion has occurred and that appropriate steps must be taken at that time to overcome the complication. Prompt return of color rather than pulse return is the important observation, since pulse return may be delayed for an hour or longer.

Two related questions posed by the editors concern the technical feasibility of TEA in aortoiliac atherosclerosis and the relative ease of performance as compared with BPG. Our only contraindication for TEA in Type I disease is the presence of preaneurysmal and degenerative changes in the aortic segment. This may be apparent on the preoperative aortograms as one or more localized dilatations in the aortic lumen. At operation, these are visible as focal areas of discrete or circumferential bulges exceeding the normal external diameter of the aorta. Aortotomy generally reveals a layer of grey liquefied material in the aortic wall. Pathologic examination of the residual media shows degenerative changes not ordinarily seen in this layer. We suspect that the natural history of this variant of the usual occlusive atherosclerotic lesion is progression to frank aneurysmal disease. Late aneurysms have appeared in only two patients in our TEA series, and both patients showed these changes at the original operation.

Calcification of the aortic wall has not been a contraindication to TEA. On numerous occasions calcification has been so dense that a satisfactory BPG was technically impossible to apply. If one applies particular care, a suitable endarterectomy plane can be accomplished.

The only technical difficulty results from perivascular inflammatory reaction, which is rarely encountered. If reasonable care is taken, this presents no real problem. The experienced surgeon usually finds little difference in the times required to perform a TEA and a BPG for Type I disease.

Type II aortoiliac atherosclerosis introduces a number of new considerations which have a substantial influence on the selection of operative method. It also introduces additional variables which influence the result of either operation and which increase the difficulty in comparing the two operations.

We have defined this group as all patients with atherosclerotic disease in the infrarenal aorta and/or common iliac arteries who have demonstrated distal lesions beyond the first 2 or 3 cm. of the external iliac arteries. This includes patients whose external iliac arteries have spotty or continuous posterior plaque formation without hemodynamically significant narrowing of the arterial lumen. Most patients in this group have arteriographically demonstrable irregularities in various segments of the femoropopliteal segments and often in the orifice of the profunda femoris arteries. Bilateral involvement is almost uniformly present, even though the obstructive lesions may be more advanced on one side and the symptoms confined to one leg at the time of the original operation.

There are wide variations in the rate of progression of the distal lesions. In our own experience, progression is more rapid in those patients whose first symptoms appear at a younger age (i.e., less than 50 years) and in women. The multiple foci of disease throughout the iliofemoral-popliteal arterial segment and the variations in rate of progression have a major impact on the durability of either operative method. As commonly performed, both operations terminate at a point proximal to the common femoral artery bifurcation and thus both become vulnerable to late failure as a result of progressive restriction of the outflow tract.

Since most patients with Type II aortoiliac atherosclerosis are susceptible to eventual occlusion of the superficial femoral arteries, the duration of patency of the profunda femoris arteries is a major factor in preserving patency of the proximal reconstructive operation. A widely patent profunda femoris collateral system sustains an adequate clinical result, even when superficial femoral disease progresses. Except for lesions at the orifice, the profunda femoris artery is usually the last artery in the leg to become involved with atherosclerosis. When disease does appear, it rarely extends beyond the second or third perforating branches. Martin,[2] Leeds,[3] Morris,[4] and their co-workers have stressed the importance of recognition of atherosclerosis in the profunda femoris artery and of operative procedures to deal with it. In our own experience, this is the most important part of the operation and often the part requiring the greatest technical skill.

In the discussion of operations for Type I disease, we listed technical approaches which we believe would compromise the long-term effectiveness of the operation. A similar list could be made of common practices in the use of TEA and BPG for Type II disease which lessen their effectiveness and durability.

1. Terminating the graft or the TEA at a convenient level in the external iliac arteries when there is palpable atherosclerosis of any degree in the distal portions of the external iliac artery.

2. Anastomosing the graft to a soft area on the wall of the common femoral artery without removing by endarterectomy any significant atheromatous involvement in other portions of the arterial wall at that site.

3. Failure to assure or develop a normal orifice into the profunda femoris artery and to remove atheromatous deposits in more distal portions of that artery.

4. Using a graft with an iliac arm of greater dimension than the outflow tract. This encourages mural thrombus within the graft subject to later disruption with thigh flexion. In general, an 8-mm. graft should be considered the maximum size for anastomosis to the common femoral artery.

5. Anastomosing the common femoral graft onto an arteriotomy which extends into the profunda femoris artery without removal of atheroma in the profunda orifice.

Review of our BPG series, now in progress, suggests that several of our late graft failures from our earlier operations are traceable to one or more of these technical errors. The published reports make little mention of these issues, and it seems highly probable that the difference in attention paid to them is a substantial cause of the wide variation in the frequency of late occlusion.

The editors have asked for an evaluation of endarterectomy with respect to the length of the arterial segment involved. They are, of course, calling attention to problems that might occur after endarterectomy of the external iliac artery. In our experience, the length of the segment is of less importance than the completeness of the endarterectomy. This view is supported by the experience of Inahara (Series G). His technique of eversion endarterectomy of the excised external iliac segment permits complete removal of the entire intimal layer. Of 147 external iliac arteries with diffuse atherosclerosis operated upon by him, there were only four in which endarterectomy could not be performed. In three of these the artery had atrophied to a fibrous cord. Inahara's report of a cumulative patency rate of 93.3 per cent at 8 to 9 years supports our belief that the endarterectomized external artery has no special predilection to late occlusion. The report of Duncan et al. (Series I) adds further support to this opinion.

Our own method utilizes the arterial stripper followed by careful palpation and inspection of the artery to make certain that there are no retained intimal fragments. We have favored this method over the eversion method because it permits preservation of the inferior epigastric and circumflex iliac arteries, two arteries which become an important source of collateral blood supply in the event of late occlusion of the iliac arteries. This method is technically feasible in approximately 85 per cent of patients with Type II disease.

A more important consideration is the relative ease with which BPG and TEA can be performed for external iliac disease. When the eversion endarterectomy technique is used, both methods require comparable operative maneuvers. The internal stripping method, however, requires a greater degree of skill and experience than the more simple BPG. Garrett et al.[5] have reported their preference for BPG operations in all patients with Type II disease. Judging from numerous personal communications with other surgeons, this now appears to be the dominant attitude in this country. Recently we have been turning more and more to BPG, frequently combined with endarterectomy of the common and profunda femoris arteries. It is apparent from both our own experience and that reported by others that extensive TEA for Type II disease should be performed only by surgeons with broad experience in endarterectomy techniques.

The critical technical factors in both operations appear in the methods of management at the distal level of the operation in the groin. If there is no palpable atherosclerosis beyond the middle third of the common femoral artery (an unusual event), a satisfactory end point for TEA can easily be obtained using a longitudinal arteriotomy. In most cases, variable degrees of abnormal intimal thickening extend into the superficial femoral artery. This is often patchy in distribution. The most satisfactory method for obtaining a suitable end point in this case is to transect the superficial femoral artery at a point of minimal disease. The TEA is then extended to that level. Anastomosis of the divided artery with fine (6–0) interrupted sutures provides a firm end point which is not vulnerable to further dissection.

The profunda femoris artery should be mobilized for at least its first 5 cm. or to the end of palpable atherosclerosis. If only an orifice lesion is present in the first 5 mm. of the artery, it usually may be removed through the common femoral arteriotomy and an adequate end point assured by direct inspection. If the atheroma extends beyond this level, attempts to remove it by blind forceps extraction invites early thrombosis from dissection beneath a loosely attached distal flap. A safer method is to transect the artery distal to the end of palpable disease and endarterectomize to that point. For extensive disease, transection may be required at intermediate points; the intima is then removed by subintimal passage of a dissecting instrument, sometimes combined with partial arterial eversion to assure completeness. In all cases requiring extensive profundoplasty, an operative arteriogram should be performed to demonstrate that an even lumen of normal caliber has been obtained.

A final statement should be made to conclude this chapter. This concerns the long-term management of patients who have undergone either reconstructive operation. The data clearly indicate that all patients are vulnerable to late failure. Following TEA, this may be caused by recurrent atherosclerosis in the endarterectomized segment. Following either operation, late closure may be the result of advancing lesions at the outflow site. In either case, impending failure may often be suspected by diminution in the femoral pulse or new bruits in the abdomen or over the groin. Demonstration of stenotic lesions by aortography at this time usually reveals correctable lesions, and appropriate operation will often forestall further difficulty. For these reasons, all patients should be followed at yearly intervals or more often.

# References

1. Staple, T. W.: The solitary aortoiliac lesion. Surgery 64:569, 1968.
2. Martin, P., Frawley, J. E., Barabas, A. P., and Rosengarten, D. S.: On the surgery of atherosclerosis of the profunda femoris artery. Surgery 71:182, 1972.
3. Leeds, F. H., and Gilfillan, R. S.: Revascularization of the ischemic limb (importance of the profunda femoris artery). Arch. Surg. 82:25, 1961.
4. Morris, G. C., Edwards, W., Cooley, D. A., Crawford, E. S., and DeBakey, M. E.: Surgical importance of the profunda femoris artery. Arch. Surg. 82:32, 1961.
5. Garrett, E. H., Crawford, E. S., Howell, J. F., and DeBakey, M. E.: Surgical considerations in the treatment of aortoiliac occlusive disease. Surg. Clin. North Am. 46:949, 1966.

# Series References

A. Humphries, A. W., Young, J. R., and McCormack, L. T.: Experiences with aortoiliac and femoropopliteal endarterectomy. Surgery 65:45, 1969.
B. Imparato, A. M., Sanoudos, G., Epstein, H. Y., Abrams, R. M., and Beranbaum, E. R.: Results in 96 aortoiliac reconstructive procedures: Preoperative, angiographic and functional classifications used as prognostic guides. Surgery 68:610, 1970.
C. Szilagyi, D. E., Smith, R. F., and Whitney, D. G.: The durability of aorto-iliac endarterectomy. Arch. Surg. 89:827, 1964.
D. Mozersky, D. J., Sumner, D. J., and Strandness, D. E.: Long-term results of reconstructive aortoiliac surgery. Am. J. Surg. 123:503, 1972.
E. Butcher, H. R., and Jaffe, B. M.: Treatment of aortoiliac arterial occlusive disease by endarterectomy. Ann. Surg. 173:925, 1971.
F. Pilcher, D. B., Barker, W. F., and Cannon, J. A.: An aortoiliac endarterectomy case series followed 10 years or more. Surgery 67:5, 1970.
G. Inahara, T.: Endarterectomy for occlusive disease of the aortoiliac and common femoral arteries. Am. J. Surg. 124:235, 1972.
H. Sawyer, P. N., Pasupathy, C. E., Fitzgerald, J., Kaplitt, M. J., Costello, M., Keates, J. R. W.,

O'Malley, G., and Lapovsky, A.: Six-year follow-up study in the use of gas endarterectomy. Surgery 72:837, 1972.

I.  Duncan, W. C., Linton, R. R., and Darling, R. C.: Aortoiliofemoral atherosclerotic occlusive disease: Comparative results of endarterectomy and Dacron bypass grafts. Surgery 70:974, 1971.

J.  Kouchoukos, N. T., Levy, J. F., Balfour, J. F., and Butcher, H. R.: Operative therapy for aortoiliac arterial occlusive disease. Arch. Surg. 96:628, 1968.

K.  Waibel, P. P., and Dunant, J. H.: Late results of aortoiliac reconstructive surgery. J. Cardiovasc. Surg. 14:492, 1973.

# Aortoiliac Occlusive Disease: Advantages of Bypass Grafting

**A. W. HUMPHRIES**

*Cleveland Clinic Foundation*

**and T. P. CORRIGAN**

*University College, Dublin, Ireland*

## Introduction

During the past two decades reconstruction of the aortoiliac arteries has become an established procedure in the treatment of ischemia of the lower limbs. Many studies have shown that long-term patency associated with symptomatic relief can be experienced by more than 75 per cent of patients following these procedures.[1-6] In addition, an in-hospital mortality of less than 5 per cent can be achieved.[1-8]

Two surgical techniques—endarterectomy and bypass graft—are available for reconstruction of the occluded aortoiliac segment. Which of the two is the better remains a matter of controversy.

The prime advantage of endarterectomy is that the procedure avoids the placement of a foreign body, whereas the basic disadvantages of endarterectomy are that the procedure is limited in scope and that it leaves behind the remnants of a vessel that has already proved itself susceptible to arteriosclerotic degeneration. The chief advantage of the graft is that the extent of diseased artery that must be bridged is essentially unlimited, while the disadvantages of grafting are that it requires the implantation of a foreign body with its attendant problems, should infection supervene, and whose suture lines may disrupt.

It is the purpose of this essay to show that bypass grafting constitutes the better overall approach.

## Comparison

We concur with the editors' introductory remarks regarding the desirability of properly controlled trials for the assessment of treatment methods.

451

Unfortunately, the available data are almost exclusively retrospective analyses of consecutive series of patients. We must base our assessment upon the published results of others and our own experience with the two procedures. We reviewed our experience with endarterectomy in 1969. Recently we have reviewed 102 cases of bypass graft for aortoiliac reconstruction done between 1967 and 1971. There are several ways in which the two procedures may be compared.

### Stress of Operation

The severity of the operation in terms of the extent of dissection, blood loss, and the time required to complete the procedure is particularly important in this group of patients, the majority of whom are in the older age group and have associated cardiopulmonary and renal disease. Gaspard and his colleagues[9] studied these points in a trial in which patients with aortoiliac occlusive disease of similar extent were randomly allocated to one or the other procedure. They found that not only was the blood requirement less in the bypass group, being 2.7 units per patient average as against 3.6 units per patient having endarterectomy, but also the average operating time was less, being 4.6 as against 5.8 hours.

In addition, they found that, of 22 patients in whom endarterectomy was attempted, the procedure had to be abandoned in 6 for technical reasons. These 6 patients then required some form of bypass graft. Failure to complete the operation in almost one-third of the patients represents a hidden high primary failure rate for the procedure. Our own experience has been that often several hours of work has been done before the endarterectomy is abandoned in favor of a bypass procedure. In these instances, the time of operation is obviously very prolonged. The inability to use endarterectomy for unexpectedly extensive disease is a strong deterrent against selection of the procedure for anything more than the most limited occlusions.

### Operative Mortality

On theoretic grounds, we would not expect to find a marked difference in the mortality rate from the two procedures, and indeed this is so, as indicated by published reports (Table 1).

#### TABLE 1. Operative Mortality

| Author | | Bypass | | Endarterectomy | |
|---|---|---|---|---|---|
| Gomes et al.,[6] | 1967 | (153)* | 4% | (75) | 3% |
| Duncan et al.,[4] | 1971 | (112) | 4% | (230) | 3% |
| Dean and Foster,[10] | 1973 | (39) | 7% | (60) | 19% |
| VanLent et al.,[3] | 1974 | (76) | 5% | (93) | 4% |
| Humphries et al.,[1] | 1969–1974 | (102) | 4% | (166) | 4% |

*Figures in parentheses indicate number of patients.

## Operative Morbidity

In contrast to the common complications of renal insufficiency, atelectasis, pneumonia, and myocardial ischemia, which should be the same in patients undergoing aortoiliac endarterectomy or bypass graft, the complication of operative infection carries different implications, depending upon the nature of the primary procedure. If infection occurs in the patient who has undergone endarterectomy, it can usually be successfully controlled by the use of suitable antibiotics, and the incidence of disruption of the arteriotomy closure is low. If infection occurs in a patient who has undergone a bypass graft, it is rarely controlled until the prosthesis, acting as a foreign body, has been removed. Such removal has, in the past, usually meant total loss of blood supply, massive gangrene, and frequently death. Although now this problem may sometimes be successfully handled by the use of extra-abdominal grafts (axillofemoral, femorofemoral), which permit removal of the infected aortoiliac or aortofemoral graft without resultant gangrene, infection of a prosthetic graft is frequently a disastrous occurrence.

Fortunately, the incidence of infected grafts is low. Szylagyi in 1972[11] reported a 1 per cent incidence of infection in bypass grafts for aortoiliac occlusions. Goldstone and Moore[12] have reported an infection rate of 2.5 per cent in 566 prostheses over a 15-year period. In that study the incidence of infection dropped from 4.1 per cent during the first 8 years to 1.5 per cent during the subsequent 7 years, the decrease being attributed to a more intensive use of prophylactic antibiotic management. It is of interest that in this study there was no difference in the incidence of infection between patients whose grafts were confined to the abdomen and those in whom they extended below the inguinal ligament into the groin. In our own series, two patients (2 per cent) developed infection. One which developed in the early postoperative period resulted in rupture of the femoral anastomosis, and the second was an incidental unexpected finding at autopsy of a patient 3 years after his aortofemoral graft. Death was from another cause.

## Early Patency

Some instances of reported early patency rates are shown in Table 2, and it may be seen that, in this respect, there is little difference between endarterectomy and bypass. Again, one must remember that some of the bypass procedures started out as endarterectomies that were abandoned in favor of the bypass for technical reasons.

The cause of early failure is usually technical in both procedures. In the case of endarterectomy, most primary failures are related to an inability to reach a spot where the endarterectomy can be terminated without leaving a significant "shelf" that can either dissect or cause thrombosis. In the case of bypass grafts, most primary failures are related to the distal anastomosis, particularly in those instances in which the graft is carried to the common femoral artery in the groin. In up to 50 per cent of cases in reported series, the superficial femoral artery is already occluded, and the distal runoff consists of only the profunda femoris and the circumflex vessels. If an adequate

TABLE 2.  Early Patency

| Author | | Bypass | | Endarterectomy | |
|---|---|---|---|---|---|
| Gomes et al.,[6] | 1967 | (153) | 96% | (72) | 96% |
| Irvine et al.,[13] | 1972 | (33) | 92% | (205) | 91% |
| Dean and Foster,[10] | 1973 | (39) | 93% | (60) | 93% |
| VanLent et al.,[3] | 1974 | (76) | 96% | (93) | 95% |
| Humphries et al.,[1] | 1969–1974 | (102) | 99% | (166) | 92% |

common femoral–profunda local endarterectomy is carried out and a proper distal anastomosis is achieved, these vessels provide adequate outflow. If not, a poor distal anastomosis will result in thrombosis of the graft and early failure.

### Late Patency

It may be seen from Table 3 that a similar patency rate may be expected for both endarterectomy and bypass during the first 5 years—perhaps slightly better in the case of grafts.

Late failure of an endarterectomy is usually caused by recurrence of arteriosclerosis, either within the endarterectomized segment or at the point of termination of the endarterectomy. Recurrence becomes more common the smaller the vessel involved and is so high in cases in which the external iliac artery has been endarterectomized that extension of an endarterectomy distal to the common iliac bifurcation has been generally abandoned. In Szilagyi's excellent follow-up studies,[17] recurrence, as demonstrated angiographically, progressed from 15 per cent at 3 years to 45 per cent at 6 years. He also noted that, once recurrence was demonstrable on arteriography, occlusion was essentially inevitable within 3 years. This progressive recurrence of the original disease has been reported by others.

The most common cause of bypass graft failures, especially when the repair is carried to the common femoral artery, is progressive arteriosclerosis distal to the area of repair. This results in a diminution in the size of the outflow tract and an increase in the peripheral resistance, thus causing slow

TABLE 3.  Late Patency

| Author | | Follow-up Period | Bypass | Endarterectomy |
|---|---|---|---|---|
| Gomes et al.,[6] | 1967 | 5-year average | | 75% |
| Gomes et al.,[6] | 1967 | 2-year average | 70% | |
| Irvine et al.,[13] | 1972 | 2-year average | 66% | 80% |
| Dickinson et al.,[14] | 1967 | 1–4 years | 92% | 82% |
| Dean and Foster,[10] | 1973 | 5 years | 85% | 65% |
| VanLent et al.,[3] | 1974 | 3 years | 84% | 84% |
| Szilagyi,[15] | 1972 | 5 years | 91% | 82% |
| Szilagyi,[15] | 1972 | 10 years | 70% | 60% |
| Perdue et al.,[16] | 1971 | 36-month average | 95% | 93% |
| Pilcher et al.,[7] | 1970 | 5 years | | 89% |
| Pilcher et al.,[7] | 1970 | 10 years | | 69% |

flow in the graft and ultimately thrombosis in situ. Progressive distal disease has uncommonly been cited as a cause of late failure following aortoiliac endarterectomy.

An additional cause of late failure of prosthetic grafts is the development of a false aneurysm, especially at the site of an end-to-side anastomosis. The incidence of false aneurysm in the groin has been reported as 2 to 3 per cent.[16-18] Since thrombosis of a false aneurysm is common, even a small one can result in a late occlusion of that limb of the graft. There was a period in 1958–59 when silk was commonly used for the suture material. Since silk loses 90 per cent of its tensile strength in the first year, false aneurysms were unnecessarily common. With Dacron suture being used, they are now far less common and are usually due to weakening of the patient's own tissue at the suture line rather than to breaking of the suture material itself.

### Reoperation

In the event of a late failure, the procedure required to manage the problem is quite different, depending upon the nature of the original procedure. If it was endarterectomy, the abdomen must be reopened and, since a second endarterectomy is usually technically impossible, some form of bypass graft must now be employed. If the original procedure was an aortofemoral graft, it is usually possible to restore patency by approaching the graft in the groin. The distal runoff can then be inspected and a local endarterectomy performed if necessary. The occluded limb of the graft may be thrombectomized by the use of a Fogarty catheter, Cannon loops, or both. This is a simple procedure when compared to a graft placement in the case of a patient who had originally undergone endarterectomy, an important point when the initial operation to be selected in these patients is being considered.

### Sexual Function

There has been little reported concerning the effect of aortoiliac surgery upon sexual function. Evaluation is difficult since there are no criteria to evaluate accurately blood flow to the genitals either before or after endarterectomy or bypass graft. In addition, the majority of these patients are in the age group in which sexual activity is less dominant in their way of life than it had previously been.

May[19] reported on this subject and found the incidence of impotence to be lower in patients whose procedure was confined to vessels proximal to the iliac bifurcation (27 per cent) than in those having aortofemoral bypass graft (45 per cent). Restoration of potency was higher (38 per cent) in those males having operations for less extensive disease (thus clearly revascularizing the hypogastric artery) than in those with extensive bypass procedures (0 per cent).

The incidence of retrograde ejaculation is directly related to the extent of dissection and to whether the nerve supply to the bladder neck sphincter is lost. This "dry" ejaculation has no effect on potency other than a psychological one.

## Discussion

As may be surmised from the preceding comparisons, the advantages of one procedure over the other are minimal. This must be the case if selection of the procedure remains a matter for controversy. However, in evaluating these points of comparison, three inequities, all of which favor endarterectomy, should be borne in mind.

1. Endarterectomy is generally reserved for patients whose disease is limited to the aorta and common iliac arteries,[3, 5, 16, 18, 21] while bypass is used in those patients with more extensive disease involving the external iliac artery and common femoral segment. This has the effect of preselecting for endarterectomy a group of patients who have disease that is readily amenable to operative correction. Szilagyi[17] indicated that, of patients with symptomatic aortiliac occlusive disease, only 25 to 30 per cent are suitable for endarterectomy proximal to the common iliac bifurcation. A similar figure is reported by Duncan,[4] who showed that, of 678 patients, only 32 per cent had disease limited to the aorta–common iliac segment. The remaining two-thirds of patients with more extensive disease must then perforce be treated with bypass graft.

2. Age has been used as a criterion for selection.[4] Bypass is frequently chosen in the older age groups in which associated disease increases the risk in the more extensive and longer endarterectomy procedure. The incidence of associated disease is high, as demonstrated by our own series in which, of 102 patients, 19 had previously documented myocardial infarcts, 9 had previous cerebrovascular disease, 7 had significant angiographically documented carotid stenosis, and 46 were hypertensive.

3. Several reported series of grafts include among the results those of homografts, Teflon, nylon, and other materials, the use of which has been abandoned because of poor results.[20-22]

## Conclusions

On the basis of our own experience and that of others with both endarterectomy and bypass graft for aortoiliac occlusive arteriosclerosis, we now use a bypass procedure in all patients unless they have uncommonly localized disease limited to the aorta and/or common iliac artery. We have made this decision for the following reasons:

1. Operative time, blood loss, and amount of dissection are less when a bypass graft is employed. These are important points when patients in the older age group, many of whom have other disease, are being operated upon.

2. Somewhat better long-term patency can be expected from bypass than from endarterectomy.

3. Bypass procedures have a wider applicability than endarterectomy. Virtually all patients are suitable for bypass, whereas only one-third are suitable for endarterectomy.

4. In the event of late occlusion, flow can often be reestablished in the case of a graft by operation limited to the groin, whereas occlusion of a previous endarterectomy generally requires reopening of the abdomen and placement of a bypass graft for correction.

The complications of infection and false aneurysm that are unique to the graft procedure are so infrequent at this time that we feel they are satisfactorily outweighed by the advantages of the procedure.

## *References*

1. Humphries, A. W., Young, J. R., and McCormack, L. J.: Experiences with aortoiliac and femoropopliteal endarterectomy. Surgery 65:48, 1969.
2. Szilagyi, D. E., Smith, R. F., Elliott, J. P., and Allen, H. M.: Long-term behavior of a Dacron arterial substitute. Ann. Surg. *162*:453, 1965.
3. VanLent, D., Kuijpers, P. J., Skotnicki, S. H., and Meyer, I.: Aortoiliac surgery: A comparative study between thromboendarterectomy and bypass. J. Cardiovasc. Surg. *15*:352, 1974.
4. Duncan, W. C., Linton, R. R., and Darling, R. C.: Aortoiliofemoral arterosclerotic occlusive disease: Comparative results of endarterectomy and Dacron bypass grafts. Surgery *70*:974, 1971.
5. Garrett, E. H., Crawford, E. S., Howell, J. F., and DeBakey, M. E.: Surgical considerations in the treatment of aortoiliac occlusive disease. Surg. Clin. North Am. 46:949, 1966.
6. Gomes, M. R., Bernatz, P. E., and Juergens, J. L.: Aortoiliac surgery—Influence of clinical factor on results. Arch. Surg. 95:387, 1967.
7. Pilcher, D. B., Barber, W. F., and Cannon, J. A.: An aortoiliac endarterectomy: Case series follow-up—10 years or more. Surgery 67:5, 1970.
8. Levinson, S. A., Levinson, H. J., Halloran, L. G., Brooks, J. W., Davis, R. J., Wolf, J. S., Lee, H. M., and Hume, D. M.: Limited indications for unilateral aortofemoral or iliofemoral vascular grafts. Arch. Surg. *107*:791, 1973.
9. Gaspard, D. J., Cohen, J. L., and Gaspar, M. R.: Aortoiliofemoral thromboendarterectomy vs. bypass graft: A randomized study. Arch. Surg. *105*:898, 1972.
10. Dean, R. H., and Foster, J. H.: Aortoiliac occlusive disease: Fifteen years' operative experience. South. Med. J. 66:813, 1973.
11. Szilagyi, D. E., Smith, R. F., and Elliott, J. P.: Infection in arterial reconstruction with synthetic grafts. Ann. Surg. *176*:321, 1972.
12. Goldstone, J., and Moore, W. S.: Infection in vascular prostheses. Am. J. Surg. *128*:225, 1974.
13. Irvine, W. T., Booth, R. A., and Myers, K.: Arterial surgery for aortoiliac occlusive vascular disease—Early and late results in 238 patients. Lancet *1*:738, 1972.
14. Dickinson, P. H., McNeill, I. F., and Morrison, J. M.: Aortoiliac occlusion. A review of 100 cases treated by direct arterial surgery. Br. J. Surg. *54*:764, 1967.
15. Szilagyi, D. E. (1972), *In* discussion of paper by Gaspard et al., 1972.[9]
16. Perdue, G. D., Long, W. D., and Smith, R. B.: Perspective concerning aorto-femoral arterial reconstruction. Arch. Surg. *173*:940, 1971.
17. Szilagyi, D. E., Smith, R. F., and Whitney, D. G.: The durability of aortoiliac endarterectomy. Arch. Surg. 89:827, 1964.
18. Moore, W. S., Cafferata, H. T., Hall, A. D., and Blaisdell, F. W.: In defense of grafts across the inguinal ligament: An evaluation of early and late results of aortofemoral bypass grafts. Ann. Surg. *168*:207, 1968.
19. May, A. G., DeWeese, J. A., and Rob, C. G.: Changes in sexual function following operation on the abdominal aorta. Surgery 65:41, 1969.
20. Minken, S. L., DeWeese, J. A., Southgate, W. A., Mahoney, E. B., and Rob, C. G.: Aortoiliac reconstruction for atherosclerotic occlusive disease. Surg. Gynecol. Obstet. *126*:1056, 1968.
21. Kouchoukos, N. T., Levy, J. F., Balfour, J. F., and Butcher, H. R.: Operative therapy for aortoiliac arterial occlusive disease—A comparison of therapeutic methods. Arch. Surg. 96:628, 1968.
22. Healey, S. J., Wheeler, H. B., Crane, C., and Warren, R.: Reconstructive operations for aortoiliac obliterative disease. New Engl. J. Med. *271*:1386, 1964.

# 20

# *Peripheral Nerve Injury — Primary versus Delayed Repair*

PRIMARY REPAIR OF INJURED
NERVES
   *by Erle E. Peacock, Jr.*

DELAYED REPAIR OF
PERIPHERAL NERVES
   *by Donald L. Erickson*

## Statement of the Problem

*The controversy relates to primary versus delayed repair of traumatically divided peripheral motor nerves and analyses of long-term results.*

Compare data on immediate repair versus delayed repair of a peripheral motor nerve in a relatively clean case with the nerve sharply and completely divided.

Compare the two techniques when a segment of nerve has been avulsed but where, with appropriate mobilization, the ends can be approximated.

In making the decision for immediate repair versus delayed repair, analyze and assign priority to the period of delay between injury and a favorable opportunity to attempt a repair, distance between the site of injury and the innervated muscles, complexity of muscular function lost, size of the nerve involved, and loss of function time. In addition, indicate the degree to which the skill of the injured person (artisan versus manual laborer) influences the choice of treatment (early or delayed).

Evaluate the importance of such factors as facilities and age of the injured person.

# Primary Repair of Injured Nerves

ERLE E. PEACOCK, JR.

*University of Arizona College of Medicine*

## *Introduction*

The first report of operative repair of a divided nerve was the description of a primary repair; so was the second report.[8] By 1893, a series of primary nerve repairs had been reported, and there seemed little possibility that controversy could ever arise over the choice of time when a peripheral nerve should be repaired.[5] Perhaps controversy would not have developed on this subject if two major events had not occurred—World War I and World War II. Large numbers of casualties with peripheral nerve injuries treated under less than optimum conditions by surgeons of varying experience and training could have been expected to produce statistics that would challenge any previous trend or established thinking. Such reports did appear and are the major reason why a controversy exists now about the proper time to repair severed nerves. The major contributors to the controversy have been the collectors and reporters of raw statistics; another factor, of course, has been a lack of critical thought on the part of surgeons. Review of prewar, war, and postwar experience leaves no doubt that primary repair of a severed peripheral nerve can produce excellent results (better than 85 per cent return of progressive Tinel's sign and motor and sensory function); the same is true, incidentally, following secondary repair.[12, 16] That either primary or secondary repair produces superior results when all other factors are equal has not been shown by any study performed on human beings. Moreover, the type of study which would be required to determine whether primary repair is better than secondary repair is not likely to be performed on human beings in the foreseeable future. Thus, a treatise designed to show the superiority of primary nerve repair over secondary repair cannot be anything more than a theoretic discourse. There are no new data to report, and preexisting data from study of human nerve injuries are of little or no scientific value. There are several reasons why this is true.

461

The most obvious reason why data from the study of human patients cannot be used to support primary or secondary nerve repair is that random selection of injuries and unbiased second-party evaluation of results (two of the most important criteria in clinical investigation) are not found in any previously reported group of patients. Apparently, control of conditions, other than time of repair, has been impossible, particularly during war. Moreover, measurement of results following nerve repair suffers from lack of reproducible end points, particularly in the evaluation of sensory function.[14] Fortunately for some patients, but unfortunately for investigators trying to assess axonal regeneration, there are a number of ways by which patients recover sensation in an anesthetic area other than by regeneration of a severed axon.[10] Electromyography and evoked axon potentials have provided a semblance of numerical end points, but again limb function, the sine qua non of motor regeneration, can be due to many factors other than axonal regeneration. The most direct appraisal of axonal regeneration — counting axons on the distal side of an anastomosis — has been virtually impossible for technical reasons. Only a cross-section of a whole nerve will suffice for axon counting, and present staining techniques for axons have not been dependable when applied to a cross-section of peripheral nerve. Longitudinal sections can be stained fairly accurately, but axoplasm is washed out too readily when a cross-section of a whole nerve is prepared for staining of axons. At present, electron microscopy is the best method for determining if axoplasm is really within an endoneural tube, but this is extremely difficult to carry out in a cross-section of a whole nerve from a human being. Although there are many reports based upon evaluation of axonal regeneration by histologic techniques, the technical problems involved in positively identifying axoplasm in whole nerve cross-sections have restricted the use of this measurement for evaluation of primary or secondary repairs.[13]

In summary, therefore, the author is of the opinion that published data do not support or weaken the case for either primary or secondary repair of a peripheral nerve when all other factors are equal. In spite of rather voluminous medical literature purporting to do so, lack of random selection of patients, lack of unbiased evaluation of neurologic results, and inaccurate laboratory techniques eliminate previous clinical reports from serious scientific consideration. Such reports either substantiate nothing except the bias of the author or show the effect of peripheral or ancillary factors, such as military conditions, surrounding wound complications, and training of the surgeon, on the results of nerve repair. The fact that results from one particular series of patients appear to favor primary or secondary repair is little more than coincidental in most such reports. Examples include the pre–World War I statistics of Howell, Huber, and Létiévant.[5,8] Howell and Huber reported 100 per cent improvement of neurologic function following primary repair of civilian nerve injuries and 88 per cent neurologic improvement following secondary repair of civilian injuries. An example of typical World War I statistics is provided by the data of Platt and Bristow, who reported 80 per cent good results following both primary and secondary repairs.[11]

The most extensive analysis of peripheral nerve injuries was conducted in the various peripheral nerve centers during and after World War II.[15] Typical of these results are those reported by Woodhall and Lyons, who found that there were only 5 per cent complete failures in peripheral nerves repaired secondarily, while there were 22.4 per cent complete failures of neurologic return in patients with peripheral nerves repaired at the time wounds were debrided.[16] Zachary and Holmes, analyzing the results of peripheral nerve repairs in British centers, reported twice as many good results following secondary repair as following primary repair.[17] The results of repair of peripheral nerve injuries in civilians after World War II have been reported by Stromberg, McFarlane, Bell, Sakellarides, and Larsen.[6, 12, 14] Typical of these reports are the data of Larsen, who found a 66 per cent incidence of return of motor function following primary repair of the nerves of the upper extremity; only 50 per cent of patients recovered motor function after secondary repair. All of these data probably are placed in proper perspective by the report of McEwan, which showed that when the results of war and civilian experiences are combined data do not seem to favor either primary or secondary repair of peripheral nerves.[9]

Before presenting the theoretic arguments supporting primary repair of peripheral nerves, it is important to recognize that secondary repairs do not mean a delay of many months or years. During World War I, primary repair meant immediate nerve repair at the time a wound was closed; delayed repair meant anastomosing the nerve several weeks after wound closure. Secondary repair meant a delay of many months or several years, so that function could be evaluated before deciding to repair a nerve. Although it is possible to recover some function months, or occasionally even years, after division of a peripheral nerve, delays of this order are not advocated. The term "primary nerve repair" denotes an immediate repair at the time of wound closure, and "secondary repair" means performing a definitive anastomosis anywhere from 3 weeks to 3 months after the wound has been closed and inflammation in surrounding tissue has subsided. Most surgeons recommend "tacking" the nerve ends together during wound closure, even though secondary definitive anastomosis is planned. Loosely tacking nerve ends together to prevent shortening of the nerve during soft tissue healing should not be confused with proper preparation of the nerve and performing a definitive anastomosis as either a primary or secondary procedure.

## Experimental Data

Good experimental evidence supporting primary repair of divided peripheral nerves can be found in an excellent study by Grabb performed in 1968.[3] All of the factors which presently are thought to influence axonal regeneration were controlled by Grabb except the time of anastomosis. The median nerve in monkeys was severed, and the results of primary immediate repair were compared with the results of a 2-week delayed repair. Electromyographic measurements in the opponens pollicis muscle were graded by an experienced observer who did not know whether the nerve had been repaired primarily or secondarily. The most critical weakness in the study was that a subjective evaluation of electrical response was necessary; reproducibility was higher than expected, however. Analysis of the grades of electrical response following primary repair resulted in superior (Grades A and B) electromyographic muscular response in the stimulated opponens pollicis muscle in all 30 primary nerve repairs. Following secondary repair in 30 monkeys, the electromyographic response was graded poor (C) in 27 monkeys and absent (D) in two others. The major criticism of this study involves the use of electromyography to assess function following nerve repair. Under the conditions of the experiment, however, primary repair of the median nerve in a monkey appeared superior to a delayed repair.

## Theoretic Arguments

With the exception of electromyographic data from a controlled experiment in monkeys, the case for primary repair of major nerves in the upper extremity has to be made on a theoretic basis. There are two theses—one based upon deduction of biologic data from wound healing experiments, the other based upon empiric observations and conclusions.

One may correctly deduce that primary repair of a peripheral nerve is most desirable because collagen synthesis and deposition by intra- and extraneural cells provide a physical barrier to axonal regeneration. Following this line of reasoning, a biologically oriented surgeon will approximate the proximal and distal endoneural tubes as soon as possible, so that axons can "jump the gap" and proceed down proper channels before endoneural scarring leads them astray or obliterates normal passageways. Not only would a delay of 2 or 3 weeks allow collagen to be deposited within and around an endoneural tube, but also the "secondary healing effect" would be at peak level, meaning that synthesis and deposition of new collagen following secondary repair would be occurring at a rate greatly accelerated over earlier periods.[7] Measurement of net collagen deposition following primary and secondary nerve repairs in guinea pigs showed an average of 26.5 μg. of hydroxyproline per mg. dry weight of nerve tissue following primary repair of the sciatic nerve, and 41.7 μg. of hydroxyproline per mg. dry weight of nerve following a 2-week delay before nerve repair. Interestingly, cutting back proximal and distal nerve ends several millimeters did not eliminate increased deposition of collagen in nerve ends following secondary anastomosis.[4]

Major objections to the argument for primary repair to anticipate collagen synthesis and deposition have been based upon morphologic changes in the cell body and the debris caused by wallerian degeneration in the distal neural tubes. Because cytoplasm clears, Nissl bodies temporarily disappear, and the location of the nucleus becomes eccentric following division of a peripheral axon, it has been suggested that synthesis of new axoplasm does not start for at least 3 weeks.[2] Therefore, an anastomosis delayed for at least 3 weeks would have marked advantage over a primary one owing to preparation of the distal endoneural tubule for instantaneous flow of axoplasm and availability of rough endocytoplasmic reticulum for new axoplasm synthesis. In considering such an argument, however, it must be remembered that, even though morphologic appearance of nerve cells in the dorsal ganglia does not appear favorable for axoplasm synthesis for several weeks, sprouting axoplasmic cylinders have been identified at the distal end of the proximal stump in a much shorter period of time.

A second theoretic disadvantage to primary repair—the appearance of lipid debris and phagocytic cells during wallerian degeneration—appears to involve a biologic and physical impediment to axoplasmic regeneration. The weakness of this argument is that debris is still present three or more weeks after injury, and there is not a whit of evidence that such debris affects the regeneration of axons in a distal endoneural tube. It must also be recognized that the same statement or reasoning can be made about collagen fibrils. Actually, regenerating axoplasm probably is more misdirected by fibrous protein than blocked by it. Because neuromas form about the same way and regeneration of axoplasm can be seen in about the same pattern in scorbutic as in normal guinea pigs, it seems most likely that neither cellular debris nor newly synthesized collagen fibrils have much to do with axonal regeneration.[4]

In summary, theoretic biology supporting primary nerve suture by giving regenerating axoplasm a head start on collagen synthesis is rather effectively counterbalanced by a similar argument favoring secondary repair. When the arguing is over, one is left with the cold realization that no data exist showing that cytoplasmic changes, distal scavenger activity to prepare a suitable runway, or local collagen synthesis is significant in recovery of distal motor and sensory function. Remarkable success following both primary and secondary nerve repairs suggests that none of the factors studied so far has a significant influence on neurologic recovery.

## Clinical Data

An occasional empiric clinical observation that supports primary repair over secondary repair is the finding of an extraordinary return of function or advancing Tinel's sign while waiting to perform a secondary repair. Most surgeons have had the disquieting experience of detecting an advancing Tinel's sign or even a proximal return of sensation in a patient in whom a secondary repair has been planned. This occurs most often after the ends of a severed nerve have been loosely tacked together by a single suture to prevent shortening. The phenomenon has occurred in the author's experience even when nerve ends have been left in 180 degrees of malrotation, so that only a tiny fraction of the cross-section of either nerve end was in contact with the other. When this happens, reluctance to re-open the wound and perform a secondary anastomosis is understandable. Valuable time is lost if procrastination continues; valuable function, which may not be regained, is lost if a secondary anastomosis is performed. Such a dilemma can be avoided by either performing the best technical anastomosis possible at the first operation (primary repair) or going back for a secondary repair so quickly that no evidence of regeneration can be detected. If the surgeon re-opens the wound early, however, many of the theoretic advantages of secondary repair may be lost; regeneration in a peripheral nerve may be detectable before all of the changes in the nerve body, distal sheath, and collagen system are theoretically favorable.

## Conclusions

Finally, the author has reasoned that analysis of all of the clinical data, all of the experimental data, and all of the theoretic biologic deductions leaves the thoughtful surgeon with the inescapable conclusion that major factors affecting regeneration of axons do not include whether a primary or early secondary anastomosis is performed. With the exception of the monkey experiments performed by Grabb, all other data seem to be reporting the effects of various clinical complications which led the surgeon to perform either a primary or secondary anastomosis in the first place and not whether a primary or secondary anastomosis affected the outcome. Such factors are a crushing versus an incisional injury, a tidy versus an untidy wound, an infected versus a contaminated wound, a skilled versus an unskilled surgeon, etc. Critical thinking and logical reasoning provide the strongest, if not the best, argument for performing a primary nerve repair. The conclusion is that, if it can be done, there does not seem to be any reason now not to perform a primary anastomosis, so why make a two-stage procedure out of what can be performed successfully in one stage? Such factors as inability to judge accurately longitudinal extent of nerve injury, inadequate soft tissue cover, lack of surgical technical ability, and excess tension are obvious contraindications to immediate repair of a peripheral nerve—regardless of theoretic factors involving axoplasmic regeneration. If no obvious contraindication to primary repair exists, however, the theoretic arguments favoring secondary repair do not seem very powerful in light of existing knowledge that primary repairs are known to produce a high incidence of good functional return. Expressed differently, controversy over whether primary or secondary nerve repair produces better functional results when obvious contraindications to primary repair do not exist seems more artifactual than real. It is probably safe to predict, therefore, that, once the real biologic, chemical, and electrical forces involved in directing regenerating axoplasm toward sensory and motor endplates are identified, the question of whether to perform a technical adjunct primarily or secondarily will no longer be controversial.

## References

1. Björkesten, G.: Suture of war injuries to peripheral nerves; clinical studies of results. Acta Chir. Scand. Suppl. *119*:1, 1947.
2. Ducker, T. B.: Metabolic factors in surgery of peripheral nerves. Surg. Clin. North Am. 52:1109, 1972.

3. Grabb, W. C.: Median and ulnar nerve suture: An experimental study comparing primary and secondary repair in monkeys. J. Bone Joint Surg. 50-A:964, 1968.
4. Hastings, J. C., and Peacock, E. E., Jr.: Effect of injury, repair, and ascorbic acid deficiency on collagen accumulation in peripheral nerves. Surg. Forum 24:516, 1973.
5. Howell, W. H., and Huber, G. C.: J. Physiol., London, 14:1, 1893.
6. Larsen, R. D., and Posch, J. L.: Nerve injuries in the upper extremity. Arch. Surg. 77:469, 1958.
7. Leonard, J. R., Madden, J. W., and Peacock, E. E., Jr.: The use of lathyrism to study secondary wound healing. Surg. Gynecol. Obstet. 133:247, 1971.
8. Létiévant, J. J.: Traité des sections nerveuses, Paris, 1873.
9. McEwan, L. E.: Median and ulnar nerve injuries. Aust. N. Z. J. Surg. 32:89, 1962.
10. Peacock, E. E., Jr.: Restoration of sensation in hand with extensive median nerve defects. Surgery 54:576, 1963.
11. Platt, H., and Bristow, W. R.: Br. J. Surg. 11:535, 1923.
12. Sakellarides, H.: A follow-up study of 172 peripheral nerve injuries in the upper extremity in civilians. J. Bone Joint Surg. 44-A:140, 1962.
13. Schröder, J. M.: Quantitative evaluation of regenerated nerve fibers. In Klunze, K., and Desmedt, J. E. (eds.): Studies on Neurovascular Diseases. Basel, S. Karger, 1975, p. 206.
14. Stromberg, W. B., McFarlane, R. M., Bell, J. L., Koch, S. C., and Mason, M. L.: Injury of the median and ulnar nerves. J. Bone Joint Surg. 43-A:717, 1961.
15. Woodhall, B., and Beebe, G. W.: Peripheral nerve regeneration. A follow-up study of 3,656 World War II injuries. Vet. Adm. Med. Monograph, Washington, D.C., Government Printing Office, June, 1956.
16. Woodhall, B., and Lyons, W. R.: Peripheral nerve injuries. I. The results of "early" nerve suture: A preliminary report. Surgery 19:757, 1946.
17. Zachary, R. B., and Holmes, W.: Primary suture of nerves. Surg. Gynecol. Obstet. 82:632, 1946.

# Delayed Repair of Peripheral Nerves

DONALD L. ERICKSON

*University of Minnesota Health Sciences Center*

## Introduction

When one considers the numerous stages of regeneration and repair that must occur sequentially to result in adequate neurologic recovery after a peripheral nerve operation, it is not difficult to understand why its outcome remains capricious. Following nerve transection, the cell body must begin preparation for axon repair, while peripherally the distal nerve stump is being cleared of useless debris by phagocytes. The nerve stumps must be approximated to allow the slowly growing axon to penetrate the distal tubules and ultimately reinnervate the end organ. Many factors beyond the surgeon's control, such as age of the patient, level of the injury, type of nerve involved, and severity of injury, will influence the ultimate result. The surgeon does, however, have a decisive role in the technical excellence of the repair as well as the timing of the repair. A controversy persists regarding the virtues of primary versus delayed nerve repair.

Respected surgeons have presented clinical series espousing primary repair, but equally qualified individuals have preferred secondary nerve suture. This debate remains unresolved because there is yet to be a well-controlled clinical series of nerve repairs using the two methods in unselected cases. Even in the absence of a controlled series, there are some generally accepted principles regarding the timing of nerve repair. Few surgeons would attempt primary repair of a nerve transected by a high-velocity missile. Conversely, the nerve accidentally transected during an operative procedure would be primarily repaired. This still leaves a large gray area, which represents the bulk of civilian nerve injuries, in which surgical judgment alone dictates the timing of the nerve repair. It is to these injuries that I will address this communication and for which I will recommend delayed nerve repair.

Prior to further discussion, we must agree on what is meant by delayed

469

nerve repair. I would prefer to use the term "two-stage nerve repair" to emphasize that there is a definitive management of the nerve stumps at the time of initial trauma as well as at the time of delayed repair. At the time of injury, it is our policy to do a careful epineural approximation, with debridement of only obviously necrotic nerve tissue, after concomitant surrounding tissue injuries have been repaired. After a delay of 2 to 4 weeks, the definitive repair is undertaken using an operating microscope to resect the stumps back to viable, normal-appearing funiculi. While we prefer a microsurgical funicular repair with 9–0 or 10–0 suture, many surgeons still perform a standard epineural repair with 6–0 or 7–0 suture. The controversy regarding funicular perineural suture or more classic epineural repair should be left for another paper. The nerve is mobilized sufficiently to allow anastomosis without tension at the suture line, and if this is impossible, autograft cables are used.

The reasons for the careful epineural repair at the first stage are as follows: (1) retraction of the nerve ends is prevented, which minimizes dissection and mobilization at the second stage; (2) nerve exposure is simplified at the second stage if the nerve is in continuity; and (3) careful epineural closure may reduce the deleterious effect on the nerve of fibroblastic activity from the surrounding traumatized tissue, although it is emphasized by Seddon[16] that most of the fibroblastic activity originates from within the nerve. I would reiterate at this time that, as we refer throughout this communication to first-stage nerve repair, we simply mean the careful epineural approximation in preparation for definitive delayed repair.

I believe it would be unreasonable to compare the results of primary and delayed nerve repair if one included all delayed repairs, regardless of how the nerve was handled primarily, how long a delay occurred prior to secondary repair, or whether the nerve was selected for delayed repair because the injury was too complex to lend itself to primary repair. The following information from published clinical series, research studies, and personal experience is presented to emphasize the pitfalls of primary repair and the advantages of delayed nerve repair.

## Clinical Data

Woodhall and Zachary[20, 21, 23] reported on military peripheral nerve injuries, and both authors emphasized the high failure rate with primary repair. In Zachary's group of 55 primary repairs, 19 underwent re-exploration, of which 6 were found to be grossly separated and 12 had dense neuromas at the suture line. Woodhall found a 50 per cent failure rate following primary repair. Although these are military injuries, two-thirds of Zachary's patients had lacerations rather than bullet wounds as the cause of nerve injury. Michon and Masse[11] compared results of the two types of repairs and found delayed repair superior. Haymaker[5] and White[19] emphasized the folly of primary repair in gunshot wounds.

Seddon[16] took a more intermediate stance, preferring delayed repair, but accepting the possibility that some nerve injuries would benefit by primary repair. He agreed that in small nerves located where delayed repair would be difficult (such as in the palm) primary repair is indicated. Sunderland[17, 18] also accepted the potential use of primary repair but established rigid criteria for its use.

Rank, Wakefield, Hueston, McEwan, and Bunnell[10, 15, 26] reported enthusiastically about the results of primary nerve repair. The one fact that continually surfaces in their papers, however, is the need to do primary repairs only in tidy wounds. Rank and Wakefield, in addition, emphasized the necessity of the availability of ideal supportive operating room help and rapid repair to avoid infection.

Some serious deficiencies in these clinical reports prevent one from establishing a firm opinion regarding the superiority of one technique over the other. Those favoring delayed repair have lumped many types of nerve injury together, including high-velocity missile injuries, which would certainly lead to many primary repair failures. Michon and Masse[11] compared primary nerve repairs performed by a variety of surgeons with delayed repairs done by themselves, which of course introduces a factor of technical differences. Larsen and Posch[9] favored primary repair but gave no statistics. Those authors who favored primary repair admittedly selected only clean wounds with sharply transected nerves and made no attempt to divide these into controlled primary and delayed series.

We are therefore presented with a large body of clinical information from which we can make no rational conclusion. Seddon sums it up candidly by stating, "If the surgeon says he is convinced of the superiority of one form of treatment, he is choosing to live by faith and not by reason." We must therefore look to other areas of information to make our decision.

## Research Information

Grabb[4] and others reported results on a controlled study of primary and delayed nerve repair in rhesus macaque monkeys. The nerves were divided by a knife or more bluntly by a hammer and anvil. Animals with primarily repaired nerves had better motor recovery. A similar study by Kline et al.[8] resulted in the same conclusions. Several items should be considered in evaluating their results. In the nerves selected for delayed repair, no attempt was made to approximate them initially to avoid retraction. Even in those nerves bluntly divided, the trauma to the nerve was very localized, and there was virtually no surrounding tissue injury. In Grabb's study, the nerves were divided at the wrist and were therefore very distal injuries. I do not believe that, based on this work, we can generalize that primary repair is superior in any but that very specific situation.

An excellent summary of the metabolic basis for nerve repair presented by Ducker[3] lends some theoretic support to delayed repair. Following axonal injury, the cell body sustains an initial insult, resulting in quiescence of axonal growth. There follows an increase in chromatolytic activity, which is interpreted as a preparation of the cell to repair that axon. This activity peaks in 2 to 3 weeks, while fibroblastic activity at the transection site proceeds at a more rapid rate and could potentially occlude the endoneural tubules before the neuron is capable of sending a new axon across the anastomosis. If one waits 2 to 3 weeks before doing the definitive nerve repair, the neuron is in a prime state to send out an axon bud with a greater chance of anastomosis penetration. The neuron does not suffer the same insult when the neuroma is resected at the time of delayed repair, because only a small amount of viable axon is resected. This short delay would then theoretically enhance nerve recovery, with little or no loss of time in reinnervation. This factor may be even more crucial in proximal nerve injuries, in which the phase of neuron recovery and regenerative preparation is even longer.

The published research on peripheral nerve injuries gives us some insight into the complex process of axon regeneration but inadequately deals with the problem of timing.

## Technical Considerations in Favor of Delayed Repair

It is impossible, at the time of initial trauma, to determine the extent of damage to proximal and distal segments. Several weeks following trauma, the demarcation between damaged and normal nerve is clearly visible, and herein rests the single most important advantage of delayed nerve repair. Having done temporary first-stage approximation in what appeared to be sharply transected nerves, I have found dense neuromas 1 or more cm. in length at the time of delayed repair 3 or 4 weeks later. When nerves have been torn or stretched, this proximal neuroma may be several centimeters long. If one attempts primary repair of such a nerve, it will surely fail. If, however, one arbitrarily resects a centimeter or more of nerve at the time of primary repair, some normal nerve may be sacrificed. Even more diastrous is the situation which results when a nerve is resected for primary repair and a failure occurs, requiring additional resection at the time of delayed repair, in turn adding to tension at the suture line, or even requiring a nerve graft to achieve continuity.

A simple but critical technical problem relates to maintaining nerve stump approximation following primary repair. The epineurium becomes progressively edematous and friable following trauma, so that tissue, seemingly sturdy several hours after transection, may have much less tensile strength on the following day, allowing disruption of the suture line. The slight thickening that occurs in the epineurium during the first several weeks after injury makes delayed repair technically easier and dehiscence less likely. Another problem related to primary repair is the reluctance of the surgeon to mobilize the nerve proximally and distally in a potentially contaminated wound. Without adequate mobilization, the anastomosis would be performed under increased tension, predisposing it to disruption and also, according to Samii,[25] to inadequate nerve regeneration.

If there is significant associated tendon or muscle injury requiring repair, one can be certain that these tissues will be incorporated in one block of scar with the nerve anastomosis. If one delays the nerve repair, anastomosis is then performed in a dry field with a minimum of surrounding acute tissue damage, so that the nerve is less likely to become densely bound to adjacent structures.

Other minor problems such as duration of tourniquet time for concomitant injuries, availability of experienced, nonfatigued operating room personnel, and presence of an experienced surgeon may all help dictate the selection of delayed nerve repair.

## VALIDITY OF TECHNICAL CONSIDERATIONS IN FAVOR OF PRIMARY NERVE REPAIR

Primary nerve repair has not been adequately demonstrated to be superior to delayed repair in humans, even in clearly transected nerves. We shall therefore review and discuss the commonly stated advantages of primary repair in an attempt to assess their validity.

1. "Primary repair is more convenient for the patient because only one operative procedure is necessary." This argument is valid only if primary repair does not fail, for if it does, the inconvenience to the patient is compounded and the ultimate result unsatisfactory. The reported high failure rates in unfavorable injuries would certainly negate this potential advantage.

2. "Primary repair avoids delay of neurologic recovery." When one considers the slow rate of axon growth, a delay of 2 or 3 weeks is insignificant. Sunderland, Tower, and Woodhall[17, 18, 20, 21, 26] have all emphasized the progressive changes in denervated muscle following nerve transection, but according to Woodhall, the reduction of motor recovery is only 1 per cent for every 3-week delay. There appear to be no deleterious effects of delay upon return of sensory function.

3. "Primary repair is technically easier because one does not need to dissect the nerve stumps from the scar that is inevitably present at the time of delayed repair." Although this is certainly true, it is that very scar tissue which may be the barrier to adequate nerve regeneration. Furthermore, if the nerve is carefully approximated initially, the exposure is technically easy at the time of delayed repair. Moreover, if the delayed repair is performed in the first 2 to 3 weeks, the scar tissue is generally not excessive.

4. "Primary repair prevents nerve retraction and the subsequent mobilization that is required for delayed repair." We agree with this concept and, for that reason, do an epineural approximation at the time of the initial injury.

5. "The opportunity for funicular matching is lost if primary repair is not done." This concept is true only if the transection is so neat that virtually no trimming of the nerves is required, because Sunderland's work has demonstrated that funicular patterns may change markedly in as little as 2 to 3 mm.

6. "One last concept regarding primary repair is that if it fails one can always do a delayed repair." The obvious defect in this plan is related to the excessive time delay required to determine the efficacy of the primary

repair. Depending on the location, some months can elapse before failure or success is determined. One could use the recording technique suggested by Kline,[7, 8] but this would require re-exposure of the nerve proximal and distal to the anastomosis some weeks after repair. If the delay lasts several months, small muscle atrophy increases and distal stump endoneural tubules shrink, reducing the likelihood of a successful recovery.

## Summary

Primary nerve repair must be reserved for only the most cleanly severed peripheral nerves, and even in those selected injuries, no one has demonstrated its superiority over delayed repair. The risk of failure with primary repair in any but simple nerve injuries remains high.

Delayed nerve repair continues to be a dependable method of restoring neurologic function in the majority of peripheral nerve injuries.

## References

1. Campbell, E. H.: The Mediterranean theater of operations. *In* Coates, J. B. (ed.): *Surgery in World War II.* Vol. II. *Neurosurgery.* Washington, D.C., U. S. Government Printing Office, 1959, pp. 231–238.
2. Davis, L., and Davis, R. A.: *Principles of Neurological Surgery.* Philadelphia, W. B. Saunders Co., 1963, pp. 491–494.
3. Ducker, T. B., Kempe, L. G., and Hayes, G. J.: The metabolic background for peripheral nerve surgery. J. Neurosurg. *30*:270, 1969.
4. Grabb, W. C.: Median and ulnar nerve suture: An experimental study comparing primary and secondary repair in monkeys. J. Bone Joint Surg. *50-A*:964, 1968.
5. Haymaker, W.: Pathology of peripheral nerve injuries. Milit. Surg. *102*:448, 1948.
6. Kahn, F. A.: Peripheral nerve. *In Correlative Neurosurgery.* 2nd ed. Springfield, Ill., Charles C Thomas, Publisher, 1969.
7. Kline, D. G., Hackett, E. R., and LeBlanc, H. J.: The value of primary repair for bluntly transected nerve injuries: Physiological documentation. In *Surgical Forum, 6th Annual Clinical Congress.* Vol. 25. Chicago, American College of Surgeons, 1974, pp. 436–438.
8. Kline, D. G., Hackett, E. R., and May, P. R.: Evaluation of nerve injuries by evoked potentials and electromyography. J. Neurosurg. *31*:128, 1969.
9. Larsen, R. D., and Posch, J. L.: Nerve injuries of the upper extremity. Arch. Surg. 77:469, 1958.
10. McEwan, L. E.: Median and ulnar nerve injuries. Aust. N.Z. J. Surg. 32:89, 1962.
11. Michon, J., and Masse, P.: Le moment optimum de la suture nerveuse dans les plaies du membre superieur. Rev. Chir. Orthop. 50:205, 1964.
12. Mullan, S.: *Essentials of Neurosurgery.* New York, Springer Publishing Co., Inc., 1961, pp. 188–191.
13. Nulsen, F. E., and Kline, D. G.: Acute injuries of peripheral nerves. *In* Youmans, J. R. (ed.): *Neurological Surgery,* Vol. 2. Philadelphia, W. B. Saunders Co., 1973, pp. 1089–1140.
14. Nulsen, F. E.: The management of peripheral nerve injuries producing hand dysfunction. *In* Flynn, J. T. (ed.): *Hand Surgery.* Baltimore, The Williams & Wilkins Co., 1966, pp. 457–481.
15. Rank, B. K., Wakefield, A, R., and Hueston, J. T.: *Surgery of Repair as Applied to Hand Injuries.* 3rd ed. Edinburgh, Livingstone, 1968.
16. Seddon, H.: *Surgical Disorders of the Peripheral Nerves.* Baltimore, The Williams & Wilkins Co., 1972.
17. Sunderland, S., and Bradley, K. C.: Denervation atrophy of the distal stump of a severed nerve. J. Comp. Neurol. *93*:401, 1950.

18. Sunderland, S., and Ray, L. J.: Denervation changes in mammalian striated muscle. J. Neurol. Neurosurg. Psychiatry 13:159, 1950.
19. White, J. C.: Timing of nerve suture in gunshot wound. Surgery 48:946, 1960.
20. Woodhall, B., and Beebe, G. W.: Peripheral nerve regeneration. (American) Veterans Administration Monograph. Washington, D.C., United States Government Printing Office, 1956.
21. Woodhall, B., and Lyons, W. R.: Peripheral nerve injuries. I. The results of "early" nerve suture: A preliminary report. Surgery 19:757, 1946.
22. Yahr, M. D., and Beebe, G. W.: Recovery of motor function. In Woodhall, B., and Beebe, B. W. (eds.): Peripheral Nerve Regeneration. Washington, D.C., United States Government Printing Office, 1956, pp. 71–97.
23. Zachary, R. B., and Holmes, W.: Primary suture of nerves. Surg. Gynecol. Obstet. 82:632, 1946.
24. Tower, S. S.: Atrophy and degeneration in skeletal muscles. Amer. J. Anat. 56:1, 1935.
25. Samii, M., and Wallenborn, R.: Experimental investigations concerning the influence of tension in the results of nerve sutures. Acta Neurochir. 27:87, 1972.
26. Bunnell, S.: Surgery of the Hand. Philadelphia, J. B. Lippincott Co., 1964.

# 21

# *Retroperitoneal Lymph Node Dissection for Testicular Tumors*

THE ROLE OF RADICAL
OPERATION IN THE
MANAGEMENT OF
NONSEMINOMATOUS GERMINAL
TUMORS OF THE TESTICLE IN
THE ADULT
*by Elwin E. Fraley, Kailash Kedia,
and Colin Markland*

THE MANAGEMENT OF TUMORS
OF THE TESTIS
*by John Blandy, Robin Chapman,
David Pollock, and Elizabeth Molland*

## Statement of the Problem

*The major questions addressed are the extent of lymph node dissection and the use of supplemental radiotherapy in various histologic types of testicular tumors — seminoma, embryonal carcinoma, and teratocarcinoma — assuming a single cell type.*

*With a palpable, recently discovered testicular mass, should an incisional or excisional biopsy be done? Describe your approach to establishing the diagnosis.*

*Do you proceed with a potentially curative radical procedure on the basis of frozen section diagnosis?*

*Analyze how the histologic character dictates the primary operation.*

*Define the role of lymphangiography in the decision about the need for node dissection.*

*Evaluate cure and morbidity statistics for radical versus conservative node dissection, comparing histologic types. Provide data.*

*Analyze data for and against use of postoperative radiation therapy with respect to each histologic type.*

*Provide data for radiotherapy as an alternative to or supplement to retroperitoneal node dissection. Should radiotherapy precede or follow node dissection?*

*Indicate bases for a decision to carry out a node dissection in the presence of a potentially solitary lung metastasis.*

# The Role of Radical Operation in the Management of Nonseminomatous Germinal Tumors of the Testicle in the Adult

ELWIN E. FRALEY,
KAILASH KEDIA,
and COLIN MARKLAND

*University of Minnesota Health Sciences Center*

Neoplasms of the testicle are classified according to their probable cell of origin—that is, germinal or nongerminal cell tumors. Over 95 per cent of testis tumors in adults are germinal cell cancers, and all are malignant. Pathologists in the United States classify germinal cell neoplasms according to four main histologic types—seminoma, teratocarcinoma, embryonal carcinoma, and choriocarcinoma. The majority of nonseminomatous tumors are either embryonal carcinoma or teratocarcinoma, or some combination thereof (mixed tumors); pure choriocarcinoma or mixed tumors of the testis which contain choriocarcinoma are rare.

There is little disagreement that seminomas should be treated by radical orchiectomy and radiation therapy, since this regimen has produced an overall cure rate of approximately 95 per cent in most series. By contrast, the proper treatment for nonseminomatous cancers is more controversial.

Although a variety of therapies has been advocated for nonseminomatous tumors, the best overall results have been obtained either by radical inguinal orchiectomy and radical retroperitoneal dissection alone or by radical orchiectomy, radical retroperitoneal dissection, and radiation (Table 1).[1-5] In most series in which operation and radiation have been employed, the radiation has been given either in selected cases postoperatively or both pre- and postoperatively as a "sandwich" technique.[4]

479

Any suspected testis tumor should be explored by using an inguinal incision. Unfortunately, the diagnosis is often established by an improper approach to the tumor. For example, in our series of 62 patients, 25 had "contaminated" scrotums which occurred when the surgeon either performed a biopsy on the testis or did an orchiectomy through the scrotum. Either of these maneuvers can contaminate the lymphatics of the scrotal skin with tumor, and these lymphatics have ubiquitous connections with the lymphatics of the abdominal wall and inguinal region. Our patients with contaminated scrotums were treated by hemiscrotectomy and superficial inguinal lymphadenectomy, as described previously.[6]

To reiterate, the proper approach to any potentially neoplastic testicular mass is through an inguinal incision, so that the spermatic cord can be isolated and occluded at the internal ring before the testis and all of its surrounding tissues are delivered into the wound. Often the diagnosis is obvious from the gross appearance of the testicle, but occasionally a frozen section must be obtained before the orchiectomy is done. Biopsy of a suspected testicular tumor must be carried out with meticulous technique, so that the inguinal region is not contaminated with tumor. If a testicular cancer is present, the cord is divided at the internal inguinal ring, and the vas deferens and spermatic vessels are ligated with permanent sutures, so that the site where the cord was transected can be identified when the spermatic vessels are removed during the subsequent retroperitoneal dissection. It is important to remove all of the cord structures from the inguinal canal, because metastases are often present in the lymphatics of the cord distal to the inguinal ring.

Usually the orchiectomy is done as soon as possible after a scrotal mass is discovered. Since the diagnosis is unknown, the patient usually has not had a thorough preoperative evaluation for cancer prior to the testicular exploration, and therefore no other treatment is carried out at the time of orchiectomy. Another reason for deferring further therapy is that any analysis of testis tumors by frozen section is unreliable because of a potential sampling error. The corollary of the preceding statement is that all testicular cancers should be examined by multiple permanent sections before deciding on treatment. If a testis cancer contains any nonseminomatous components, it must be treated as a nonseminomatous tumor.

Once the orchiectomy has been completed—if the patient does not have a pure seminoma, a pure choriocarcinoma, or widespread metastases—he is evaluated more extensively to determine whether a transthoracic retroperitoneal dissection should be done. The most important preoperative radiographic procedure in terms of staging a testis cancer is chest tomography, since the lungs are one of the common sites of extranodal metastases. Moreover, it is essential to obtain an intravenous urogram for two reasons: (1) the urogram may show displacement of both the ureter and the normal kidney axis if multiple retroperitoneal metastases are present; and (2) it may be necessary to remove the ipsilateral kidney as part of the en bloc dissection if extensive metastases are present; therefore, the condition of the contralateral kidney must be known preoperatively. We do not do lymphangiography because it has hazards, and even if it suggests multiple metastases, radical operation is done provided the patient does not have widespread cancer. A patient with

**TABLE 1.** Overall Survival with Nonseminomatous Germinal Cell
Testicular Neoplasms (Stage A and B) Treated with Radical Orchiectomy
Plus Radical Retroperitoneal Lymph Node Dissection
with or without Radiation and/or Chemotherapy

| | | Survival | |
| Series | Number of Cases | Number | Per Cent |
|---|---|---|---|
| Maier et al.[1] | 213 | 125 | 59 |
| Skinner and Leadbetter[2] | 57 | 42 | 74 |
| Staubitz et al.[3] | 65 | 57 | 87 |
| Nicholson et al.[4] | 35 | 29 | 83 |
| Walsh et al.[5] | 64 | 53 | 83 |

tumor localized to the testicle has Stage A disease; if the retroperitoneal nodes are positive, the disease is Stage B; and if widespread metastases or metastases outside the retroperitoneum above the diaphragm are present, the cancer is Stage C.

Because excellent results have been obtained in the treatment of non-seminomatous tumors by operation alone or by operation and radiation (Table 1), we have treated all patients with Stage A and B teratocarcinomas, embryonal carcinomas, or mixed tumors by radical operation. We do not advocate radical operation for pure choriocarcinoma, because no therapy has proved effective, probably because these tumors metastasize early by blood vessels. However, mixed tumors containing choriocarcinoma were treated like any other nonseminomatous tumors. As will be discussed, patients with positive retroperitoneal nodes also received postoperative radiation.

We prefer the high transthoracic approach to the retroperitoneum, because it is the technique which gives the most adequate exposure of the aorta and vena cava proximal to the renal vessels.[7] The chest and diaphragm should be opened using an eighth or ninth rib incision, which is carried medially across the ipsilateral rectus; the contralateral rectus also is partially divided. Another incision is made lateral to the ipsilateral rectus from the inguinal region to the midportion upper incision—a so-called T incision. It is necessary to begin the dissection above both renal vascular pedicles so as to obtain an adequate proximal margin on the tissues which may contain tumor. The tissues that are removed are the ipsilateral adrenal gland, the ipsilateral perirenal fat, the lymphatics and sympathetics from both sides of the great vessels down to the level of the inferior mesenteric artery, and the ipsilateral lymphatics and sympathetic tissues down to the level of the bifurcation of the common iliac vessels. Thus, a bilateral lymphadenectomy is carried out from the crus of the diaphragm down to the inferior mesenteric artery, and then a unilateral dissection is done on the side of the primary tumor. The ipsilateral adrenal gland is removed because the periadrenal lymphatics are not an uncommon site for metastases. The retroperitoneal spermatic lymphatic and blood vessels also must be removed completely, and their distal transected ends can be identified if nonabsorbable sutures were used to ligate the cord structures at the time of orchiectomy. Thus, it is more appropriate to use the appellation "retroperitoneal dissection" than "retroperitoneal lymphadenectomy" to describe this operation.

We have performed 62 operations for nonseminomatous tumors using this technique, and Skinner and Leadbetter[2] and Donohue[8] have reported 100 additional patients treated in essentially the same way without an operative death. The most likely explanation for the low death and complication rate in these series is that the majority of the patients are otherwise healthy men between 18 and 35 years of age. The most significant postoperative morbidity involves the sterility of the patients because they do not ejaculate. However, all of our patients are potent, and all experience satisfactory orgasms. We have shown that the aspermia in these patients is not due to retrograde ejaculation, as previously thought, but rather is caused by extirpation of the ipsilateral lumbar sympathetics, which we have postulated interferes with seminal vesical contraction and transport of semen into the prostatic urethra.[9] There are no other detailed reports on sexual function in patients who have had this operation, even though it has been written repeatedly that these patients are impotent postoperatively.

In our series of 62 patients, 54 have been followed from 2 to 7 years, with an overall survival rate of 92 per cent (Table 2). Of these patients 28 had negative nodes and 26 had positive nodes. All patients with negative nodes were treated by operation alone, and not one has developed recurrent tumor. Staubitz reported an 85 per cent survival rate in patients with negative nodes treated by operation alone,[3*] and Donohue[8] also has achieved over 90 per cent survival in patients with Stage A and B disease treated by operation alone or by combined operation, radiation, and, in some instances, chemotherapy. The patients in both of these series have been followed for 2 or more years. Although there is no clear statement on this issue elsewhere in the literature, these data suggest that radical orchiectomy and radical retroperitoneal dissection are sufficient treatment for patients with histologically negative nodes. We believe that it is important to avoid radiating these patients for four reasons. First, since patients with Stage A disease treated by either pre- or postoperative radiation or both have a less satisfactory survival than our patients treated by operation alone, it is conceivable that radiation may be detrimental in patients with negative nodes. Second, as was pointed out by Nicholson et al.,[4] there is some indication that young patients who receive extensive radiation have an increased incidence of other tumors that develop subsequently.[10, 11] Third, in Donohue's[8] series of 46 patients fol-

---

*A 2-year survival figure is important, because nonseminomatous testicular tumors treated by operation very rarely recur after 2 years.[12]

**TABLE 2.    Two-Year or More Survival of Patients with Nonseminomatous Germinal Cell Tumors of the Testes – University of Minnesota Experience**

| Series | Number of Cases | Survival | |
|---|---|---|---|
| | | Number | Per Cent |
| Overall survival | 54 | 49 | 92 |
| With negative nodes | 28 | 28 | 100 |
| With positive nodes | 26 | 21 | 81 |

lowed for over 2 years, there were two deaths from late complications of radiation in patients who were tumor-free. A similar experience has been reported by Nefzger and Mostofi,[12] who showed that 24 patients who died between 2 and 17 years after treatment of nonseminomatous germinal cell testicular tumors died from the effects of radiation. Finally, it is our clinical impression that radiation combined with operation produces more morbidity than either treatment alone.

All patients with positive nodes in our series were treated with radiation therapy beginning 4 to 6 weeks postoperatively. The mediastinum and left supraclavicular region were treated first with a total of 4500 R. After the mediastinal radiation was completed, the patient was given 4000 R. to the retroperitoneum and ipsilateral common iliac and inguinal nodes. For the most part, none of our patients with positive nodes received chemotherapy unless he subsequently developed widespread metastatic disease. If these patients required chemotherapy, this was done in collaboration with the Medical Oncology Service, and the types of drugs, dosage schedules, and other pertinent data have been reported.[13] The overall 2-year or more survival rate in patients with positive nodes operated on for cure in our series was 81 per cent (Table 2). All of these patients are apparently disease-free.

Although we use postoperative radiation in patients with positive nodes, there are no data to prove that survival is enhanced. However, now that some centers are treating these patients by operation alone, several important questions with respect to the selection of candidates for additional treatment may soon be resolved. For example, results from the "operation only" group may show that patients with one or two microscopic metastases should not be given postoperative radiation. Furthermore, the results in patients treated by operation alone may demonstrate that patients with positive nodes from one type of tumor are at greater risk than those with a different histologic type and thus may be better candidates for multimodal therapy. Data from the London Hospital[14, 15] suggest that teratocarcinomas are more radiosensitive (Table 3).

Of course, nonseminomatous testicular tumors have been treated by other methods. For example, there is enough evidence to show that radical orchiectomy alone is associated with only a 30 to 50 per cent overall survival;[2] orchiectomy alone is not considered proper therapy. Another possible treatment would combine orchiectomy and chemotherapy, but there are neither data nor any logical reasons to suggest that this form of treatment should be considered. The results of treatment consisting of radical orchiectomy and radiation alone are not as satisfactory as those obtained with either orchiectomy and radical operation alone or orchiectomy, retroperitoneal dissection, and radiation. However, there are some individuals who still argue in favor of treating at least certain of these tumors with only radical orchiectomy and radiation; therefore, the merit of this point of view is examined in more detail.

None of the major cancer centers in the United States is treating nonseminomatous testicular cancers or mixed tumors by orchiectomy and radiation as the sole treatment. One of the largest series of patients treated by this regimen has been reported from the London Hospital,[14] as summarized in

TABLE 3.   Two-year Survival Stages I and II Teratomas of the Testicle Treated by Radiation Therapy—London Hospital Series

| Terminology | | Available | Two-year Survival | Lost to Follow-up by 2 Years | Four Years | Lost to Follow-up by 4 Years |
|---|---|---|---|---|---|---|
| *British* | *American* | | | | | |
| MTA | Embryonal carcinoma: undifferentiated | 10 | 4/10 | 0 | 3/9 | 1 |
| MTIA | Teratocarcinoma | 30 | 25/28 | 2 | 18/24 | 6 |
| MTIB | Embryonal carcinoma: better differentiated | 13 | 3/12 | 1 | 1/10 | 3 |
| TD | Teratoma | 2 | 0/1 | 1 | 0/1 | 1 |
| Unclassified | | 21 | 13/12 | 0 | 10/21 | 0 |
| Total | | 76 | 45/72 (overall survival 63%) | 4 | 32/65 (overall survival 49%) | 11 |

Table 3. However, it is impossible to consider the London Hospital series without a discussion of the differences in classification of testicular tumors by pathologists from England and the United States. In brief, both groups agree that germinal cell tumors can be divided into seminomatous and non-seminomatous groups, but the British classify all nonseminomatous germinal tumors as teratomas, which they further subdivide on the basis of the degree of differentiation present in the most differentiated portion of the tumor.

If we assume that the tumors which the British classify as MTIA (malignant teratoma intermediate anaplastic) are at least roughly equivalent to teratocarcinomas (U.S.), then the reported 83 per cent 2-year survival rate for these tumors suggests that radiation therapy can produce a satisfactory survival rate in this subgroup of nonseminomatous tumors. However, if the same patients are examined with respect to 4-year survival, 18 of 24, or 75 per cent of the patients who were available for assessment, survived. Whether this last figure reflects true survival is impossible to determine, since six patients with MTIA had been lost to follow-up after 4 years. Assuming that four of the patients who were not available for assessment died of their cancers, the 4-year survival rate for MTIA treated by radiation and orchiectomy would have been 20 of 28, or 71 per cent. As was stated previously, it is unusual for patients with Stage A or B nonseminomatous testicular tumors treated by retroperitoneal dissection who are free of disease for at least 2 years to develop subsequent metastases. In fact, Nefzger and Mostofi[12] showed that, in a series of 273 patients who were treated for nonseminomatous germinal cell testicular tumors and who survived 2 years, the chance of living an additional 15 years was almost exactly the same as that of a normal population of men of the same age. Furthermore, in our own series, the longest survival of any patient who died of his disease following treatment was 20 months. Thus, it may be that the patients with MTIA who died after 2 to 4 years had their tumors arrested only temporarily by radiation and that the 4-year survival reflects more accurately the efficacy of radiation therapy in these patients.

To summarize the early results from the London Hospital, the overall 2-

year survival was 63 per cent, and the 4-year survival was 49 per cent (Table 3). Again, this last figure makes no allowance for the 11 patients who were lost to follow-up. Assuming that two-thirds of the 11 patients died of their tumors, the overall 4-year survival in this series would have been 48 per cent.

It should be emphasized that the results of the London Hospital series presented in Table 3 were obtained in patients treated since 1927. Obviously, the techniques of radiation therapy have been improving steadily, and the results of modern approaches may be more satisfactory. Furthermore, follow-up in many of these patients was difficult because of World War II. A more recent analysis of data from the same institution was presented by Chapman et al.,[15] who reported on a group of patients with clinical Stage A MTIA treated with orchiectomy and radiation after 1950. In contrast to the earlier report,[14] there were 37 patients with Stage A disease, all of whom were followed 5 years or more, with a crude survival of 89 per cent. There were no survival statistics presented on clinical Stage B MTIA tumors, even though there were three patients cited as having Stage B tumors. If none of the patients with Stage B tumors survived their disease, then the 5-year survival for MTIA Stage A and B treated by radiation only would have been 33 of 40, or 82.5 per cent. This figure is very close to the 4-year survival (75 per cent) reported earlier (Table 3).[14] The figures which have been reported for Stage A and B teratocarcinoma treated by operation alone or by operation and radiation show an 85 per cent 2- to 5-year survival (Table 4). The report by Chapman et al. also did not discuss the difficulty involved in accurately staging testis tumors if a retroperitoneal dissection is not done. Chapman[15] did imply, however, that lymphangiography was a reliable method of detecting retroperitoneal metastases, a contention that has never been proved and one with which we disagree.

It is interesting to review other series of nonseminomatous testicular tumors treated by orchiectomy and radiation alone, because they do not report survivals comparable to those reported from the London Hospital.[16,17,18] For example, in a recent report by Kenny and associates,[18] the 4-year survival of patients with Stage A and B teratocarcinoma was 4 of 11, or 36 per cent, and an earlier paper by Vechinski et al.[17] reported a 5-year survival of 42 per cent (5 of 12) in these patients. In fact, Kenny et al. reported better 5-year survival in Stage A and B embryonal carcinoma—12 of 20, or 60 per cent—which, of course, is better than the results obtained by them for teratocarcinoma.

TABLE 4.   Two- to 5-year Survival of Patients (Stage A and B) with Teratocarcinoma Treated with Orchiectomy Plus Radical Retroperitoneal Lymphadenectomy Alone or with Radiation

| Series | Number of Cases | Survival | |
|---|---|---|---|
| | | Number | Per Cent |
| Skinner and Leadbetter[2] | 36 | 29 | 80 |
| Walsh et al.[5] | 41 | 36 | 85 |
| Staubitz et al.[3] | 11 | 11 | 100 |
| University of Minnesota | 11 | 10 | 90 |

Our analysis of the data from the London Hospital and elsewhere has led us to the following conclusions: (1) there is now no justification for treating nonseminomatous testicular cancers by radiation alone; (2) excellent results have been obtained by treating clinical Stage A teratocarcinomas (MTIA) by radiation alone in England, but these results have not been duplicated by others; (3) the overall survival rate for both Stage A and Stage B teratocarcinomas treated primarily by retroperitoneal dissection is slightly better than that obtained by radiation alone if compared with the English data, but the results obtained with operation are much better than those obtained with radiation alone by others;[16,17,18] and (4) the exact role of radiation in the treatment of teratocarcinomas (MTIA) would be easier to determine if there were a uniform international system for classifying testicular cancers, so that results of various therapies could be compared on a worldwide basis. Consequently, we believe that a joint commission of urologic surgeons, radiation therapists, and pathologists consisting of representatives from at least the United States and Great Britain should be established to review the massive data already available and, if indicated, to design a prospective study to determine whether, in fact, a subgroup of nonseminomatous testicular cancers exists that can be treated as effectively by radiation as by operation.

Finally, the role of operation in the management of Stage C disease must be considered. If a patient presents with multiple lung metastases, he is given chemotherapy selected on the histology of the primary tumor. However, if a patient with an embryonal cancer has a solitary lung metastasis, he is treated first with chemotherapy (usually mithramycin*).[13] If the lung metastasis disappears or at least stops growing, we then excise either the site of the metastasis or the lesion itself; if no additional metastases appear within 3 months, a radical retroperitoneal dissection is done. The rationale for this therapy is that, although chemotherapy may control lung metastases, the cancer may persist in the retroperitoneal nodes. If a patient presents with teratocarcinoma, we prefer to resect the metastases, and if the metastases are primarily teratocarcinoma and not some other type of tumor, the patient is given triple drug therapy.[13] Again, if no additional metastases develop, a radical retroperitoneal dissection is done. An aggressive approach to therapy also is used in patients who develop lung metastases following retroperitoneal dissection. For example, we have one patient who developed a single metastasis in each lung postoperatively. Both of these metastases were excised, and he has survived 2½ years while receiving long-term chemotherapy. In fact, we have three patients with Stage C disease who are long-term survivors treated aggressively by multimodal therapy. Leadbetter[19] also reported good results using combined therapy for patients with a limited number of lung metastases.

There are no urologic neoplasms that have shown a more dramatic improvement in survival as a result of aggressive operative treatment than nonseminomatous germinal cell cancers of the testis. The overall cure rate in these tumors, excluding pure choriocarcinoma, now approaches 90 per cent. The best results in the treatment of these neoplasms as a whole have been

---

*Pfizer, Inc., New York, New York.

obtained by radical retroperitoneal dissection either alone or combined with radiation. In our series, radical operation alone has produced a 100 per cent 2-year or more survival for early or Stage A disease, and results from other series suggest that Stage A tumors can be treated by operation alone.[3, 8] In contrast, the precise role of postoperative radiation therapy in the treatment of patients with positive retroperitoneal lymph nodes (Stage B) has yet to be defined. The most significant morbidity of retroperitoneal dissection is that a proper operation usually produces a loss of ejaculation. Those who advocate using orchiectomy and radiation therapy alone in these tumors have not obtained overall survival figures to support their position. Furthermore, many of the reasons which have been advanced against radical retroperitoneal dissection, to the effect that these patients are impotent or that a thorough lymphadenectomy cannot be done or that the results of radical surgery are poor, are not correct. It now appears that the proponents of radiation therapy have retreated somewhat from advocating that all patients with nonseminomatous testicular tumors should be treated by radiation, and at least the English are now suggesting that only the MTIA or teratocarcinomas should be treated in this manner. However, whether it will be possible to identify a subgroup of nonseminomatous testicular tumors, such as teratocarcinomas (U.S.) or MTIA (British), that can be treated by orchiectomy and radiation alone as effectively as by radical operation is not known. In our opinion this question will not be resolved until a uniform system for classifying these tumors is adopted and until the studies such as those suggested in this chapter are carried out. Treatment of patients with advanced or Stage C disease requires a multidisciplinary effort by urologic surgeons, medical oncologists, radiation therapists, and, on occasion, thoracic surgeons.

ACKNOWLEDGMENTS: We are indebted to Seymour Levitt (Radiation Therapy), B. J. Kennedy (Medical Oncology), and Richard Varco (Thoracic Surgery) and their associates, who have contributed to the care of the patients with testicular cancer as reported herein.

# References

1. Maier, J. G., VanBuskirk, K. E., Sulak, M. H., et al.: An evaluation of lymphadenectomy in the treatment of malignant testicular germ cell neoplasms. J. Urol. 101:356, 1969.
2. Skinner, D. G., and Leadbetter, W. F.: Surgical management of testis tumors. J. Urol. 106:84, 1971.
3. Staubitz, W. J., Early, K. S., Magoss, I. V., and Murphy, G. P.: Surgical management of testis tumor. J. Urol. 111:205, 1974.
4. Nicholson, T. C., Walsh, P. C., and Rotner, M. B.: Lymphadenectomy combined with preoperative and postoperative cobalt 60 teletherapy in the management of embryonal carcinoma and teratocarcinoma of the testis. J. Urol. 112:109, 1974.
5. Walsh, P. C., Kaufman, J. J., Coulson, W. F., and Goodwin, W. E.: Retroperitoneal lymphadenectomy for testicular tumors. J.A.M.A. 217:309, 1971.
6. Markland, C., Kedia, K., and Fraley, E. E.: Inadequate orchiectomy for patients with testicular tumors. J.A.M.A. 224:1025, 1973.
7. Fraley, E. E., Markland, C., and Kedia, K.: Treatment of testicular tumors. Minn. Med. 56:593, 1973.

8. Donohue, J. P.: Unpublished data.
9. Kedia, K. R., Markland, C., and Fraley, E. E.: Sexual function following high retroperitoneal lymphadenectomy. J. Urol. *114*:237, 1975.
10. Arseneau, J. C., et al.: Non-lymphomatous malignant tumors complicating Hodgkin's disease. Possible association with intensive therapy. New Engl. J. Med. *287*:1119, 1972.
11. Senyszyn, J. J., Johnston, A. D., Jacox, H. W., and Chu, F. C. H.: Radiation induced sarcoma after treatment of breast cancer. Cancer *26*:394, 1970.
12. Nefzger, M. D., and Mostofi, F. K.: Survival after surgery for germinal malignancies of the testis. I. Rates of survival in tumor groups. Cancer *30*:1225, 1972.
13. Blackard, C. E., and Fraley, E. E.: Drug therapy of genitourinary cancer. Part I: Tumors of the testes and prostate. Drug Therapy *2*:40, 1972.
14. Blandy, J. P., Hope-Stone, H. F., and Dayan, A. D.: Tumors of the testicle. *In* William Heinemann Medical Books Limited, London, 1970.
15. Chapman, R. H., Blandy, J. P., Hope-Stone, H. F., Pollock, D., and Dayan, A. A.: Identification of a favorable group of teratomas. Proc. R. Soc. Med. *66*:1045, 1973.
16. Host, H., and Stokke, T.: The treatment of malignant testicular tumors at the Norwegian Radiation Hospital. Cancer *12*:323, 1959.
17. Vechinski, T. O., Jaeshke, W. H., and Vermund, H.: Testicular tumors. An analysis of 112 consecutive cases. Am. J. Roentgenol. *95*:494, 1965.
18. Kenny, G. M., Wildermuth, O., Werner, G. A., Block, W. D., and Simons, C. E., Jr.; Radiation therapy: Testicular tumors. J. Urol. *112*:495, 1974.
19. Skinner, D. G., Leadbetter, W. F., and Wilkins, E. W., Jr.: The surgical management of testis tumors metastatic to lung: A report of 10 cases with subsequent resection of from one to seven pulmonary metastases. J. Urol. *105*:275, 1971.

# The Management of Tumors of the Testis

JOHN BLANDY,
ROBIN CHAPMAN,
DAVID POLLOCK,
and ELIZABETH MOLLAND
*The London Hospital*

## Introduction

There is no longer any room for argument about how to remove a testicular tumor: it should be taken out through an incision in the groin, and the spermatic cord should be ligated at the internal inguinal ring. To remove a tumor through a scrotal incision invites inguinal and scrotal recurrence and is a mistake tantamount to negligence. Nor is there any dispute among surgeons all over the world as to the correct management of seminomas; it is agreed that after an inguinal orchiectomy, the retroperitoneal nodes should be treated with radiotherapy. Choriocarcinomas are so rare and so serious that nobody knows how they should be treated. Mature or differentiated teratomas are also so uncommon that none of us can justifiably claim that one form of therapy is better than another. But there remain the majority of those germinal cell tumors which are not pure seminomas; we give them the generic name "teratoma" following the original description of Chevassu,[7] while others prefer to call them "nonseminomas." The patient who develops one of these tumors in Britain or Scandinavia will undergo inguinal orchiectomy and then have a course of radiotherapy to his retroperitoneal nodes. In most centers in North America, he will undergo a retroperitoneal node dissection. The tumors are similar, the patients the same sort of men, the surgeons all intelligent men of goodwill; how does this odd situation come about?

Ten years ago, we set out to enquire whether or not we ought to change our treatment policy at The London Hospital and again begin to perform radical retroperitoneal node dissection for teratomas, an operation abandoned here in the 1930's.[4, 19] At the end of an exhaustive study of the case material gathered over the years, we came to the conclusion that radical node dissection had nothing to offer in the treatment of teratocarcinoma Group IV of

489

Dixon and Moore.[18] At that time we saw too few of the embryonal cell carcinomas (Group III) to draw any useful conclusion. Nor was it reasonable to make very much of the difference in survival we had found in the small numbers studied at that time. The comparison had been made in retrospect, the slides were evaluated by a pathologist not trained in the U.S.A.F.I.P. system, and the patients had been treated at different times by surgeons on different sides of the Atlantic. Nevertheless, the results gave us no justification for embarking again on a policy of node dissection.

The rationale for node dissection in teratoma is based upon three premises: (1) that nonseminomas are insensitive to radiation; (2) that operative dissection can remove all the affected lymphatics and lymph nodes; and (3) that the results of node dissection are better than those of radiation. It may be useful to consider these premises in some detail.

## The Radioinsensitivity of Nonseminomas

In the early days of radiotherapy, when the sources of radiation and the method of calculating the dose were in their infancy, only seminomas seemed to shrink up after being irradiated, and the notion got around that nonseminomas were insensitive. This idea was soon shown to be mistaken,[2, 17] but in accordance with the well-established principle of the Bellman,* frequent repetition more than made up for want of evidence.[14, 15, 16] In North America it became customary to refer to these tumors as radioinsensitive, an idea which led logically to the need to remove their lymphatic catchment area by operation. In Europe, on the contrary, it soon became commonplace to see large teratomatous metastases melt away with radiotherapy, and in many centers the survival rate for nonseminomas with orchiectomy and radiation began to approach that for seminomas.[6, 29] Whether or not there was a place for operative dissection of the nodes in some kinds of teratoma remained a question to be decided. What was certain, however, was that the first premise—the radioinsensitivity of teratomas—was false.

## The Feasibility of Removing All the Affected Nodes

When Jamieson and Dobson[20] made their classic study of the lymphatic drainage of the testis, they had in mind the current vogue for radical orchiectomy for tumor. They observed that, if the operative excision were to be successful, it was necessary for the surgeon to:

... strip the aorta and vena cava, the common iliac vessels, the proximal third or so of the internal iliac vessels and the upper part of the spermatic vessels on either side, of all the cellulo-fatty tissue lying on, around, and between them, from the level of the renal vessels downwards.

---

*"What I tell you three times is true." The Bellman: "The Hunting of the Snark," Fit 1, line 4. Lewis Carroll, 1876.

Some thought this such a tall order as to be operatively impossible. Others thought it quite feasible, at least in their hands. By many it was seriously suggested that this bilateral dissection could be accomplished through a unilateral approach. When Tavel et al.[31] set out to accomplish this operation in the cadaver, in which for once relaxation was complete, hemostasis no problem, and time no object, they found that they could only remove two-thirds of the nodes in question. Today, as surgeons begin to doubt their ability to remove every microscopic focus of tumor with their well-trained hands, it has become customary to justify radical operation on the grounds of the removal of "bulk" tumor, invoking if not fully understanding an immunologic concept which is probably quite unsound in regard to the numerical populations of tumor cells involved.

## Comparison of Results of Operation Versus Radiotherapy

Any such theoretical arguments would be disproved if it could be shown that a patient were more likely to be cured if his nodes were removed operatively than if they were irradiated. To make this comparison, however, it is necessary to be quite sure that the same kind of tumor is being treated in the same stage of pathologic spread. At present, in the absence of any prospective, well-controlled studies, the best we can do is to examine the statistics published by different centers, and this examination must give proper attention to known important sources of error. First, one finds that different *classifications* are in use in different centers and that confusion is often confounded by the use of terms such as "embryonal carcinoma" and "teratocarcinoma," which can be applied to quite different entities. Second, quite different systems of *staging* are used by the advocates of radiotherapy and the advocates of radical operation. Third, there is no universal agreement on the method of expressing the survival after treatment. Finally, the case for radical operation is often obfuscated by giving radiation to patients whose lymph nodes, on dissection, are found to contain tumor.

However, since we are not all speculative surgeons but operative ones and must decide on the best method of treatment for the young man with a teratoma, we have to make the best of the data, however imperfect, which are available. So it behooves us to take great care that we have made allowances for the more important of these sources of error.

### ERRORS ARISING FROM DIFFERENCES IN HISTOLOGIC CLASSIFICATION

There are two distinct problems here. First, there seems to be a discrepancy in the proportion of cases which are labeled "seminoma" in different centers. In most North American series, in which radical operation is the rule for nonseminomas, one finds that the proportion of germinal tumors labeled as seminoma is about 40 per cent, whereas in Europe, the proportion runs about 55 to 60 per cent.[1] One possible reason for this difference may be that there are some very undifferentiated tumors which are interpreted as being seminomas by one group of pathologists and as being anaplastic embryomas by another. If this is the case, and the prognosis for the embryomas is much worse than that for the seminomas, then to include in the seminoma category a batch of embryomas by mistake ought to make the survival figures for the seminomas substantially worse in the radiotherapy series. (In fact, as we see later, they seem to be universally about the same.)

The second problem in classification is that in Britain we have been using the T.T.P.R. system,[8] whereas in North America it has been customary to follow the classification devised by the U.S.A.F.I.P.[10] Mostofi and Price[23] have recently denied that it is possible to correlate these two systems; however, on rescrutinizing 105 available cases in The London Hospital Institute of Pathology, we found that in roughly 9 out of 10 instances "teratocarcinoma-with-embryoma, Group IV" matches the category MTI (formerly called MTIA by Collins and Pugh), while every one of the 49 "embryonal carcinomas, Group III" falls into the category MTU (which combines the old subgroups MTIB and MTA) (Table 1).

It would of course be better if a pathologist from the U.S.A.F.I.P. were to scrutinize our material, since subjective errors in interpretation of Mostofi and Price's fascicle may well have crept into our analysis. Such a scrutiny would, of course, be welcome.

## ERRORS ARISING FROM DIFFERENT METHODS OF STAGING

While there is general agreement that tumors confined to the testis are in Stage 1, those with metastases below the diaphragm in Stage 2, and those with pulmonary or hematogenous spread in Stage 3, there are very considerable differences in the accuracy of staging, since such different diagnostic criteria are used in evaluating the stage. When cases are treated by radiotherapy, the presence of tumor in the retroperitoneal nodes can only be surmised. One may try to feel the lesions under anesthesia, but one can only palpate a lump when it is very big. One may try to detect them by the way they displace the kidneys or the ureters in the excretion urogram, but this does not reveal small deposits. A lymphangiogram may reveal metastases, but it does not reliably detect small collections of tumor and may entirely

TABLE 1.   Comparison of British T.T.P.R. and
U.S.A.F.I.P. Classifications

|  | MTI | MTU | TD | Total |
|---|---|---|---|---|
| Teratocarcinoma with embryonal carcinoma | 49 | 0 | 0 | 49 |
| Embryonal carcinoma | 0 | 49 | 0 | 49 |
| Teratoma, immature | 4 |  |  | 4 |
| Teratoma, mature | 1 |  | 2 | 3 |
| Total | 54 | 49 | 2 | 105 |

fail to reveal large deposits, particularly when the tributary lymphatics have been blocked. Clinical Stage 1 cases must include a substantial number of men in whom laparotomy and retroperitoneal node dissection would reveal tumor in the nodes. Indeed, up to 50 per cent of nonseminomas are found to show tumor in the specimen which is removed.[3, 13, 24, 26, 27, 28] In many of these patients in clinical Stage 1, the nodes are found at operation to be fixed and irremovable or to extend above the diaphragm, so that the case is assigned to Stage 3. The proportion of these operatively incurable cases varies in the literature from 10 to 27 per cent of all men explored.[12, 13, 24] Since there are likely to be such enormous differences in the stage which the tumors have reached in series treated by radiotherapy alone and in those treated by retroperitoneal dissection, comparisons of survival results in terms of Stage 1 or Stage 2 are meaningless and misleading. Even the palpability of a paraaortic mass is not a useful criterion, since the mere fact that a mass can be felt does not mean that it is inoperable or might not be cured by operative removal alone. Only a prospective comparison will help us arrive at an answer.

## ERRORS IN METHODS OF PRESENTING RESULTS OF TREATMENT

An unfortunate error has crept into the conventional wisdom about testicular tumors; it is repeatedly stated that 2- or 3-year survivals are valid tests of cure. Statistics collected at The London Hospital since 1927, though not necessarily complete, reveal again and again the existence of the risk of delayed recurrence of testicular tumors.[1] We have seen delayed recurrence of all kinds of testicular tumor even after 20 years. This is no new phenomenon in cancer, and it is surprising to us to learn that in other centers none of the patients who have lived 2 years ever gets run over by a bus or dies from some other disease, and we find it hard to credit the guarantee of immortality which is implicit in some statistics purporting to show a 100 per cent survival after one or other form of treatment. Many of the patients in our practice have moved house, gone to jail, emigrated, or died of other diseases. Our statistics would be considerably improved if we discounted these factors. It has seemed more honest, however, to provide crude survival figures and, when comparing one form of treatment with another, to think in terms of at least 5 years and preferably 10; indeed, as we get older, we find this ideal term for the follow-up seems to get longer.

## ERRORS ARISING FROM SUPPLEMENTARY RADIOTHERAPY

In most series which advocate node dissection, it has been the practice for a patient who is found to have cancer in the nodes, which are removed by retroperitoneal dissection, to be given supplementary radiation.[22] Even Skinner and Leadbetter[28] used it in 8 out of 14 cases, and Castro[5] found recurrence inevitable unless such radiotherapy was given.

There are logical difficulties here; if patients are to be subjected to retroperitoneal node dissection because the tumors are supposed to be radioinsensitive, it is difficult to explain why radiotherapy is expected to do good if tumor is found in the nodes which have been removed. Equally, if one believes that it is possible to get all the affected tissue out by operation, then why give radiotherapy afterward?

Only Staubitz et al.[30] escape this objection, and it must be admitted that their results are astonishingly good, though their numbers are small. As many as 10 of the 12 patients with embryomas found to have operable metastases at laparotomy survived 5 years without radiotherapy, results which are unique in the literature.

## Examination of The London Hospital Results

Against this background we have examined the results obtained by inguinal orchiectomy followed by radiotherapy along the lines previously described.[1] For this analysis we used a simplified version of the Collins and Pugh system in 289 germinal cell tumors (Table 2). In this simplified version we did not make a separate category for those tumors in which seminoma occurred in combination with teratoma, because in our previous studies we had found that the prognosis of these men followed the behavior of the teratomatous element. Again, because in our previous study we found that the outlook of the two subgroups MTIB and MTA were indistinguishably bad,[1] we have combined them in a single category—MTU (undifferentiated), a change accepted now by the British Testicular Tumour Panel and Registry.[25]

It should be pointed out that in our material 55.6 per cent of the men had seminomas—a higher proportion than usually reported in North American series—opening us to the charge that we have mistakenly included some uniformly anaplastic embryomas in our seminoma category. (We do not think this is the case, but in any event if it were, it ought to strengthen, not weaken, the rationale for radiotherapy on the lines explained above.) In fact, the survival figures for seminoma are no worse than those obtained in other contemporary centers (Table 3 and Figure 1), and they would be improved if we doctored them so as to give corrected survival rates rather than the crude survivals reported here.

Granted the possibility of an error in the proportion of seminoma versus teratoma, if we now turn to examine the results of treatment in the non-

TABLE 2. Classification of 289 Germinal Cell Tumors

| Lesion | Number | Per Cent |
|---|---|---|
| Seminoma | 161 | 55.6 |
| Malignant teratoma, intermediate | 67 | 23.2 |
| Malignant teratoma, undifferentiated | 56 | 19.4 |
| Teratoma, differentiated | 4 | 1.4 |
| Teratoma, trophoblastic | 1 | 0.4 |
| Total | 289 | 100 |

TABLE 3.   Seminoma

| Clinical Stage[*] | Years | < 1 | 1 | 2 | 3 | 4 | 5 |
|---|---|---|---|---|---|---|---|
| 1 | Surv. | 105 | 104 | 98 | 91 | 83 | 80 |
| | No. | 105 | 104 | 101 | 98 | 93 | 90 |
| | CSR % | 100 | 100 | 97 | 93 | 89 | 89 |
| 2 | Surv. | 38 | 29 | 25 | 21 | 15 | 15 |
| | No. | 38 | 35 | 35 | 35 | 35 | 25 |
| | CSR % | 100 | 83 | 72 | 60 | 43 | 43 |
| 3 | Surv. | 18 | 6 | 2 | 1 | 1 | 1 |
| | No. | 18 | 17 | 17 | 16 | 16 | 16 |
| | CSR % | 100 | 35 | 12 | 7 | 7 | 7 |

[*]Staging as defined by Blandy et al.[1]

seminoma patients, we observe a striking difference in the survival of those with intermediate and those with undifferentiated teratomas (Figure 2 and Table 4). Once more, we could falsify our crude survival rates by eliminating the handful of men who got lost or died of another cause.

In view of the substantial agreement between our interpretation of Mostofi and Price's system and the Collins and Pugh system (Table 1), it is not surprising that the 5-year survivals for Group IV and Group III teratomas show an equally marked difference (Table 5 and Figure 2).

Two conclusions may be drawn at this stage from these findings, however crude and imperfect they may be. First, one can no longer regard all nonseminomas as being radioinsensitive. Second, it is now evident that there is a huge difference in malignancy between these two groups of nonseminomas, however they are classified. What now gives us cause for concern is the accusation that we have neglected a possible therapeutic benefit in the treatment of our MTU patients, because they were not offered retroperitoneal node dissection. Of the 20 such patients in clinical Stage 1, we would probably have found inoperable metastases or nodes above the diaphragm in 3 or 4 of them and positive nodes in half the specimens removed

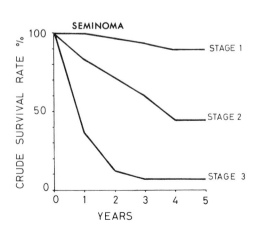

*Figure 1.* Crude survival rates (per cent) in 161 seminomas according to clinical stage at presentation. Seminomas were treated by inguinal orchiectomy and radiation.

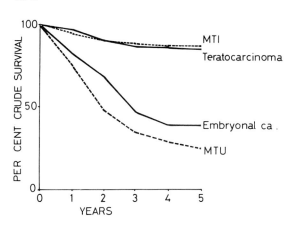

*Figure 2.* Crude survival rates (per cent) in nonseminomas. MTI/teratocarcinoma and MTU/embryonal carcinoma presenting in clinical Stage 1 (without obvious metastases) and treated by inguinal orchiectomy and radiation.

from the other 16. This would leave us with perhaps 8 men in a "surgical" Stage 1, who would be possible candidates for a 5-year survival. There were 5 survivors, so we might have claimed a 62 per cent survival. Such playing with small numbers of statistics gathered in retrospect is unlikely to solve any problems, but it does show that the difference in survival which is found in these groups of teratomas may be due not to the histologic grade of the tumor but to its pathologic stage of spread. Even at the time of presentation (Table 6), many more of the MTU cases have developed advanced metastases, and this would suggest that they are tumors with an inherently greater tendency to spread by the bloodstream, to spread early, and to spread rapid-

**TABLE 4.   Nonseminomas: Crude 5-Year Survivals (British Classification)**

|       | Clinical Stages | Years | <1 | 1 | 2 | 3 | 4 | 5 |
|-------|-----------------|-------|-----|------|-----|-----|-----|-----|
| MTI   |     | Surv.  | 49  | 45   | 43  | 41  | 39  | 38  |
|       | 1   | No.    | 49  | 47   | 47  | 46  | 44  | 43  |
|       |     | CSR%   | 100 | 95   | 92  | 89  | 89  | 89  |
|       |     | Surv.  | 10  | 5    | 3   | 3   | 3   | 2   |
|       | 2   | No.    | 10  | 10   | 7   | 7   | 7   | 6   |
|       |     | CSR%   | 100 | 50   | 43  | 43  | 43  | 33  |
|       |     | Surv.  | 8   | 1    | 0   | 0   | 0   | 0   |
|       | 3   | No.    | 8   | 8    | 7   | 7   | 7   | 6   |
|       |     | CSR%   | 100 | 12.5 | 0   | 0   | 0   | 0   |
| MTU   |     | Surv.  | 28  | 21   | 13  | 8   | 6   | 5   |
|       | 1   | No.    | 28  | 28   | 27  | 23  | 21  | 20  |
|       |     | CSR%   | 100 | 75   | 48  | 35  | 29  | 25  |
|       |     | Surv.  | 10  | 7    | 4   | 2   | 2   | 2   |
|       | 2   | No.    | 10  | 10   | 6   | 5   | 5   | 5   |
|       |     | CSR%   | 100 | 70   | 67  | 40  | 40  | 40  |
|       |     | Surv.  | 18  | 1    | 0   | 0   | 0   | 0   |
|       | 3   | No.    | 18  | 18   | 18  | 17  | 14  | 13  |
|       |     | CSR%   | 100 | 5    | 0   | 0   | 0   | 0   |

**TABLE 5.** Nonseminomas: Crude 5-Year Survivals (U.S.A.F.I.P. System)

|  | Clinical Stages | Years | <1 | 1 | 2 | 3 | 4 | 5 |
|---|---|---|---|---|---|---|---|---|
| Teratocarcinoma and embryonal | 1 | Surv. | 34 | 31 | 29 | 27 | 26 | 25 |
|  |  | No. | 34 | 32 | 32 | 31 | 30 | 29 |
|  |  | CSR% | 100 | 97 | 91 | 87 | 87 | 86 |
|  | 2 | Surv. | 8 | 4 | 3 | 3 | 3 | 2 |
|  |  | No. | 8 | 8 | 7 | 7 | 7 | 5 |
|  |  | CSR% | 100 | 50 | 43 | 43 | 43 | 40 |
|  | 3 | Surv. | 7 | 1 | 0 | 0 | 0 | 0 |
|  |  | No. | 7 | 7 | 7 | 6 | 6 | 6 |
|  |  | CSR% | 100 | 14 | 0 | 0 | 0 | 0 |
| Embryonal cancer | 1 | Surv. | 23 | 18 | 13 | 7 | 5 | 5 |
|  |  | No. | 23 | 22 | 19 | 15 | 13 | 13 |
|  |  | CSR% | 100 | 82 | 68 | 47 | 39 | 39 |
|  | 2 | Surv. | 10 | 7 | 4 | 2 | 2 | 2 |
|  |  | No. | 10 | 10 | 8 | 6 | 6 | 6 |
|  |  | CSR% | 100 | 70 | 50 | 33 | 33 | 33 |
|  | 3 | Surv. | 16 | 1 | 0 | 0 | 0 | 0 |
|  |  | No. | 16 | 16 | 16 | 15 | 12 | 12 |
|  |  | CSR% | 100 | 6 | 0 | 0 | 0 | 0 |

ly. Looking through the records of these patients, we invariably find that they developed pulmonary or osseous metastases and that these deposits usually appeared within a few months of the discovery of their tumors.

## The Place of Node Dissection

Our figures show that there is virtually no indication for retroperitoneal node dissection in seminoma or in teratocarcinoma-MTI-Group IV tumors. It

**TABLE 6.** Nonseminomas: Clinical Stages at Time of Presentation

|  |  | Stages | | | |
|---|---|---|---|---|---|
|  |  | 1 | 2 | 3 | Total |
| MTI | No. | 49 | 10 | 8 | 67 |
|  | % | 73.2 | 14.9 | 11.9 | 100 |
| TEC Gp. IV | No. | 34 | 8 | 7 | 49 |
|  | % | 69.4 | 16.3 | 14.3 | 100 |
| MTU | No. | 28 | 10 | 18 | 56 |
|  | % | 50 | 17.8 | 32.2 | 100 |
| Embr. Gp. III | No. | 23 | 10 | 16 | 49 |
|  | % | 44.7 | 21.3 | 34.0 | 100 |

is possible that node dissection may be appropriate in MTU-Group III-embryomas, but this is a question which only a properly controlled prospective trial can answer. Some surgeons have suggested that one should do a node dissection in order to obtain accurate staging information. It is difficult to see how such an operation could be justified if it did not materially improve the chances of survival. Perhaps in time better experience and expertise with lymphangiography will eliminate even this argument.[21]

In The London Hospital it is our practice to reserve node dissection for those patients in whom, after radiotherapy, the retroperitoneal tumor does not go away and in whom hematogenous metastases have not appeared. Persistent retroperitoneal tumor is determined by the finding of a palpable mass, by lymphangiogram, or by the finding of lateral displacement of the kidneys on X-ray study. This is a very small proportion indeed, and it includes an occasional patient in whom the retroperitoneal metastasis from an undifferentiated nonseminoma, after radiation, leaves only a shell of well-differentiated mature teratoma in the nodes—a phenomenon reported by Smithers et al.[29] and by Dees[9] after radiation and chemotherapy, respectively.

## Conclusions

We need to join forces if we are to make any progress in this matter. Testicular tumors are uncommon enough for it to be possible for every nonseminoma to be examined by an impartial panel of pathologists equally versed in all the various classifications. It should not be too difficult to arrange a prospective clinical trial, statistically controlled, randomized, and uninfluenced by surgical prejudice or faith. In our view such a trial ought to be restricted to the bad teratomas, the MTU-embryoma-Group III cases, for we can see no possible ethical justification (at present) for node dissection in the better differentiated teratocarcinomas. Until such a trial is started—and we would be glad to participate—node dissections will not be performed in The London Hospital.

ACKNOWLEDGEMENTS: This study refers to patients under the care of the surgeons of The London Hospital; these patients were treated by the radiotherapists Dr. Shanks, Dr. Hope-Stone, and Dr. Mantell. We are grateful for their permission to report these results.

## References

1. Blandy, J. P., Hope-Stone, H. F., and Dayan, A. D.: *Tumours of the Testicle*. London, William Heinemann Medical Books, 1970.
2. Boden, G., and Gibb, R.: Radiotherapy and testicular neoplasms. Lancet 2:1195, 1951.
3. Bradfield, J. S., Hagen, R. O., and Ytredal, D. O.: Carcinoma of the testis: An analysis of 104 patients with germinal tumors of the testis other than seminoma. Cancer 31:633, 1973.
4. Cairns, H. W. B.: Neoplasms of the testicle. Lancet 1:845, 1926.

5. Castro, J. R.: Lymphadenectomy and radiation therapy in malignant tumors of the testicle other than pure seminoma. Cancer 24:87, 1969.
6. Chapman, R. H., Blandy, J. P., Hope-Stone, H. F., Pollock, D., and Dayan, A. D.: Identification of a favourable group of teratomas. Proc. R. Soc. Med. 66:1045, 1973.
7. Chevassu, M.: *Tumeurs du Testicule*. Thèse de Paris 193. Paris, G. Steinheil, 1906.
8. Collins, D. H., and Pugh, R. C. B. (Eds.): Classification and frequency of testicular tumours. Br. J. Urol. (Suppl.) 36:1, 1964.
9. Dees, J. E.: Metastatic embryonal cell carcinoma of testis: An apparent 8-year cure. J. Urol. 110:90, 1973.
10. Dixon, F. J., and Moore, R. A.: Testicular tumors. Cancer 6:427, 1953.
11. Dixon, F. J., and Moore, R. A.: Tumors of the male sex organs. In A.F.I.P. Atlas of Tumor Pathology. VIII, 31B and 32. Washington, D.C., U.S. Government Printing Office, 1952.
12. Dowd, J. B.: Surgery of testicular tumors. Surg. Clin. North Am. 42:779, 1962.
13. Ekman, H., Giertz, G., Jönsson, G., and Notter, G.: Tumours of the testicle: A report from Sweden on combined surgico radiotherapeutic treatment. Thirteenth Congr. Int. Soc. Urol. 1:26, 1964.
14. Friedman, M.: Supervoltage roentgen therapy at Walter Reed General Hospital. Surg. Clin. North Am. 24:1424, 1944.
15. Friedman, M.: Tumors of testis: Relation of histogenic classification to radiosensitivity and prognosis. In Proceedings of the New York Pathological Society, April 27, 1950, pp. 33–41.
16. Friedman, M.: Superior value of supervoltage irradiation in special situations: Carcinoma of mouth and carcinoma of testis. Radiology, 67:484, 1956.
17. Gordon-Taylor, G., and Wyndham, N. R.: On malignant tumours of the testicle. Br. J. Surg. 35:6, 1947.
18. Hope-Stone, H. F., Blandy, J. P., and Dayan, A. D.: Treatment of tumours of the testis. Br. Med. J. 1:984, 1963.
19. Howard, R. J.: Malignant disease of the testis. Practitioner 79:794, 1907.
20. Jamieson, J. K., and Dobson, J. F.: The lymphatics of the testicle. Lancet 1:493, 1910.
21. Maier, J. G., and Schamber, D. T.: The role of lymphangiography in the diagnosis and treatment of malignant testicular tumors. Am. J. Roentgenol. 114:482, 1972.
22. Maier, J. G., and Sulak, M. H.: Radiation therapy in malignant testis tumors: Part II. Carcinoma. Cancer 32:1217, 1973.
23. Mostofi, F. K., and Price, E. B.: Tumors of the male genital system. In A.F.I.P. *Atlas of Tumor Pathology* 2nd Series, Fascicle 8. Washington, D.C., U.S. Government Printing Office, 1973.
24. Patton, J. F., Seitzman, D. N., and Zone, R. A.: Diagnosis and treatment of testicular tumors. Am. J. Surg. 99:525, 1960.
25. Pugh, R. C. B. (1973): Comment after Chapman et al. (1973) q.v.
26. Richardson, J. F., and LeBlanc, G. A.: Treatment of testicular tumors: Analysis of 135 cases with 5-year follow up. J. Urol. 93:717, 1965.
27. Robson, C. J., Bruce, A. W., and Charbonneau, J.: Testicular tumors: A collective review from the Canadian Academy of Urological Surgeons. J. Urol. 94:440, 1965.
28. Skinner, D. G., and Leadbetter, W. F.: Surgical management of testicular tumors. J. Urol. 106:84, 1971.
29. Smithers, D. W., Wallace, E. N., and Wallace, D. M.: Radiotherapy for patients with tumours of the testicle. Br. J. Urol. 43:83, 1971.
30. Staubitz, W. J., Early, K. S., Magoss, I. V., and Murphy, G. P.: Surgical management of testis tumor. J. Urol. 111:205, 1974.
31. Tavel, F. R., Osius, T. G., Parker, J. W., Goodfriend, R. B., McGonigle, D. J., Jassie, M. P., Simmons, E. L., Tobenkin, M. I., and Schulte, J. W.: Retroperitoneal node dissection. J. Urol. 89:241, 1963.

# 22

# Treatment with Radiotherapy of Metastatic Carcinoma in a Cervical Lymph Node from a Hidden Primary*

A RADIOTHERAPEUTIC
APPROACH TO THE PATIENT
WITH CANCER IN THE CERVICAL
NODES AND AN UNKNOWN
PRIMARY LESION
*by David G. Smith*

---

*An accompanying article on Radical Neck Dissection for Metastatic Carcinoma in a Cervical Lymph Node was to have been included here, but the manuscript was not received in time for publication.

## Statement of the Problem

*The problem discussed is that of the patient who has been found to have undifferentiated carcinoma in a cervical lymph node after an extensive work-up revealed no primary lesion.*

*Given the situation that a cervical lymph node biopsy shows undifferentiated carcinoma on frozen section and no primary lesion has been found in a thorough preoperative investigation, provide data for the point of view that a radical neck dissection should be done. Describe the follow-up routine. Consider the same questions for metastatic adenocarcinoma and squamous cell carcinoma in the neck with the primary unknown.*

*Define the statistical basis for a bilateral lymph node dissection for involved cervical lymph nodes with no identifiable primary. Provide survival data.*

*Analyze the role of radiation therapy in these situations. Compare results of radiation, radiation plus neck dissection, and neck dissection alone for unilateral and bilateral cervical node metastases without an apparent primary lesion.*

# A Radiotherapeutic Approach to the Patient with Cancer in the Cervical Nodes and an Unknown Primary Lesion

DAVID G. SMITH

*University of Minnesota Health Sciences Center*

## Introduction

The problem presented by the patient with cancer in the cervical nodes and an unknown primary lesion is one which has generated a significant amount of commentary and no consensus regarding proper treatment. This condition, found in 3 to 10 per cent of patients presenting with metastatic cancer in cervical lymph nodes,[1, 2, 3] has been dealt with in various ways. Certain authors favor an operative approach primarily,[1, 4, 5, 6] while others prefer a radiotherapeutic approach.[7, 8] Other groups suggest various combinations of operation and radiotherapy as the best treatment.[9, 10, 11, 12, 13]

All patients with cervical lymph node metastases from an occult primary tumor do not present identical situations with respect to diagnosis and treatment. A patient with a single, small, mobile node in the subdigastric area, or one in whom all palpable disease has been removed at the time of biopsy, does not present the same therapeutic problem as one with multiple ipsilateral or bilateral nodes. The latter situation represents a considerably more difficult problem in control. Similarly, supraclavicular lymph node involvement is associated with a poorer prognosis than is upper cervical nodal involvement. This difference arises from the high incidence of primary disease below the clavicle in the former circumstance. Adenocarcinoma in cervical nodes will certainly cause the investigator to pursue a different approach than will squamous cell or undifferentiated carcinoma. In the former, one suspects a primary in the salivary glands or thyroid or an infraclavicular origin. In the latter, the likely site for the occult primary lesion would be the

503

nasopharynx, oropharynx, hypopharynx, supraglottic larynx, or intraoral cavity.

Many discussions are addressed to the question of therapy for nodal disease and essentially disregard immediate treatment for the primary lesion. Such an approach is, in my judgment, faulty because of the poor prognosis associated with delayed discovery of a primary lesion.[5, 7, 10, 13] If the primary is never discovered, it appears that the patient's prognosis is better.[5, 9, 11, 13]

To arrive at a rational treatment plan, two separate questions must be answered: 1. What is to be done about the primary? 2. How are the neck metastases best treated?

Generally, when an adult patient presents with a painless mass in the neck, a thorough search for a primary malignant lesion is required. This includes a full ENT examination, with direct laryngoscopy, nasopharyngoscopy, esophagoscopy, and bronchoscopy, and biopsies of all suspected mucosal areas. When no worrisome areas are found, "blind biopsies" of the nasopharynx, tonsil, base of the tongue, and hypopharynx are indicated. Other recommended examinations include radiographs of the sinuses, soft tissue studies of the neck, and tomograms of the lung, even if the routine chest film is within normal limits. An iodine-131 scan of the thyroid and a parotid sialogram are other possible diagnostic procedures. A barium esophogram with an upper gastrointestinal series, barium enema, and intravenous pyelogram is advised.

Several authors have cautioned against removal of the cervical mass as the primary diagnostic procedure.[4, 5, 11] Rather, a biopsy with a small-caliber needle is advocated. If these diagnostic procedures leave the site of the primary lesion in doubt, the following treatment plan is proposed.

## Treatment of the Primary Lesion

By definition, the location of the primary is unknown. How can we treat it? And indeed, can we do so with certainty, inasmuch as a primary lesion is never discovered in many of these cases?[1, 7, 9, 10] However, a primary lesion is subsequently discovered in a significant proportion of cases, and remarkable similarity in site and frequency is apparent in the published series[1, 2, 7, 8, 9, 11, 12] (Table 1). When the histopathologic diagnosis is squamous or undifferentiated carcinoma in cervical nodes, primary lesions are found most frequently in the mucosa of the nasopharynx, oropharynx (including palatine tonsil and base of tongue), hypopharynx (including pyriform sinus), and supraglottic larynx. Those advocating a purely operative approach to this situation must of necessity withhold treatment to these potential primary sites of involvement and follow an expectant course, hoping to discover the primary lesion in a stage early enough for subsequent control.

I believe, however, that irradiation to these potential primary sites offers a reasonable alternative to the operative approach for the following reasons:

1. The smaller the nest of malignant cells, the smaller the dose of radiation necessary to eradicate it.[2]

2. The smaller the primary lesion, the greater the chance of cure with irradiation.[14, 15]

3. If the primary lesion can be prevented from appearing at a later time, the patient will enjoy a better prognosis.[5, 9, 11, 13]

One of the best controlled series reported a primary lesion subsequently appearing in 20 per cent of those treated operatively (21 of 104 cases) but in only 6 per cent of those treated with irradiation (3 of 52 cases).[13] For those primary lesions in the radiation failure group, an insufficient dose of irradiation may have been given. In this same series, those individuals developing a primary above the clavicle had a 31 per cent chance of living 3 years, whereas those without subsequent development of a primary in the head and neck area had a 58 per cent chance of living 3 years. These data present a strong case for an initial attempt to eradicate the primary lesion with irradiation in hopes of preventing its subsequent appearance.

It is certainly true that, if the primary lesion is subsequently discovered in the head and neck region, definitive treatment can be applied with expectation of cure in a significant percentage of cases.[9, 13] However, it seems logical to expect that an attempt to eradicate the primary lesion with irradiation in its minute, undetectable state at the time of initial diagnosis holds greater promise of success than later treatment of a larger, grossly obvious lesion.

Certain authors have discouraged the use of irradiation to the potential sites of occult primary lesions because of its side effects. "We prefer not to maximize radiation therapy treatment to produce just a few more patients free of cancer if the alternative is to make all treated patients uncomfortable because of severe dryness."[13] I do not agree with this viewpoint.

## Treatment of the Neck Nodes

How is the neck best treated? The size, number, location, character, and histology of the involved lymph nodes will all influence the choice. Many recommend radical neck dissection in selected patients with cervical node metastases from an unknown primary lesion.[1, 4, 5, 6, 9, 13] The Memorial Hospital experience demonstrated a 32 per cent 5-year survival in patients primarily treated by radical neck dissection. A 15 per cent 5-year survival after radical neck dissection was reported from Michigan.[5]

A report from Roswell Park Hospital noted a 30 per cent 4-year tumor-free rate in a group of patients treated primarily with irradiation.[7] Radical neck dissection was considered unsuitable in 80 per cent of these patients because of advanced neck involvement. These data do not clearly demonstrate a significant advantage for irradiation or operation in the treatment of this condition.

Jesse advocates radical neck dissection as the only treatment in the following situations: (1) a single movable node in the submaxillary triangle or subdigastric area; (2) a single movable node in the midjugular area.[9]

Fletcher believes a cervical node less than 3 cm. in diameter receiving 7000 rads followed by nodal disappearance at the end of treatment has been

## TABLE 1.

| Number of Primary Lesions Later Found | Location of Primary | | Results | |
|---|---|---|---|---|
| | | | *Primary Found* | *Primary Not Found* |
| 38/123 (31%) | Supraglottic — larynx | 9 | 31% 5-yr. determinate | 32% 5-yr. determinate |
| | Nasopharynx — | 8 | | |
| | Base tongue — | 5 | | |
| | Tonsil — | 4 | | |
| | Hypopharynx — | 2 | | |
| 15/61 in life 6/61 at autopsy (35%) | Nasopharynx — | 1 | Combined survival — 8% 3-yr. | |
| | Hypopharynx — | 2 | | |
| | Tonsil — | 1 | | |
| | Hard palate — | 1 | | |
| | Lung — | 6 | | |
| | Breast — | 2 | | |
| | Cervix — | 1 | | |
| | Ovary — | 1 | | |
| 42/103 (41%) | Thyroid — | 11 | 3/7 nasoph. alive 1.5 – 7 yr. 3/5 tonsil alive 1–11 yr. | 16 pt. surviving 1½–11 yr. |
| | Nasopharynx — | 7 | | |
| | Tonsil — | 5 | | |
| | Base tongue — | 2 | | |
| | Esophagus — | 1 | | |
| | Below clavicle — | 9 | | |
| 48/127 (38%) | Oropharynx ⎫ Nasopharynx⎭ | 11 | 12/48 3-yr. survival (25%) | 32/79 3-yr. survival (40%) |
| | Thyroid — | 9 | | |
| | Larynx ⎫ Hypopharynx⎭ | 4 | | |
| | Miscel. head & neck — | 5 | | |
| | Lung — | 10 | | |
| | GI — | 5 | | |
| | Miscel. below clavicle — | 4 | | |
| 8/33 in life 7/33 at autopsy (45%) | Nasopharynx — | 4 | 3/15 alive 30 months | 10/18 alive & disease-free at 4 yr. |
| | Pharynx — | 2 | | |
| | Antrum — | 1 | | |
| | Lip — | 1 | | |
| | Lung — | 2 | | |
| | Pancreas — | 2 | | |
| | Breast — | 1 | | |
| 22 (33%) | Nasopharynx — | 2 | Overall 3-yr. survival 33% | |
| | Supraglottic larynx — | 3 | | |
| | Other head & neck — | 3 | | |
| | Thyroid — | 1 | | |
| | Lung — | 4 | | |
| | Kidney — | 2 | | |
| | Stomach — | 2 | | |
| 19 (18%) | Nasopharynx — | 5 | 0% 5 yr. survivors | 16/87 5-yr. survival (18%) |
| | Floor mouth — | 1 | | |
| | Lip — | 1 | | |
| | Parotid — | 2 | | |
| | Lung — | 6 | | |
| | Breast — | 1 | | |
| | Stomach — | 1 | | |
| | Colon — | 1 | | |

| Reporting Institution | Number of Patients | Nodal Involvement | | | Histopathology | | | Treatment | | |
|---|---|---|---|---|---|---|---|---|---|---|
| | | Single Level & No Resid. Tumor | Mult. Nodes | Bilat. & Fixed | Squamous | Undiff. | Adeno. | Surg. | RT | Combin. |
| Memorial 1950–64 (Barrie, Knapper, Strong) | 123 | 75/136 Neck | 61/136→ | | 104→ Miscel. = 8 | | 11 | 125 | 7 | 18 |
| Middlesex Engl. 1954–68 (Probert) | 61 | 18 p. 29 p. | < 20 sq. cm. > 20 sq. cm. | | 15 Miscel. = 8 | 16 | 11 | | 58 (10 pt. – chemotherapy) | 3 |
| Mayo Clinic 1945–54 (Comess, Beahrs, Dockerty) | 103 | | | | 43 | 7 ←31→ | 17 | Primarily operative series | | |
| M.D. Anderson 1952–62 (Jesse, Neff) | 127 | | | | 60 Miscel. = 20 | 27 | 20 | 76 | 18 | 18 |
| Roswell Park 1950–57 (Marchetta, Murphy, Kovaric) | 33 | 67% had mass 5-cm. diameter | | | 6 | 27 | | | 33 | |
| Stanford 1958–70 (Fu, Stewart, Bagshaw) | 67 | 18 | 27 | 12 | 35 | 21 | 11 | 6 | ←52→ | |
| Michigan 1953–69 (Winegar, Griffin) | 106 | | | | 47 Miscel. = 3 | 36 | 17 | 18 | 58 (Chemotherapy – 18 or no therapy) | 12 |

given definitive treatment.[2] Jesse obtained equal results in treating early neck disease with either neck dissection or radiation therapy.[9] Hanks et al. reported a 26 per cent 5-year survival rate in patients with advanced neck disease associated with various primary lesions treated with irradiation alone.[16]

Most authors agree that when multiple ipsilateral nodes, posterior cervical nodes, or bilateral or fixed nodes are involved, irradiation should form an integral part of treatment in order to prevent recurrence in the treated neck.[2, 5, 7, 9] Strong reported that 54 per cent of patients with positive cervical nodes and 71 per cent of patients with multiple level positive nodes developed local recurrences after neck dissection alone.[17] He also found a low preoperative irradiation dose (2000 R./week) to reduce significantly the incidence of local recurrence in a controlled prospective study.[17]

An additional justification for the use of irradiation in this disease is documented in a study from M. D. Anderson Hospital.[9] They reported a 16 per cent incidence of contralateral neck disease in patients treated by radical neck dissection alone and a complete absence of subsequent contralateral extension when the patient was treated with irradiation either alone or in combination with operation. These data reinforce the concept of irradiation, at doses considerably less than needed to eradicate palpable disease, for control of microscopic deposits of tumor cells.

## Conclusions and Recommendations

1. Radiation should be considered the primary modality of treatment for squamous or undifferentiated metastases to the neck, because it may prevent the later appearance of a primary lesion, may control or contribute to control of the ipsilateral neck disease, and may prevent the appearance of new disease in the contralateral neck.

2. Patients with a histopathologic diagnosis of squamous or undifferentiated carcinoma without residual disease in the neck after biopsy or those presenting with a single lymph node less than 3 cm. in diameter in the subdigastric, midjugular, submaxillary, or upper posterior cervical areas should be treated with irradiation alone. Opposing lateral portals covering the potential sites of a primary lesion (nasopharynx, oropharynx, hypopharynx, and larynx) are carried to a moderate dose, in the range of 5000 to 6000 rads, with the expectation of control of the primary lesion. The lower neck is treated with a similar dose from an anterior portal. If palpable neck disease is originally present, the dose to that area must be raised to 6500 to 7500 rads, with the larger doses prescribed for the larger nodes.

3. Patients with a histopathologic diagnosis of squamous cell or undifferentiated carcinoma presenting with nodal disease of greater than 3 cm. diameter and with multiple ipsilateral, bilateral, or fixed nodes should be given combined treatment. The patient is treated initially with irradiation portals covering potential primary sites as defined above, plus the lower neck, to a prescribed dose of 5000 to 6000 rads. This is followed after a suit-

able rest interval (4 to 6 weeks) by radical neck dissection for removal of residual disease. If radical neck dissection is not feasible, areas of palpable disease must be treated with 7000 rads or more. This radiation dose would be expected to control the occult primary lesion and prevent recurrence of disease in both the ipsilateral and contralateral nodes.

4. Patients presenting with a histopathologic diagnosis of adenocarcinoma should be evaluated for the presence of salivary gland, thyroid, or infraclavicular primaries. Irradiation may play a role in control of extensive disease not adequately treated by operation alone or as a palliative measure.

5. Patients presenting with supraclavicular nodal disease will likely be found to have an infraclavicular primary lesion, and palliative therapy only is indicated. The prognosis is poor.

It is hoped that by means of an aggressive treatment approach to this problem that employs irradiation as the primary therapy, the results can be improved beyond the 10 to 40 per cent survival figures currently being reported.

# References

1. Barrie, J. R., Knapper, W. H., and Strong, E. W.: Cervical nodal metastases of unknown origin. Am. J. Surg. *120*:466, 1970.
2. Fletcher, G.: *Textbook of Radiotherapy.* 2nd ed. Philadelphia, Lea & Febiger, 1973, pp. 174–197.
3. Martin, H., and Morfit, H. M.: Cervical lymph node metastasis as the first symptom of cancer. Surg. Gynecol. Obstet. 78:133, 1944.
4. MacComb, W.: Diagnosis and treatment of metastatic cervical cancerous nodes from an unknown primary site. Am. J. Surg. *124*:441, 1972.
5. Winegar, L. K., and Griffin, W.: The occult primary tumor. Arch. Otolaryngol. 98:159, 1973.
6. Doberneck, R. C.: Diagnosis and treatment of the solitary mass in the neck. Am. Surg. *40*:181, 1974.
7. Marchetta, F. C., Murphy, W. T., and Kovaric, J. J.: Carcinoma of the neck. Am. J. Surg. *106*:974, 1963.
8. Probert, J. C.: Secondary carcinoma in cervical lymph nodes with an occult primary tumor. A review of 61 patients including their response to radiotherapy. Clin. Radiol. *21*:211, 1970.
9. Jesse, R. H., Perez, C. A., and Fletcher, G. H.: Cervical lymph node metastasis from an unknown primary. Cancer *31*:854, 1973.
10. Jesse, R. H., and Neff, L. E.: Metastatic carcinoma in cervical nodes with an unknown primary lesion. Am. J. Surg. *112*:547, 1966.
11. Martin, H., and Romieu, C.: The diagnostic significance of a "lump in the neck." Postgrad. Med. *11*:491, 1952.
12. Fu, K. K., Stewart, J. R., and Bagshaw, M. A.: Cervical node metastases from occult primary sites. Rocky Mt. Med. J. *70*:31, 1973.
13. Fletcher, G.: *Textbook of Radiotherapy.* 2nd ed. Philadelphia, Lea & Febiger, 1973, pp. 325–332.
14. *Ibid.,* pp. 812–887.
15. Shukovsky, L. J.: Dose time volume relationships in squamous cell carcinoma of the supraglottic larynx. Am. J. Roentgenol. *108*:27, 1970.
16. Hanks, G. E., Bagshaw, M. A., and Kaplan, H. S.: The management of cervical lymph node metastasis by megavoltage radiotherapy. Am. J. Roentgenol. *105*:74, 1969.
17. Strong, E. W.: Preoperative radiation and radical neck dissection. Surg. Clin. North Am. *49*:271, 1969.
18. Comess, M. S., Beahrs, O. H., and Dockerty, M. B.: Cervical metastasis from occult carcinoma. Surg. Gynecol. Obstet. *104*:607, 1957.

# 23

# Management of Symptomatic Hiatus Hernia

MEDIAN ARCUATE REPAIR FOR
HIATUS HERNIA AND
GASTROESOPHAGEAL REFLUX
   *by Lucius D. Hill*

OBJECTIVES AND INDICATIONS
FOR ANTIREFLUX OPERATION
   *by Sidney Cohen*

HIATUS HERNIA AND
GASTROESOPHAGEAL REFLUX
   *by Lawrence DenBesten*

## Statement of the Problem

*Two questions are to be dealt with: (1) under what circumstances should a hiatus hernia be repaired; and (2) what operative procedure should be done?*

*What is the natural history of hiatus hernia with mild chronic esophagitis? With moderately severe esophagitis?*

*Analyze objective data with regard to success of medical treatment of esophagitis associated with hiatus hernia. Provide evidence for the benefits of nonoperative measures that include weight loss, elevating the head of the bed, and antacids. In a large series of such patients treated nonoperatively, what is the frequency of bleeding, persistent esophagitis, and esophageal stricture? Analyze available information about benefits provided by mechanical dilation of strictures.*

*What data define the best operation for correcting the complications of hiatus hernia? For special circumstances, what are the alternative but acceptable operations? Do you favor a thoracic or an abdominal operative approach and why?*

*Document the bases used to select patients for operation. Symptoms? X-ray? Manometry? Esophagoscopy? Biopsy? Acid Perfusion Test?*

*For the technique of operation, discuss the importance of (1) the intra-abdominal position of the gastroesophageal junction; (2) construction of a flap, valve mechanism; (3) fixation of the gastroesophageal junction; (4) approximation of the crus; and (5) acid-reducing procedures, such as vagotomy plus pyloroplasty or antrectomy.*

# Median Arcuate Repair for Hiatus Hernia and Gastroesophageal Reflux

LUCIUS D. HILL

*University of Washington School of Medicine, Seattle*

Esophageal hiatus hernia, once considered a rarity, is now recognized as one of the most common disorders of the upper gastrointestinal tract in man. Radiologists at this center demonstrate a hiatus hernia in 12 per cent of upper GI tract x-rays. The diagnosis is more common than the combined incidence of active duodenal and gastric ulcer. With advanced age, the incidence of hiatus hernia increases.

Ninety-six per cent of herniations through the esophageal hiatus are of the sliding variety. The remainder are paraesophageal hernias. A small percentage of sliding hernias have a paraesophageal component and are combined hernias. An additional small group of patients have an incompetent lower esophageal sphincter and have reflux without a demonstrable hernia. If these four groups are considered, the problem of hiatus hernia and gastroesophageal reflux is indeed large. Development of new instrumentation, including manometry and pH determination, has led to better understanding of the pathophysiology of this common disorder. The majority of symptoms associated with hiatus hernia are related to gastroesophageal reflux, but there are some patients with a competent lower esophageal sphincter who develop symptoms from incarceration and displacement of the viscus into the chest. An incompetent lower esophageal sphincter allows reflux to occur, leading to esophagitis. Esophagitis, in turn, produces the classic symptoms of sliding hiatal hernia—heartburn and esophageal pain; reflux with overflow into the tracheobronchial tree produces respiratory symptoms.

The most important factor in gastroesophageal reflux and hiatus hernia is the competence of the lower esophageal sphincter. The gastroenterologist has challenged the surgeon by posing the question of whether or not operation can truly restore sphincter competence and thereby solve the problem of reflux over the long term. In this chapter we show that the surgeon can indeed restore sphincter competence.

Another important question to be answered is whether or not medical management can influence sphincter competence to the extent that reflux

513

can be prevented and sphincter pressure improved. With a problem as common as hiatus hernia, medical management should be tried, and indications for operative intervention should be strict to prevent needless operations. On the other hand, allowing a patient to continue on medical management until ulceration with bleeding or stricture formation occurs is unfortunate. The problem is then converted from one that is relatively simple to manage to a problem that can be difficult, with increased morbidity and mortality.

Many patients with a small hiatus hernia and a low-normal sphincter pressure may have only occasional reflux and may suffer from intermittent heartburn for years without serious damage to the esophagus. Such patients can be handled medically without serious complications. On the other hand, the patient with a grossly incompetent sphincter, which allows acid to bathe the lower esophagus over long periods of time, develops severe heartburn. This can become troublesome, despite medical management, to the point that the individual cannot lead a normal life. Gross incompetence of the lower esophageal sphincter with free reflux produces severe esophagitis. Untreated severe esophagitis leads to ulceration, bleeding, and stricture. In this series, 14 per cent of patients were operated upon for stricture, and 2.5 per cent of patients had discrete ulceration with or without stricture. Ten per cent developed bleeding with chronic anemia.

The medical program that should be tried in all cases includes elevation of the head of the bed, frequent administration of antacids, and advising the patient to refrain from eating before going to bed and to lose weight, when indicated. In an analysis of objective data regarding the effectiveness of medical treatment, Behar et al.[1] found in 12 patients that, regardless of symptomatic and objective response to medical management, mean resting lower esophageal sphincter pressure (LESP) and gastroesophageal reflux remained unchanged after 1 year of continuous treatment. In addition, the response of the LES to increased intra-abdominal pressure showed no improvement. These objective data indicate that, while medical management may control symptoms, it has no effect on the underlying problem of an incompetent resting LES and gastroesophageal reflux. Regardless of the quality of medical treatment, these abnormalities persist.

Analysis of our data indicates that approximately 85 per cent of patients with hiatus hernia either are asymptomatic or can be controlled by medical management. This would indicate that medical management is effective in controlling symptoms in the majority of patients with hiatus hernia. Fifteen per cent of patients on medical management, however, developed symptoms or complications serious enough to require operation.

The most common indication for operation is intractability to medical management. This means the patient has severe, incapacitating symptoms which preclude his being a productive citizen, even after a thorough trial on medical management. Those patients who show no remission of symptoms over a period of time or who develop complications on medical management should be evaluated for operation.

A second indication for operation is esophagitis. The development of esophagitis can be detected by x-ray, esophagoscopy, and biopsy. If the esophagitis is mild and the patient has not been on medical management, there is no indication for operation. If esophagitis persists or worsens on medical management, or if ulceration and bleeding develop, operation should be considered.

A third indication for operation is stricture, with or without ulceration. While this indication has accounted for 14 per cent of patients operated upon in the author's series, the development of stricture and ulceration indicates that the patient has been carried too long on conservative management. Esophagitis is the consequence of continued reflux, whether it is acid or alkaline. Repeated bathing of the esophageal mucosa over long periods of time with hydrochloric acid and enzymes can cause histologic alterations in the esophageal mucosa, which have been best described by Pope.[2] Macroscopic evidence of reflux is seen on esophagoscopy. These changes consist of erythema, friability, and, ultimately, ulceration. By the time shallow ulceration develops, esophagitis becomes visible on esophageal x-rays. A number of patients who have no macroscopic evidence of esophagitis have microscopic changes—thickening of the basal layer of the squamous cell lining, with the dermal pegs reaching toward the luminal surface. In advanced esophagitis, the dermal pegs actually reach the luminal surface. When these dermal pegs containing the nerve plexus contact the acid secretion in the esophageal lumen, severe pain and symptoms of heartburn ensue.

Esophageal stricture, ulceration, and bleeding are obvious indications for operation. The mortality rate for operation in the presence of stricture in our hands is approximately six times the mortality rate for operation for primary hiatus hernia. Such statistics make a forceful argument for repair of hiatus hernia before stricture develops. Another indication for operation is pulmonary aspiration producing damage to the tracheobronchial tree and lungs. Reflux with overflow into the tracheobronchial tree produces chronic obstructive pulmonary disease and even lung abscess. Approximately 20 per cent of patients operated upon in this series had significant respiratory complications. This symptom is a particularly important one to correct. The patient with heartburn relieved by antacids will continue to have respiratory problems if there is reflux with overflow into the trachea. Nocturnal coughing and asthmatic-like attacks should alert the physician to the presence of nocturnal aspiration.

In selecting patients for operation, the history and physical examination should uncover the preceding indications. Further tests, however, are mandatory to confirm the presence or absence of reflux and determine the status of the lower esophageal sphincter. In our experience, the most important test has been combined pH and manometry. We consider this to be a routine part of the preoperative work-up. The first report of pre- and postoperative pH and pressure studies emanated from this laboratory in 1961.[3] This study of 103 patients evaluated by pH and manometry was begun in 1957 and conducted simultaneously with the work of Tuttle and Grossman.[4] We have now employed these tests in over 5000 patients with a variety of esophageal disorders. These tests allow for detection of reflux with greater accuracy than any other means, including x-ray. More importantly, manometry defines the status of the lower esophageal sphincter. A lower esophageal sphincter pressure below 10 mm. Hg generally indicates an incompetent sphincter. A sphincter pressure greater than 30 mm. Hg in a patient complaining of esophageal pain raises the question of esophageal spasm rather than incompetence of the lower esophageal sphincter. The length of the lower esophageal sphincter can also be measured. Our data suggest that an adequate sphincter pressure distributed over a longer length, up to 4 cm., represents a more competent sphincter than when the pressure is distributed over a short distance. A high, spiking pressure distributed over a few millimeters has occasionally been associated with failure to prevent reflux in response to increased intra-abdominal pressure. Other tests, including the water siphon test and the Bernstein test, are used infrequently in preoperative evaluation. The Bernstein test consists of dripping 0.10 normal HCL into the esophagus, which will produce heartburn in the presence of esophagitis, whereas a control drip of saline will produce no symptoms. The 24-hour pH monitoring test is also valuable in determining sphincter competence.

The pH plus manometry test is simple and safe. With this test, two types of reflux can be determined. The milder form of reflux, or *induced reflux*, occurs only on forceful maneuvers intended to overcome the barrier pressure of the sphincter. *Free reflux* occurs simply upon the patient's assuming the supine position, or even spontaneously, and is detected by a change to an acid pH in the esophagus without forceful maneuvers. Free reflux indicates a grossly incompetent sphincter. In addition to the status of the sphincter, manometry will also uncover motility disorders of the esophagus which may cause esophageal pain, mimicking heartburn. Other studies of value are gastrointestinal x-rays, which give further indication of the size of the hernia and the presence of reflux. Finally, it is important to determine whether or not the patient has a duodenal ulcer, gastric outlet obstruction, or other problems in the stomach or duodenum that interfere with gastric drainage and that will compromise an antireflux procedure.

Esophagoscopy is very commonly employed preoperatively in order to determine the status of the esophageal mucosa, particularly if there is a question of esophagitis. If there is any doubt about the presence of carcinoma, esophagoscopy is mandatory. Biopsy to rule out malignancy and to determine the extent of esophagitis is indicated.

After the studies are completed, the selection of an operation should be based on the following parameters:

1. The ability of the operation to correct the underlying problem—namely, the incompetent lower esophageal sphincter.

2. Prevention of hernia recurrence over a period of years and maintenance of competence of the sphincter over the long term.

3. The technical ease with which the operation can be performed.

4. The mortality, morbidity, and complication rate of the operation.

5. Its reproducibility and results in other hands.

Our preference for operative management of hiatus hernia has been a median arcuate posterior gastropexy, which begins with reduction of the hernia and dissection of the preaortic fascia and median arcuate ligament, followed by freeing of the greater curvature of the cardia of the stomach. The greater curvature is freed in order to allow rotation of the stomach, so that the posterior aspect of the stomach can be visualized and the anterior and posterior cut edges of the phrenoesophageal bundle and the gastrohepatic omentum can be demonstrated. The esophageal hiatus is closed loosely so that a finger can be readily inserted alongside the esophagus. The celiac axis is identified and the median arcuate ligament dissected out. A Goodell dilator is placed underneath the median arcuate ligament to protect the aorta and celiac axis. Sutures are then taken to anchor the phrenoesophageal bundle to the preaortic fascia and median arcuate ligament (Figure 1). Further sutures are taken to imbricate the phrenoesophageal bundle in order to place tension on the collar sling musculature and thereby narrow the esophageal introitus and strengthen the lower esophageal sphincter mechanism. These sutures in the anterior and posterior cut edges of the phrenoesophageal and gastrohepatic bundles are taken in a manner that carefully avoids the vagus trunks. As these sutures are tied, the tension placed on the collar sling musculature automatically accentuates the cardioesophageal angle and recreates an elongated flap valve that can be palpated through the wall of the stomach. These maneuvers are designed to recreate and accentuate the normal anatomy and function of the gastroesophageal junction.

Even though the operation appeared to be technically satisfactory, in our early experience 4 to 5 per cent of patients continued to demonstrate reflux in the absence of a recurrent hernia. Of these, 2 per cent had free

*Figure 1.* The anterior and posterior phrenoesophageal bundles have been visualized by rotating the stomach anteriorly. A Goodell dilator is placed beneath the median arcuate ligament, and a posterior suture is placed to anchor the gastroesophageal junction to the preaortic fascia and median arcuate ligament.

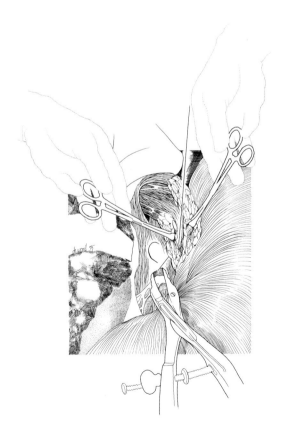

reflux with symptoms. Every effort should be made to ensure that function has been restored and reflux will not continue. In order to give the surgeon additional evidence at operation that the sphincter function has been improved, we began 1½ years ago to measure the barrier pressure intraoperatively. This is done by having a nasogastric tube in the stomach at the time of operation. To this tube is attached a polyethylene catheter with a side opening 8 cm. from the tip of the tube. The polyethylene tube is, in turn, attached to a transducer and recorder, which allows the surgeon to readily measure the LESP before and after repair.* The introitus of the esophagus is calibrated, as discussed above, by placement of the sutures, imbricating the lesser curvature until the introitus of the esophagus is tight around the NG tube. As the sutures are tied, the nasogastric tube, which serves as a sensing device, is passed up and down across the sphincter, and pressures are recorded. This maneuver is continued until the pressure is around 40 to 50 mm. Hg, which will produce a postoperative pressure of around 20 to 25 mm. Hg (Figure 2). In the first 60 patients operated upon using intraoperative manometry, the mean sphincter pressure before repair was 9 mm. Hg and following repair was 41.4 mm. Hg. This is a key maneuver in the operation.

Postoperatively in 54 patients tested, the mean LESP has been 20 mm. Hg, which is well above normal. It is noteworthy that the length of the sphincter can also be measured by intraoperative manometry. The mean length of the sphincter in the first 60 patients operated upon was 2 cm. prior to repair and increased to a mean of 3.6 cm. following repair. A control group of 12 patients with no known esophageal disease was studied with intraoperative manometrics. The mean LESP in this group was 17 mm. Hg, with a range of 12 to 40 mm. Hg. In no patient of the first 60 studied did free reflux

---

*The device used to measure lower esophageal sphincter pressure during operation is manufactured by Physio Control Corp., Seattle, Washington.

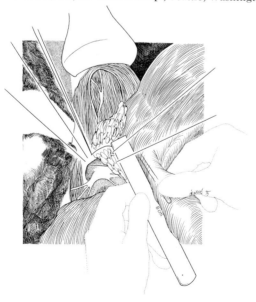

*Figure 2.*   The imbricating sutures have been placed in the anterior and posterior phrenoesophageal bundles, anchoring them to the median arcuate ligament. As these are tied down, measurement of the sphincter pressure is obtained with a sensing device in place to ensure that the sphincter pressure has been elevated to above the normal level.

*Figure 3.* This calibration, or narrowing of the esophageal introitus or cardia, occurs automatically with the tying of the sutures that have been placed in the anterior and posterior phrenoesophageal bundles. As they are tied, tension is placed on the collar sling musculature, automatically narrowing the esophageal introitus. This can be palpated very nicely by invaginating the stomach wall and palpating along the nasogastric tube that is in place. The flap valve that has been accentuated and re-created can be detected along the nasogastric tube. Measurement of the sphincter pressure gives objective evidence that the valve has been strengthened so that the sphincter competence will be restored.

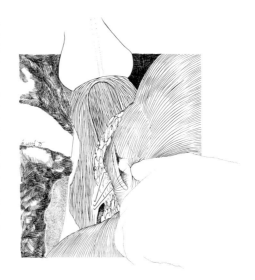

occur. In one patient, induced reflux could be produced with forceful respiratory maneuvers. This patient, however, was asymptomatic. This study indicates that sphincter competence had been restored. Intraoperative manometry can improve the accuracy of the antireflux operation, regardless of the technique employed. It is simple and safe, and adds approximately 15 minutes to the operation time.

The median arcuate repair is done through an abdominal approach, since dissection of the preaortic fascia and median arcuate ligament can best be accomplished through this approach rather than through a thoracic incision. In the presence of stricture and recurrent hernia, the chest should be prepared, however, so that a counterincision can be made in the thorax if additional freeing up of the esophagus is required. Careful inspection of the pylorus for pyloric stenosis or duodenal ulcer can best be carried out from an abdominal approach. Should the patient have a duodenal ulcer or pyloric stenosis of sufficient degree to compromise gastric drainage, vagotomy and pyloroplasty can be added to the operation. Unless these conditions exist, however, vagotomy and pyloroplasty add nothing to a well-done antireflux operation. The most important step in the antireflux procedure is correction of the incompetent lower esophageal sphincter. This requires meticulous and careful calibration of the cardia around a small tube that is no larger than a No. 18 nasogastric tube (Figure 3). This raises the LESP to above normal, as described previously.

One can argue about the merits of the cardioesophageal angle and the flap valve arrangement. Butterfield[5] showed in autopsy specimens that the current antireflux procedures, including the Belsey, Nissen, and posterior gastropexy, produce flap valves that prevent reflux in the cadaver, even after resection of the lower esophagus. This one-way flap valve obviously assists the sphincter in its work and appears to operate whether the valve is in the chest or abdomen. An intra-abdominal segment of the esophagus is theoretically important, since this portion of the esophagus enjoys the support of positive intra-abdominal pressure. It is difficult to document this concept with hard data, however. In the living subject, in contrast to the autopsy material studied by Butterfield, the function of the lower esophageal sphincter is complex. The living subject must use the esophageal sphincter in swallowing a large bolus of food. This opening and closing of the esophagus must be accomplished without loss of competence, so that the gastroesophageal junction is more than a dead one-way flap valve. It is an intricate functioning mechanism that maintains constant tone, preventing reflux, and at the same time is capable of allowing the passage of a large bolus. This sphincter mechanism is, in our opinion, the single most important factor in the prevention of reflux.

Restoration of sphincter function, therefore, is the sine qua non for success in an antireflux operation. A dead one-way flap valve will inevitably deteriorate with time. The normal sphincter maintains its strength and competence throughout life. A normal sphincter not only maintains a resting pressure of 15 to 20 mm. Hg but also responds to increased intra-abdominal pressure by a rise in sphincter pressure that is greater than the intragastric pressure. This is expressed by $\frac{\Delta S}{\Delta G} > 1$. A similar response occurs with the administration of pentagastrin, which also results in $\frac{\Delta S}{\Delta G}$ being greater than one. In this regard the study of Lipschutz et al.[6] is very important. Previous reports by Behar et al.,[1] Cohen and Harris,[7] and others have indicated that the antireflux operation restores the resting LES pressure but that the responsiveness of the sphincter to increased intra-abdominal pressure remains unchanged. These studies suggest that the sphincter mechanism in the hiatus hernia patient is abnormal and that no operative procedure will restore normal sphincter response. The report of Lipschutz et al. clearly refutes these contentions. Lipschutz and co-workers studied 15 patients, 8 of whom had posterior gastropexy and 7 of whom had the Belsey procedure. Following operation, the LESP was increased from 5.4 mm. Hg to 16.5 mm. Hg with the posterior gastropexy and to 12.2 mm. Hg after the Belsey repair. In addition, there was improvement in the pressure response to abdominal compression and to pentagastrin administration. Before operation, the increment in gastric pressure exceeded the increment in LES pressure and response to straight leg raising, producing a $\frac{\Delta S}{\Delta G}$ ratio of 0.67±0.02.

The $\frac{\Delta S}{\Delta G}$ ratio increased to 1.62 after the Hill gastropexy and to 1.47 after the Belsey transthoracic repair. The difference between the preoperative and postoperative values is highly significant. The postoperative response was similar to the normal LES response to abdominal compression. Similar improvement marked the peak sphincter response to pentagastrin administration, which increased from 17.2 mm. Hg to 35.5 after the Hill repair and to 41.7 after the Belsey repair. Lipschutz and co-workers concluded from their data that the Hill repair and Belsey repair resulted in both clinical improvement and a restoration of lower esophageal sphincter function to normal. Of the seven patients who had the Belsey procedure, one had recurrent herniation shortly after operation. There were no recurrences among patients who had the posterior gastropexy. The follow-up was from 1 to 4 years. This important study shows that a posterior gastropexy, when properly done, increases the resting LESP and prevents reflux. In addition, it restores the neural (increased intra-abdominal pressure) and humoral (pentagastrin) stimulation to normal. After these procedures, the LES responds as a normal sphincter. This report, therefore, indicates that the sphincter in hiatus hernia is not an abnormal sphincter, as suggested by previous studies, but is a normal sphincter that has been displaced. With restoration of its normal anatomic position, it will resume normal function.

The mortality rate of posterior gastropexy in 511 patients operated on for primary hiatus hernia has been 0.39 per cent. There were two deaths. One patient had a myocardial infarction and the other a bleeding gastric ulcer. The complications and morbidity of the procedure largely evolve around the so-called "gas bloat" syndrome, or gastric dilatation, which has developed in approximately 12 per cent of patients. In most of these patients, the syndrome has been mild and transient. In about 3 per cent of patients, air trapping has been marked and severe. Air trapping can be caused by the undetected presence of pyloric stenosis or by previous duodenal ulcer with scarring not appreciated at operation. The pylorus should be carefully inspected at operation. Damage to the vagus nerve from sutures along the lesser curvature may also produce gastric dilatation. Care is taken to avoid both the anterior and posterior vagus trunks. Generally, air trapping subsides after a period of 1 to 2 months. In about 2 per cent of these patients, dilatation to relieve esophageal stenosis has been required. These same patients experience dysphagia from repair that is too tight. This, again, is transient but may require one to three dilatations. With intraoperative manometrics, hopefully, these complications can be avoided. A sphincter pressure of 60 mm. Hg or more at the time of operation indicates that the esophageal introitus has been rendered too tight; the sutures should be loosened at that time to avoid postoperative dysphagia. Damage to the celiac axis is a potential hazard of dissection of the median arcuate ligament but has been largely avoided by protecting the artery with an instrument inserted between the artery and the median arcuate repair.

To be of value an operation should be reproducible in other hands. Median arcuate repair has been employed with good results by several surgeons, including Skinner,[9] Csendes and Larrain,[10] Lipschutz,[6] and others. A significant report in this regard is that of Thomas et al.,[11] who employed posterior gastropexy in 79 patients. Early in their experience, these authors had eight patients with persistent herniation who were symptomatically improved. With refinement in their technique, Thomas and co-workers had no recurrent herniation in 79 patients over a 2½-year period. Forty-two of these patients were chronic alcoholics, and 15 had neuropsychiatric problems. These excellent results, as well as those achieved by Lipschutz, Larrain, and others, indicate that the median arcuate repair, when properly performed, is a reproducible operation. It is noteworthy that, in the report by Lipschutz et al., the LESP did not decrease over a period of 4 years. Thomas and co-workers likewise concluded that reflux was corrected in their patients studied by pH and manometry tests. A recent report by Demeester et al.[12] included 45 patients done by the Belsey, Hill, and Nissen procedures, with 15 patients in each group. In this report the posterior gastropexy was performed over a No. 30 French tube with no apparent effort to calibrate the cardia properly. This indicates an apparent lack of appreciation of the necessity to calibrate accurately the esophageal introitus in order to restore resting LESP and function. If one is to label an operation "posterior gastropexy," it is important that the key part of the operation not be left out.

We have had an opportunity to study patients as long as 10 years postoperatively and find that reflux does not occur in a well-performed gastropexy. In addition to five documented anatomic recurrences over the past 10 years, approximately 4 per cent of patients developed signs of recurrent reflux after 4 to 5 years. The majority of these patients remained symptomatically improved and had reflux only with forceful respiratory maneuvers. It is predicted that, with intraoperative manometry and the production of a sphincter pressure that is higher than normal, even with some deterioration in LESP over the years, the sphincter will remain competent. It is important the the length of the sphincter is also increased by posterior gastropexy. In the 60 patients studied, the sphincter length was increased from 1.5 to 3.6 cm. A long sphincter performs more effectively than does a short sphincter which produces a normal pressure distributed over an insufficient length.

## Reflux Strictures

The most severe complication of reflux esophagitis is stricture formation. The controversy surrounding benign stricture has misled surgeons into employing large resectional procedures with high mortality and morbidity for a benign disease. The term "Barrett's short esophagus" has unfortunately been applied to this entity, because the tubular esophagus below the stricture is often lined with gastric epithelium and is mistaken for stomach. This unfortunate term has also misled surgeons into believing that the gastroesophageal junction is well above the diaphragm and that the esophagus is grossly shortened. Careful manometric studies of the esophagus indicate that the strictures in reflux esophagitis occur at the squamocolumnar junction, that the gastric epithelium may be present all the way up to the aortic arch, and that the esophagus is rarely, if ever, shortened. That portion of the gullet between the stricture and the stomach has all of the manometric characteristics of the esophagus despite its columnar epithelial lining.

In our first report of 36 patients with esophageal stricture,[13] 25 had stricture high in the esophagus, up to and above the aortic arch. Even in the presence of these high strictures, the gastroesophageal junction can be brought down below the diaphragm and a simple posterior gastropexy or other antireflux procedure performed. Following a successful antireflux operation, the strictures heal with surprising rapidity. Dilatation at operation and one to two postoperative dilatations suffice to open up the obstruction. Our series of strictures now numbers 96 patients, and the findings are essentially the same as in the first report. It is imperative in these patients that the sphincter be restored to its normal function; otherwise, reflux will continue and the stricture will not heal. The failure to perform an adequate antireflux procedure has led some surgeons to believe that antireflux procedures are not sufficient in the presence of a stricture. Composite studies in postoperative patients, including radiographic, pathologic, esophagoscopic, manometric, and pH studies, indicate clearly the true nature of these strictures. Even the high strictures occur at the squamocolumnar junction, with columnar epithelium lining the esophagus below the stricture. The tubular gullet, from a level of the stricture downward, has all the manometric characteristics of the esophagus. The sphincter mechanism, when replaced below the diaphragm, resumes its normal function and prevents reflux. The operation is done through the abdomen, but the chest is prepared for a counterincision to expose the esophagus, if necessary. Patients who have undergone previous esophageal operations with perforation have iatrogenic shortening of the esophagus. In such cases it may be necessary to do a plication procedure in the chest, which does not restore function and anatomy to normal but is preferable to a resectional procedure with substitution of the colon or jejunum. The term "short esophagus" is inaccurate. The lower esophageal sphincter is the functional dividing line between the esophagus and the stomach, and if the term "short esophagus" is to be used, it must be demonstrated that the distance between the esophageal inlet and the sphincter is shortened. To our knowledge, no such demonstration of short esophagus has been presented, even in the presence of severe reflux strictures. Whereas the patient with lye or corrosive stricture may develop shortening, it has not been demonstrated that gastroesophageal reflux appreciably shortens the esophagus. Therefore, in patients with reflux strictures, the surgeon should consider a simple antireflux procedure rather than a resectional procedure. The findings of our original report have now been confirmed by Hall and Thomas, Hall, and Haddad,[11] Csendes and Larrain,[10] Naef,[14] Safaie-Shirazi,[17] and most recently by Herrington,[15] who reported 17 consecutive patients treated by simple antireflux procedure with healing of the strictures.

## Paraesophageal Hernia

True paraesophageal hernias constitute around 4 per cent of herniations in the esophageal hiatus.[16] It is important to distinguish true paraesophageal hernia from sliding hernia, as the pathophysiology is entirely different. In the true paraesophageal hernia, the esophagus lies in its normal position, fixed posteriorly with a normal functioning sphincter mechanism. Reflux does not occur, and the stomach simply rolls up in the chest through the enlarged esophageal hiatus. Pressure and pH studies indicate a normally functioning esophagus and a normally functioning sphincter. The displaced stomach may become incarcerated or may be the site of ulcer formation with bleeding and pressure symptoms.

Incarcerated paraesophageal hernia is an operative emergency.[18] In the true paraesophageal hernia, as long as the entire stomach is dislocated into the posterior mediastinum, incarceration does not occur. When the fundus becomes distended and prolapses out of the posterior mediastinum through the esophageal opening into the abdomen, obstruction occurs at the esophageal, midgastric, and duodenal levels. Incarceration becomes irreducible, except by operative intervention, if not relieved promptly. If a nasogastric tube can be inserted and the stomach decompressed, the patient can be operated upon electively. If decompression cannot be accomplished because of obstruction, the patient should be taken to the operating room immediately. The mortality rate in the group of patients with incarceration that could not be decompressed was 50 per cent in our hands; two patients died of cardiac arrest during the induction of anesthesia. Operation should be strongly considered in the good-risk patient with true paraesophageal hernia, particularly when symptomatic, because of the constant threat of incarceration as well as ulceration in a displaced stomach.

Operative repair of paraesophageal hernia differs from that of sliding hernia because the esophagus is in its normal location and well fixed. Therefore, simple reduction of the hernia and closure of the large esophageal hiatus is all that is necessary to restore anatomy and function to normal. To tear down the moorings of the esophagus and repair the hernia posteriorly simply predisposes the patient to a sliding hernia which may be more troublesome than the paraesophageal hernia. The surgeon must be absolutely certain that the hernia is a true paraesophageal one, however, for if there is a sliding component, the hernia is then a combined sliding and paraesophageal one and must be treated as a sliding hernia. The recurrence rate following repair of paraesophageal hernia should approach 0. The long-term results in 39 patients have been excellent.

## Recurrent Hernia

The management of recurrent hernia has received very little attention. We previously reported an experience with 63 patients referred with recurrent hiatus hernias.[19] This series has now expanded to 105 patients. At the time of repair of these hernias, an effort was made to determine the type of previous procedure and why it failed. The Allison procedure was the most common, and it failed because sutures were taken through the anterior portion of the phrenoesophageal membrane, which seldom holds over the long term. Two common factors were present in most of the patients, regardless of the type of procedure employed. First, the surgeon failed to anchor the stomach in its infradiaphragmatic position, which allowed for the development of recurrent herniation. Second, there appeared to be no deliberate effort to calibrate the cardia to correct reflux. Fixation sutures were not employed, were improperly placed, or were placed in tissue that did not hold. Even though the stomach had been anchored below the diaphragm, the cardia was still patulous, allowing three to four fingers to be placed up into the esophagus. At reoperation these patients had a median arcuate repair with careful attention to calibration of the cardia. Follow-up on recurrent herniation now extends to nearly 12 years, with a mean follow-up of 6.3 years. The mortality rate in this group is 2.9 per cent, which is over six times the mortality rate of primary repair of hiatus hernia, and emphasizes that the optimal time to repair a hernia is at the first operation.

The complications that have occurred in dealing with both recurrent hernia and stricture are related to the inability to recreate a lower esophageal sphincter. In part, this failure has been due to destruction of the sphincter by multiple operations. In these patients calibration of the cardia must be carried higher than usual, with additional imbricating sutures carried high on the lesser curvature. This creates a longer flap valve that is not a normal sphincter but is the best that can be accomplished in the presence of a destroyed sphincter. In the presence of stricture and recurrent hernia, the diseased and adherent gastroesophageal junction is particularly prone to perforation. There have been three perforations in this series, one of which was recognized immediately and resutured. Two patients suffered late perforations 2 to 3 days postoperatively, possibly related to the inadvertent passage of a nasogastric tube. These are exceedingly grave complications. One of these patients died as a result of the perforation, and the other survived after a prolonged hospital course.

## Summary and Conclusions

Hiatus hernia is now recognized as one of the most common gastrointestinal abnormalities in man. The majority of patients can be treated medically, and the criteria for operation should be strict. Otherwise, needless procedures will be performed. An attempt should be made to manage all patients medically; when it becomes obvious that they have failed to respond, operation should be recommended before complications, particularly ulceration, bleeding, and stricture, develop. The mortality rate and results from operation of primary hiatus hernia are good as long as a meticulous effort is made to recreate the normal anatomy and function. The mortality rate in procedures for stricture and recurrent herniation, however, is six times the mortality rate in primary hiatus hernia. This indicates that the best time to repair a hiatus hernia is at the first operation and before complications develop. A simplified antireflux procedure with dilatation will correct reflux strictures of the esophagus.

With modern instrumentation and techniques it is possible to measure objectively what has been accomplished with antireflux procedures. It is clear that a properly done antireflux procedure restores resting LESP. It also restores the normal sphincter responsiveness to neural and humoral stimulation. With the further additions of intraoperative manometrics, the antireflux operation should rank among the most effective and accurate procedures in the surgeon's armamentarium. The morbidity and mortality should be as low as 1 per cent. The recurrence rate with posterior gastropexy reported worldwide is now around 1 per cent. The worldwide recurrence rate with the Nissen procedure varies from 3 per cent[1] to 9 per cent.[19] The worldwide recurrence rate with the Belsey procedure, however, appears to between 11 per cent and 14 per cent.[20]

## *References*

1. Behar, J., Biancani, P., Spiro, H. M., and Storer, E. H.: Effect of an anterior fundoplication on lower esophageal sphincter competence. Gastroenterology 67:209, 1974.
2. Pope, C. E.: Recognition and management of gastro-esophageal reflux. Viewpoints on digestive diseases, Vol. 4, No. 1, January, 1972.
3. Hill, L. D., Chapman, K. W., and Morgan, E. H.: Objective evaluation of surgery for hiatus hernia and esophagitis. J. Thorac. Cardiovasc. Surg. *41*:60, 1961.
4. Tuttle, S. G., and Crossman, M. I.: Detection of gastroesophageal reflux by simultaneous measurement of intraluminal pressure and pH. Proc. Soc. Exp. Biol. Med. 98:225, 1958.
5. Butterfield, W. C.: Current hiatal hernia repairs; similarities, mechanisms and extended indications—An autopsy study. Surgery 69:910, 1971.
6. Lipschutz, W. H., Eckert, R. J., Gaskins, R. D., Blanton, D. E., and Lukash, W. M.: Normal lower esophageal sphincter function after surgical treatment of gastroesophageal reflux. New Engl. J. Med. *291*:1107, 1974.
7. Cohen, S., and Harris, L. D.: Hiatus hernia and esophageal reflux. New Engl. J. Med. *284*:1053, 1971.
8. Woodward, E. R., Rayl, J. E., and Clarke, J. M.: Esophageal hiatus hernia. Curr. Probl. Surg., Dec., 1970, pp. 1–62.
9. Skinner, D. B., Belsey, R. H., Hendrix, T. R., and Zuidema, G. D.: *Gastroesophageal Reflux and Hiatus Hernia.* Boston, Little, Brown and Company, 1972.
10. Csendes, A., and Larrain, A.: Effect of posterior gastropexy on gastroesophageal sphincter pressure and symptomatic reflux in patients with hiatal hernia. Gastroenterology 63:19, 1972.
11. Thomas, A. N., Hall, A. D., and Haddad, J. K.: Posterior gastropexy: Selection and management of patients with symptomatic hiatus hernia. Am. J. Surg. *126*:148, 1973.
12. Demeester, T. R., Johnson, L. F., and Kent, A. H.: Evaluation of current operations for the prevention of gastroesophageal reflux. Ann. Surg. *180*:511, 1974.
13. Hill, L. D., Gelfand, M., and Bauermeister, D.: Simplified management of reflux esophagitis with stricture. Ann. Surg. *172*:638, 1970.
14. Naef, A. P. and Savary, M.: Conservative operations for peptic esophagitis with stenosis in columnar lined lower esophagus. Ann. Thorac. Surg. *13*:543, 1972.
15. Herrington, J. L., Wright, R. S., Edwards, W. H., and Sawyers, J. L.: Conservative surgical treatment of reflux esophagitis and esophageal stricture. Ann. Surg. *181*:552, 1975.
16. Hill, L. D., and Tobias, J. A.: Paraesophageal hernia. Arch. Surg. 96:735, 1968.
17. Safaie-Shirazi, S., Zike, W. L., Anuras, S., Condon, R. E., and DenBesten, L.: Nissen fundoplication without crural repair. Arch. Surg. *108*:424, 1974.
18. Hill, L. D.: Incarcerated paraesophageal hernia—A surgical emergency. Am. J. Surg. *126*:286, 1973.
19. Hill, L. D.: An effective operation for hiatal hernia: An eight-year appraisal. Ann. Surg. *166*:681, 1967.
20. Woodward, E. R.: Discussion of evaluation of current operations for the prevention of gastroesophageal reflux. Ann. Surg. *180*:511, 1974.
21. Skinner, D. B., Belsey, R. H., Hendrix, T. R., and Zuidema, G. D.: *Gastroesophageal Reflux and Hiatus Hernia.* Boston, Little, Brown and Company, 1972.

# Objectives and Indications for Antireflux Operation

SIDNEY COHEN

*The University of Pennsylvania School of Medicine*

## Introduction

The reflux of gastric contents into the esophagus produces a clinical syndrome which is manifest by the symptoms of heartburn and the sequelae of esophagitis, stricture, or peptic ulcer of the esophagus. The operative treatment of gastroesophageal reflux is directed toward restoring the competence or strength of the lower esophageal sphincter (LES), the major factor in the prevention of reflux. It has been shown that certain operative procedures can effectively improve LES strength and thus restore gastroesophageal competence. Although effective antireflux operations have been devised, there is yet considerable disagreement as to the mechanism of action and the indications for these procedures. Many patients still undergo unnecessary operation for poorly defined symptoms of a hiatus hernia and not for the designated objective of the operation—the prevention of gastroesophageal reflux.

It is the purpose of this article to discuss the appropriate use of antireflux operation in the management of gastroesophageal reflux. Three specific areas will be covered: (1) the mechanism of gastroesophageal competence and the clinical significance of a sliding hiatus hernia; (2) the diagnosis and documentation of gastroesophageal reflux and its sequelae; and (3) the appropriate indications for, and possible modes of action of, certain antireflux operations.

## Pathogenesis of Gastroesophageal Reflux: Does a Hiatus Hernia Constitute a Clinical Entity?

During the past 25 years, a sliding hiatus hernia achieved recognition as the "masquerader of the upper abdomen."[1] Clinicians were convinced that a hiatus hernia was the causative factor in the etiology of gastroesophageal reflux and other unexplainable symptoms referable to the upper abdomen and chest. During this era, operation was directed toward repairing the hiatus hernia. The erroneous concept of the relationship of gastroesophageal reflux to a hiatus hernia has been difficult to change. However, the present approach to the medical and operative therapy of gastroesophageal reflux and its sequelae no longer allows the clinician to maintain this erroneous impression. It will only lead to improper patient management and inaccurate selection of patients for operative intervention. Three lines of evidence support the contention that the recognition (or, by inference, the correction) of a hiatus hernia is of no clinical significance.

### Lack of Correlation Between Hiatus Hernia and Symptoms of Gastroesophageal Reflux

In patients undergoing an upper gastrointestinal x-ray evaluation, heartburn, regurgitation, belch, and other symptoms attributed to a hiatus hernia showed no correlation with the x-ray presence of a hiatus hernia.[2, 3] In large series of patients with symptoms or complications of gastroesophageal reflux, a hiatus hernia may be absent in 30 to 55 per cent of patients.[3, 8] Thus, a large proportion of patients with the symptoms of gastroesophageal reflux have no demonstrable hiatus hernia, and the symptoms of reflux do not correlate with the radiographic diagnosis of a hiatus hernia.

### The Frequency of a Sliding Hiatus Hernia

The frequency of hiatus hernia in x-ray studies is directly dependent upon the effort of the radiologist. In several large series, when aggressive maneuvers are used to demonstrate a hiatus hernia, the frequency increases from 10 to 20 per cent at age 20 to 30, up to 40 to 60 per cent at age 50 to 60, and 60 to 90 per cent at age 70.[9-13] In a smaller series of young individuals, the frequency was 33 per cent. The high frequency of hiatus hernia, especially in older patients, without a concomitant rise in the frequency of gastroesophageal reflux is strong evidence against any etiologic significance of a hiatus hernia.

### Lower Esophageal Sphincter Competence as the Prime Factor in the Prevention of Gastroesophageal Reflux

The symptoms of gastroesophageal reflux can be correlated with the intrinsic strength of the physiologic lower esophageal sphincter (LES).[3-6] The competence of the LES is an intrinsic factor of the sphincter muscle itself, independent of surrounding pressure (i.e., positive intra-abdominal pressure versus negative intrathoracic pressure), placement above or below the diaphragm, and supporting structures.[15, 16]

The current concept of the pathophysiology of gastroesophageal reflux centers about the basal tone of the LES and abnormalities in the two major adaptive responses of the LES—the responses to changes in intra-abdominal pressure and feeding.[11-20] Although the pathogenesis of LES incompetence has not been entirely clarified, three important observations have been made. First, the incompetent LES responds poorly to changes in intra-abdominal pressure.[3, 15-19] Second, the incompetent LES responds abnormally to endogenous stimuli known to release gastrin.[20] Third, the basal LES tone is reduced in patients with gastroesophageal reflux whether or not a hiatus hernia is present.[3, 16] The abnormalities in basal LES pressure and the two adaptive sphincter mechanisms are the findings that best explain the pathogenesis of gastroesophageal reflux. The incompetent LES is probably not a result of primary smooth muscle failure, since sphincter competence may be restored by pharmacologic or operative means. An abnormality in the neurohumoral regulation of the sphincter and a disruption of the mechanical properties of the LES muscle are the most likely causes of LES incompetence.

The concept of a sphincter abnormality as the cause of gastroesophageal reflux is of major importance in the diagnosis and management of this disorder. The diagnosis of gastroesophageal reflux no longer depends upon finding a hiatus hernia on x-ray.[21-25] The treatment of gastroesophageal reflux, whether medical or operative, is directed toward restoring intrinsic LES tone.

## Diagnosis of Gastroesophageal Reflux

The symptom of heartburn indicates gastroesophageal reflux and serves as the clinical standard upon which most objective measures of reflux are validated.[3-6] Heartburn is a specific symptom for gastroesophageal reflux and should not be interpreted as a nonspecific symptom of many gastrointestinal diseases. Heartburn is defined as a retrosternal burning pain which travels in the oral direction and is made worse by eating, bending, or lying down. Postural regurgitation of gastric contents into the mouth is another important symptom of gastroesophageal reflux.

Objective studies of gastroesophageal competence have been difficult to interpret. Since competence at the gastroesophageal junction is a function of the intrinsic LES, measurement of LES pressure provides a direct assessment of competence. The normal LES pressure is above 12 mm. Hg. In patients with symptomatic gastroesophageal reflux, an LES pressure below 10 mm. Hg has been recorded in 80 to 100 per cent of patients.[3-6, 26]

Standard radiographic studies show gastroesophageal reflux in only 10 to 25 per cent of symptomatic patients.[27, 28] More vigorous radiographic techniques, such as the water siphon test and the acid-barium swallow, may be more sensitive tests for diagnosing gastroesophageal reflux, but false-positive results are so high as to make the procedures valueless.[2, 26] The water siphon test and the acid-barium swallow show an overall poor correlation with symptomatic gastroesophageal reflux.

The Bernstein test, or acid perfusion test of the esophagus, is a sensitive means of reproducing the symptom of heartburn.[4, 26, 29] It is of value in confirming the clinical impression of heartburn, but it is of little use in distinguishing chest pains of multiple etiologies. Acid reflux studies using a pH probe in the esophagus may be worthwhile, providing the artifact of placing exogenous acid into the stomach is not introduced.[4-6] Without exogenous acid, the positive yield decreases from the very sensitive 90 per cent level. False-positive results also decrease when exogenous acid has been excluded.

Despite the availability of clinical tests for the evaluation of patients with gastroesophageal reflux, they may not be frequently used because they are costly, inaccurate, and difficult to perform. The approach to each patient should be individualized. In a given patient with clinical symptoms of gastroesophageal reflux, an upper gastrointestinal x-ray with cineesophagography should be performed. The x-ray will provide a clear assessment of esophageal function, give information as to the radiographically identifiable complications of gastroesophageal reflux, and help in excluding other complicating or treatable disorders. Esophageal function is assessed as to the presence of normal progressive primary peristaltic waves. The function is best observed in the prone position. It is essential to evaluate peristalsis in all patients with gastroesophageal reflux secondary to suspected scleroderma. Free gastroesophageal reflux may be seen on tilting the patient and is a valuable finding. More vigorous maneuvers to demonstrate reflux or a hiatus hernia add little to the clinical management of a given patient.

The need to perform esophagoscopy with biopsy and cytology in a patient with uncomplicated gastroesophageal reflux is unresolved. Certainly any stricture, hemorrhage, or esophageal ulcer requires endoscopic evaluation. Additionally, if the patient responds poorly to initial medical management, endoscopy is indicated. If the patient has uncomplicated gastroesophageal reflux and responds well to initial medical treatment, endoscopy may be deferred.

In a clinical situation in which a patient has a confusing history, further diagnostic studies beyond x-ray and endoscopy may be indicated. The Bernstein test may be most helpful in this setting. In the majority of patients, the diagnostic evaluation need not progress past this point. In a limited number of patients, esophageal manometry may be of significant diagnostic and therapeutic importance. Esophageal manometry may be used as an ancillary or supporting diagnostic study to demonstrate the presence of LES incompetence in a suspected case of gastroesophageal reflux. Most importantly, esophageal manometry should be used as a preoperative study in all patients with gastroesophageal reflux in whom no clear-cut complication of the reflux is present. Thus, a patient should not be submitted to an antireflux operation to restore LES competence unless it is certain that LES incompetence exists. The presence of a normal LES pressure should make one suspect the clinical diagnosis of gastroesophageal reflux.

# Objectives of Operation in the Treatment of Gastroesophageal Reflux

Operation for the treatment of gastroesophageal reflux has had two objectives. First, most operations have been aimed at effective restoration of gastroesophageal competence. Second, some operative procedures have been directed at diminishing gastric acid secretion.[30-32] At present, most clinicians would agree that the major aim of operation in patients with gastroesophageal reflux should be the restoration of gastroesophageal competence. Acid-reducing procedures have little usefulness except in a secondary role, and even as such they may be detrimental. It has been shown that vagotomy may compromise LES function in the basal state and especially in response to changes in intra-abdominal pressure.[17, 18, 33] The possible beneficial effect of reducing gastric acid secretion may be outweighed by a negative effect on an already incompetent sphincter. Antrectomy may also diminish sphincter function by its concomitant reduction in serum gastrin. Although a clear-cut relationship between basal serum gastrin and sphincter pressure has not been established, there are well-documented cases of severe gastroesophageal reflux following antral resection.[15] Currently, no role for either vagotomy or antrectomy has been established in the treatment of gastroesophageal reflux.

In recent years, several operations have received impressive endorsement in the medical literature.[34-40] These operations have as their primary goal the restoration of gastroesophageal competence. The operative procedures are not hiatus hernia repairs, since they may be performed in the presence or absence of a hiatus hernia. To prevent confusion, these procedures should be called antireflux operations, not hiatus hernia repairs. The latter connotes an operative procedure that has no valid claim to a pathophysiologic mechanism. Indeed, it should be obvious by this time that "hiatus hernia repairs" have historically been dismal failures. The newer antireflux operations are an interesting family of operations that have as their prime objective the restoration of LES competence.[34-36, 39, 40] The mechanics of each procedure will be discussed by my surgical colleagues. Each operative procedure has several key features that the proponent of the operation considers most important to the success of the procedure. The mechanism by which the operation restores sphincter competence is not established despite these hypotheses.

In general, the antireflux operations are felt to work through several mechanisms: (a) establishment of a long intra-abdominal segment of esophagus; (b) approximation of the diaphragmatic crura; (c) fundoplication; (d) fixation of the esophagus below the diaphragm; and (e) miscellaneous other explanations. Actually, these are objectives of the operation rather than mechanisms whereby LES competence is restored. I feel that antireflux operation restores LES competence by altering the mechanical properties of the circular muscle of the LES.[41] All muscle, including the circular muscle of the LES, has specific mechanical properties as defined by length-tension and force-velocity curves.[41, 42] These curves indicate that LES muscle contracts maximally in response to neural and hormonal stimuli at considerably less passive stretch than muscle from the adjacent stomach or esophagus. When stretched in excess of its length of optimal response, the muscle contracts poorly to these stimuli. It is possible that antireflux operation restores LES muscle to a length at which it can better respond to neurohumoral stimulation. This hypothesis would explain why simple hiatus hernia repairs have had little beneficial effect in restoring LES competence.

Another hypothesis is that fundoplication creates a new distal sphincter owing to the characteristics of the plicated fundic circular muscle.[43] Fundic muscle may have a sensitivity to neurohumoral stimulation similar to that of the LES muscle. When plicated around the distal esophagus, it may create a sphincter mechanism which supports the existing LES. The change in LES pressure in response to neurohumoral stimuli and the ability to relax or open with swallowing are functions retained by the postoperative but now competent LES. The presence of these functions indicates that operation has not simply created a flap-valve or a mechanical barrier. In summary, antireflux operation works by restoring the competence of the LES. The mechanism by which LES competence is improved is not entirely clear.

## Indications for Antireflux Operation

Although seemingly effective antireflux operations have been described, the indications for these procedures have not been established. Operation (whether it be antireflux operation, at present, or hiatus hernia operation, as in the past) is greatly overused. The difficulty in the selection of patients for operation is twofold. First, in most cases the indications for operation are based upon the subjective interpretation of the clinician, who may be biased or erroneous in his evaluation of the patient's symptoms or the significance of certain "objective" findings. Second, even in patients with documented sequelae of gastroesophageal reflux, the response to operation versus different forms of medical therapy has not been evaluated in a controlled manner. Thus, the subjectivity in selecting patients for operation and the absence of good objective studies have allowed a wide use of operation.

At present, it seems that there are four indications for antireflux operation in patients with gastroesophageal reflux. These indications, shown in Table 1, are self-explanatory. Each indication, with the exception of intractability of symptoms, is an objective finding which has been clearly shown to be a sequela of gastroesophageal reflux. Stricture, peptic ulcer of the esophagus, and hemorrhage secondary to erosive esophagitis are conditions that can be diagnosed by either x-ray or esophagoscopy. Although each patient's management is to be individualized, I would use the objective sequelae as indications for antireflux operation if no contraindications exist and if the patient has had some reasonable attempt at medical management. Intractability of symptoms is an indication for operation which is to be used only after certain provisions have been satisfied. First, the symptoms are clearly those of gastroesophageal reflux (heartburn or postural regurgitation of gastric con-

TABLE 1.  Valid Indications for Antireflux Operation

---

Peptic stricture of the esophagus
Peptic ulcer of the esophagus
Hemorrhage secondary to erosive esophagitis
Intractable symptoms plus:
   Incompetent LES by manometry
   Positive Bernstein test
   Free reflux (not a water siphon test) on radiography

---

tents). Vague, nonspecific symptoms in a patient with a hiatus hernia are not an acceptable indication for surgery. Second, there should be some established objective evidence that LES incompetence is present: demonstration of an incompetent LES (pressure less than 10 mm. Hg) by manometry; free reflux in the Trendelenburg position on x-ray (not the water siphon test); or a positive Bernstein test. Third, intractability by present definition should include a trial of specific pharmacologic agents shown to increase LES tone. Thus, operation should be performed only in those patients with sequelae of gastroesophageal reflux or in patients with intractable symptoms of reflux who have objective evidence of LES incompetence.

In Table 2 are shown several conditions which have been excessive, or even erroneous, indications for operation. Many of the indications for operation in this category stem from the naive and false implication of the sliding hiatus hernia as the "masquerader of the upper abdomen."[1] Based on recent studies, it is clear that a hiatus hernia is not a clinical entity and should not be treated as such. "Hiatus hernia" is probably the single most overstated incorrect indication for operation. Iron deficiency anemia in a patient with hiatus hernia is not an indication for operation unless one is certain that the bleeding is secondary to gastroesophageal reflux. This is to be distinguished from proven junctional ulceration seen in patients with a true paraesophageal hernia. In the patient with a sliding hiatus hernia, one should demonstrate gastrointestinal blood loss by stool examination, gastroesophageal reflux by manometry or x-ray, and biopsy evidence of esophagitis. Fulfillment of these requirements would limit operation in patients with unexplained anemia.

The two additional indications for operation—globus hystericus and pulmonary disease—are also overstated. Globus is an hysterical symptom which bears no relationship to gastroesophageal reflux. This symptom alone is not an indication for operation. Chronic pulmonary disease and asthma are common conditions that are frequently seen in the absence of gastroesophageal

TABLE 2.  Poorly Documented or Erroneous Indications
for Antireflux Operation

---

Unexplained abdominal or thoracic symptoms in a patient with a sliding hiatus hernia
Unexplained iron deficiency anemia in a patient with a hiatus hernia
Globus hystericus as a manifestation of cricopharyngeal spasm due to gastroesophageal reflux
Chronic pulmonary disease and asthma secondary to aspiration, secondary to gastroesophageal
  reflux

---

reflux. Likewise, gastroesophageal reflux is a common disorder. The clinician must be absolutely certain that the occurrence of two frequently observed conditions are causally related. An association does not necessarily mean a cause-and-effect relationship has been established. The increased use of pulmonary disease as an indication for operation is probably invalid.

The indications for operation, as discussed above, are for the patient with idiopathic gastroesophageal reflux. In patients with gastroesophageal reflux of a specific etiology, the indications for operation are even less well established. The causes of gastroesophageal reflux of specific etiology are: (a) pregnancy, (b) chalasia of infancy, (c) scleroderma, (d) iatrogenic.

Reflux of a significant degree occurs in one-third to one-half of all pregnant women. The condition is usually transient, and surgery is not indicated. Chalasia of infancy is a condition that has been operated upon in many cases. The condition is probably secondary to slow maturation of sphincter function, and many infants should outgrow this condition if untreated.[44] Many of the antireflux operations performed in infants are probably unnecessary. The striking operative success in infants is most likely related to this condition becoming a nondisease with age. There is no evidence that chalasia of infancy is related to adult idiopathic gastroesophageal reflux.

Scleroderma is an interesting condition whereby the LES becomes markedly incompetent in a patient with poor to absent distal esophageal peristalsis. The esophagus becomes markedly inflamed, and strictures develop rapidly. Gastroesophageal reflux with esophagitis and stricture formation has been the major clinical feature in some patients with scleroderma. Antireflux operation may serve an important role in the management of these individuals.[45] Available operative data in this group are encouraging and should be followed carefully. Antireflux operation may represent a major advance in the management of this otherwise untreatable disease. The suggestion that the esophageal stricture in scleroderma may be resected is an outdated concept.[46] Antireflux operation and vigorous dilatation seem to constitute the most rational approach in a patient with scleroderma with a peptic esophageal stricture.

## References

1. Harrington, S. W.: Various types of diaphragmatic hernia treated surgically. Report of 430 cases. Surg. Gynecol. Obstet. 86:735, 1948.
2. Stilson, W., Sanders, I., and Gardner, G.: Hiatal hernia and gastroesophageal reflux. Radiology 93:1323, 1969.
3. Cohen, S., and Harris, L.: Does hiatus hernia affect competence of the lower esophageal sphincter. New Engl. J. Med. 284:1053, 1971.
4. Ismail-Beigi, F., Horten, P., and Pope, C.: Histological consequences of gastroesophageal reflux in man. Gastroenterology 58:163, 1970.
5. Haddad, J.: Relation of gastroesophageal reflux to yield sphincter pressures. Gastroenterology 58:175, 1970.
6. Pope, C.: A dynamic test of sphincter strength: Its application to the lower esophageal sphincter. Gastroenterology 52:779, 1967.
7. Palmer, E.: The hiatus hernia–esophagitis–esophageal stricture complex. Am. J. Med. 44:566, 1968.

8. Texter, E. C., Jr., VanDerstappen, G., Chejfec, G., et al.: Criteria for the diagnosis of hiatal hernia. Arch. Intern. Med. *110*:827, 1962.

9. Wolf, B., Brahms, S., and Khilnami, M.: The incidence of hiatus hernia in barium meal examination. J. Mt. Sinai Hosp. 26:598, 1959.

10. Kramer, P.: Does a sliding hiatus hernia constitute a distinct clinical entity? Gastroenterology 57:442, 1969.

11. Stein, G., and Finkelstein, A.: Hiatal hernia: Roentgen incidence and diagnosis. Am. J. Digest. Dis. 5:77, 1960.

12. Tumen, H., Stein, G., and Shlansky, E.: X-ray and clinical features of hiatal hernia. Gastroenterology 38:873, 1960.

13. Pridie, R.: Incidence and coincidence of hiatus hernia. Gut 7:188, 1966.

14. Dyer, N., and Pridie, R.: Incidence of hiatus hernia in asymptomatic patients. Gut 9:696, 1968.

15. Cohen, S., and Harris, L.: The lower esophageal sphincter. Gastroenterology 63:1066, 1972.

16. Wankling, W., Warrian, W., and Lind, J.: The gastroesophageal sphincter in hiatus hernia. Can. J. Surg. 8:61, 1965.

17. Lind, J., Warrian, W., and Wankling, W.: Responses of the gastroesophageal junctional zone to increases in abdominal pressure. Can. J. Surg. 9:32, 1966.

18. Lind, J. F., Cotton, D., Blanchard, R., et al.: Effect of thoracic displacement and vagotomy on the canine gastroesophageal junctional zone. Gastroenterology 56:1078, 1969.

19. Lind, J., Crispin, J., and McIver, D.: The effect of atropine on the gastroesophageal sphincter. Can. J. Physiol. Pharmacol. 46:233, 1968.

20. Lipshutz, W., Gaskins, R., Lukash, W., and Sode, J.: Pathogenesis of lower esophageal sphincter incompetence. New Engl. J. Med. 289:182, 1973.

21. Hiebert, C.: Primary incompetence of the gastric cardia. Am. J. Surg. *119*:365, 1970.

22. Field, P., and Stalker, M.: Incompetence of the cardiac sphincter without radiologic demonstration of hiatus hernia. Can. J. Surg. *11*:412, 1968.

23. Stiles, Q., and Henry, W.: Acid reflux esophagitis with and without demonstrable hiatus hernia. Am. Surg. 30:442, 1964.

24. Hiebert, C., and Belsey, R.: Incompetency of the gastric cardia without radiologic evidence of hiatal hernia. J. Thorac. Cardiovasc. Surg. 42:352, 1961.

25. Olsen, A., Schlegel, J., and Payne, W.: The hypotensive gastroesophageal sphincter. Mayo Clin. Proc. 48:165, 1973.

26. Benz, L., Hootkin, L., Marguiles, S., Donner, M., Cauthorne, R., and Hendrix, T.: A comparison of clinical measurements of gastroesophageal reflux. Gastroenterology 62:1, 1972.

27. Pope, C.: Viewpoints. *In* Digest. Dis. *4*:1, 1972.

28. Battle, W., Nyus, L., and Bombeck, C.: Gastroesophageal reflux: Diagnosis and treatment. Ann. Surg. *177*:560, 1973.

29. Bernstein, L., and Baker, L.: A clinical test for esophagitis. Gastroenterology *34* 760, 1958.

30. Herrington, J.: Treatment of esophageal hiatal hernia. Arch. Surg. 84:379, 1962.

31. Silber, W.: Augmented histamine test in the treatment of symptomatic hiatal hernia. Gut *10*:614, 1969.

32. Squire, B., Glick, S., and Benn, A.: Maximal acid output and oesophagitis in hiatus hernia. Thorax 23:683, 1968.

33. Crispin, J., McIver, D., and Lind, J.: Manometric study of the effect of vagotomy on the gastroesophageal sphincter. Can. J. Surg. *10*:299, 1967.

34. Csendes, A., and Larrain, A.: Effect of posterior gastropexy on gastroesophageal sphincter pressure and symptomatic reflux in patients with hiatal hernia. Gastroenterology 63:19, 1972.

35. Lind, J., Burns, C., and MacDougall, J.: Physiological repair for hiatus hernia—manometric study. Arch. Surg. *91*:233, 1965.

36. Behar, J., Biancani, P., Spiro, H., and Storer, H.: Effect of anterior fundoplication on lower esophageal competence. Gastroenterology 67:209, 1974.

37. Hill, L.: An effective operation for hiatal hernia: An eight year appraisal. Ann. Surg. *166*:681, 1967.

38. Baue, A., and Belsey, R.: The treatment of sliding hiatus hernia and reflux esophagitis by the Mark IV technique. Surgery 62:396, 1967.

39. DiMarino, A. J., Rosato, E., Rosato, F., and Cohen, S.: Improvement in lower esophageal sphincter pressure following surgery for complicated gastroesophageal reflux. Ann. Surg. *181*:239, 1975.

40. Lipshutz, W. H., Gaskins, R. D., Lukash, W. M., and Sode, J.: Pathogenesis of lower esophageal sphincter incompetence. New Engl. J. Med. 289:182, 1973.

41. Lipshutz, W., and Cohen, S.: Physiological determinants of lower esophageal sphincter function. Gastroenterology *61*:16, 1971.

42. Cohen, S., and Green, F.: The mechanics of esophageal muscle contraction; evidence for an inotropic effect of gastrin. J. Clin. Invest. 52:2029, 1973.
43. Siewert, R., Jennewein, H. M., and Waldeck, F.: Mechanism of action of fundoplication. Proceedings of the Fourth International Symposium on Gastrointestinal Motility. Session II, 143. Vancouver, Mitchell Press, Ltd., 1974.
44. Cohen, S.: Developmental characteristics of lower esophageal function: A possible mechanism for infantile chalasia. Gastroenterology 67:252, 1974.
45. Henderson, R. D., and Pearson, F. G.: Surgical management of esophageal scleroderma. J. Thorac. Cardiovasc. Surg. 66:686, 1973.
46. McLaughlin, J. S., Roig, R., and Woodruff, M. A. F.: Surgical treatment of strictures of the esophagus in patients with scleroderma. J. Thorac. Cardiovasc. Surg. 61:641, 1971.

# Hiatus Hernia and Gastroesophageal Reflux

LAWRENCE DENBESTEN

*The University of Iowa College of Medicine*

## Introduction

The esophagus is intended as a conduit to convey materials from the pharynx to the stomach. A complex distal sphincter ordinarily isolates it from corrosive gastric contents. The sphincter can relax to allow eructation or emesis. Gastric contents are quickly cleared from the esophagus by reflex peristaltic movements before damage occurs. Failure of this sphincter may lead to reflux of gastric contents, resulting in esophagitis manifested clinically as pyrosis and substernal pain. Progression of symptoms, hemorrhage, dysphagia, or obstruction secondary to stricture finally bring the patient to the physician. Perspectives on the natural history, preferred methods of patient evaluation, and effective treatment of gastroesophageal reflux are difficult to extract from a diffuse literature heavily laced with the mystical and anecdotal.

## Current Knowledge

The current status of our knowledge of reflux esophagitis and hiatus hernia fall into areas of *documented data, controversial data,* and *no data.*

### Documented Data

The incidence of hiatus hernia at random postmortem or careful radiographic examination in patients over 40 years of age approaches 30 per cent.[1,2] Fifteen to 20 per cent of patients with reflux have no hiatus hernia,[1,3] and 60 to 70 per cent of patients with hiatus hernia have no reflux.[2] Anatomic (crural) repair alone results in 50 per cent recurrence of the hernia and 15 to 20 per cent recurrence of symptoms.[4,5,6] Treatment of reflux by the various flap-valve operations (Belsey,[7] Hill,[8] Nissen[9]) is 95 per cent effective.

537

### Controversial Data

The importance of adding crural repair to valve operations is strongly supported[10] and contested.[11, 12] The importance of fixing the esophagogastric junction below the diaphragm is also vigorously supported[10] and contested.[11, 12, 13] The reported frequency of morbidity and valve operation has ranged from 10 per cent[12] to 50 per cent.[4]

### No Data

No data from prospective studies are available on the natural history of peptic esophagitis, the importance and effectiveness of modalities of medical treatment, or the incidence of stricture and significant hemorrhage in treated and untreated patients.

# Medical Treatment of Reflux Esophagitis

The medical treatment of reflux esophagitis mingles the practical and the mystical. Sliding (axial) hiatus hernia without reflux requires no treatment. Paraesophageal hiatus hernia is an operative problem. Symptoms range from mild postprandial fullness due to entrapment of food in the intrathoracic stomach to severe left upper abdominal, chest, and shoulder pain from incarceration. The threat of strangulation and perforation of the herniated stomach, with a predicted mortality of 50 per cent, makes operative repair of the hernia mandatory at almost any age.

Nonoperative treatment of reflux esophagitis is based on two therapeutic modalities: (1) altering the materials refluxed (frequent and even hourly antacids); and (2) decreasing the frequency with which the esophagus is bathed by gastric contents (elevation of the bed on 9-inch blocks, weight loss, wearing loose clothing, and avoiding food for 2 hours prior to retiring). Clearly, these modalities of therapy have their bases in empiricism and tradition and have never been evaluated by prospective studies. However, the effectiveness of nonoperative treatment can be derived by inference. As previously noted, 30 per cent of patients on barium contrast x-rays of the upper gastrointestinal tract, or at postmortem examination, have a hiatus hernia, and 30 to 40 per cent of these have reflux. To derive the total population with reflux, one must include the 20 per cent of patients with reflux who have no hiatus hernia. If data on the incidence of reflux are assumed to apply mainly to the population over 40 years of age, then 3.3 million people in the United States have gastroesophageal reflux. Although the frequency of operation for the treatment of medically intractable reflux esophagitis is unknown, it is probably safe to say that the vast majority of patients with reflux either fail to develop symptoms or are managed by combinations of self- and medically directed nonoperative treatment.

Maximum benefit from medical treatment of reflux esophagitis depends on the rigidity with which patients adhere to treatment. Weight reduction, considered important by many clinicians, has never been evaluated prospectively and is difficult to attain. The frequent association of obesity with reflux esophagitis, together with an occasional anecdotal report that healing of esophagitis occurred coincident with weight reduction, appears to be the basis of this long accepted therapeutic recommendation. Antacids, preferably liquid, should be given hourly (6 A.M. to 12 A.M.), with an additional dose at 3 A.M. during acute phases of esophagitis. The entire bed (not head only) should be elevated 6 to 9 inches, probably for life. After symptoms subside, antacids should be given between meals, at bedtime, and at any time symptoms are perceived. The lower esophageal pressure in the cat decreases during induced esophagitis and returns to normal with healing.[21] Humans with esophagitis exhibit disorganized contractions in the distal esophagus when bathed with acid.[22, 23] With healing, these disorganized responses to acid stimulation are replaced by sweeping peristaltic waves which quickly remove acid and reestablish a neutral intraesophageal pH (unpublished personal data). Adherence to rigid therapy is spotty, at best, after acute symptoms subside; reestablishment of reflex clearing of the esophagus of acid after healing of esophagitis and continued bed elevation are the two factors which limit the frequency of recurrent esophagitis in the patient with reflux.

## Complications of Reflux Esophagitis

The complications of gastroesophageal reflux include persistent symptomatic esophagitis, stricture, and hemorrhage. Approximately 25 per cent of patients with significant reflux treated by physicians come to operation.[14] Of the indications for operation, persistent symptomatic reflux refractory to treatment after 6 months accounts for 65 per cent of patients, an additional 25 per cent have early or late neglected strictures,[15] and 10 per cent have had previous severe hemorrhage.[16] Approximately 90 per cent of strictures of the distal esophagus have a clear history of peptic esophagitis[15, 17] diagnosed for 6 months to 7 years ($\overline{X}$, 26 months before operation). There is no correlation between the severity of symptoms and the likelihood of stricture formation,[14] and available data suggest that 25 per cent of patients with narrowing of the esophagus and reflux will go on to develop a stricture with medical treatment alone.[15] Fibrosis secondary to reflux rarely, if ever, involves the submucosa and muscle wall of the esophagus. Repeated dilatation may result in minute lacerations of the mucosa and cause spread of the fibrotic process to the entire wall of the esophagus. On the other hand, the limited involvement of the esophageal wall by the fibrotic process explains the usual excellent results of dilatation if further injury from reflux is prevented. Dilatation as a primary mode of therapy for distal esophageal strictures secondary to reflux esophagitis should be reserved for the very elderly or medically debilitated patient, since most will go on to develop a more rigid and elongated stricture, and dilatation itself encourages reflux.[18] Preoperative or intraoperative dilatation of strictures complemented by an antireflux procedure and followed by dilatations until the caliber of the esophagus has stabilized in 6 to 9 months will usually result in essentially normal esophageal function thereafter.[12, 14]

# Criteria for Selection of Patients for Operative Management

### Symptoms

Patients with symptoms of pyrosis, substernal pain, and dysphagia refractory after 4 to 6 months of vigorous medical treatment should be encouraged to have operative treatment unless concurrent medical problems make operation hazardous. The observation that there is poor correlation between the degree of symptoms and the likelihood of peptic esophagitis and stricture must be kept in mind. The patient who awakens daily with gastric contents on his pillow or who has chronic aspiration pneumonia in spite of bed elevation is probably an urgent candidate for operation.

### X-Ray

Properly executed barium contrast studies of the distal esophagus will identify more than 90 per cent of patients with reflux. When an esophagram is done without special attention to the distal esophagus, hiatus hernia is diagnosed in 1 to 3 per cent of random patients. However, when the study is done with abdominal compression and the patient in the prone position, 30 per cent of patients have demonstrated hiatus hernia, about 40 per cent of whom have reflux. The water siphon test,[19] done by having the patient sniff and sip water while in the prone position with barium in the stomach, is positive in 30 to 40 per cent of normal patients and should be discarded. Studies with acid barium also miss up to 40 per cent of patients with reflux and are positive in an equal number of normal patients.

### Manometry

Although a population of patients with gastroesophageal reflux will have a mean lower esophageal sphincter pressure which is statistically lower than normal, this test has minimal application in the evaluation of the individual patient except as a research tool. Some patients with reflux have lower esophageal sphincter pressures greater than 15 mm. Hg as compared to gastric pressures. Many with pressures less than 10 mm. Hg have no other evidence of reflux.

### Esophagoscopy and Biopsy

This examination, using a modern flexible endoscope, is mandatory in evaluating patients with reflux. Reflux can often be seen during examination, the presence and gross degree of esophagitis can be recorded, and biopsy can be carried out. The biopsy may show thickening of the basal layer of the mucosa from its normal 2 to 4 cells to 6 to 8 cells, together with elongation of the dermal pegs. These changes probably result from chronic mucosal insult by acid gastric chyme and correlate with pain sensation during acid perfusion. Microscopic changes may progress to polymorphonuclear cell infiltration into the submucosa, and on to frank ulceration, or to replacement of epithelium with columnar epithelium containing parietal cells.

## Acid Perfusion

Alternate perfusion of the distal esophagus with room temperature saline and 0.1 normal HCl at a constant rate will reproduce symptoms in almost 100 per cent of patients with reflux esophagitis if the acid perfusion is continued up to 20 minutes. In clinical practice this test is reserved for use in patients presenting with symptoms compatible with esophagitis, but without gross esophagitis, or with microscopic changes limited to thickening of the basal layer of the mucosa and deepening of the dermal pegs.

## Acid Reflux

After the instillation of 300 ml. of 0.1 normal HCl into the stomach, the distal esophageal pH will be less than 4 in 85 per cent of patients with symptomatic esophageal reflux. This test has been difficult to interpret in our hands, and we have abandoned it for all but research purposes. Most consistent results are obtained if the test is carried out as follows: After 300 ml of 0.1 normal HCl has been placed in the stomach, the distal esophageal pH is monitored in the resting prone position, during straining (Valsalva), straight leg raising, bending over, and deep breathing. Execution of the various maneuvers is difficult to repeat accurately, and a negative study is of little significance. When the test is positive, careful barium contrast x-rays will almost always show clearly documented reflux.

# Operative Treatment of Reflux Esophagitis

### Criteria of Successful Operative Treatment

Criteria of successful operation for the treatment of reflux esophagitis should include the following: (1) absence of symptoms of pyrosis, substernal pain, and dysphagia; (2) absence of reflux; (3) healing and subsequent absence of esophagitis; (4) minimal new morbidity resulting from operation. Relief of symptoms should be complete. Those patients with severe esophagitis without symptoms will, of course, notice little change after operation. Symptomatic dysphagia may be due to early stricture, and these patients may continue to have sticking of food in the distal esophagus until the stricture stabilizes with repeated dilatations. The absence of reflux is important, since the distal esophagus seldom, if ever, becomes inflamed without reflux of gastric contents. The absence of reflux must be established by careful barium x-ray contrast studies and pH monitoring of the distal esophagus. Absence of esophagitis postoperatively, as assessed by esophagoscopy and biopsy, is probably most important from the physician's perspective, since esophagitis is the etiology of the severe complications of reflux.

Crural repair of the hiatus hernia, with its 50 per cent recurrence of the hernia and 15 to 20 per cent recurrence of symptoms and signs of reflux esophagitis, is being abandoned by most surgeons. It has no application to those patients with reflux esophagitis and no hernia, and clinicians are gradually accepting incompetence of the gastroesophageal junction as the primary lesion in reflux esophagitis. Those who continue to do crural repair defend this position on the basis of the 80 to 85 per cent symptomatic relief of symptoms and the morbidity after valve operations, the reported incidence of which ranges from 10 to 50 per cent. Final resolution of these two positions must await data on the frequency with which patients made asymptomatic by crural repair eventually develop stricture, bleeding, or late symptoms because of continuing reflux. Data on the true incidence and severity of morbidity following careful valve operations are of equal importance.

### Management of Stricture

In our experience nearly all strictures less than 5 cm. in length can be dilated preoperatively, followed by a valve operation and repeated dilatations in the postoperative period. Postoperative dilatations should be done frequently enough to prevent repeated trauma and healing by scar formation. This often requires weekly dilatations beginning at 2 weeks after operation and continued with decreasing frequency until no residual stricture is present, usually 6 months after operation.

The very infrequent long stricture which cannot be dilated under direct vision during operation or the midesophageal stricture presents a different problem. We treat these distal esophageal strictures by a combination Thal operation to which is added a Nissen fundoplication. For this procedure the esophageal hiatus is opened to 7 to 8 cm., and the repair is placed in the chest, above the diaphragm. Midesophageal strictures secondary to reflux are best treated by resection of the stricture and distal esophagus. Continuity is reestablished using a left colon segment, remembering that 25 per cent will develop a stricture at the distal anastomosis in spite of good medical therapy.[15]

### Operative Approach

The choice of abdominal or thoracic approach depends on personal preference plus the degree of one's concern with conditions which often occur concurrent with reflux esophagitis. We generally prefer the abdominal route. This route allows careful assessment or treatment of the 10 to 15 per cent of patients who also have duodenal ulcer[2,6,15] and the 20 per cent who have cholelithiasis.[6]

## Operative Technique

The problem in medically refractory reflux esophagitis is caused by reflux of corrosive substances through an incompetent lower esophageal sphincter. Successful operative management requires an operation which prevents reflux, has a minimum of side effects, and gives consistent results in the hands of the average trained gastrointestinal surgeon. We have adopted the Nissen fundoplication[9] as our standard operation for treatment of reflux esophagitis. This procedure depends for its success on the creation of a flap-valve at the gastroesophageal junction. The standard operation is carried out as follows: The gastroesophageal junction is identified, encircled with a Penrose drain, and mobilized from the mediastinum to obtain a 6-cm. segment of esophagus. The gastrohepatic ligament is divided between clamps up to the left gastric artery (this vessel, although usually preserved, may be divided if required technically). Short gastric vessels are divided if the high attachment of the spleen interferes with plication. With a No. 40 Hurst dilator through the gastroesophageal junction, a 5-cm. segment of esophagus is encircled by the fundus of the stomach. Six to 8 nonabsorbable sutures are taken through the edges of the stomach wrapped around the esophagus, including esophageal muscle in each suture to prevent displacement of the fundoplication onto the stomach. The adequacy of the fundoplication to prevent reflux is evaluated intraoperatively with a "water test."[20] The Hurst dilator is replaced by a nasogastric tube through which 300 ml. of saline is instilled into the stomach. The nasogastric tube is then withdrawn to a point just above the fundoplication. With the pylorus occluded, pressure is exerted on the stomach. If a competent valve has been created, no saline will enter the esophagus above the fundoplication. Approximation of the crura and fixation of the gastroesophageal junction to maintain an intra-abdominal position of the gastroesophageal junction[10] add nothing to the short- or long-term effectiveness of the antireflux valve. In a recent study of 61 patients operated upon for reflux esophagitis, 30 had crural repair added to Nissen fundoplication; 31 did not. The cure rate was identical between the two groups of patients.[12] Fundoplication carried out in the postmortem room[13] and at the operating table has regularly demonstrated the effectiveness of the antireflux valve alone in preventing reflux. Fundoplication can be carried out in the face of a short esophagus, placing the repair in the mediastinum. If the size of the hiatus corresponds closely to the size of the plication, the hiatus should be either enlarged or closed to prevent herniation and incarceration of the repair in the hiatus. In practice, we usually do a crural repair because of concern that the fundoplication may become incarcerated in the dilated hiatus.

Acid-reducing procedures, such as vagotomy plus pyloroplasty, should not accompany fundoplication unless they are indicated for the treatment of a second, and probably unrelated, acid peptic diathesis of the distal stomach or duodenum. Acid-reducing procedures add nothing to the treatment of reflux esophagitis and incur a 15 per cent risk of dumping and diarrhea.

We have found the Nissen fundoplication more than 90 per cent effective in the treatment of reflux esophagitis. Although Belsey, Hill, and other antireflux procedures are probably equally effective when carefully performed, we have found the Nissen fundoplication an effective operation yielding consistent results in the hands of both staff and trainees.

# References

1. Bombeck, C. T., Helfrich, G. B., and Nyhus, L. M.: Planning surgery for reflux esophagitis and hiatus hernia. Surg. Clin. North Am. 50:29, 1970.
2. Pridie, R. B.: Incidence and coincidence of hiatus hernia. Gut 7:188, 1966.

3. Hiebert, C. A., and Belsey, R.: Incompetency of the gastric cardia without radiologic evidence of hiatal hernia. J. Thorac. Cardiovasc. Surg. 42:352, 1961.
4. Woodward, E. R., Thomas, H. F., and McAlhany, J. C.: Comparison of crural repair and Nissen fundoplication in the treatment of esophageal hiatus hernia with peptic esophagitis. Ann. Surg. 173:782, 1971.
5. Brintnall, E. S., Blome, R. A., and Tidrick, R. T.: Late results of hiatus hernia repair. Am. J. Surg. 101:159, 1961.
6. Allison, P. R.: Hiatus hernia: (A 20-year retrospective survey). Ann. Surg. 178:273, 1973.
7. Baue, A. E., and Belsey, R. H. R.: Treatment of sliding hiatus hernia and reflux esophagitis by the Mark IV technique. Surgery 62:396, 1967.
8. Hill, L. D.: Management of recurrent hiatal hernia. Arch. Surg. 102:296, 1971.
9. Nissen, R.: Gastropexy and "fundoplication" in surgical treatment of hiatal hernia. Am. J. Digest. Dis. 6:954, 1961.
10. Wilkins, E. W., Jr., and Skinner, D. B.: Surgery of the esophagus. New Engl. J. Med. 278:824, 1968.
11. Anderson, H. N., May, K. J., Steinmetz, G. P., et al.: The lower esophageal intrinsic sphincter and the mechanism of reflux: Experimental observations supporting a new concept. Ann. Surg. 166:102, 1967.
12. Safaie-Shirazi, S., Zike, W. L., Anuras, S., Condon, R. E., and DenBesten, L.: Nissen fundoplication without crural repair. A cure for reflux esophagitis. Arch. Surg. 108:424, 1974.
13. Butterfield, W. C.: Current hiatal hernia repairs: Similarities, mechanisms, and extended indications — an autopsy study. Surgery 69:910, 1971.
14. Gastroesophageal reflux. A panel by correspondence. Arch. Surg. 108:16, 1974.
15. Raptis, S., and Milne, D. M.: A review of the management of 100 cases of benign stricture of the oesophagus. Thorax 27:599, 1972.
16. Smith, L. C., and Bradshaw, H. H.: Esophageal hiatal hernia. Surg. Gynecol. Obstet. 109:230, 1959.
17. Vogt-Moykopf, I., Daum, R., Zeidler, D., and Greiner, C.: Conservative therapy of benign esophageal stenosis and its complications. Chirurg 44:63, 1973.
18. Rayl, J. E., and Balison, J. R.: Management of longitudinal stricture resulting from reflux esophagitis. Ann. Thorac. Surg. 15:439, 1973.
19. Crummy, A. F.: The water test in the evaluation of gastroesophageal reflux: Its correlation with pyrosis. Radiology 87:501, 1966.
20. Safaie-Shirazi, S.: Competency test after fundoplication for treatment of reflux esophagitis. Arch. Surg. 110:221, 1975.
21. Eastwood, G. L., and Higgs, R. H.: Experimental esophagitis in cats affects lower esophageal sphincter competence. Clin. Res. 22:602A, 1974.
22. Olsen, A. M., and Schlegel, J. F.: Motility disturbances caused by esophagitis. J. Thorac. Cardiovasc. Surg. 50:607, 1965.
23. Garabedian, M.: Uses of esophageal manometry and acid perfusion in the study of gastroesophageal reflux and hiatal hernia. Surg. Clin. North Am. 51:589, 1971.

# 24

# Hyperthyroidism— Operative Versus Nonoperative Treatment

THE TREATMENT OF
HYPERTHYROIDISM

> by H. Taylor Caswell,
> Willis P. Maier,
> and George P. Rosemond

NONOPERATIVE MANAGEMENT
OF HYPERTHYROIDISM

> by John B. Stanbury
> and Earle M. Chapman

## Statement of the Problem

*The cost, morbidity, and efficacy of these two approaches are considered.*

What is the frequency of permanent remission after thyroid blocking agents? After how long a therapeutic trial? Discuss their side effects, severity, and frequency. Discuss the expense of the nonoperative regimen, including the cost of the medication, doctor's time, and repeated laboratory tests. What is the time frame required for control of Graves' disease with antithyroid drugs? How well and how often can the toxic nodule be managed with antithyroid drugs?

What patients should not be subjected to radioiodine treatment of hyperthyroidism? On what basis? What are the data regarding eventual development of clinical hypothyroidism? Following radioiodine therapy, maintenance thyroid medication is required by what percentage of the patients?

Compare operative morbidity for Graves' disease with that for toxic nodular goiter. Provide data on short- and long-term frequency of hypothyroidism. Indicate incidence of thyroid crises and persistent hyperthyroidism and recurrent nerve injury. Compare costs of operative and nonoperative management.

If recurrence follows an operation for hyperthyroidism, what mode of therapy do you choose? On what basis?

# The Treatment of Hyperthyroidism

H. TAYLOR CASWELL,
WILLIS P. MAIER,
and GEORGE P. ROSEMOND

*Temple University Health Sciences Center*

At present, there are three methods available for definitively treating patients with diffuse toxic goiter (Graves' disease) and toxic nodular goiter. These are (1) subtotal thyroidectomy, (2) radioactive iodine administration, and (3) long-term antithyroid drug therapy.

The ideal treatment of hyperthyroidism is one which has the following attributes: (1) prompt control of the disease and no requirement for multiple applications, (2) minimal morbidity and mortality, (3) a low incidence of post-treatment hypothyroidism, (4) a low incidence of recurrent disease, and (5) a reasonable and acceptable cost. Treatment should be chosen on the basis of what is best for the individual patient. The patient's age, sex, physical condition, socioeconomic status, type of hyperthyroidism, and emotional stability all play a role in making this decision.

## Radioactive Iodine

Widespread use of radioactive iodine in the treatment of thyrotoxicosis began in approximately 1950. It appeared to satisfy the requirements of the ideal treatment. It does not require hospitalization in most cases, is relatively inexpensive, and avoids an operative procedure. With the passage of time, it became apparent that patients treated with radioactive iodine displayed a disturbing incidence of post-treatment myxedema. The development of myxedema was cumulative, reaching a level of 40 to 70 per cent 10 years post-treatment.[1, 2] Even those patients followed for 15 years after [131]I therapy did not show evidence of any plateau in the cumulative increase in myxedema (2 per cent a year). These results were obtained with the so-called "high dose" of radioactive iodine. Myxedema is an insidious chronic

547

disease with serious cardiovascular complications combined with loss of mental acuity, which plays a role in the patient not seeking medical care. Twenty-five to 40 per cent of patients treated with radioactive iodine require multiple doses of the drug.[3, 4] This means continuing and recurrent illness, with the risk of thyroid storm if pregnancy occurs or in the event of severe intercurrent illness, and requires meticulous follow-up in patients who are notoriously unreliable and unstable emotionally.

Patients with toxic nodular goiter who are in an older age group than those with Graves' disease require much higher doses of radioactive iodine for control. Patients with large goiters who are thyrotoxic are not well suited to treatment with radioactive iodine because of the need for multiple doses.

As a result of the high incidence of post-[131]I hypothyroidism, the use of so-called "low-dose" [131]I therapy was initiated. The dosage employed in this regime is approximately one-half of that originally used. Cevallos et al.[5] reported on a group of 102 patients treated with low-dose radioactive iodine, with a mean interval of follow-up of 66 months. These patients were given a 4-month course of potassium iodide after radioactive iodine therapy to "facilitate" the efficiency of treatment. The mode of action of potassium iodide used in this manner has not been clarified. When the potassium iodide was discontinued, 27 of the patients who had become clinically euthyroid had reappearance of thyrotoxicosis. Twelve of these who were given a second dose of radioactive iodine became euthyroid. Fifteen of the patients were given a second course of potassium iodide, resulting in euthyroidism in 12 of these patients; two patients from this group required an additional dose of [131]I. The permanence of euthyroidism occurring after a second course of potassium iodide has not been established. At the end of 5.5 years of the follow-up study, the authors reported an incidence of myxedema of 26 per cent. This is a lower incidence of hypothyroidism post-[131]I treatment than that seen with the previously widely used "high dose."

Rapoport et al.,[6] however, treating 85 patients with low-dose radioactive iodine, followed for 12 to 16 months, who were given antithyroid drugs post-[131]I treatment, found that 54 per cent of these patients were hyperthyroid on withdrawal of the antithyroid drugs. These authors concluded that the large number of patients still experiencing hyperthyroidism 1 year after therapy makes use of low-dose radioactive iodine no more advantageous than use of antithyroid drugs alone. They conclude that low-dose radioactive iodine treatment as administered in their protocol is an unsatisfactory method of treating hyperthyroidism.

At the present time, there is no evidence that the treatment of thyrotoxicosis with radioactive iodine results in an increased incidence of thyroid carcinoma, leukemia, or genetic defects in infants born to women subsequent to their treatment. Thyroid carcinoma has been reported following radioactive iodine therapy. Radioactive iodine therapy can result in nodular goiter when used in adolescence. It has been recommended by some that [131]I should not be used in younger age groups except for special reasons. It should not be used in a thyrotoxic pregnant female because of the potential damage to the fetal thyroid.

Radioactive iodine is a treatment of choice in patients who are questionable operative risks, primarily because of cardiovascular pulmonary disease. It is also the treatment of choice in patients who cannot be rendered euthyroid prior to operation with the use of antithyroid drugs and/or propranolol, in patients refusing operation, and in those patients who develop recurrent hyperthyroidism after subtotal thyroidectomy because of the risk of recurrent nerve injury or parathyroid deprivation at the second operation.

## *Operative Treatment*

Subtotal thyroidectomy in the treatment of thyrotoxicosis carries the disadvantage of requiring an operative procedure. The major complications are those of recurrent nerve injury and inadvertent removal of the parathyroid glands. Using modern operative techniques which demand identification of the parathyroid glands and the recurrent laryngeal nerves, these complications should never occur. The risk of operation should be approximately that of endotracheal anesthesia.[3, 8] Operative technique also includes leaving 7 to 9 g. of thyroid tissue on each side of the trachea in order to minimize the development of postsurgical hypothyroidism. The Cooperative Thyrotoxicosis Therapy Follow-Up Study,[4] reporting on 5221 patients who were surgically treated, noted an incidence of postoperative hypothyroidism of 25 per cent. Caswell and Maier,[7] reporting on 136 patients who were treated operatively for thyrotoxicosis, with a mean interval since operation of 8 years, noted a 10 per cent incidence of postoperative hypothyroidism and a 7 per cent incidence of recurrent hyperthyroidism. Olsen et al.[8] found a 25 per cent incidence of postoperative hypothyroidism and a 7 per cent incidence of recurrent hyperthyroidism. In both of these series, postoperative hypothyroidism developed during the first year after operation, and there was no evidence of a cumulative increase in the development of myxedema, as has been reported with the use of radioactive iodine.[4] The fact that hypothyroidism occurring after a subtotal thyroidectomy is evident in the first postoperative year makes it much more likely that the diagnosis will be established and proper treatment initiated before serious effects of myxedema can occur and prior to the development of the insidious and subtle changes in mental alertness which tend to prevent the patient from returning for follow-up examination.

Before subtotal thyroidectomy is carried out, the patient must be rendered euthyroid in every instance. Our method consists of administration of adequate doses of methimazole (Tapazole), starting with 80 to 100 mg. per day in the average patient with Graves' disease. The medication is continued at this level for 4 weeks or until the patient is unquestionably euthyroid clinically and has a normal $T_4$. At this time, methimazole administration is discontinued, and the patient is given 10 drops of Lugol's iodine twice daily for 14 days, at the conclusion of which time operation is performed. The average postoperative hospital stay is 3 to 4 days. Recently, the beta adrenergic blocking agent propranolol[9] has been used in preoperative preparation of patients with thyrotoxicosis. We have limited the use of this drug to those patients whose emotional disturbance, family situation, or economic status is such that they cannot be relied upon to take antithyroid drugs as outpatients. We have also employed it in patients who have developed drug reactions to the antithyroid drugs. The patients prepared with propranolol have been hospitalized, and the dose of the drug has varied between 80 and 260 mg. per day, depending on the patient's response. The daily dose of the drug is increased each 24 hours until all clinical evidence of hyperthyroidism has disappeared and the patient is considered euthyroid. The $T_4$ level, of course, remains elevated. Subtotal thyroidectomy is carried out, and propranolol administration is continued postoperatively in the same fashion as it was preoperatively. Daily $T_4$ determinations are used as an indication for discontinuing the drug. It is usually necessary to continue treatment for 5 to 7 days postoperatively. Propranolol can also be used in the treatment of thyroid storm.

No patient in whom a euthyroid state cannot be established preoperatively should be considered for subtotal thyroidectomy. If this rule is rigidly adhered to, postoperative thyroid storm does not occur. If euthyroidism cannot be established prior to operation, then the patient should be treated with radioactive iodine or long-term antithyroid drugs.

Operation is particularly effective in patients with toxic nodular goiter in whom the hyperfunctioning nodule can be excised and normal thyroid tissue remains without risk of postoperative hypothyroidism. It is our opinion that subtotal thyroidectomy is the treatment of choice for most patients with Graves' disease or toxic nodular goiter who are good operative risks and who can be brought to a euthyroid state with either antithyroid drugs or propranolol prior to operation.

## Long-term Antithyroid Drug Therapy

The basis for treatment of thyrotoxicosis with long-term antithyroid drugs is that prolonged control of the disease (12 to 18 months) will result in a permanent remission when the drugs are discontinued. This method has the advantage of not requiring an operative procedure; hypothyroidism after cessation of treatment is not a problem; morbidity is principally that of drug reaction (8 per cent); and control of the symptoms of hyperthyroidism is prompt. Cost is at a reasonable and acceptable level. Despite these positive attributes, it is the least desirable method of treatment of hyperthyroidism in most cases, primarily because of the high incidence of relapse after discontinuance of the drug (50 to 89 per cent).[10, 11]

The original reports on the use of antithyroid drugs as a definitive method of treating hyperthyroidism began in the 1960's. Remission rates averaging 50 to 60 per cent after 12 to 18 months of treatment were reported.[10] Most papers which reported a 70 per cent remission rate with the use of antithyroid drugs were based on results in patients who were followed for 1 year or less after discontinuing the drugs, which must be considered an inadequate period of time on which to base any conclusion on the incidence of remission.

Clinical experience with patients treated by this method has not substantiated the high remission rate of 50 per cent[11] which was originally reported. Patients with large goiters are almost certain to show relapse when treated by this method. The antithyroid drugs have the potential for causing major drug reactions, the most serious of which is bone marrow depression. A most cooperative patient is required to ensure the fact that the drug is taken regularly and that the patient reports for the required clinical and laboratory examinations at appointed intervals. Recurrence of hyperthyroidism is most disappointing to a patient who has taken drugs for a year and a half, only to find that the symptoms of his original disease are recurring. Wartofsky[11] reported a remission rate of only 11 to 17 per cent (83 to 89 per cent relapse) in 44 patients treated with long-term antithyroid drugs and noted the steady decline in remission rates reported in the 1950's and 1960's as compared to the present time. He presents the hypothesis that this may be due to an increase in the amount of dietary iodine over this period of time. Long-term antithyroid drug treatment has been recommended in the management of adolescent Graves' disease because of the supposed higher chance of permanent remission in these younger patients. This has not been substantiated, and the disadvantages of long-term antithyroid drug therapy noted in adults apply to adolescents as well. Recurrent thyrotoxicosis in 70 per cent of children followed for 2 years after long-term antithyroid drug therapy has been reported.[12]

Long-term antithyroid drugs have a specific indication for use in patients with thyrotoxicosis. They should be used as the initial treatment in hyperthyroid patients with small and nonpalpable goiters. There is clinical evidence that this group of patients has a higher remission rate after discontinuing the antithyroid drugs than that group of patients with larger glands. They are also used, in combination with thyroid replacement therapy, by some in controlling thyrotoxicosis during pregnancy. They are used together with adrenal corticosteroids and thyroid replacement in patients with Graves' disease and progressive exophthalmos.

## Costs of Treatment

The expenses involved in the treatment of hyperthyroidism with either [131]I, subtotal thyroidectomy, or long-term antithyroid drugs are not excessive by present standards. The following costs are estimated and apply to our immediate geographic area. Third-party payers usually cover the expense of inpatient treatment. Outpatient costs for office visits and laboratory work and drugs may or may not be paid by the insurers. Initial radioactive iodine uptake and scan and $T_4$ are carried out with all three methods and cost approximately $75.00.

### Radioactive Iodine

Treatment is usually carried out on an outpatient basis. The average cost of one dose of radioactive iodine is approximately $250.00. Subsequent office visits and laboratory work over a period of 1 year would average $200.00, for a total of $450.00.

Necessity for a second dose of radioactive iodine (25 to 40 per cent of patients) and subsequent office and laboratory costs would double this figure to approximately $900.00.

### Subtotal Thyroidectomy

Office visits and laboratory studies for approximately 6 weeks preoperatively would average $60.00. Antithyroid drug preparation would cost approximately $10.00. A total of 4 days of hospitalization would be approximately $600.00. The operative fee would be approximately $350.00 to $500.00, for a total cost of $1000.00 to $1200.00.

### Long-term Antithyroid Drug Therapy

This is usually carried out on an outpatient basis. Office visits of one time per month for 18 months would average $270.00. Laboratory studies during this period would average $100.00 and drug costs approximately $100.00, for a total of $470.00.

Due to the high rate (50 to 80 per cent) of recurrent thyrotoxicosis following cessation of treatment, the cost of subsequent treatment with either radioactive iodine or operation in this group of patients must be added to the estimated total of $470.00.

## Summary

The methods of treating hyperthyroidism and the importance of individualizing treatment have been discussed. The relative merits of the use of radioactive iodine, subtotal thyroidectomy, and long-term antithyroid drugs in the treatment of hyperthyroidism have been compared.

Subtotal thyroidectomy after adequate preparation of the patient is felt to be the preferred treatment in the majority of cases of hyperthyroidism. It is superior to treatment with radioactive iodine in the incidence of permanent hypothyroidism and to treatment with both radioactive iodine and long-term antithyroid drugs in the requirement for additional treatment because of recurrent or continuing disease.

## References

1. Dunn, J. T., and Chapman, E.: Rising incidence of hypothyroidism after radioactive-iodine therapy in thyrotoxicosis. New Engl. J. Med. 271:1037, 1964.
2. Nofal, M. M., Beierwaltes, W. H., and Patno, M. E.: Treatment of hyperthyroidism with sodium iodide I[131]: A 16-year experience. J.A.M.A. 197:605, 1966.
3. Caswell, H. T., Robbins, R. R., and Rosemond, G. P.: Definitive treatment of 536 cases of hyperthyroidism with I-131 or surgery. Ann. Surg. 164:257, 1966.

4. Becker, D. V., McConahey, W. M., Dobyns, B. M., Tompkins, E., Sheline, G. E., and Workman, J. B.: The results of radioiodine treatment of hyperthyroidism—A preliminary report of the thyrotoxicosis therapy follow-up study. Abstract. Presented at the 6th International Goiter Conference in Vienna, 1971.
5. Cevallos, J. L., Hagen, G. A., Maloof, F., and Chapman, E. M.: Low-dosage I[131] therapy of thyrotoxicosis (diffuse goiters). (A five-year follow-up study.) Medical intelligence. New Engl. J. Med. 290:141, 1974.
6. Rapoport, B., Caplan, R., and DeGroot, L. J.: Low-dose sodium iodide I[131] therapy in Graves' disease. J.A.M.A. 224:1610, 1973.
7. Caswell, H. T. and Maier, W. P.: Results of surgical treatment for hyperthyroidism. Surg. Gynecol. Obstet. 134:218, 1972.
8. Olsen, W. R., Nishiyama, R. H., and Graber, L. W.: Thyroidectomy for hyperthyroidism. Arch. Surg. 101:175, 1970.
9. Lee, T. C., Coffey, R. J., Mackin, J., Cobb, M., Routon, J., and Canary, J. J.: The use of propranolol in the surgical treatment of thyrotoxic patients. Ann. Surg. 177:643, 1973.
10. Hershman, J. M., Givens, J. R., Cassidy, C. E., and Astwood, E. B.: Long-term outcome of hyperthyroidism treated with antithyroid drugs. J. Clin. Endocrinol. Metab. 26:803, 1966.
11. Wartofsky, L.: Low remission after therapy for Graves' disease. J.A.M.A. 226:1083, 1973.
12. Hayles, A. B., and Chaves-Carballo, E.: Diagnosis and treatment of exophthalmic goiter in children. Clin. Pediatr. 6:681, 1967.

# Nonoperative Management of Hyperthyroidism

JOHN B. STANBURY

*Massachusetts Institute of Technology*

and EARLE M. CHAPMAN

*Harvard Medical School*

## Introduction

Operative intervention was the only effective form of therapy for thyrotoxicosis prior to 1940. Practicing surgeons gained a high degree of skill in dealing with the disorder, which affects perhaps 3 per cent of all people during their lives.[1] Many contributions to the literature recorded the low complication rates of operative thyroidectomy learned through experience, but even in the most practiced hands and in the most respected clinics, complications still occurred; the complication rates in community hospitals whose surgeons undertook procedures for which they were less well-trained were rarely, if ever, published.

The treatment of thyrotoxicosis underwent a complete renovation with the introduction into clinical therapeutics of the antithyroid drugs and radioiodine just over 3 decades ago. In most clinics today, operation for thyrotoxicosis is reserved for limited categories of patients for whom special considerations favor operative over medical management. Is this therapeutic revolution justified by theory, fact, and experience? It appears so, and in the following paragraphs we offer the supporting arguments.

## Management of Thyrotoxicosis with Antithyroid Drugs

In virtually all instances, thyrotoxicosis can be controlled by inhibition of hormone synthesis with one of the thiourylene derivatives, such as methimazole, propylthiouracil, or carbimazole. Once a diagnosis is established, treatment can begin at once, with the expectation of significant improvement within 2 to 3 weeks.

Such a program seems simple and effective, but there are limitations.

555

Complications arising from the use of these drugs have been variably reported in between 3 and 45 per cent of those treated.[2] Most commonly, these are skin rash, drug fever, adenitis, and falling hair, but occasionally leukopenia, jaundice, and even agranulocytosis associated with pharyngitis have necessitated omission of the drug. Fortunately, fatalities are very rare. Although it is often possible to shift to another antithyroid drug without recurrence of toxicity, this may not be the case, and most patients are justifiably reluctant to continue with drugs after a significant toxic reaction.

Another frequent undesired effect is the increase in goiter size. Although thyroxine in doses of 0.2 mg. or more daily may halt the process, it seldom shrinks the goiter, and it may confuse patient evaluation which uses an assay for the plasma $T_4$. Also, the use of iodide combined with drug therapy feeds the production and storage of hormone. In fact, an important observation on drug therapy comes from Scotland, where Alexander et al.[3] observed that recurrence after prolonged therapy may be suppressed by iodine deficiency and promoted by even the iodide of iodized salt or thyroxine.

A further disadvantage of antithyroid drug therapy is the continuing close surveillance which is required, not only for evaluation of adherence to the regime and maintenance of a normal metabolic state, but also for attention to possible toxic responses, such as granulocytopenia.

The principal impediment to the universal use of antithyroid drugs for thyrotoxicosis is the high relapse rate after medication is stopped. Perhaps the puzzling fact is not so much the high relapse rate as the fact that permanent remission ever occurs, because there is no reason to suppose that the medication strikes at the root cause of the disease. It is, in effect, only symptomatic treatment.

Although predictions concerning which patients would develop permanent remissions were unreliable with early suppression tests, the recent experience of Hales is encouraging. In 1968 Hales et al.[4] reported on the radioiodine uptakes during the first 15 minutes after I.V. injection before and while taking antithyroid drug and before and during attempted suppression with $T_4$. The results divided patients into three groups: (1) the 15-minute uptake fell on antithyroid drug alone; only 1 in 26 patients had recurrence; (2) the results were intermediate; and (3) neither the uptake fell nor was the gland suppressed with $T_4$; 13 of 26 patients had recurrence after long treatment. They concluded that definitive treatment should be offered the patients in this last group.

Although for many years the permanent remission rate resulting from an antithyroid drug regime for a year or more was estimated at about 50 per cent,[5] the critical analysis by Wartofsky[6] in 1973 has shaken the faith of those using benign neglect in following their patients on and after drug therapy. He used the Codman "end result" method in a very closely followed group of 44 patients. Remissions occurred in only 17 per cent of those treated longer than 12 months. None of the patients with goiters of more than 50 g. had a remission. Most relapses occurred within 24 months of cessation of therapy, and he suspected that increased iodine intake may have been a precipitating factor. Confirmation of his observations might lead to changes in the criteria for patient selection for the three principal types of therapy.

It has long been realized that the single toxic nodular goiter does not respond well to drug therapy and that, in older patients or in those with goiters of 60 g. or larger at any age, relapse is almost inevitable, even after prolonged treatment.

The present ideal use of the antithyroid drugs is in young persons with disease of short duration and a small diffuse goiter. The drug may be effective if given in one large daily dose or in divided amounts, as is so often inconveniently advised. Occasionally, doses up to 1000 mg. of propylthiouracil daily have been necessary to control resistant glands.

Children and young adults whose thyrotoxicosis apparently follows some definable emotional turmoil or situational problem seem likely to obtain a permanent remission. The eyes usually improve on drug therapy, and progressive exophthalmos is no more promoted by antithyroid drugs than by operative or radioiodine treatment or by the natural history of the disease. Fortunately, less than 3 per cent of all patients develop severe eye signs. Unfortunately, we do not know the cause, prevention, or cure of this disorder.

## Management of Thyrotoxicosis with Radioactive Iodine

During the 30 years since radioactive iodine has been readily available for the treatment of thyrotoxicosis, there have been reservations regarding its safety in the minds of those using this form of treatment. Virtually everyone is agreed that radioiodine would otherwise be the ideal form of treatment, and indeed it has been used successfully in hundreds of thousands of patients. The treatment is simple, quick, effective, and relatively inexpensive. Hypothetical and real complications have impeded its universal adoption as the primary resource in the treatment of thyrotoxicosis. They merit individual consideration.

### $^{131}I$ Therapy and Leukemogenesis

A United States Public Health thyrotoxicosis therapy follow-up was started by the National Center for Radiological Health in 1961 in order to assess the incidence of leukemia in hyperthyroid patients treated by radioactive iodine as compared to the incidence in patients treated differently. In 1968[7] it reported 36,000 patients from 26 medical centers, of whom about 22,000 were treated with $^{131}I$ and about 14,000 were treated otherwise. The incidence of leukemia in patients treated with radioactive iodine and in those treated operatively did not differ.

Thus, no present evidence indicates an increased risk of leukemia in those who receive therapeutic doses of radioactive iodine.

### $^{131}I$ and Carcinogenesis

Radiation causes cancer. Prior x-radiation into the head and neck region is a well-established cause of cancer of the thyroid, not only in children but also in adults.[8] There was also an increase in nodular goiter and in cancer among those who received heavy radiation at the time of the bombings at Hiroshima and Nagasaki.[9] After these bombings, 20,000 persons have been followed closely for thyroid carcinoma by the Atomic Bomb Casualty Commission and the Japanese National Institute of Health. This has revealed 74 proven cases. Of these, 40 were diagnosed on clinical examination, and 34 were found only at autopsy; it was decided that in no case diagnosed at autopsy could the cancer have been diagnosed during life by usual procedures. The benign course of this type of cancer, which was papillary in pattern, is attested by the fact that 34 of the 40 are still living, and in only one case was death attributable to thyroid carcinoma.

Those receiving accidental exposure in 1954 following a test bomb explosion near the island of Rongalap in the mid-Pacific have been exhaustively studied.[10] The report of 1970 estimated that the thyroids of 3- to 4-year-old children received 700 to 1400 rads from $^{131,132,133,135}$I. Twenty-one of 67 people exposed showed thyroid abnormalities; 3 lesions were malignant, 16 were benign nodules, and 2 thyroids were atrophic. It was concluded that the risk of thyroid cancer was not different than after x-ray irradiation. None of the 21 died of thyroid cancer.

The same university clinics group that studied leukemia after therapeutic radioiodine reported in 1974 that they had found 86 malignant thyroid neoplasms among 34,684 patients.[11] After these data were exhaustively analyzed, the conclusion was reached that there was no increased risk of thyroid cancer after radioiodine therapy. An explanation offered is that the replicative capacity of the thyroid cell is damaged by therapeutic doses of radioactive iodine. These patients received at least 4000 to 7000 rads to the thyroid and 5 to 25 rads to the whole body. Such doses are not comparable to the very high whole-body doses (100+) from the bombing exposures.

An interesting and unexpected statistic from this thyrotoxicosis therapy follow-up study was the occurrence of neoplasia 5 years or more after the treatment; in the drug series the incidence was 0.3 per cent, while for the radioiodine-treated group it was 0.08 per cent. This indicates that the occurrence of cancer after radioiodine therapy is actually less than that after drug therapy. While cancer of the thyroid can be induced in some strains of rats by use of $^{131}$I alone, the most effective technique is by use of $^{131}$I in an animal also given a goitrogenic drug or a carcinogen.[12]

The fact remains that, with 35 years of experience in the use of radioactive iodine, evidence is lacking that this form of therapy carries an increased risk of thyroid cancer. It may decrease it.

It might be argued that one should look to the long-term history of patients who have received test doses of radioactive iodine in the past in order to see whether their experience might be different. These small doses may not have damaged the replicative capacity of cells and yet have had a carcinogenic effect. Calculation of the risk factors for the doses presumably received indicates that, if one extrapolates from what is known about carcinogenesis in man and rat, many thousands of such patients would need to be surveyed before one could hope to see a significant difference in tumor incidence when compared to a control group. Interpretation of any possible result would be compounded by the additional difficulty that at least some of those patients who received test doses with radioactive iodine in the past would have been studied because there was already a suspicion of thyroid disease.

### Hypothyroidism Following Radioiodine Therapy

It is extraordinary that nearly 20 years elapsed between the introduction of radioiodine into clinical therapeutics and the appreciation of its propensity for causing late hypothyroidism.[13] Estimates vary widely, but most physicians now agree that almost 50 per cent of all patients successfully treated in this way will eventually develop some degree of hypothyroidism.[14] The incidence figures have been uncertain because of the difficulty in clinical appraisal of borderline hypothyroidism and the confusing problem of patients with low plasma $T_4$ levels but normal plasma $T_3$ concentrations. After an initial incidence of 6 to 10 per cent in the first year after treatment, there is a continual increment of approximately 2 per cent of patients per year who become hypothyroid, and so far there seems to be no leveling off in the curve.[15] This late effect of radiation is considered to be the result of damage to the thyroid cells which becomes significant only as, in time, the cells are called upon to undergo division, at which point they die. The reaction is dose-related. Patients receiving high doses have twice the incidence of those receiving doses of radioiodine half as large.

Attempts have been made to reduce the apparent incidence of hypothyroidism by reducing the initial dose of radioiodine and by restraint in substitution therapy in the first wave of hypothyroidism that occurs when the cells are stunned or are suppressed by oral iodide. The patients have been maintained temporarily on an antithyroid drug[16] or on iodide in an endeavor to keep them comfortable while the slowly developing radiation effect reduces innate thyroid function to tolerable levels.[17] While there is evidence that these programs of reduced dosage have also reduced the incidence of later hypothyroidism, they have by no means eliminated the problem. Thus, in the series of Hagen et al.,[17] after 19 months, 6 per cent of the patients were hypothyroid, and after 5 years, 24 per cent were hypothyroid, which is less than in other series reported.

Patients who become hypothyroid require replacement medication for the remainder of their lives. The difficulty which this entails for the patient is something which has to be decided on an individual basis, but it is perhaps a small price to pay for so effective a treatment as radioiodine. The principal risk is that the patient will voluntarily discontinue the medication and develop myxedema, which, if neglected, can be a serious medical disorder and even life-threatening.

### [131]I and Genetic Damage

The genetic damage which might result from radioactive iodine treatment could be extremely difficult to detect. Most of the mutational events which might occur would probably be recessive in character, i.e. single gene defects. The probability that a subsequent random mating would give a homozygote child would be exceedingly small. Identifying a defective child as arising from use of [131]I in the parentage would require a remote radiation history, and the event would have to be considered against the natural occurrence of such an event. Thus the possibility of detecting single gene damage resulting from radiation, in view of the radiation dose and the well-known genetic effects of radiation, seems beyond possibility at present. Alternatively, one could examine for the appearance of major genetic damage, such as chromosomal breaks, or events which would be detectable in the heterozygote (dominance). Nonlethal damage of this kind is highly unlikely, but should it occur, the event would require measurement against the natural occurrence of such genetically damaged individuals.

We know of only two attempts that have been made to search for genetic defects in children born of treated parents. Dr. Paul Starr, with an early experience in treating 73 children (56 females and 17 males) with larger than present dosages, recently reported that 111 children had been born of these parents.[18] Among them, two had minor defects. It seems significant that most of the mothers had been made hypothyroid by their treatment.

In 1968 we began a pilot study to search for genetic defects and recalled over 200 children above 3 years of age born of treated mothers and 20 of treated fathers.[19] The incidence of defects found was the same as in the general public. Among the karyotypes made on 41 of these children, one was abnormal (XYY). The Atomic Bomb Casualty Commission[20] found no increase in major congenital abnormalities, stillbirths, or infant mortality in persons born of parents exposed to doses of radiation much greater than the whole-body radiation dose of 5 to 25 rads received from therapeutic doses of [131]I now employed. Thus, transmission of genetic damage has not been documented in patients treated with radioiodine for thyrotoxicosis, but neither has it been excluded.

The question has been raised regarding the fertility of radiation-treated women and men and has not been fully answered, in part because of the difficult statistical problems which are involved. Nevertheless, sterility has not been a significant complaint among those treated with radioiodine, and at least a casual inspection of the available experience indicates that these persons are normally fertile (Table 1).[19]

Pregnancy is an absolute contraindication to radioiodine treatment. There have been at least five pregnant patients who have been treated with large doses of radioiodine who have given birth to cretinous infants[21, 22] and a larger number whose offspring have been normal after the smaller doses now used for thyrotoxicosis.[23] Radioiodine should never be given unless the possibility of pregnancy has been fully eliminated.

Thyroid storm has been reported in patients following radioiodine therapy. In order to avoid this complication, it would perhaps be wise to pretreat a patient with severe thyrotoxicosis and nutritional depletion with an antithyroid drug, possibly beta sympathetic blockade, and nutritional repletion prior to radioiodine therapy.

Some patients with thyrotoxicosis respond slowly or incompletely to the initial dose, although there is probably no such thing as failure if enough

TABLE 1.   Reproductive History of 103 Women*

|  | Full-Term Children | Premature Children | Miscarriages |
|---|---|---|---|
| Before [131]I | 174 | 11 | 28 |
| After [131]I | 142 | 10 | 27 |

*From Chapman, E. M.: Choice of treatment for hyperthyroidism. Missouri Med. 68:21, 1971.

radioiodine is given. Those patients who have severe disease or who are severely depleted would not be good candidates for a therapeutic program which involves a long delay in recovery. In such an instance, it would be wise to follow the radioiodine administration with small doses of potassium iodide (5 drops daily = 250 mg. iodine) beginning 10 to 14 days later. One could then test and perhaps re-treat some months later, depending on indications at that time. In this way the morbidity attendant upon a slow response to the radioiodine could be minimized.

A concern with radioiodine is its possible danger in the treatment of childhood and adolescent thyrotoxicosis. It is often stated that the thyroid cell of the young person is more susceptible to the carcinogenic effect of radiation than is the adult cell. Proof for this hypothesis seems to be lacking, and there is no convincing evidence that radioiodine in children or adolescents has any particular deleterious effect as compared to the adult.[24] As a result of these considerations, an increasing number of physicians have been using radioiodine in the treatment of childhood and adolescent thyrotoxicosis without noteworthy complications.[25, 26]

It is appropriate to add a word about the cost of radioiodine therapy. The cost for the isotope itself is only a few dollars. Maintenance of a laboratory with equipment is also not expensive if there is even a modest patient flow. Thus, in most clinics the total charge including physician time and support service is only a fraction of the expense involved in hospitalization and operative care.

## The Management of Thyrotoxicosis by Operation

There has recently been a resurgent interest in operation for thyrotoxicosis as a result of the high incidence of hypothyroidism following radioiodine therapy on the one hand, and the high relapse rate following discontinuance of antithyroid medication on the other. The specter of late effects of radiation in provoking cancer or genetic defects in the descendants of those treated has also influenced recent thinking. Moreover, there is professional dissatisfaction with the sharp decline in the number of patients operated upon in the past decade, because this has impaired the educationally profitable experience for those in training programs, especially in teaching hospitals. In recent times, few surgeons have become experts in thyroid surgery.

Let us probe the validity of these arguments. Is the high incidence of hypothyroidism after treatment a telling feature? The incidence of hypothyroidism in operatively treated patients was formerly reckoned on comparatively short-term follow-up, but in 1970 Hedley[27] from Great Britain, using the methodology of the U.S.P.H. Follow-up Study, first revealed the rising incidence of late hypothyroidism after operation. The rate had reached 37 per cent in patients operated upon 2 to 21 years previously. Thus, insofar as late hypothyroidism is concerned, the end results are not very different between the two methods of ablation.

The fears of carcinogenesis have not been substantiated by the passing years, as we have seen, and the fears of genetic defects in future generations have to be balanced against the here-and-now hazards of the operation, especially in children.[28] Operation on the thyroid carries a tangible set of risks. In young persons, even the early postoperative rate of hypothyroidism has been high (35 per cent). In our series (Table 2), the recurrence rate was 5 per cent, and temporary or permanent hypoparathyroidism occurred in 10 per cent of patients. In addition, there have been the rare complications of cardiac arrest, hemorrhage, infection, and injury to the recurrent laryngeal nerves. The patient deserves a choice based on the facts.

Some physicians are unwilling to use radioiodine in children or women who have not completed their families. However, over 300 persons under 18 years of age who were treated in the United States have been recently reviewed by the Cleveland Clinic Group.[25] They believe that [131]I is now the most reasonable treatment for hyperthyroidism due to Graves' disease in children and adolescents.

Finally, we cannot support a point of view that would have us return to a form of therapy in order that more physicians could be trained for that form of treatment; this is a "Catch-22" argument. Nor can we accept the recent statement that operative treatment is the "standard by which other treatment methods are measured."[29] Arrogant nonsense.

### Special Situations Favoring Operative Treatment

There can be no doubt that operation is a highly satisfactory form of therapy for the patient with thyrotoxicosis associated with special situations who is well-prepared by informed consent[30] and appropriate medication. For example, the patient who is emotionally concerned about the carcinogenic or genetic effects of radiation and who has not responded to antithyroid drugs would be a suitable candidate for operative treatment.

TABLE 2.  Comparison of Results of Radioiodine and Operative Therapy at the Massachusetts General Hospital in Children 8 to 18 Years of Age

| Mode of Therapy | Number of Cases | Hypothyroid | | Recurrence Rate | |
|---|---|---|---|---|---|
| | | Number of Patients | Per Cent | Number of Patients | Per Cent |
| Operative | 61 | 20 | 33 | 3 | 5 |
| Radioiodine | 30 | 8 | 26 | 1 | 3 |

Operation is indicated for the patient at the midtrimester of pregnancy with thyrotoxicosis which is not readily amenable to drug treatment.[31] Fortunately, the number of such patients is remarkably small.

Although the single, toxic, autonomous nodule may be treated successfully with doses of radioactive iodine larger than those used for diffuse goiters,[32] the response may be slow, and the residual inactive thyroid needs to be maintained in the suppressed state with oral thyroxine. The persistence of a unilateral goiter may require operation.

Thyrotoxicosis often occurs late in the course of multinodular goiter, and although it is sometimes controlled with either antithyroid drugs or radioiodine over a prolonged period, the persistence of nodules and the chronicity of disease favor operation. Such treatment also removes a lingering suspicion that one or more nodules may be malignant. In these patients, thyroid storm is almost never a problem, and hypothyroidism rarely occurs as even a late complication.

## Summary

In virtually all instances, Graves' disease can be controlled easily and effectively with radioiodine. There are no established serious complications, and the costs to the patients both financially and in terms of disability are minimal compared to those of operation.

Thyrotoxicosis can also be controlled with antithyroid drugs, but they have the disadvantage that the majority of patients have recurrent thyrotoxicosis when the medication is discontinued. Radioiodine may always be used for such failures.

Earlier concerns for carcinogenesis and leukemogenesis after radioiodine treatment have not materialized. It is virtually impossible to assess objectively any possible long-term genetic damage, but search for effects in the children of patients treated with radioiodine has so far revealed none. The principal failing of $^{131}$I therapy is the rate of late hypothyroidism, but in this respect, it is not very different from operation. If it occurs, it is easily treated with replacement medication.

Operation may be the preferred form of therapy for thyrotoxicosis in those patients who have toxic nodular goiters or in those who have glands suspected of malignant change. It may be preferred in the rare pregnant patient who cannot be managed by medical means.

## References

1. Tunbridge, W. M. G., and Evered, D.: The prevalence of thyroid disorders in an English community. Proc. 7th Int. Thyroid Conf., Boston, Mass. Int. Congress Series No. 361. Princeton, Excerpta Medica, 1975, p. 101.
2. Amrhein, J. A., Kenny, F. M., and Ross, D.: Granulocytopenia, lupus-like syndrome, and other complications of propylthiouracil therapy. J. Pediatr. 76:54, 1970.
3. Alexander, W. D., Harden, R. M., Koutras, D. A., and Wayne, E.: Influence of iodine intake after treatment with antithyroid drugs. Lancet 2:866, 1965.

4. Hales, I., Stiel, J., Reeve, T., Heap, T., and Myhill, J.: Prediction of the long-term results of antithyroid drug therapy for thyrotoxicosis. ATA Meeting, 1968, p. 998.
5. Hershman, J. M., Givens, J. R., Cassidy, C. E., and Astwood, E. B.: Long-term outcome of hyperthyroidism treated with antithyroid drugs. J. Clin. Endocrinol. Metab. 26:803, 1966.
6. Wartofsky, L.: Low remission after therapy for Graves' disease. J.A.M.A. 226:1083, 1973.
7. Saenger, E. L., Thoma, G. E., and Tompkins, E. A.: Incidence of leukemia following treatment of hyperthyroidism. J.A.M.A. 205:855, 1968.
8. Refetoff, S., Harrison, J., Karanfilski, B. T., Kaplan, E. L., DeGroot, L. J., and Bekerman, C.: Thyroid carcinoma after irradiation to the neck in infancy and childhood. New Engl. J. Med. 292:171, 1975.
9. Parker, L. N., Belsky, J. L., Yamamoto, T., Kawamoto, S., and Keehn, R. J.: Thyroid carcinoma after exposure to atomic radiation. Ann. Intern. Med. 80:600, 1974.
10. Conard, R. A., Dobyns, B. M., and Sutow, W. W.: Thyroid neoplasia as a late effect of exposure to radioactive iodine in fallout. J.A.M.A. 214:316, 1970.
11. Dobyns, B. M., Sheline, G. E., Workman, J. B., Tompkins, E. A., McConahey, W. M., and Becker, D. V.: Malignant and benign neoplasms of the thyroid in patients treated for hyperthyroidism. J. Clin. Endocrinol. Metab. 38:976, 1974.
12. Doniach, I.: Experimental thyroid tumours. In Smithers, Sir David (ed.): Neoplastic Disease at Various Sites. Vol. VI: Tumours of the Thyroid Gland. Edinburgh, E. & S. Livingstone, 1970, p. 73.
13. Chapman, E. M., and Maloot, F.: The use of radioactive iodine in the diagnosis and treatment of hyperthyroidism: ten years' experience. Medicine. 34:293, 1955.
14. Burke, G., and Silverstein, G. E.: Hypothyroidism after treatment with sodium iodide [131]I. J.A.M.A. 210:1051, 1969.
15. Cevallos, J. L., Hagen, G. A., Maloof, F., and Chapman, E. M.: Low-dosage [131]I therapy of thyrotoxicosis. New Engl. J. Med. 290:141, 1974.
16. Wilson, G. M., and Smith, R. N.: Clinical trial of different doses of [131]I in treatment of thyrotoxicosis. Br. Med. J. 1:129, 1967.
17. Hagen, G. A., Ouellette, R. P., and Chapman, E. M.: Comparison of high and low dosage levels of [131]I in the treatment of thyrotoxicosis. New Engl. J. Med. 277:559, 1967.
18. Starr, P., Jaffe, H. L., and Oettinger, L. J.: Later results of [131]I treatment of hyperthyroidism in 73 children and adolescents: 1967 follow-up. J. Nucl. Med. 10:586, 1969.
19. Chapman, E. M.: Choice of treatment for hyperthyroidism. Missouri Med. 68:21, 1971.
20. Hollingsworth, J. W.: Delayed radiation effects in survivors of the atomic bombings. New Engl. J. Med. 263:481, 1960.
21. Fisher, W. D., Voorhess, M. L., and Gardner, L. I.: Congenital hypothyroidism in infant following maternal [131]I Therapy. J. Pediatr. 62:132, 1963.
22. Green, H. G., Gareis, F. J., Shepard, R. H., and Kelley, V. C.: Cretinism associated with maternal sodium iodide [131]I therapy during pregnancy. Am. J. Dis. Child. 122:247, 1971.
23. Hamburger, J. I.: Northland Thyroid Lab., Southfield, Mich., Personal communication.
24. Doniach, I.: Aetiological consideration of thyroid carcinoma. In Smithers, Sir David (ed.): Neoplastic Disease at Various Sites. Vol. VI: Tumours of the Thyroid Gland. Edinburgh, E. & S. Livingstone, 1970, p. 55.
25. Safa, A. M., Schumacher, P., and Rodriguez-Antunez, A.: Long-term follow-up results in children and adolescents treated with radioactive iodine ([131]I) for hyperthyroidism. New Engl. J. Med. 292:167, 1975.
26. Hayek, A., Chapman, E. M., and Crawford, J. D.: Long-term results of treatment of thyrotoxicosis in children and adolescents with radioactive iodine. New Engl. J. Med. 283:949, 1970.
27. Hedley, A. J., Flemming, C. J., Chesters, M. I., Mitchie, W., and Crooks, J.: Surgical treatment of thyrotoxicosis. Br. Med. J. 1:519, 1970.
28. Saxena, K. M., Crawford, J. D., and Talbot, N. B.: Childhood thyrotoxicosis: A long-term perspective. Br. Med. J. 2:1153, 1964.
29. Caswell, H. T., and Maier, W. P.: Letter: The treatment of Graves' disease. J.A.M.A. 227:939, 1974.
30. Deterling, R. A.: Surgical training on the private patient and the matter of informed consent. Tufts Health Sci. Rev. 4:9, 1974.
31. Herbst, A. L., and Selenkow, H. A.: Hyperthyroidism during pregnancy. New Engl. J. Med. 273:627, 1965.
32. Horst, W., Rosler, H., Schneider, C., and Labhart, A.: 306 Cases of toxic adenoma. J. Nucl. Med. 8:515, 1967.

# 25

# *The Appropriate Operation for Gastric Ulcer*

PROXIMAL GASTRIC (PARIETAL
CELL) VAGOTOMY WITHOUT
DRAINAGE FOR ALL BENIGN
GASTRIC ULCERS
   *by Harold Burge*

THE OPERATIVE MANAGEMENT
OF GASTRIC ULCER
   *by M. Michael Eisenberg*

## Statement of the Problem

*The discussion centers on the problem of possible malignancy in an ulcerating gastric lesion and how this potential influences the conduct of the operation. It also deals with the long-term results of resection versus vagotomy with or without a drainage procedure.*

*Give your analysis of the discriminant reliability of x-ray studies, endoscopy, and cytology in the differential diagnosis of benign and malignant gastric ulceration.*

*How long do you delay operation if these studies are negative for malignancy? If the ulcer does not completely heal and remain healed in a patient who is middle-aged and hypochlorhydric? Young and with normal acid secretory capacity? Young and with cancer not excluded?*

*What operation is used for a proximal one-third ulcer? Middle one-third ulcer? Distal one-third ulcer? Do you always, never, or sometimes do an open biopsy of a gastric lesion? What is your operative plan if the ulcer is on the high lesser curvature and you are uncertain as to possible malignancy?*

*Analyze the long-term results of resection as compared with vagotomy and drainage or parietal cell vagotomy with respect to patient satisfaction, dumping, other postprandial symptoms, weight loss, anemia, and ulcer recurrence.*

*If resection is to be favored, should it be accompanied by vagotomy, and, if so, under what circumstances? Cite data to support your answer.*

# Proximal Gastric (Parietal Cell) Vagotomy Without Drainage for All Benign Gastric Ulcers[*]

HAROLD BURGE

*Charing Cross Hospital, London, England*

## *Benign Lesser Curve Ulcer*

Two hypotheses compete today to explain the etiology of benign lesser curve gastric ulcer:

1. The ulcer is caused by gastric retention. To this we must probably add one or more genetic factors, for we know that genetic factors are important in the etiology of duodenal ulcer. Dragstedt[5,6] has always taught—and there is much in his own experimental work to support this view—that the ulcer is in fact caused by an augmented hormonal phase of gastric acid secretion directly due to the retention.

2. The ulcer is caused by reflux of the duodenal contents through the pylorus into the stomach. This refluxing fluid is supposed to give rise to an area of gastritis in which a benign gastric ulcer forms. Those who support this view apply it to juxtacardiac as well as to mid–lesser curve ulceration. They have made little or no attempt to date to state the cause of the reflux.

### THE RETENTION HYPOTHESIS

#### *Gastric Retention from Duodenal Disease*

For at least 50 years surgeons have known that, when duodenal ulceration becomes so advanced that it produces duodenal stenosis and gastric retention, a benign ulcer may be found on the lesser gastric curve. Indeed, such ulceration may in time lead to an hourglass stomach. Figure 1 could hardly illustrate this more clearly. Probably all surgeons agree that in these circumstances the lesser curve ulcer is caused by the retention. If this is true, let us assume that all benign lesser curve ulcers are caused by gastric retention, for why should we expect more than one cause of lesser curve

---

[*]The editors wish to acknowledge A. H. Amery, Consultant Surgeon, Frimley Park Hospital, Frimley, Surrey, England, for his assistance in preparing this article for publication.

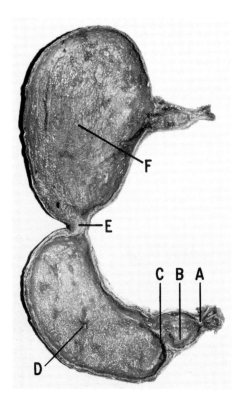

*Figure 1.* A, Duodenal stenosis; B, distended obstructed duodenal duct; C, the pylorus widely open from obstruction and therefore allowing reflux; D, distended obstructed antrum; E, hourglass stomach from chronic lesser curve ulcer; F, obstructed and distended upper stomach.

ulcer? The pursuit of this assumption will lead us into an interesting field, not only with regard to the cause of gastric ulcer but also with regard to its operative treatment. In the presence of benign lesser curve ulcer and duodenal ulcer, many surgeons would perform vagotomy, expecting the operation, if complete on the esophagus, to cure the duodenal disease as well as the lesser curve ulcer which is secondary to it. The operation of choice today in these circumstances would be proximal gastric (parietal cell) vagotomy without drainage. A drainage operation is added only if severe organic duodenal stenosis makes it necessary. There is good evidence now that this is true and that proximal gastric vagotomy without drainage, not gastric resection, is the operation of choice for patients with lesser curve benign ulcer.

Gastric retention from organic duodenal disease is, except in very advanced cases, *transient* due to spasm and edema. When the active phase of the disease passes, these features are not present, and the stomach empties normally in spite of some degree of fibrotic narrowing. We all know this from experience. In this way we explain not only the transient though recurrent nature of gastric retention from duodenal disease but also the transient and recurrent nature of lesser curve gastric ulcer.

Duodenal ulceration is present in some 30 per cent of all lesser curve gastric ulcers and is, therefore, if this hypothesis is correct, the cause of 30 per cent of all lesser curve ulcers.

Many workers have noted the high incidence of gastric retention in patients with lesser curve gastric ulcers since Carman published his paper in

TABLE 1.   Retention in Gastric Ulcer

| | | |
|---|---|---|
| Carman[3] | 1917 | — |
| Emery and Monroe[7] | 1931 | 50% |
| Bull[2] | 1935 | 25% |
| Feldman[8] | 1946 | — |
| Dragstedt[5] | 1959 | 80% |

1917. Table 1 lists five authors who recorded this association over the years. Many others, of course, did so too. Accepting this association of lesser curve ulcer and retention, some workers have sought the cause of the retention (Table 2). Note that pyloric muscle hypertrophy, pylorospasm, and inhibition of (antral) peristalsis were all noted many years ago. As we shall see later, these were important observations not understood in those times but certainly understood today.

It is important to realize that duodenal ulcer is generally accepted as an ulcer occurring in the duodenum, the site of duodenitis. Pathologically the lesion is essentially a duodenitis and not a duodenal ulcer. Duodenitis causes spasm and edema as well as gastric retention if the pathologic condition is close to the pylorus.

### Gastric Retention from Pyloroantritis (Figures 2, 3, and 4)

Every patient with benign lesser curve ulcer, no matter how high on the lesser curve, has a prepyloric gastritis. This has been proved many times (Magnus, 1936); there is also a pyloritis, and every patient with pyloroantritis has a duodenitis (Schrager, Spink, and Mitra, 1967). No wonder then that Konjetzny (1936) regarded this mucosal disease as extending from the prepyloric stomach to the duodenum across the pylorus and used the term "gastroduodenitis."

The pathology and radiology of this benign disease of the distal stomach and pylorus were well documented in the past by many workers. The basic features described are:

1. A "primary" mucosal pathology.

2. Spasm of the pyloric and prepyloric area.

3. Muscle hypertrophy of the prepyloric and pyloric muscle, usually asymmetrical.

4. Diminished and sometimes almost absent peristalsis in the diseased prepyloric stomach.

The gastric retention in pyloroantritis arises from each of these fea-

TABLE 2.   Cause of Retention

| | | |
|---|---|---|
| Stone and Ruggles[14] | 1932 | Pyloric hypertrophy and pylorospasm |
| Bull[2] | 1935 | Inhibition of gastric peristalsis |
| Golden[9] | 1937 | Pylorospasm |
| Feldman[8] | 1946 | Pyloric hypertrophy |
| Dragstedt[5] | 1959 | Inhibition of gastric peristalsis |

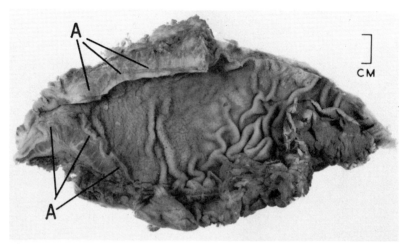

*Figure 2.* Pyloroantritis. The mucosa of the antrum is quite abnormal and the prepyloric lumen stenosed. The muscle of the prepyloric stomach is thickened. So too is the pyloric muscle. There is stenosis of the pyloric canal.

tures—from pylorospasm, from pyloric muscle hypertrophy, and from diminished antral peristalsis.

If we then conclude that lesser curve gastric ulcer is always secondary to gastric retention, persistent or transient, due to duodenal pyloroantritis and that this disease of the distal stomach and duodenum is cured by vagotomy, then vagotomy must cure all lesser curve ulcers as long as the stomach after operation is without retention. Moreover, the operation of choice will be proximal gastric (parietal cell) vagotomy without drainage. This is the only form of vagotomy which preserves the innervation and therefore the motor function of the prepyloric stomach. In the presence of *severe* organic stenosis at the pylorus or in the duodenum, a pyloroplasty must then, but only then, be added. My own studies confirm that vagotomy does cure lesser curve gas-

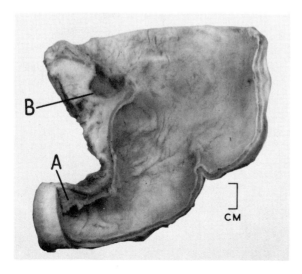

*Figure 3.* A, The typical asymmetrical muscular hypertrophy of pyloroantritis. B, A chronic lesser curve gastric ulcer. The whole prepyloric stomach is grossly narrowed from organic disease. No wonder Boas in 1898 used the term "stenosing gastritis."

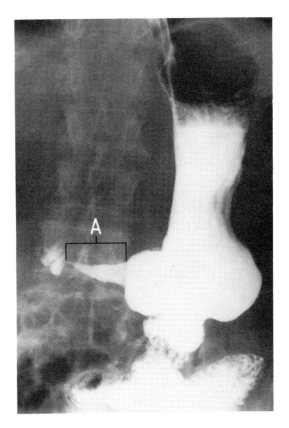

*Figure 4.* A, Typical prepyloric narrowing on x-ray examination. Usually, however, this narrowing is present but not so severe. Gastric retention is usually present.

tric ulcer, and proximal gastric (parietal cell) vagotomy without drainage is the method of choice. These studies performed since 1962 have recently been published (1974).[1] Johnston and his colleagues[10] have studied and recently published the results of proximal gastric vagotomy without drainage for gastric ulcer.

Finally, we may say that it does not matter what blocks the pylorus. A piece of string in the dog, as Dragstedt has shown, or a carcinoma in man (Figure 5) will produce gastric retention and lesser curve ulcer.

## THE REFLUX HYPOTHESIS

Those who support this hypothesis regard the lesser curve ulcer as nothing more than an ulcer occurring in an area of gastritis due to the reflux of duodenal content through the pylorus into the stomach. We know that such reflux is much more common in gastric ulcer patients than in normal people. Surgeons who support this hypothesis usually advise gastric resection and not vagotomy for lesser curve gastric ulcer.

Indeed, gastric resection does cure benign lesser curve ulcer, though recurrent lesser curve ulcer may occur after a Billroth I resection when there is gastric retention from too small a stoma.

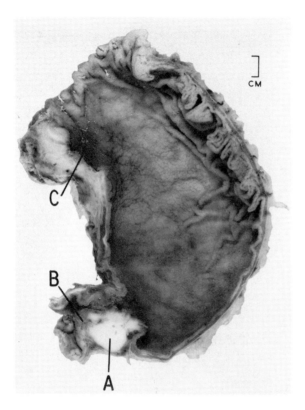

*Figure 5.* *A, B,* Carcinoma blocking the pylorus. *C,* Chronic lesser curve ulcer.

However, there are several objections to this hypothesis:

1. A low gastric resection, either Billroth I or Billroth II, done *below* a high lesser curve ulcer cures the ulcer (the Kelling-Madlener operation), yet the reflux after such a low resection must be more free than before the operation. This fact is an obvious and important objection to the reflux hypothesis, which cannot be answered by those who support it.

2. No attempt is made at gastric resection for lesser curve ulcer to define the limits of the so-called "reflux gastritis," and reflux must continue after the operation.

3. The retention hypothesis, based as it is on the concept of a duodenal pyloroantritis (or a gastroduodenitis, as Konjetzny called it), explains the common reflux in gastric ulcer. Mitral stenosis and mitral regurgitation occur in the heart because of disease of the valve and its neighboring structures. So, too, the duodenal pyloroantritis always present in lesser curve gastric ulcer causes disturbance of pyloric function and allows reflux. The picture we see here is identical to that of the cardiac state. Indeed, it has been claimed that when the gastric ulcer heals the reflux commonly disappears (Cocking and Grech, 1973). This, of course, we would expect in a transient attack in a patient as yet without severe fibrotic disease. Should the ulcer be advanced and fibrotic, the reflux would of course persist. Figure 6 shows the rigid, open yet stenosed, eccentric pyloric canal in a gastric resection specimen taken from a patient with a high juxtacardiac ulcer and gastric retention. Its exact similarity to a diseased mitral valve is quite apparent.

4. There seems to be no reasonable claim put forward to show that the reflux hypothesis leads to proximal gastric (parietal cell) vagotomy without drainage as the operation of choice for benign lesser curve ulcer.

## Benign Prepyloric Gastric Ulcer

### THE DUODENAL PYLOROANTRITIS HYPOTHESIS

Here again the duodenal pyloroantritis hypothesis regards duodenal pyloric and prepyloric ulcers as ulcers occurring in this mucosal disease, which is cured by vagotomy. The operative treatment, therefore, of duodenal, pyloric and prepyloric ulcers is proximal gastric (parietal cell) vagotomy, preferably without drainage. We now know from many years experience that vagotomy is curative of benign pyloric and prepyloric ulcers, as it is of duodenal ulcers, and that the operation of choice is proximal gastric vagotomy without drainage.

### THE REFLUX HYPOTHESIS

The reflux hypothesis as in mid or high lesser curve ulcer regards the prepyloric ulcer as a lesion occurring in a mucosa gastritic from reflux. Its exponents usually advise gastric resection, although the patient is still left with the same but more severe reflux, which still presumably causes gastritis. Nevertheless, gastric resection does cure benign prepyloric ulcer in spite of the postoperative reflux.

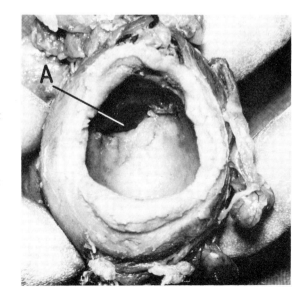

*Figure 6.* A, The eccentric, deformed, rigid, stenosed, yet open pylorus of severe pyloroantritis. That duodenogastric reflux can occur in this disease is obvious. The situation resembles mitral valve disease. This patient had gastric retention and a juxtacardiac gastric ulcer.

## *The Problem of Cancer*

Most surgeons today would agree that our problem with regard to malignancy is to differentiate between a primary benign gastric ulcer and a primary carcinoma. The problem of malignant change in a benign ulcer hardly arises.

Those who support gastric resection and not vagotomy *only* because of the risk of overlooking malignancy would seem to be at fault for several reasons. A problem arises only in the doubtful cases. How should these be managed?

1. By a thorough knowledge of x-ray appearances of malignant and benign gastric ulceration. Very seldom in the hands of experienced radiologists and clinicians is there doubt.

2. By waiting for some weeks. If a lesion is malignant, little is lost by waiting a few weeks and then repeating the x-ray studies. Not infrequently, the patient may be saved from having any operation at all. If the lesion is malignant, the prognosis hardly changes by such a short delay.

3. By fiberoptic biopsy. As in biopsies of esophageal lesions, a negative finding is valueless, for the biopsy forceps may not have found the true pathologic lesion. The biopsy forceps presently used in the fiberoptic endoscope is very small indeed. Often a specimen is too small for the pathologist to be certain of an accurate diagnosis. Only a *definite, undoubted* positive report of malignancy is helpful. Then and only then does there cease to be a problem.

4. By operative findings. As we have seen, a problem only arises in the *doubtful* ulcer. Then the surgeon must open the stomach and take a good large biopsy specimen from the edge of the ulcer in one or more quadrants. If he uses a frozen section, then this will only be of value if the pathologist is prepared to make a report which leaves *no doubt* about the nature of the lesion. Then the surgeon will perform a high resection if the ulcer is malignant or a vagotomy if it is benign.

If the pathologist is not willing to guarantee a correct diagnosis, then the surgeon should close the opening in the stomach and perform a vagotomy, preferably, as we have seen, a proximal gastric (parietal cell) vagotomy without drainage. He will then await the result of the paraffin section a few days later.

If the paraffin section proves the ulcer benign, then nothing more needs to be done. If it is malignant, then an extensive cancer resection should be performed.

Above all, two mistakes must be avoided and can be avoided if the advice above is taken:

1. A radical gastric resection must not be done for an ulcer thought to be malignant but later in the resected specimen shown to be benign. This is perhaps the greatest error that can be made in gastric surgery.

2. A gastric resection must not be done only a little above a *doubtful* ulcer which later proves to be malignant on paraffin section. This operation is inadequate and invites recurrence. A vagotomy should initially be done, then a radical resection later well above the lesion.

# The Use of an Intraoperative Test for Completeness of Nerve Section on the Esophagus

We know that recurrent duodenal ulceration following vagotomy of any type done for duodenal disease is due to incomplete vagotomy on the lower esophagus. Such recurrences have been reported in some 5 to 20 per cent of cases.[2] We know this recurrence can be prevented by the use of the electrical stimulation test at the time of operation to prove completeness of nerve section. Some 30 per cent of lesser curve ulcers are associated with and presumably secondary to duodenal disease. Certainly in such cases an intraoperative test is essential. If vagotomy cures, as it does gastric ulcer, presumably its completeness on the esophagus is always important.

The principle of the Burge electrical stimulation test is shown in Figure 7, and the Burge vagotometer is shown in Figure 8.

The principle of the test is simple. A circular electrode is placed around the lower esophagus, and the intragastric pressure is recorded. Even the smallest intact nerve causes a rise in intragastric pressure which is easily seen on the inflation meter and also on the pen recorder. Figure 9 shows a very incomplete vagotomy test in which the rise of pressure is approximately 20 mm. of water. However, this test must be used to a sensitivity of 1 mm. of water. Figure 10 shows the completed vagotomy being tested. There is then no risk of recurrent ulceration.

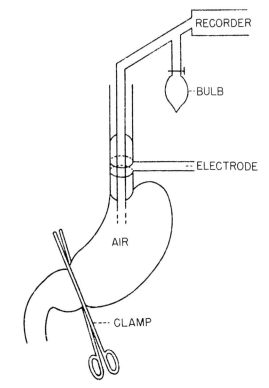

*Figure 7.* Principle of the Burge electrical stimulation test.

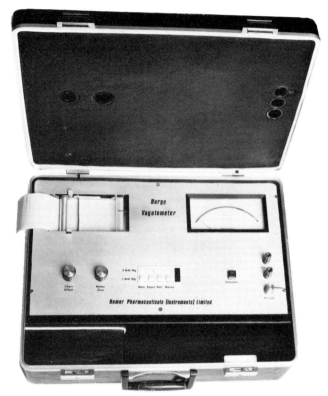

*Figure 8.*   Burge vagotometer.

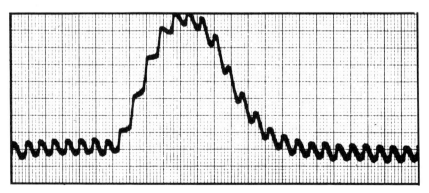

*Figure 9.*   Incomplete vagotomy.

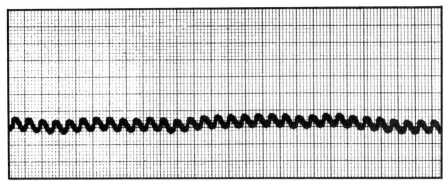

*Figure 10.* Complete vagotomy.

# References

1. Amery, A. H., Cox, P., and Burge, H.: Vagotomy for benign lesser curve gastric ulcer. Chir. Gastroenterol. (Eng. Edit.), 8:11, 1974.
2. Bull, H. C. H.: *X-Ray Interpretation.* London, Oxford University Press, 1935, p. 196.
3. Carman, R. D.: Roentgen diagnosis of concurrent gastric and duodenal ulcer. Am. J. Roentgenol. *4*:552, 1917.
4. Cocking, J. B., and Grech, P.: Pyloric reflux and the healing of gastric ulcers. Gut *14*:555, 1973.
5. Dragstedt, L. R.: A concept of pathogenesis of gastric and duodenal ulcer. Md. Med. J. 8:98, 1959.
6. Dragstedt, L. R., and Woodward, E. R.: Gastric stasis, a cause of gastric ulcer. Scand. J. Gastroenterol. 5(Suppl. 6):243, 1970.
7. Emery, E. S., and Monroe, R. T.: Am. J. Roentgenol. 25:51, 1931.
8. Feldman, M.: Clin. Radiol. *1*:509, 1946.
9. Golden, R.: Antral gastritis and spasm. J.A.M.A. *109*:1497, 1937.
10. Johnston, D., Humphrey, C. S., Smith, R. B., and Wilkinson, A. R.: Treatment of gastric ulcer by highly selective vagotomy without a drainage procedure: An interim report. Br. J. Surg. 59:787, 1972.
11. Konjetzny, G. E.: Das Krankheitsbild der Gastro-Duodenitis. Med. Klin. 32:473, 1936.
12. Magnus, H. A., and Rodgers, H. W.: St. Bartholomew's Hospital Reports Vol. LXXI, 1936.
13. Schrager, J., Spink, R., and Mitra, S.: The antrum in patients with duodenal and gastric ulcers. Gut 8:497, 1967.
14. Stone, R. S., and Ruggles, H. E.: Am. J. Roentgenol. 27:193, 1932.

# The Operative Management of Gastric Ulcer

M. MICHAEL EISENBERG

*University of Minnesota Health Sciences Center*

The evolution of attitudes in the operative approach to the management of gastric ulcer is dynamic and at present remains incomplete. Controversy surrounding the importance of gastric carcinoma as a dominant factor in the decision to operate on gastric ulcer, for example, has smoldered for more than half a century. At present, however, sophistication in diagnosis by means of radiographic study, gastric analysis, cytology, and flexible endoscopy with biopsy and an improved appreciation of epidemiologic patterns with regard to both the incidence of gastric ulcer and the response of gastric ulcer to medical management have all contributed to a shift in balance in the decision-making apparatus.

The question of just how important gastric malignancy is in terms of its overall impact upon the judgment of whether to operate or not remains open. Precise data on the incidence of gastric carcinoma in gastric ulcerating lesions are lacking, but it seems reasonable to conclude that a figure of 3 to 7 per cent is appropriate,[1, 2, 3] although up to 15 per cent and higher has been reported.[4] Whether or not benign lesions ever undergo malignant degeneration is not nearly so important to the examining physician as is the question of the possible malignant status of the ulcer with which he is now confronted.

In the recently reported Veterans Administration cooperative study on 638 cases of gastric ulcer, neoplasms were found in 25, or 3.9 per cent. While four of the malignancies were missed on initial evaluation, the errors in diagnosis represent only 0.6 per cent of all patients examined, for an overall accuracy rate of 99.4 per cent. Based on these data and other similar information, it does not seem plausible to recommend surgery for all gastric ulcers solely because of the oft repeated exhortation that only examination of the entire specimen can conclusively rule out carcinoma, though this is true. Moreover, there is no real evidence that the overall longevity of patients with carcinoma, delayed in therapy, is significantly altered. Ruling on the status of possible malignancy in a gastric lesion is, nonetheless, an essential feature of proper operative management.

## *Preoperative Evaluation*

Preoperative distinction between benign and malignant lesions using currently available techniques is very accurate, and the operating surgeon in the vast majority of cases will know in advance the precise nature of the lesion with which he is dealing. The following represents a review of the standard diagnostic regimen by which all of our patients are evaluated prior to surgery for gastric ulcer.

### Radiology

In an evaluation of radiologic diagnosis alone, Strandjord and co-workers[5] reported a correct diagnosis of cancer made in 78 per cent of 283 cases of gastric ulcer. In 6 per cent an undecided diagnosis was made, and in 16 per cent the wrong diagnosis was made. Amberg,[6] in a review of 35,396 x-ray reports on 21,783 patients, found 861 cases of carcinoma of the stomach. False-positive diagnoses were present in 7.8 per cent and false-negative diagnoses in 8.4 per cent. Mitty and co-workers[7] reported a 91 per cent accuracy rate in 155 patients who were studied with upper GI tract x-ray or abdominal complaints. Hennig and Harvey,[8] in a review of 1250 gastric lesions, found that 19 out of 150 resectable cancers were not diagnosed preoperatively, for an accuracy rate of 88 per cent. X-ray alone, therefore, while extremely valuable and perhaps the most commonly used screening technique, has an accuracy rate of no better than 80 to 90 per cent.

### Gastroscopy

The use of gastroscopy in the diagnosis of various lesions of the stomach has met with a considerable degree of success and enthusiasm since the first practical design of a flexible gastroscope in 1932 by Schindler. (The Schindler scope was, paradoxically, considered flexible — previous ones were less so.) The relative value of gastroscopic examination in the diagnosis of carcinoma of the stomach has been described by Villako.[9] Forty-three patients with gastric neoplasms were investigated using gastroscopy and x-ray. All were subsequently operated upon, and the diagnosis was confirmed in all but one case. This type of data, although encouraging, was reported on the basis of now obsolete techniques for gastroscopic evaluation of stomach lesions. It is reasonable to conclude that those methods provided a 70 to 85 per cent accuracy rate. There is testimony but no hard data suggesting that, with improved training and widespread use of the fiberoptic endoscope coupled with biopsy, substantial improvement in accuracy is now available. Although endoscopically controlled biopsy is far from perfect in terms of accuracy in "sampling" the lesion, current experience based on personal communication with mature endoscopists suggests that the achievement of precise diagnoses is, in fact, improving.

### Gastric Analysis

Gastric analysis (with or without combined cytologic study) finds its greatest usefulness in differentiating benign from malignant gastric lesions in those patients who are shown to be incapable of secreting hydrochloric acid in response to histamine or pentagastrin stimulation. About 70 per cent of patients with gastric carcinoma are histamine or pentagastrin fast achlorhydric.[10] If, in fact, a patient with gastric ulcer can be shown to be incapable of producing acid, diagnosis of gastric carcinoma is virtually assured, although there are very rare exceptions (personal experience from our own lab [1 case/3000]). A response to stimulation, with the production of acid, does not, however, rule out carcinoma.

The degree to which a patient responds to parietal cell stimulation also has value in terms of ascertaining a rough estimate of the virulence of benign peptic ulcers.[11, 12] For example, in a patient with combined gastric and duodenal ulcer, we anticipate a normal or greater than normal response to stimulation. In a patient with garden variety gastric ulcer and no duodenal lesion, we anticipate a normal or low secretory response. Patients with prepyloric gastric ulcers, lesions which tend to have acid *secretory* patterns more characteristic of duodenal rather than corpus gastric ulcer, have *clinical* patterns which also emulate duodenal ulcer. We can make use of these data to contribute in the decision as to whether or not to add parasympathetic denervation (vagotomy) to our operative management of gastric ulcer.[13, 14]

## Exfoliative Cytology

A variety of procedures have been devised whereby carcinoma cells are obtained by means of gastric lavage. Antral abrasive balloons, brushes, high-pressure fluid streams, lavage with papain, chymotrypsin, and simple lavage with saline have all been reported in the literature.[15, 16, 17] Saline alone has been found to offer the same degree of yield and accuracy as any of the more complicated lavage solutions and is the technique which we use.[18, 19]

While there is no general agreement as to the overall value of cytologic techniques when compared with x-ray and gastroscopic examination, the reports have been for the most part encouraging (Table 1). Ross et al. reported an accuracy rate of 71 per cent.[18] Cytology has been shown to have

TABLE 1.   Accuracy in Diagnosis of Malignancy in Gastric Ulcer (Selected Reports)

| | | |
|---|---|---|
| Gastroscopy | Arnold et al.[47] | 95.3% |
| | Villako[9] | 83.7% |
| Cytology (when positive) | Arnold et al.[47] | 97.7% |
| | Nieburgs et al.[48] | 80.0% |
| | Ross et al.[18] | 71.0% |
| X-ray | Amberg[6] | 83.8% |
| | Arnold et al.[47] | 92.7% |
| | Ross et al.[18] | 67.5% |
| | Strandjord et al.[5] | 78.0% |
| | Villako[9] | 86.0% |

its highest degree of accuracy in that group of patients in whom x-ray is also definitive. In cases in which the radiologist misses the diagnosis, the cytologic error, however, may be as high as 38 per cent. In a study of 2500 patients, it was found that the best diagnostic material came from small gastric lesions and those confined to the mucosa.[20] The debris from the larger lesions increased diagnostic error substantially. In summation, therefore, cytologic techniques are very accurate when positive for malignancy. False-positive studies are very rare. When negative, however, the accuracy rate may fall to approximately 70 per cent.

### Overall Analysis of Preoperative Study

While the individual techniques for establishing or ruling out the diagnosis of gastric carcinoma do not appear in and of themselves sufficiently accurate for the surgeon to rely upon (perhaps 70 to 90 per cent correct), *combination of the techniques* of cytology and x-ray, gastroscopy and x-ray, or x-ray, cytology, gastroscopy, and gastric analysis is most impressive (almost 100 per cent accurate) (Table 2). We feel confident, therefore, that the preoperative distinction between benign and malignant lesions, using currently available techniques, is extremely precise and that the surgeon will know in advance, in the vast majority of cases, the potential for malignancy of the lesion with which he is dealing.

## The Pathogenesis of the Benign Gastric Ulcer

Du Plessis has stated that "gastric ulceration is not a single disease, but the result of a variety of conditions which lower gastric mucosal resistance, allowing peptic ulceration to occur. When deciding on the surgical treatment of ulcer it is therefore necessary to determine the basic abnormality, because the treatment must be directed at the primary cause."[21] Gastric ulcer is, in fact, a protean disease, and the exact cause or causes remain indistinct. Until recent years, most of the data in the literature concerning the usefulness of various operations for gastric ulcer have lumped the lesion together with duodenal ulcer under a common heading of "peptic ulcer." There have been serious attempts to differentiate gastric ulcer from duodenal ulcer and, further, to categorize separate types of gastric ulcer. For example, while we are

**TABLE 2.   Accuracy of Combined Techniques**

| | | |
|---|---|---|
| Cytology and x-ray | Ross et al.[18] | 85% |
| Gastroscopy and x-ray | Villako[9] | 100% |
| X-ray, cytology, and gastroscopy | Strandjord et al.[5] | 94% |
| X-ray, cytology, secretory analysis, and endoscopy | Littman[49] | 99.4% |

generally aware that approximately 75 per cent[22] of chronic benign gastric ulcers may exist as a single entity, it is now also recognized that up to 40 per cent[23] of gastric ulcers may be associated with healed or active duodenal ulcer disease. Whether or not there is a sequential cause and effect relationship between preexisting duodenal ulcer and the subsequent development of gastric ulcer is at present undetermined. Other gastric ulcers, although isolated, appear to be related to the chronic ingestion of anti-inflammatory drugs, such as aspirin, colchicine, steroids, indomethacin, and others. Although some gastric erosions may be associated with stress (such as may be incurred in sepsis, extensive burns, head injuries, and other central nervous system damage), for the most part these are acute superficial mucosal lesions which, should the primary underlying systemic problem be successfully managed, usually do not require surgery. Management of these lesions is beyond the scope of this discussion. Finally, some distinction has been made of late between corpus gastric ulcers, that is, ulcers lying on the junction between the antrum and the parietal cell border, and those which have been termed prepyloric (within 1 to 2 cm. of the antral-duodenal junction). The latter appear to act both pathophysiologically and clinically as duodenal ulcers.[50]

Although from a theoretic and intellectual point of view, distinction between the specifics in the pathogenesis of these various lesions is interesting and perhaps potentially important, from a practical point of view, operative management tends to overlap. Still, it is desirable to delineate, when possible, identifiable elements in the pathogenesis of individual lesions and, if possible, to tailor the operative approach in a way such that the underlying cause is rectified. With these thoughts in mind, a brief review, highly selective in nature, of three hypotheses in the pathogenesis of gastric ulcer is appropriate.

### The Dragstedt Hypothesis

It was observed by Dragstedt that, of 131 patients who underwent truncal vagotomy alone, 5 developed gastric ulcer in the postoperative period, while in a series of more than 800 patients with duodenal ulcer treated by vagotomy and a drainage procedure, no gastric ulcer developed.[24] These observations were further supported by a series of experimental laboratory trials and formed the basis for the concept that, while duodenal ulcer may be based on a hypersecretion of acid gastric juice due to hyperactivity of the central nervous system, mediated by way of the vagus nerves, gastric ulcer is related to hypergastrinemia during the digestive phase of acid secretion. It has been stated that the antrum is primarily responsible in the pathogenesis of these lesions. Antral stasis, with excessive release of gastrin secondary to food ingestion, has been invoked as the primary cause of gastric ulcer.

Skillman has emphasized several important contradictions in this thesis.[25] While there is some overlap with normal acid secretory patterns, the majority of patients with benign gastric ulcer tend to produce less than normal amounts of acid; hypergastrinemia has not been proved in patients with classic benign gastric ulcer; three-fourths of patients with gastric ulcer (i.e., those who do not have an associated healed or active duodenal lesion) cannot be demonstrated by radiographic or motility techniques to have gastric stasis; pernicious anemia with histamine-fast achlorhydria has been shown to be associated with severe hypergastrinemia, but benign gastric ulcer does not accompany this syndrome. Finally, correction of "stasis" with a drainage procedure alone does not cure the ulcer.[14, 26, 27] Still, the hypothesis deserves attention and may have validity in that group of patients with evidence of some outlet obstruction, as seen in old duodenal ulcer disease.

### The Davenport-Du Plessis Hypothesis

A second concept of the pathogenesis of gastric ulcer, brought forth in recent years and now gaining considerable credence, is based on relationships between the gastric mucosal barrier, back diffusion of acid, bile reflux, gastritis, and pyloric sphincter dysfunction. Data have accumulated which suggest that, in many patients, the reflux of bile and pancreatic juice into the stomach may be causally related to the development of chronic gastritis and, subsequently, the development of gastric ulcer. Du Plessis[28] noted that, of 75 stomachs resected for gastric ulceration, 65 displayed chronic gastritis extending from the pylorus for a variable distance proximally. The chronic gastritis in these cases was much more extensive and severe than that noted in 18 cases of duodenal ulcer. The gastric ulcer was always found in the area affected by chronic gastritis; the authors believed this to be the predisposing factor in these cases. They suggested that chronic gastritis is due to reflux of duodenal contents through the pylorus. Concentrations of bile-acid conjugates in the fasting gastric aspirates of patients with gastric ulcer were noted to be abnormally high. Although the authors acknowledged that duodenal reflux does not account for all gastric ulcers, they suggested that, in some cases of duodenal ulcer, reflux is excessive and that this may account for the gastric ulcers that follow duodenal ulceration in the absence of pyloric outlet obstruction. They concluded that the refluxing fluid probably acts by interfering with the protective layer of mucus and by allowing acid and pepsin free access to the mucus membrane. This also helps to explain why the ulcer is usually on the proximal edge of the affected mucosa.

Delaney and co-workers,[29] in a review of the literature and based in part on animal experimental studies of their own design, reported that, while the motor abnormality that leads to excessive regurgitation of duodenal contents into the stomach is not understood, the propulsive peristaltic waves in the antrum are significantly less vigorous in patients with gastric ulcer than in normal controls. They also concluded that gastritic changes seem to be a prerequisite, though not the sole cause, of gastric ulcer.

The role of acid secretion in the development of regurgitation gastritis remains unclear. It has been pointed out that bile alone definitely does not cause the mature lesion, and it appears that elements of pancreatic juice may, in fact, play a more important role.

The Dragstedt hypothesis of hypersecretion of acid gastric juice due to antral stasis has been difficult to justify in view of the observation that most patients with unobstructed benign gastric ulcer tend to secrete normal or less than normal amounts of acid. Davenport,[30] however, has suggested that the *apparent* hyposecretion may be related to excessive loss of hydrogen ion as a result of "back-diffusion" into gastric mucosa, the intregity of which is diminished or destroyed by a defective permeability barrier. In investigations designed to study the effect of a variety of agents (aspirin, ethanol, bile, and pancreatic juice), he suggested that the lipoprotein layer of cell walls damaged by these agents permitted increased permeability of the stomach to acid.[31, 32, 33] Clinical evidence, in large measure corroborating this concept, lends further support to the concept that an abnormal gastric mucosal barrier may be at least one important factor in the pathogenesis of benign chronic gastric ulcer.

### The Oi Hypothesis[34, 35, 36]

Oi, in a series of three carefully executed and extremely important studies reported in 1959 but generally ignored by surgeons until the very recent past, examined the location of 170 gastric ulcers localized to the stomach alone and an additional 50 gastric ulcers associated with duodenal ulcer. He emphasized that the fundic and the pyloric gland tissues form at their interface a junctional zone which constitutes a *locus minoris resistentiae* (area of decreased resistance), and he suggested that the pathogenesis of gastric ulcer is closely related to this local congenital factor. He showed that all of the 170 gastric ulcers occurred in the pyloric gland area, at most 1.5 cm. (0.32 cm. average) from the border zone. Further, in an examination of 114 operative specimens, he observed that duodenal ulcer occurred in 99.3 per cent of the cases within 2 cm. from the border of the pyloric antrum and the duodenal mucosa. Finally, in a single spectacular case involving gastric, duodenal, and esophageal ulcer in the same specimen, all three occurred at the junction of two different tissues. He concluded that the location of virtually all peptic ulcers is closely related to the *locus minoris resistentiae* of congenital origin in an area which corresponds to the nonparietal cell tissue and which may be exposed most strongly to acid gastric juice.

These are key observations and of considerable potential importance to the operating surgeon. They imply, for example, that, while the junctional zone may vary from patient to patient and in fact has been shown to migrate cephalad during the course of aging, *the location of the gastric ulcer on or near the lesser curvature of the stomach usually delineates the upper border of the non–acid-secreting portion of the stomach and may represent a useful landmark for the operating surgeon in the performance of resective procedures.*

It is apparent from the cumulative literature on the subject that all three of these hypotheses have merit and that, while the data currently available do not yet fully satisfy careful critical analysis, they emphasize that gastric ulcer is a much more complex disease than previously appreciated and that operative management of these lesions can be aided by a more sophisticated appreciation of some of the fundamentals of pathogenesis. For the purposes of the present discussion, it is convenient to start with an assumption that, in patients with pyloric stenosis due to old or active duodenal ulcer disease, Dragstedt's theory may be appropriate. It is also reasonable to assume that, for some—though not all—other gastric ulcers, the bile reflux theory may have merit. Finally, utilizing the information available to us from Oi's studies, we now have, in combination with the other available data, a working hypothesis for the pathogenesis of most gastric ulcers and can proceed with operative management accordingly.

## Operation for Gastric Ulcer

The ideal operative procedure for the management of gastric ulcer should include (1) zero mortality, (2) zero recurrence rate, (3) zero morbidity, and (4) perfect differentiation between benign and malignant disease. While no operation meets all of these criteria, their achievement, nonetheless, represents a worthy goal.

Many operations for gastric ulcer have been used in clinics throughout the world for the past 80 or 90 years. These include wedge resection; gastroenterostomy and pyloroplasty; total gastrectomy; extensive subtotal gastrectomy (66 to 90 per cent); vagotomy and a drainage procedure; vagotomy and limited gastric resection (50 per cent); selective vagotomy with either a drainage procedure or limited gastric resection; antrectomy (30 to 35 per cent) (Kelling-Madlener); highly selective vagotomy with drainage; and highly selective vagotomy without drainage. The variety of operations have all, during past years, featured aspects which recommended their widespread use. The majority, however, have fallen into disuse based primarily on changes in operative "fashion," disappointment in morbidity, mortality, and recurrence rates, or the introduction of improved techniques. Although pockets of the world continue to advocate some of the lesser known procedures, in general, only two or three survive in widespread use today, and one or two additional procedures, recently introduced, fall into the realm of experimental clinical trials. I will emphasize and consider in some detail vagotomy (truncal or selective) with drainage; vagotomy (truncal or selective) with limited gastric resection; extensive or limited subtotal gastrectomy without vagotomy; and highly selective vagotomy with or without drainage.

### Vagotomy (Truncal or Selective) with Drainage

The use of truncal or selective vagotomy with drainage in the management of *duodenal* ulcer has proved to be a very effective approach.[37] However, it is now becoming apparent that fundamental differences in both the pathophysiology and clinical patterns of benign gastric ulcer make this operation substantially less effective for the isolated gastric lesion (i.e., those not associated with duodenal ulcer). Although there are several reports in the literature with follow-ups of from 2 to 17 years reporting both low mortality and recurrence rates, other studies report an alarmingly high recurrence of from 14.3 to 35.7 per cent in 7 years or less.[26, 27, 38, 39] Moreover, our current understanding and interpretation of the pathophysiology and clinical patterns of gastric ulcer suggest that vagotomy and drainage will not satisfactorily correct the underlying defects. Finally, since reported results of clinical experience do not support this approach, we have abandoned it.

### Subtotal Gastrectomy or Antrectomy

Accuracy in diagnosis of malignancy and its very low incidence in the population with gastric ulcer no longer make extensive gastric resection a mandatory procedure. Total gastrectomy or extensive subtotal gastrectomy (75 per cent or greater) is curative of gastric ulcer but is too large a procedure for the benign lesion. In addition it carries an unacceptably high rate of morbid complications. The incidence of dumping and/or difficulty in maintenance of body weight is closely correlated with the extent of gastric resection.[40] Following total gastrectomy, patients almost invariably dump. In gastric resection of 66 to 75 per cent, the percentage of dumping varies, but an incidence of at least 40 to 50 per cent is probable in carefully evaluated patients.[41] Following limited (50 per cent) gastric resection ("antrectomy"), dumping occurs in approximately 20 per cent of patients.[42]

In view of the fact that partial gastric resection with Billroth I reconstruction carries with it an extremely low mortality (0 to 2.9 per cent) and low recurrence (0 to 4.4 per cent) in from 1 to 25 years of follow-up, gastric resection to include the antrum and the ulcer appears to offer safe, reliable, and attractive therapy for benign gastric ulcer.[27, 43, 44]

### Vagotomy and Resection

The addition of truncal or selective vagotomy to limited (50 per cent) gastric resection (antrectomy) is used by some surgeons under certain specific circumstances. The precise rationale and physiologic basis for adding vagotomy to antrectomy are vague and at present unsupported by clear-cut clinical data. Although hypersecretion is uncommon in corpus gastric ulcer, normal or low-normal amounts of acid may be "excessive" in these patients. There is no reason to believe that the addition of parasympathetic denervation of the stomach decreases the quality of results in terms of recurrence or significantly increases mortality. There is some evidence, nevertheless, that alteration in bowel habit and/or changes in biliary and pancreatic secretory function may be the price paid, without significant improvement in cure rate.[38] Further discussion appears below.

### Highly Selective (Parietal Cell) Vagotomy With and Without Drainage

Finally, highly selective vagotomy (vagotomy limited to the parietal cell mass, with innervation to the antrum left intact) is currently being used with or without pyloroplasty in the form of randomized clinical trials in a number of operative centers throughout the world for duodenal and/or gastric ulcers.[45, 46, 51, 52, 53, 54, 55] The reported data are inconsistent in terms of effectiveness of the operation, and there is no reason at this time to advocate its use, either with or without drainage. This is not to say that future experience may not prove it to be the most valuable procedure yet devised. If it can be shown that highly selective vagotomy brings with it the same level of control as other currently used procedures while minimizing or eliminating morbidity and mortality, more enthusiasm can be engendered for it than is now possible.

## The Current Approach for Operation for Gastric Ulcer

### The Decision to Operate

Based on the above observations and with full acknowledgment of the fact that the pathogenesis of benign gastric ulcer and its ideal operative therapy are not yet fully understood or clarified by hard data, the following represents an outline of our current approach to operative management.

From a practical standpoint, the vast majority of these patients are referred to the surgeon by internists and gastroenterologists because the various criteria for satisfactory response to tests of healing have not been met. (1) All of our patients are evaluated prior to a recommendation for surgery by x-ray, endoscopy with biopsy, gastric analysis, and cytology. Unless all four of these modalities establish the benignancy of the lesion, immediate operation is recommended. (2) If there is no evidence of neoplasm but the patient has failed a single test of healing (usually 50 per cent decrease in the size of the crater by endoscopy and x-ray within 6 weeks and complete or virtually complete healing within 12 weeks using standard medical therapy of antacids, anticholinergics, diet, sedation, and a varying term of hospitalization), immediate operation is recommended. (3) If the patient has sustained a single episode of hemorrhage requiring transfusion, a prolonged test of healing is not advocated, and immediate operation is recommended. (4) If a patient has satisfactorily completed a test of healing but has developed a recurrence, immediate operation is recommended. Over 50 per cent of patients whose ulcers satisfactorily heal will experience recurrence within 2 years and up to 80 per cent in 5 years. *These criteria for immediate operation, in our judgment, encompass the vast majority of patients with chronic benign gastric ulcer.*

### The Operation

We use one of two operative procedures to manage the benign gastric ulcer: limited subtotal gastrectomy (approximately 50 per cent) to include the ulcer and most or all of the antrum; and truncal vagotomy and limited subtotal gastrectomy (approximately 50 per cent) to include the ulcer and all or most of the antrum.

LIMITED SUBTOTAL GASTRECTOMY. If the patient has a benign gastric ulcer satisfactorily established by preoperative evaluation, does not have a normal or hypernormal acid secretory state, does not have associated duodenal ulcer, is not dependent upon ulcerogenic drugs for other systemic disease (chronic arthritis, ulcerative colitis, regional enteritis, gout, etc.), and is not a chronic alcoholic, we prefer limited subtotal gastrectomy to include the ulcer and the antrum. This provides us with a total biopsy of the lesion, conclusively establishing the benignancy of the ulcer. This operative approach also eliminates Oi's *locus minoris resistentiae* and furthermore removes the area of decreased resistance due to the presence of the lesion or scar of the lesion. Although the operation cannot be claimed to reduce bile and pancreatic reflux, it does remove the most susceptible areas for injury. Finally, this eliminates the target organ hypothesized by Dragstedt's theory of antral stasis and furthermore improves gastric emptying in the presence of outlet obstruction. Based on extensively reported data as well as on our own experience, this approach can be expected to bring about a virtually perfect cure rate with an extremely low mortality. Recurrence rate under these circumstances is small (0 to 4.4 per cent), although there is an occasional report out of this range. Morbidity in terms of dumping and weight loss is minimal and acceptable.

LIMITED SUBTOTAL GASTRECTOMY WITH VAGOTOMY. If the patient has an associated duodenal ulcer, a prepyloric (1 to 2 cm. proximal) ulcer, or a high-normal or hypersecretory acid pattern, or if he is a chronic alcoholic, is dependent upon ulcerogenic drugs, or is a juvenile, we routinely add truncal vagotomy to limited gastric resection (including the ulcer). This approach encompasses all of the beneficial aspects of limited gastric resection alone and affords added protection in terms of control of acid by parasympathetically denervating the stomach. Unfortunately, there are not yet hard data available either to endorse conclusively this approach or to justify clearly the possibility of added morbidity (change in bowel habits, possible biliary or pancreatic dysfunction), which may be the price of a "gratuitous" vagotomy. We feel, however, that our attitude is warranted on the basis of theoretic physiologic grounds; the subsequent appearance of data which either support or contradict this rationale will color future management.

BILLROTH I VERSUS BILLROTH II RECONSTRUCTION. It is now apparent, based on data from a number of clinics, that there is no significant difference in terms of postoperative morbidity, recurrence, or mortality between Billroth I and Billroth II reconstruction of the gastrointestinal tract following subtotal gastrectomy. In the majority of patients with gastric ulcer, the duodenum is essentially normal. Because of simplicity of technique (one less suture line) and suggestive—though inconclusive—evidence of somewhat improved iron and protein absorption with the Billroth I reconstruction, we use it when technical considerations permit.

## Summary and Conclusions

Benign gastric ulcer is a complex disease, the pathogenesis of which is only partially understood. Differentiation between benignancy and malignancy in the lesion is important but, with currently available techniques, is virtually assured preoperatively. We recommend operation for the vast majority of patients with proven benign chronic gastric ulcer, and we attempt to tailor the operation to the pathogenesis as we currently understand it. For most patients with chronic benign gastric ulcer, limited (50 per cent) subtotal gastrectomy to include resection of the ulcer is the procedure of choice. Truncal vagotomy is added in a group of patients under certain specific criteria which have been outlined. The Billroth I reconstruction is preferred.

## *References*

1. Wenger, J., Brandborg, L. L., and Spellman, F. A.: Gastroenterology 61:598, 1971.
2. Paustion, F. F., Stein, G. N., Young, J. F., Roth, J. L. A., and Bockus, H. L.: Gastroenterology 38:155, 1960.
3. Flood, C. A.: Am. J. Digest. Dis. 6:555, 1961.
4. Runyeon, W. K., and Hoerr, S. O.: Gastroenterology 32:415, 1957.
5. Strandjord, N. M., Moseley, R. D., Jr., and Schweinefus, R. L.: Radiology 74:442, 1960.
6. Amberg, J. R.: Am. J. Digest. Dis. 5:259, 1960.
7. Mitty, W. F., Jr., Rousselot, L. M., and Grace, W. J.: Am. J. Digest. Dis. 5:249, 1960.
8. Hennig, G. C., and Harvey, H. D.: Ann. Intern. Med. 50:43, 1959.
9. Villako, K. P.: Klin. Med. (Wien) 37:69, 1959.
10. Hitchcock, C. R., Sullivan, W. A., and Wangensteen, O. H.: Gastroenterology 29:621, 1955.
11. Kronborg, O.: Gut 15:714, 1974.
12. Dinstl, K.: Surg. Gynecol. Obstet. 128:77, 1969.
13. Grassi, G.: Personal communication, 1974.
14. Woodward, E. R., Eisenberg, M. M., and Dragstedt, L. R.: Am. J. Surg. 113:5, 1967.
15. Panico, F. G., Papanicolaou, G. N., and Cooper, W. A.: J.A.M.A. 143:1308, 1950.
16. Rosenthal, M., and Traut, H. F.: Cancer 4:147, 1951.
17. Rubin, C. E., and Benditt, E. P.: Cancer 8:1137, 1955.
18. Ross, J. R., McGrath, J. M., Crozier, R. E., and Rohart, R. R.: Gastroenterology 34:24, 1958.
19. Eisenberg, M. M., and Woodward, E. R.: Arch. Surg. 87:810, 1963.
20. Schade, R. O. K.: Br. Med. J. 1:743, 1958.
21. du Plessis, D. J.: Am. Gastroenterol. Assoc. Post-Grad. Course Proceedings 20–1, 1974.
22. Aagaard, P.: Acta Chir. Scand., Suppl. 318, 1963.
23. Rumball, J. M.: Gastroenterology 61:622, 1971.
24. Dragstedt, L. R., Camp, E. H., and Fritz, J. M.: Ann. Surg. 130:843, 1949.
25. Skillman, J. J.: Surgery 76:515, 1974.
26. Kraft, R. O., Fry, W. J., and Ranson, H. K.: Arch. Surg. 92:456, 1966.
27. Stemmer, E. A., Zahn, R. L., Hom, L. W., and Connally, J. E.: Arch. Surg. 96:588, 1968.
28. du Plessis, D. J.: Lancet 1:974, 1965.
29. Delaney, J. P., Cheng, J. W. B., Butler, B. A., and Ritchie, W. P., Jr.: Gut 11:715, 1970.
30. Davenport, H. W.: Gut 6:513, 1965.
31. Davenport, H. W.: Gastroenterology 46:245, 1964.
32. Davenport, H. W.: Proc. Soc. Exp. Biol. Med. 126:657, 1967.
33. Davenport, H. W.: Gastroenterology 59:505, 1970.
34. Oi, M., Oshida, K., and Sugimura, S.: Gastroenterology 36:45, 1959.
35. Oi, M., and Sakurai, Y.: Gastroenterology 36:60, 1959.
36. Oi, M., and Oshida, K.: Gastroenterology 36:57, 1959.
37. Eisenberg, M. M., Woodward, E. R., Carson, T. J., and Dragstedt, L. R.: Ann. Surg. 170:317, 1969.
38. Duthie, H. L.: Gut 11:540, 1970.
39. Farris, J. M., and Smith, G. K.: Surg. Clin. North Am. 46:329, 1966.
40. Woodward, E. R.: *The Postgastrectomy Syndromes*. Springfield, Ill., Charles C Thomas, Publisher, 1963.
41. Jordan, G. L., Jr., Bolton, B. F., and DeBakey, M. E.: J.A.M.A. 161:1605, 1956.
42. Cox, A. G., Spencer, J., and Tinker, J.: *In* Williams, J. A. (ed.): *After Vagotomy*. Chapt. 9, p. 119. New York, Appleton-Century-Crofts, 1969.
43. Harvey, H. D.: Surg. Gynecol. Obstet. 113:191, 1961.
44. Walters, W., Lynn, T. E., and Mobley, J. E.: Gastroenterology 33:685, 1967.
45. Johnston, D.: Gut 15:748, 1974
46. Hedenstedt, S.: Scand. J. Gastroenterol. 8(Suppl. 20):10, 1973.
47. Arnold, W. T., Hampton, J., Olin, W., Glass, H., and Carruth, C.: J.A.M.A. 173:1117, 1960.
48. Nieburgs, H. E., Werther, J. L., Hollander, F., and Janowitz, H. D.: Am. J. Digest. Dis. 5:63, 1960.
49. Littman, A.: Gastroenterology 61:567, 1971.
50. Johnson, H. D.: Lancet 2:515, 1957.
51. Holle, F., and Hart, W.: Med. Klin. 62:441, 1967.
52. Holle, F.: Personal communication, 1974.
53. Johnston, D., Humphrey, C. S., Smith, R. B., and Wilkinson, A. R.: Brit. J. Surg. 59:787, 1972.
54. Johnston, D., Lyndon, P. J., and Smith, R. B.: Gut 14:825, 1973.
55. Hallenbeck, G.: Personal communication, 1975.

# 26

# Operative Treatment for Carcinoma at the Esophagogastric Junction

ONE-STAGE RESECTION AND
RECONSTRUCTION FOR
CARCINOMA OF THE
ESOPHAGOGASTRIC JUNCTION

by W. Spencer Payne and
Philip E. Bernatz

ADENOCARCINOMA AT THE
ESOPHAGOGASTRIC JUNCTION

by Edward W. Humphrey and
Thomas E. Kersten

## Statement of the Problem

The controversy deals, in the main, with the amount of esophagus and stomach which should be removed in a patient with an adenocarcinoma or a squamous cell carcinoma present at the gastroesophageal junction. It examines, too, the various operative approaches and considers the character of the node dissection.

Discuss cell type as a determinant of the extent of the esophagectomy, including both radiologic and scope lengths. Is spread into the esophageal submucosa a function of histologic type? Give data relating recurrence rate at the suture line to the extent of esophagectomy.

Discuss palliative esophagogastrectomy for obstructing or nonobstructing but incurable lesions. Provide any data which show prolonged survival and/or improved quality of life.

For carcinoma at the esophagogastric junction, how much stomach should be removed distal to the gross lesion? What is the extent of intra-abdominal node dissection? Give data supporting your decisions.

Describe and defend your preference for reconstitution of the gastrointestinal tract.

# One-Stage Resection and Reconstruction for Carcinoma of the Esophagogastric Junction

W. SPENCER PAYNE
and PHILIP E. BERNATZ

*Mayo Clinic and Mayo Foundation*

It is difficult to be dogmatic regarding the treatment of a condition such as carcinoma of the esophagogastric junction, in which causes remain unknown, early diagnosis is elusive, and all current therapies are unsatisfactory. Nonetheless, much that is known about this condition provides a rational and compassionate basis for management.

## Nonresective Therapy

The natural history of untreated carcinoma of the esophagogastric junction is that approximately 25 per cent of patients are dead within 6 months of onset of symptoms, 75 per cent are dead within a year, and 90 per cent are dead within 18 months. The average duration of survival of untreated patients is approximately 8 months. Palliative treatment in the form of esophageal intubation and feeding gastrostomy provides no significant prolongation of survival. Radiation therapy can provide significant palliation but rare cure. Its use at the esophagogastric junction is restricted to the uncommon cases of squamous cell carcinoma, in which it relieves esophageal obstruction in less than half of instances. Moertel and associates[12] have shown significant prolongation of survival of patients with inoperable or nonresectable adenocarcinoma of the stomach and cardia after combined 5-fluorouracil and radiation therapy, but long-term control by this means has not been achieved.

593

## *Operative Management*

Classic resective procedures that are directed to the wide local removal of the primary neoplasm and regional lymph nodes (esophagogastrectomy) provide 3-year and 5-year survivals of 21 and 12 per cent, respectively[5] (Table 1). We restrict resective operation almost wholly to patients whose gross neoplasm can be incorporated in a single en bloc operative specimen. At our institution, patients with distant metastasis or fixed local lesions have not generally been subjected to operative ablation. Although the intent of resection is cure, resection too often proves to be palliative though not an insignificant benefit for many patients. The present universal inability to define accurately the stage of malignancy precludes a more precise selection of patients for operative cure. Nonetheless, resection under the circumstances currently definable achieves the best cure rate for the few and provides significant palliation and prolongation of survival. Unsatisfactory as overall results are at this time, some form of palliation of the esophageal obstruction should be provided for patients whose tumors are advanced and incurable, and similar palliation and possible cure for those with less advanced neoplasms. Further, strategies of treatment must be well-defined not only in

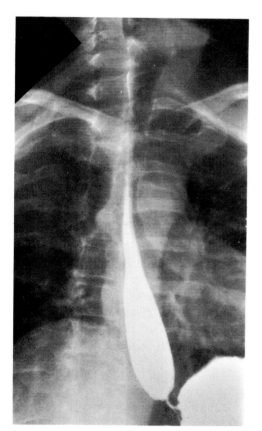

*Figure 1.* Well-localized annular lesion at esophagogastric junction. Esophagoscopy revealed Grade 4 adenocarcinoma, 18 inches from incisor teeth. This type of lesion is suitable for esophagogastrectomy, as illustrated in Figure 2. Equally satisfactory tumor-free margins and functional results can be obtained using the techniques shown in Figures 4 and 6.

terms of factors that are known to influence the course of disease but also in terms of introducing new methods or the study of combinations of different modalities in a prospective manner. Thus, we are currently involved in prospective randomized studies that are designed to provide more specific knowledge regarding treatment of this tragic disease.

We have employed three basic operations in treating carcinomas of the esophagogastric junction, irrespective of the type of epithelial malignancy encountered. However, more than 90 per cent of the cancers are adenocarcinomas of gastric epithelial origin, and less than 10 per cent are squamous carcinomas of esophageal origin. The selection of the operation for carcinoma of the esophagogastric junction depends on certain anatomic considerations as well as on the individual preference of the operating surgeon. Thus, when a small gastric neoplasm minimally involves the esophagus and stomach (Figure 1), a left thoracic or left thoracoabdominal incision provides adequate exposure for partial esophagogastrectomy with esophagogastrostomy[8] (Figure 2). Pyloroplasty usually is performed concurrently, since resection of the esophagus necessarily involves resection of vagal trunks, with resultant impairment of gastric emptying.

When the neoplasm involves the proximal part of the stomach exten-

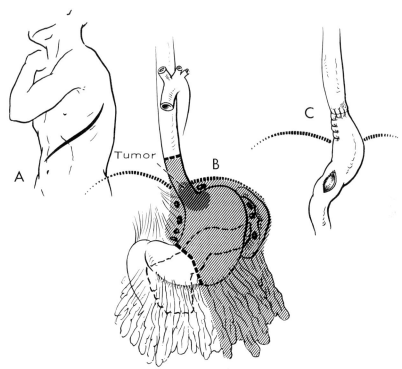

*Figure 2.* Technique of esophagogastrectomy for well-localized cancer of the esophagogastric junction. *A,* Left thoracoabdominal incision. *B,* Shaded area indicates tissues to be resected. *C,* Reconstruction by esophagogastrostomy end-to-end with pyloroplasty. (From Ellis, F. H., Jr.: Surgical aspects of malignant lesions of the esophagogastric junction. *In* ReMine, W. H., Priestley, J. T., and Berkson, J. (eds.): *Cancer of the Stomach.* Philadelphia, W. B. Saunders Co., 1964, pp. 127–140.)

sively and the esophagus rather minimally (Figure 3), or when the patient has had a previous antrectomy, the combination of total gastrectomy, splenectomy, and omentectomy with partial distal esophagectomy is preferred. This usually requires a left thoracoabdominal incision, though a simultaneous upper abdominal and right thoracic incision may be required occasionally. While various esophagointestinal anastomoses have been employed, reconstruction probably is best effected by a long-limb Roux-Y or less frequently by a similar length of jejunum interposed between esophagus and duodenum[16] (Figure 4).

When carcinoma of the esophagogastric junction extends largely upward to involve several inches of the lower thoracic part of the esophagus (Figure 5), as it most often does, an adequate margin of normal esophagus above the neoplasm is best obtained by a combined upper abdominal and right thoracic procedure[9] (Figure 6). This permits transabdominal pyloroplasty, splenectomy, and liberation of the stomach on a vascular pedicle of right gastric and right gastroepiploic vessels. The separate right thoracotomy permits the liberation and resection of the distal two-thirds of the esophagus and proximal third of the stomach, so that esophagogastrostomy can be effected at or above the level of the azygos vein. An attempt is made to prevent esophageal reflex with a gastroplasty (modified Nissen) whenever possible.

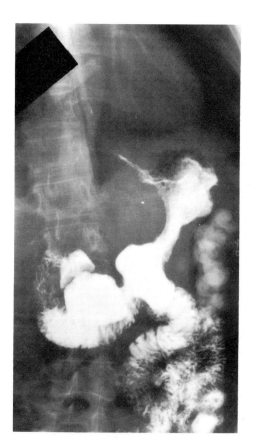

*Figure 3.* Esophagus and stomach in patient with extensive proximal gastric neoplasm and minimal involvement of distal esophagus. Esophagoscopy revealed Grade 4 adenocarcinoma, 19 inches from incisor teeth. This type of neoplasm is particularly suitable for total gastrectomy and reconstruction by the methods illustrated in Figure 4.

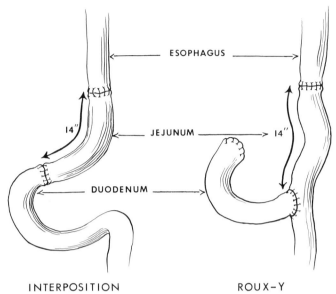

INTERPOSITION                    ROUX-Y

*Figure 4.*   Methods of reconstruction after total gastrectomy, omentectomy, and splenectomy with partial esophagectomy in patients with extensive proximal gastric neoplasm. A 14- to 18-inch isoperistaltic segment of jejunum prevents bile esophagitis whether operation is effected as an interposition (*left*) or as a Roux-Y (*right*). (From Payne, W. S.: Esophageal reflux ulceration: Causes and surgical management. Surg. Clin. North Am. *51*:935, 1971.)

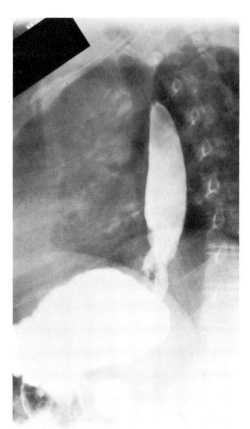

*Figure 5.*   Grade 4 adenocarcinoma with minimal gastric involvement by extension up the distal esophagus for approximately 2 inches. Endoscopy revealed that the proximal end of the tumor could be visualized 16 inches from the upper incisor teeth. This type of malignancy lends itself best to resection as illustrated in Figure 6.

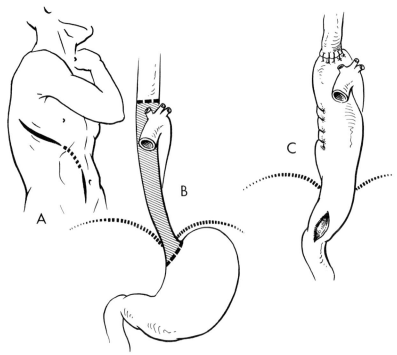

*Figure* 6.   Technique favored for cancer of esophagogastric junction in which neoplasm extends cephalad from the cardia up the esophagus. *A*, Incision in upper midline of abdomen to liberate proximal portion of stomach and to effect splenectomy and pyloroplasty. Right thoracotomy is performed for resection of involved part of thoracic esophagus and cardia. *B*, Shaded areas indicate just portion of esophagus to be resected. A portion of the lesser curvature and fundus of stomach also must be resected with the esophageal specimen. This creates a tube of greater curvature of stomach with a right gastroepiploic vascular pedicle and effects removal of left gastric lymph nodes with specimen. *C*, Esophagogastrostomy done high in thorax. (From Ellis, F. H., Jr.: Treatment of carcinoma of the esophagus and cardia. Proc. Staff Meet. Mayo Clin. 35:653, 1960.)

Each procedure is designed to provide a proximal and distal line of resection that not only is free of tumor involvement but also provides at least a 4-cm. margin of normal tissue proximal and distal to the neoplasm. Additionally, each procedure provides for the resection of the left gastric nodes and lymph node–bearing tissues along the lesser curvature of the stomach, resection of nodes and tissue associated with the short gastric vessels and proximal omentum and the splenic hilus, and resection of nodes and tissue in the mediastinum adjacent to the esophagus.

Of special concern has been a distressingly high mortality rate (10 per cent) associated with almost all operations for cancer of the cardia. When the usual age of patients with cancer of the esophagogastric junction is considered, it is perhaps not surprising that half of the deaths have been from degenerative cardiovascular disease, thromboembolism, and associated obstructive lung disease.

In the past, nearly half of these deaths (approximately 5 per cent) have been related to a leaking intrathoracic esophageal anastomosis. Some surgeons have sought to avoid this complication by placing the esophageal anastomosis outside the thorax, where leakage is less likely to be fatal. We believe that fatal anastomotic failure generally can be avoided. The incidence of leakage can be minimized by assuring a good blood supply of structures at the site of anastomosis and, as suggested by Maillard et al.,[11] by increasing the use of end-to-side anastomosis when it does not compromise tumor-free margin. Recent experience[17] indicates that fatal leakage of intrathoracic anastomoses can be further minimized. Total parenteral alimentation for 14 days or more after the early postoperative roentgenographic identification of anastomotic leakage provides sufficient healing for an oral diet to be resumed without catastrophic results in almost all incidences. Thus, we believe not only that a single-stage operation with an intrathoracic anastomosis provides optimal operative extirpation of neoplasms at the esophagogastric junction but also that such a procedure can be done with a total operative mortality rate of less than 10 per cent. Finally, the operative procedures described provide reasonably satisfactory digestive comfort and nutrition. If the neoplasm is small, well-localized, and confined to esophagogastric junction, esophagogastric anastomosis often can be performed end-to-side, with the incorporation of a competence-restoring plication of stomach about the distal esophagus, as suggested by Bombeck et al.[1] A Roux-Y gastric drainage procedure is occasionally necessary to relieve intractable bile esophagitis after low esophagogastrectomy with end-to-end esophagogastrostomy.[17] Because the blood supply of the gastric remnant in these patients is almost entirely dependent on the right gastric and right gastroepiploic vessels, the duodenum must be transected just distal to the pylorus and the site of the pyloroplasty, the distal end of the duodenum must be closed, and the long limb of the Roux-Y loop must be anastomosed to the pyloric end of the stomach without disturbing nutrient vessels. High esophagogastrostomy of the Ivor Lewis type[9] is rarely complicated by digestive distress or bile reflux. This procedure provides the best function and is the one that is done in most of our patients with carcinoma of the esophagogastric junction.

## Discussion

Any operative ablative procedure for malignancy should take advantage of frozen-section pathologic techniques to assure that the lines of resection are free of tumor involvement. Although the techniques provide such assurance, all too often the microscopic tumor-free margin is considerably less than the intraoperative in situ assessment of 4 cm.

Shrinkage is so geat in esophageal specimens that it is virtually impossible to reconstruct meaningful measurements, especially on the esophageal portion of the specimen. Nonetheless, tumor-free margins, both proximal and distal, are obtained in approximately 95 per cent of operative specimens by the procedures described. We have seen secondary submucosal esophageal nodules and actual satellite tumor ulcerations near adenocarcinomas and squamous cell carcinomas of the esophagogastric junction. Both cell types are capable of submucosal lymphatic penetration remote from the gross primary. We have not sought to extend resections beyond a microscopic tumor-free margin in the presence of extensive nodal metastatic involvement or transmural penetration of the tumor.

Thus, evidence for extensive circumferential spread is thought to preempt any curative advantage gained by extending the linear tumor-free margins. This seems to be supported by survival data (Table 1), which clearly are related to the presence or absence of nodal involvement. More than 90 per cent of patients who have undergone resection experience unobstructed swallowing for the duration of their survival. Recurrent obstruction, when it occurs, is usually late in the course of the disease and is usually associated with signs of distant spread. Tumor-free margins cannot be correlated with such recurrent esophageal obstruction, and this suggests that operative procedures are ineffective in eradicating mediastinal disease in the presence of transmural and extensive nodal involvement. Thus, while we support the concept that residual tumor at the site of resection invites anastomotic recurrence, we would add that the apparent absence of such residual tumor does not preclude residual mediastinal disease from effecting late malignant esophageal obstruction. Our experience suggests that residual mediastinal disease is more often responsible for so-called anastomotic recurrences than is a failure to have a tumor-free margin at the time of resection.

We have little experience with intentional palliative resection of carcinoma of the esophagogastric junction in the presence of hepatic or other definable distant metastasis. We are convinced that such patients are all incurable by current methods and that the anticipated duration of survival (8 months) probably does not justify elaborate palliation of dysphagia. For these patients, we attempt some less difficult but reasonably effective form of

TABLE 1. Five-year Survival Rates After Resection for Carcinoma of Cardia (Mayo Clinic, 1946–1963)*

| Pathologic findings or procedure | Number of patients | Five-year survival | |
|---|---|---|---|
| | | Number | Per cent |
| Squamous cell carcinoma | | | |
| Negative lymph nodes | 11 | 6 | 55 |
| Positive lymph nodes | 13 | 2 | 15 |
| Palliative | 1 | 0 | 0 |
| Adenocarcinoma | | | |
| Negative lymph nodes | 67 | 18 | 27 |
| Positive lymph nodes | 171 | 13 | 8 |
| Palliative | 52 | 1 | 2 |
| Lost to follow-up | 7 | — | — |
| Total | 322 | 40 | 12 |

*Data from Gunnlaugsson, G. H., Wychulis, A. R., Roland, C., et al.: Analysis of the records of 1,657 patients with carcinoma of the esophagus and cardia of the stomach. Surg. Gynecol. Obstet. 130:997, 1970.

palliation for esophageal obstruction (short of resection). Chief among these are palliative intubation,[2, 18] esophageal bougienage, and local bypass,[7] as well as irradiation and chemotherapy.[12] We seldom employ feeding gastrostomy because it provides no palliation for dysphagia but merely provides an alternate route for alimentation. Thus, the patient continues to struggle with the problem of eliminating salivary secretions and recurrent respiratory aspiration unless esophageal obstruction can be relieved by nonoperative means.

Obviously, the amount of esophagus and stomach to be resected beyond a tumor-free margin is unclear. Logan[10] suggests that radical extirpation of stomach and esophagus with adjacent distal pancreas and periaortic nodes (even when fixed) may provide significant improvement in results. As Logan has noted, however, the disease is so complex that it is difficult to evaluate the mechanism by which the prognosis for these patients is modified by the treatment employed.

Nonetheless, evidence favors a one-stage resection and reconstruction for carcinoma of the esophagogastric junction, using relatively low-risk reconstructive procedures.[3, 4, 6, 10] The role of irradiation therapy as a preoperative or postoperative adjunct is less clear. Nakayama[14] advocated preoperative irradiation and refined methods for reducing the time and morbidity during the period of treatment. Unfortunately, there is no general agreement with Nakayama's enthusiastic reports of increased survival. Part of the problem centers around a failure to define cell type as well as anatomic location and stage in reference to adjunctive modalities. Even the Clinical Staging System for Carcinoma of the Esophagus, developed by the American Joint Committee for Cancer Staging and End Results Reporting (October, 1973), has stated that "the behavior pattern of nonsquamous cell carcinoma did not differ [in their material] sufficiently from that of squamous cell carcinoma to justify the development of classification schemes for different histologic types." However, they caution that the stage classification proffered is based entirely on preoperative findings—clinical, roentgenographic, and endoscopic—with the provision that operative and pathologic findings can be added later as supplementary data. Thus, it appears that radiation therapy, as a potent and effective modality, may have a role in the management of certain esophageal tumors[13, 15] but an uncertain role in the management of usual lesions at the esophagogastric junction.

Meanwhile, we hope to have the wisdom to apply the methods currently available to take advantage of the biologic behavior of the tumor, as best we can define it, and to provide comfort during the remaining life time of those afflicted with carcinoma of the cardia. We believe that modest-risk, one-stage resection and reconstruction are essential features of these potentially curative, but more often palliative, operations.

# References

1. Bombeck, C. T., Coelho, R. G. P., and Nyhus, L. M.: Prevention of gastroesophageal reflux after resection of the lower esophagus. Surg. Gynecol. Obstet. 130:1035, 1970.
2. Duvoisin, G. E., Ellis, F. H., Jr., and Payne, W. S.: The value of palliative prostheses in malignant lesions of the esophagus. Surg. Clin. North Am. 47:827, 1967.

3. Fisher, R. D., Brawley, R. K., and Kieffer, R. F.: Esophagogastrostomy in the treatment of carcinoma of the distal two-thirds of the esophagus: Clinical experience and operative methods. Ann. Thorac. Surg. 14:658, 1972.

4. Groves, L. K., and Rodriguez-Antúnez, A.: Treatment of carcinoma of the esophagus and gastric cardia with concentrated preoperative irradiation followed by early operation. Ann. Thorac. Surg. 15:333, 1973.

5. Gunnlaugsson, G. H., Wychulis, A. R., Roland, C., et al.: Analysis of the records of 1,657 patients with carcinoma of the esophagus and cardia of the stomach. Surg. Gynecol. Obstet. 130:997, 1970.

6. Humphrey, C. R., and Cliffton, E. E.: Carcinoma of the distal part of the esophagus and carcia of the stomach. Surg. Gynecol. Obstet. 127:737, 1968.

7. Johnson, C. L., and Clagett, O. T.: Palliative esophagogastrostomy for inoperable carcinoma of the esophagogastric junction. J. Thorac. Cardiovasc. Surg. 60:269, 1970.

8. Kirklin, J. W., and Clagett, O. T.: Some technical aspects of esophagogastrectomy for carcinoma of the lower part of the esophagus and cardiac end of the stomach. Surg. Clin. North Am. 31:959, 1951.

9. Lewis, I.: The surgical treatment of carcinoma of the oesophagus: with special reference to a new operation for growths of the middle third. Br. J. Surg. 34:18, 1946.

10. Logan, A.: The surgical treatment of carcinoma of the esophagus and cardia. J. Thorac. Cardiovasc. Surg. 46:150, 1963.

11. Maillard, J. N., Launois, B., De Lagausie, P., et al.: Cause of leakage at the site of anastomosis after esophagogastric resection for carcinoma. Surg. Gynecol. Obstet. 129:1014, 1969.

12. Moertel, C. G., Childs, D. S., Jr., Reitemeier, R. J., et al.: Combined 5-fluorouracil and supervoltage radiation therapy of locally unresectable gastrointestinal cancer. Lancet 2:865, 1969.

13. Moseley, R. V.: Squamous carcinoma of the esophagus. Surg. Gynecol. Obstet. 126:1242, 1968.

14. Nakayama, K.: Pre-operative irradiation in the treatment of patients with carcinoma of the oesophagus and of some other sites. Clin. Radiol. 15:232, 1964.

15. Parker, E. F., Gregorie, H. B., Jr., Arrants, R. E., et al.: Carcinoma of the esophagus. Ann. Surg. 171:746, 1970.

16. Payne, W. S.: The long-term clinical state after resection with total gastrectomy and Roux loop anastomosis. In Smith, R. A., and Smith, R. E. (eds.): Surgery of the Oesophagus: The Coventry Conference. New York, Appleton-Century-Crofts, 1972, pp. 23–28.

17. Payne, W. S.: Unpublished data.

18. Sanfelippo, P. M., and Bernatz, P. E.: Celestin-tube palliation for malignant esophageal obstruction. Surg. Clin. North Am. 53:921, 1973.

# Adenocarcinoma at the Esophagogastric Junction

EDWARD W. HUMPHREY

*Veterans Administration Hospital, Minneapolis, Minnesota*

and THOMAS E. KERSTEN

*University of Minnesota Health Sciences Center*

Adenocarcinoma involving the cardioesophageal junction, which may be primary in either the stomach or esophagus, is often difficult to classify as to its exact site of origin. It seems important to separate this tumor from both squamous cell carcinoma of the esophagus and adenocarcinoma of the corpus and antrum of the stomach, for there may be differences in the biologic activity and patterns of extension of these tumors.[5] Fortunately, adenocarcinoma of the cardioesophageal junction is not a common lesion. In an 8-year period, only 15 patients had a resection with an attempt for cure at the Minneapolis Veterans Hospital, compared to a total of 60 squamous cell carcinomas of the esophagus and 82 adenocarcinomas of the body and antrum of the stomach.

The operative treatment of these tumors varies greatly from one surgeon to another, and the evidence supporting any one approach as superior is not convincing. Certain principles of therapy can, however, be formulated: (1) the procedure selected should offer the patient the greatest opportunity for long-term survival; (2) the risk of the operation should be at a minimum; and (3) the reconstruction should provide the patient with an adequate conduit for swallowing that not only is relatively free of long-term complications but also will not obstruct early in the course of the disease in those patients who are not cured of their carcinoma. In the past, palliation for this and other carcinomas has been equated with a prolongation of life, but this is specious reasoning. There is little evidence that differences in survival between groups of patients with cancer resected or not resected represent anything more than selection of these patients by the initial extent of their disease. Palliation in other terms is, however, possible. The ability to swallow for the major portion of a patient's remaining life represents for most a true gain.

603

## *Extent of the Resection*

For most resectable carcinomas of the cardioesophageal junction, the surgeon has two choices: he may do a partial resection of the esophagus and place the subsequent anastomosis in the chest, or he may do a total thoracic esophagectomy and place the anastomosis in the neck. There is no evidence that a larger gastrectomy contributes to an increase in survival. A margin of 5 cm. distal to the gross tumor has been adequate to provide tumor-free margins both in this series and in others.[8] However, following the commonly used operation of partial gastrectomy and partial esophagectomy, residual tumor in the esophageal remnant has been a frequent problem. While the ability of a squamous cell carcinoma of the esophagus to spread for long distances in the submucosa is well known evidence indicates that an adenocarcinoma may have an equal tendency to spread upward in the esophagus. The consensus in the past has been that a margin of 5 cm. proximal to the gross tumor was sufficient, but there is a strong possibility that such a margin is inadequate to routinely remove the local tumor. Hankins et al.[3] reported on a series of adenocarcinomas involving the lower esophagus, from which 13 patients had a partial esophagectomy with an esophagogastrostomy. Ten of these 13 patients had tumor left behind. Of the 25 patients with carcinoma of the cardioesophageal junction who underwent a resection with the intent of cure reported by Block and Lancaster, 8, or 32 per cent, had tumor in the proximal line of resection of the esophagus. In the series of adenocarcinoma of the cardioesophageal junction reported by Magill and Simmons,[6] 12 per cent of patients had tumor left at the proximal line of resection. An additional number required another resection because of tumor at the line of the first resection. Twenty-five of 106 patients with high gastric carcinomas undergoing resection who were reported by Inberg and Scheinin[4] were shown to have cancer invasion present at the line of excision. At this institution, one of nine patients who had a partial esophagectomy for adenocarcinoma at the cardioesophageal junction had tumor at the proximal line of resection 6 cm. above the gross tumor mass, and a second had tumor within 2 mm. of the esophageal resection line 5 cm. from the gross tumor.

The argument has been advanced that the prognosis for patients with this malignancy is so poor that the principal effort of the surgeon should be directed toward palliation rather than cure, and therefore an increase in the extent of the operation would not be warranted. Surely, no one can guarantee that a greater effort to remove all the local tumor will result in a larger number of long-term survivors, yet it is difficult to accept the argument that this disease inherently carries an insignificant potential for cure, when it is based on data from series in which less than a complete excision of the known carcinoma has been accomplished. The only significant difference between a partial esophagectomy and a total thoracic esophageal resection is the necessity for creating a cervical esophagostomy and the resection of an additional 5 cm. of esophagus in the latter. This may be done without redraping or changing the patient's position. Except for possible damage to the recurrent laryngeal nerves, this procedure offers little increased risk to the patient. The important modification necessitated by a total thoracic esophagectomy occurs with the reconstruction. Because a gastric tube often may not have the required length to reach into the neck, the colon must commonly be used for a conduit, and its placement may require another operation.

## Lymph Node Dissection

There is much testimony but little evidence that a significant improvement in overall survival of a group of cancer patients results from a lymph node dissection. The evidence that is available, such as that from studies of carcinoma of the breast, shows that the contribution of a lymph node dissection, though demonstrable, is minor. The cure of patients having carcinoma of the cardioesophageal junction with spread to lymph nodes is so rare as to be anecdotal. No statistically valid study is possible. Yet most surgeons are impressed by memories of individual patients with other types of cancer who have survived for long periods of time following removal of histologically positive nodes.

The primary lymph drainage areas from the cardioesophageal junction are to nodes around the celiac axis artery, in the pulmonary ligament as it is reflected on to the esophagus, and in the hilus of the spleen. There is little disagreement about the removal of the first two of these lymph node areas, for the removal is associated with little increase in morbidity, but the removal of those nodes near the spleen requires the resection of the tail of the pancreas along with the spleen, and this does contribute to the operative risk. For this reason, it has seemed advisable to do a concurrent splenectomy only in those patients with tumor involving a portion of the greater curvature of the stomach. Even this surrender to tradition must be relegated to intuition rather than evidence.

## Reconstruction

The restoration of deglutition following a resection of the primary tumor may be done using a tube fashioned from the greater curvature of the stomach, a segment of jejunum, or some portion of the colon. There are significant advantages and disadvantages to each method, but if gastroesophageal continuity can be restored, no one method is so clearly superior that its use should dictate the extent of the primary resection.

If an esophagogastrostomy is performed at the same operative intervention as the resection, it can be done either through the left chest, utilizing a thoracoabdominal incision, or by a separate thoracotomy incision, or a right lateral thoracotomy. Although it is possible to do an anastomosis through the left chest at the level of the aortic arch, the limits of exposure are such that it is usually done no higher than the pulmonary veins. The much better exposure through a right thoracotomy will allow an anastomosis at the maximum height reached by a gastric tube, usually at or just above the azygos vein. This procedure can be done in one stage and is a major advantage, for the patient's total hospitalization and cost will be less than for types of delayed reconstruction. It has, however, several disadvantages. First, the length of the gastric tube may limit the esophageal resection to one less than ideal. Second, recurrence of carcinoma at the line of resection is relatively common. This represents a major cause of morbidity in the preterminal stage of this disease. Inberg and Scheinin[4] reported that malignant stenosis of the esophageal anastomosis was "fairly frequent in this kind of surgery." They performed a repeat resection in eight patients with such a recurrence. Of nine patients undergoing a partial esophagectomy and esophagogastrostomy for this carcinoma at the Minneapolis Veterans Hospital, seven died of their disease at periods of from 6 to 37 months following operation. At autopsy, five had recurrent carcinoma at the anastomosis. Third, with the anastomosis intrathoracic, an anastomotic leak, relatively common, is a principal cause for the high mortality rate associated with this operation. Hankins et al.[3] reported that 5 of 17 patients undergoing resection for adenocarcinoma of the esophagus developed a fatal anastomotic leak. Magill and Simmons[6] found a 21 per cent anastomotic leak incidence after esophagogastrostomy or esophagojejunostomy. Fifty-six per cent of these patients died within 3 months.

Gastroesophageal regurgitation has been a difficult complication for many patients. Creation of a valve by intussusception of the esophagus into the stomach is reported to alleviate much of this problem. Experience is still limited. The method, however, requires a greater length of the stomach tube as related to residual esophagus.

The use of a jejunal segment interposed to restore gastroesophageal continuity seems to have little advantage over a direct gastroesophagostomy. The length that can be obtained is usually no more than and often less than that of the stomach itself. It requires two additional anastomoses, and the blood supply is less reliable.

A reconstruction utilizing the colon is usually performed at a second stage some weeks following the gastrectomy and esophagectomy. This delay and a second operative procedure are an inconvenience to the patient and represent an increased total hospitalization. It may, however, be an advantage for the mostly elderly and debilitated group of patients to have the operative time divided into two shorter episodes. In a series of 30 cases of carcinoma of the esophagus operated on at this institution utilizing a one-stage esophagectomy and esophagogastrostomy prior to 1959, the 30-day postoperative mortality rate was 33 per cent. The ensuing 18 cases were done from 1959 to 1962 employing a two-stage reconstruction, with a mortality rate of 17 per cent. For the last 10 years, the postoperative mortality rate in 69 patients has been 12 per cent.

Following a total thoracic esophagectomy, the colon is placed either retrosternally or subcutaneously. The retrosternal position requires less length and averts the development of the ventral hernia which often occurs with the subcutaneous placement, but in some situations, such as the presence of a permanent tracheostomy, a previous sternotomy, or a question concerning the adequacy of blood supply to the colon, subcutaneous placement is advisable.

Either the right or the left colon may be utilized as a conduit, but preference should be given to the right colon if possible. Since it is placed in an isoperistaltic manner, the periodic spasms which plague those patients with a left colon interposition are avoided. However, the length of right colon available at times is not adequate to reach the neck, and in these instances the left colon is a useful substitute. Because the marginal artery of Drummond between the middle colic and left colic arteries is very constant and the marginal artery of the right colon is not, the blood supply to the left colon is more reliable, and the length available from the left colon and sigmoid is almost always sufficient to reach the pharynx if necessary. After 6 months to a year, colon spasms usually become less frequent, and antispasmodics such as dicyclomine hydrochloride will control them. The left colon was used for 10 of the last 25 consecutive colon interpositions done at this institution, because the surgeon believed that either the right colon was too short or the blood supply was inadequate. In each instance the length of available colon was sufficient to reach into the neck, and the blood supply was adequate for healing of the esophagocolostomy. In contrast, 4 of the 15 right colon interpositions failed because of necrosis of the colon adjacent to the esophageal anastomosis.

Although anastomotic leak is no less frequent after esophagocolostomy in the neck, the consequences are less dangerous than if a leak occurs in the thorax. If an anastomotic stricture occurs, revision is a relatively minor operative procedure. In the six patients undergoing this operation for an adenocarcinoma of the esophagogastric junction at this institution, there has been no instance of a recurrence of the carcinoma at the anastomosis.

## Operative Procedure

The abdomen is explored first. If a resection for cure is potentially possible, the lymph nodes surrounding the celiac axis are dissected free, and the left gastric artery is divided. The cardia of the stomach and, if necessary, the spleen are mobilized. An attempt is then made to bring all of the gross tumor below the diaphragm. If this can be done, a pyloroplasty is made, the abdomen is closed, and the right thorax is entered. After the stomach is delivered into the chest, it is divided distal to the left gastric artery, and a tube is constructed from the greater curvature of the stomach. The esophagus is divided at the level of the azygos vein, usually at least 7 cm. above the gross tumor, and an esophagogastrostomy is done.

At the time of the laparotomy, if all of the gross tumor cannot be brought below the diaphragm, a gastrostomy and pyloroplasty are made, the abdomen is closed, and the right thorax is entered via the sixth rib. The entire thoracic esophagus is mobilized. The stomach is divided below the left gastric artery and 5 cm. distal to the gross carcinoma, is closed, and is returned to the abdomen. The esophagus is divided in the apex of the chest, and an end-on cervical esophagostomy is constructed anterior to the right sterno-cleidomastoid muscle. Three or 4 weeks later, the abdomen is re-entered, and the colon interposition is created utilizing an end-to-end cervical esophagocolostomy and an end-to-side cologastrostomy.

## Palliation

If it is accepted that no local therapeutic maneuver directed at the cancer will prolong the life of a patient not cured, then palliation in the context of the present discussion can be defined as restoration of the pleasure of eating and drinking, plus control of such symptoms as bleeding. Although irradiation is a valuable method for restoring deglutition in patients with squamous cell carcinoma of the esophagus, it is of little value to those with an adenocarcinoma. Here, the only frequently successful method is resection with restoration of gastroesophageal continuity. The decision to undertake this type of resection in an incurable patient weighs the possible duration and improved quality of life against the risk of the procedure and the length and cost of hospitalization. It would seem inadvisable to undertake such a procedure in a patient with a predicted survival of less than 6 months.

Various attempts have been made to treat unresectable carcinomas in this region with some type of bypass, but the risks have been high and the overall palliation questionable. In one such series,[2] only 51 per cent of the patients had a good functional result. Other forms of therapy for the unresectable tumor have been equally unsuccessful. A gastrostomy does little except to make home care easier. The various intraesophageal tubes have been rather unsatisfactory. Cancer chemotherapy in the past, although associated with a temporary regression in approximately 20 per cent of patients with a gastric carcinoma, has contributed little to the overall solution because of the short duration and small number of these regressions. Hopefully, newer drugs or combinations of older drugs, such as 5-fluorouracil and methyl CCNU, will be more successful.

## References

1. Block, G. E., and Lancaster, J. R.: Adenocarcinoma of the cardioesophageal junction. Arch. Surg. 88:852, 1964.
2. El-Domeiri, A., Martini, N., and Beattie, E. J.: Esophageal reconstruction by colon interposition. Arch. Surg. 100:358, 1970.
3. Hankins, J. R., Cole, F. N., Attar, S., Frost, J. L., and McLaughlin, J. S.: Adenocarcinoma involving the esophagus. J. Thorac. Cardiovasc. Surg. 68:148, 1974.
4. Inberg, M. V., and Scheinin, T. M.: The surgery of oesophageal and high gastric carcinoma. Ann. Chir. Gynaecol. Fenn. 58:197, 1969.
5. MacDonald, W. C.: Clinical and pathological features of adenocarcinoma of the gastric cardia. Cancer 29:724, 1972.
6. Magill, T. G., and Simmons, R. L.: Resection of cardio-esophageal carcinoma. Arch. Surg. 94:865, 1967.
7. Ong, G. B.: Resection and reconstruction of the esophagus. Curr. Prob. Surg., September, 1971.
8. Paulino, F., and Roselli, A.: Carcinoma of the stomach. Curr. Prob. Surg., December, 1973.

# 27

# Diet and Drugs versus Operative Treatment for Hyperlipidemia

PRESENT STATUS OF TREATMENT
OF HYPERLIPIDEMIA
by Basil M. Rifkind and Robert I. Levy

PARTIAL ILEAL BYPASS OPERATION
IN THE MANAGEMENT
OF THE HYPERLIPIDEMIAS
by Henry Buchwald

## Statement of the Problem

*The disputants discuss cost, morbidity, efficacy, potential longevity benefits, and patient long-term acceptance of these two approaches to the reduction of serum lipids in subjects less than 50 years old with history of myocardial infarction and persistent hyperlipoproteinemia.*

*Analyze data on relative effectiveness and potential statistical significance of diet and drug-induced reduction of serum lipid levels for each type of hyperlipidemia. Compare these results with those of partial ileal bypass operation alone and of the operative procedure plus diet. List hazards and morbidity, early and late, of the operation. Provide all incidence figures.*

*Discuss significant undesirable side effects of lipid-reducing drugs.*

*Analyze available evidence indicating that alteration in serum cholesterol or lipids will arrest or reverse the progression of the atherosclerotic process.*

# Present Status of Treatment of Hyperlipidemia

**BASIL M. RIFKIND**
and **ROBERT I. LEVY**

*National Heart and Lung Institute, National Institutes of Health*

In a sense, the debate on the definitive merits of ileal bypass compared to conventional diet and/or drug therapy for certain forms of hyperlipidemia is premature. Although there is substantial evidence relating hyperlipidemia to coronary heart disease (CHD) risk, and there is no doubt that appropriate therapy can partially or totally correct most forms of hyperlipidemia, it has not yet been proved in man that lowering elevated blood lipid levels is of specific benefit for the prevention or regression of CHD. Until this is established, much of the debate is more theoretic than real. In this chapter we shall briefly review the main disorders involving elevated plasma lipids, discuss our therapeutic preferences, and, most importantly, review the case for lipid-lowering by whatever means.

The major plasma lipids are cholesterol, triglyceride, and phospholipids. Only the first two need be measured in diagnosing and managing most hyperlipidemias. These lipids are insoluble in aqueous media such as plasma and circulate in the form of lipoproteins. Four families of lipoproteins are usually distinguished (Table 1). The function of the lipoproteins is, to some extent, reflected by their rather constant lipid composition (Table 2).

**TABLE 1.** Alternative Classifications of Plasma Lipoprotein Families

| Electrophoresis[*] | Density Class (Preparative Ultracentrifuge) | Density |
|---|---|---|
| Chylomicrons | Chylomicrons | <0.95 |
| Pre-beta | Very low density (VLDL) | 0.95 – 1.006 |
| Beta | Low density (LDL) | 1.006 – 1.063 |
| Alpha | High density (HDL) | 1.063 – 1.021 |

[*]On paper or agarose gel.

611

TABLE 2.   Typical Percentage Composition by Weight of Each
Plasma Lipoprotein Class

|              | Chylomicrons | VLDL | LDL | HDL |
|--------------|:------------:|:----:|:---:|:---:|
| Cholesterol  | 5            | 13   | 43  | 18  |
| Triglyceride | 90           | 65   | 10  | 2   |
| Phospholipid | 4            | 12   | 22  | 30  |
| Protein      | 1            | 10   | 25  | 50  |

HDL = high density; LDL = low density; VLDL = very low density.

The chylomicrons transport exogenous (dietary) triglyceride; the very low density lipoproteins (VLDL) transport triglyceride of endogenous (mainly hepatic) origin; the low density lipoproteins (LDL) normally carry 60 to 70 per cent of the total plasma cholesterol; the high density lipoproteins (HDL) are lipid-poor and protein-rich but carry a small and sometimes clinically significant amount of cholesterol (30 to 85 mg. per 100 ml.).

The chylomicrons are formed in the intestinal endothelium and reach the systemic circulation via the thoracic duct. Their removal from the circulation depends on the activity of a group of lipolytic enzymes. VLDL are predominantly formed in the liver and are probably removed from the blood in a manner similar to the chylomicrons. The catabolism of VLDL involves the loss of triglycerides and selective removal of surface apoproteins, resulting in the formation of LDL through the formation of a short-lived intermediate lipoprotein form. LDL appear to be largely derived from VLDL catabolism. The fate of LDL is unclear.

Since equal degrees of hypercholesterolemia and/or hypertriglyceridemia may result from elevation of different plasma lipoproteins, it is advantageous to translate hyperlipidemia into hyperlipoproteinemia. Fredrickson, Levy, and Lees described five patterns or types of lipoprotein increase (Table 3).[1, 2] Each of these may be *secondary* to a variety of disorders, some common (Table 4); each may also occur as a *primary*, often genetically determined, abnormality, so-called familial hyperlipoproteinemia. This classification has been widely adopted and has been of considerable use. It has been somewhat eroded by the anticipated demonstration of heterogeneity in the system and will eventually be replaced by a classification based on specific biochemical defects.

TABLE 3.   Main Types of Hyperlipoproteinemia

| Type | |
|:----:|---|
| I   | Chylomicrons in fasting plasma |
| II  | Increased LDL concentration without (IIa) or with (IIb) a VLDL increase |
| III | Presence of intermediate lipoprotein form ("floating" beta; d < 1.006) |
| IV  | VLDL increase only |
| V   | Chylomicrons and VLDL increase in fasting plasma |

**TABLE 4.  Some Causes of Secondary Hyperlipoproteinemia**

Diet
Hypothyroidism
Nephrosis
Obstructive liver disease
Alcoholism
Myeloma
Macroglobulinemia
Diabetic acidosis
Pancreatitis
Glycogen storage disease

## *Main Features of Primary Hyperlipoproteinemia*[1,2]

### TYPE I

The severe chylomicronemia characterizing this disorder is secondary to absence or defective activity of the enzyme lipoprotein lipase, leading to impairment of chylomicron removal from the plasma. The disorder is inherited as an autosomal recessive. Severe hypertriglyceridemia results with little or only moderate hypercholesterolemia. Attacks of acute abdominal pain with or without overt pancreatitis, hepatosplenomegaly, eruptive xanthomas, and lipemia retinalis are the clinical features. Recurrent attacks of pancreatitis may lead to chronic pancreatitis and its sequelae. Death may occur from acute hemorrhagic pancreatitis.

### TYPE II

An increased concentration of LDL constitutes the Type II pattern. It is subdivided into Types IIa and IIb, depending on whether a VLDL increase is also present (Table 3). The former leads to hypercholesterolemia without hypertriglyceridemia, the latter to an increase of both lipids. Recent studies suggest that impaired removal of LDL from the plasma, secondary to defective binding of LDL to cell membranes, is the underlying abnormality in the classic familial form which is inherited as an autosomal dominant disorder with complete penetrance and early expression.[3] Type II may be asymptomatic or lead, through lipid deposition, to tendon and tuberous xanthomas and, more importantly (especially in males), to accelerated vascular disease. The risk of CHD is greatly enhanced in Type II subjects.

### TYPE III[4]

This uncommon, but by no means rare, disorder is being recognized with increasing frequency. Its diagnostic chemical abnormalities are a lipoprotein of beta mobility but of density <1.006, (so-called "floating beta") and a VLDL cholesterol:plasma triglyceride ratio of >0.3.[5] Both hypercholesterolemia and hypertriglyceridemia usually occur.

The explanation for the excess concentrations of the intermediate lipoprotein form is still uncertain; both overproduction and impaired degradation of VLDL have been postulated. Though Type III is clearly familial and several family members may be affected, the mode of inheritance is unclear. The clinical features of Type III include the frequent occurrence of tendinous, tuberous, tuberoeruptive, and palmar planar xanthomas, as well as accelerated coronary and peripheral vessel disease. Obesity, impaired glucose tolerance, and hyperuricemia are frequent accompaniments.

## TYPE IV

The only lipoprotein to be increased in Type IV is VLDL. This results, in about 80 per cent of subjects, in hypertriglyceridemia of slight or moderate degree without hypercholesterolemia. In the remainder, the hypertriglyceridemia is of sufficient severity to be accompanied by slight to moderate hypercholesterolemia. There are probably multiple causes for the primary Type IV pattern. Nevertheless, it is distributed in many kindred along autosomal dominant inheritance lines with expression in late childhood or early adult life.

Overproduction and impaired utilization of VLDL have both been held to be responsible for the increased lipoprotein concentration. Eruptive xanthomas occasionally occur. Although the frequency with which atherosclerotic disease complicates the primary Type IV pattern is quite unclear, it is not unusual to encounter individuals with premature CHD or more widespread arterial complications. Obesity, impaired glucose tolerance, and hyperuricemia are frequently present.

## TYPE V

Increased concentrations of VLDL and chylomicrons are found in the fasting plasma of the Type V subject. Both triglyceride and cholesterol are elevated, the former especially. The disorder is frequently familial when it shows an autosomal dominant mode of inheritance with delayed penetrance, especially in females. The underlying defect is obscure; postheparin lipolytic activity is normal here as in Type IV and in contrast with Type I. Recurrent attacks of abdominal pain with or without pancreatitis, hepatosplenomegaly, eruptive xanthomas, and lipemia retinalis often occur in adult subjects, frequently accompanied by obesity, impaired glucose tolerance, and hyperuricemia. The occurrence of accelerated atherosclerosis has not been firmly established.

# Risk of Vascular Disease in Hyperlipidemic Subjects

In describing the clinical features of the primary types of hyperlipoproteinemia, allusion has been made to the predisposition to CHD and other forms of atherosclerotic disease with which certain of them are associated. However, such a relationship does not rest solely on clinical experience. It is the product of a variety of observations, the most convincing of these being the various prospective studies such as those at Framingham and elsewhere.[6, 7] These population studies generally agree that plasma cholesterol levels directly relate to the subsequent development of CHD; to that extent, cholesterol constitutes a major risk factor for the disease. Although the greatest risk is experienced by those subjects with the highest cholesterol levels, it should be emphasized that, within the range of cholesterol levels encountered in these studies of affluent populations, no level is totally immune. The studies nicely complement numerous cross-sectional observations in which higher cholesterol levels were found in CHD as compared to control subjects. The situation with respect to triglyceride is unclear. While many cross-sectional studies have also found triglyceride to be higher in CHD subjects, the few prospective studies which have been conducted in this area are in disagreement. Carlson and Böttiger found triglyceride to be an independent risk factor for CHD,[8] but Wilhelmsen et al. did not;[9] both studies were conducted in Sweden. Since plasma total cholesterol is closely correlated with LDL and fasting triglyceride with VLDL, it can be inferred from such studies that the Type II pattern carries an increased risk of CHD but that the situation is unclear for the Type IV.

The increased risk of Type II subjects has been confirmed by Stone et al., who compared Type II male and female subjects with their normal siblings and found a strikingly higher cumulative prevalence of fatal and nonfatal CHD events in the former.[10]

# Benefits of Hypolipidemic Therapy

The treatment of hyperlipidemia may be of definite advantage to some subjects. The partial or total correction of the hyperchylomicronemia of Types I and V hyperlipoproteinemia will abort and prevent the recurrence of their acute abdominal attacks of pain. The various xanthomas that may occur in each of the hyperlipoproteinemias will regress and disappear with appropriate therapy. For example, resolution of the large tuberoeruptive lesions of Type III is consistently observed on treatment. Improvement of tendinous lesions is, however, harder to achieve.

Such benefits clearly involve only a small number of subjects and are trivial as compared to what might be achieved through the successful treatment or prevention of atherosclerotic vascular disease, especially coronary artery disease. The morbidity and mortality from CHD are staggering. Approximately 1.25 million heart attacks occur each year in the United States, and in 1972 they claimed almost 700,000 lives. An estimated 3.94 million Americans have a history of heart attack and/or angina pectoris. Such statistics have provided a powerful impetus to explore the prevention or treatment of CHD by correction of the major CHD risk factors: hypercholesterolemia, hypertension, and cigarette smoking. With respect to hypercholesterolemia, consideration has been given to reducing the lipid levels of both hyperlipidemic subjects and the whole population. Many clinical trials of lipid-lowering therapy have been conducted to evaluate whether such strategies are worthwhile. They have employed diet and/or drug measures for subjects with (secondary prevention) or without (primary prevention) clinical CHD. Eighteen completed or continuing trials of cholesterol-lowering were evaluated by Cornfield and Mitchell in 1969.[11] They observed that study results were not in agreement, there being positive and negative findings with respect to their impact on CHD. For those studies reporting positive effects, there was considerable variation in their magnitude. They concluded that "despite a very considerable scientific effort and some tantalizing suggestive results, we have no clear-cut, generally accepted, answer to the question of whether cholesterol lowering measures can affect coronary disease."

Numerous reasons were held to account for the inconclusiveness of results to date. Some of these are inherent in conducting trials of CHD prevention and will be discussed shortly. Others are products of faulty study design and analysis. Several important secondary prevention studies have been reported since then. Three of them administered clofibrate to CHD subjects irrespective of their cholesterol levels. Two of these, conducted in the United Kingdom, reported a significant reduction in cardiac mortality in subjects with a history of angina at entry with or without myocardial infarction.[12, 13] Benefits were less evident for subjects with a prior myocardial infarction only. Unfortunately, these findings were not corroborated in the recently reported Coronary Drug Project (CDP), which observed no evidence of significant efficacy of clofibrate with regard to total or cause-specific mortality, even in subgroups of the study population, such as those with a prior history of angina.[14]

The CDP similarly evaluated other lipid-lowering drugs, nicotinic acid, a high- and low-dose estrogen, and D-Thyroxine (DT4). All but nicotinic acid and clofibrate had to be discontinued during the study because of toxicity.[14-17] Nicotinic acid also failed to improve mortality rates but did produce a lower incidence of nonfatal myocardial infarction.

The design and analysis of these three secondary prevention studies range from good to excellent. Nonetheless, their contrasting findings and the relatively modest cholesterol-lowering that was achieved in the CDP (clofibrate, 6.5 per cent; nicotinic acid, 9.9 per cent) still cast doubt about what can legitimately be deduced regarding the efficacy of lipid-lowering in the secondary prevention of CHD.

New reports of well-conducted primary prevention studies are scarce. Miettinen and his colleagues reported a trial of cholesterol-lowering diet in two Finnish mental hospitals over 12 years, utilizing a crossover but non–double-blind design.[18] In men, they observed a considerable and significantly reduced CHD mortality. Cornfield et al. have drawn attention to certain inadequacies of this study, such as its nonrandomized nature and indications of differences in the population studies in the two periods at each hospital.[19]

Several well-designed and ambitious primary prevention trials are presently in progress. The World Health Organization (WHO) is sponsoring a double-blind, randomized, collaborative European study of clofibrate in hypercholesterolemic males.[20] The NHLI-sponsored collaborative LRC program is evaluating cholestyramine therapy in males with Type IIa hyperlipoproteinemia, utilizing a double-blind, randomized, and stratified design. Lipid-lowering is one of the several interventions employed in the NHLI-supported Multirisk Factor Intervention Trial.

A further recent impetus toward implementation of these major endeavors is the limited but dramatic observation that the occasional substantial correction of hyperlipidemia in Type II homozygotes by portacaval shunting or plasmapheresis may be accompanied by decreased angina, improved coronary angiographic appearances, decrease or disappearance of arterial bruits and aortic valve murmurs, and diminished aortic valve gradients.[21, 22]

## Treatment[23-26]

The first objective of treatment is to lower elevated lipoprotein levels into or as near the normal range as possible.[25, 26] Correction of secondary hyperlipoproteinemia usually merely involves treatment of the primary disorder. Treatment of primary hyperlipoproteinemia is based on the selection of diet and/or drug therapy directed toward decreasing production or increasing removal of the lipoprotein fraction(s) elevated in a given subject, i.e., according to lipoprotein type.

The chylomicronemia of Type I is treated with a severe fat-restricted diet supplemented by medium chain triglyceride, which does not require chylomicron formation for absorption. Such treatment results, within days, in a clearing of the lipemia with an associated correction of the hyperlipidemia, cessation of the abdominal attacks, and regression of the hepatosplenomegaly and eruptive xanthomas. Maintenance of a sufficiently low triglyceride level will prevent recurring abdominal problems. No drug is known to be of use in Type I.

Correction of the combined chylomicronemia and VLDL increase of Type V is often effected by reduction to ideal weight, followed by a maintenance regimen which restricts both fat and carbohydrate. Alcohol is strictly forbidden. These measures alone may achieve triglyceride levels sufficiently lowered to prevent recurrent abdominal attacks. Nicotinic acid may be used as additional therapy if necessary, provided that hyperuricemia or hyperglycemia does not contraindicate its use. Progestational agents, such as norethisterone acetate, are useful in the female.

A low-cholesterol (<300 mg. per day), high-P:S (2:1) diet is an effective means of lowering the high LDL levels in Type II subjects. The diet is thought to increase the rate of LDL removal. Strict adherence, as in the metabolic ward, usually reduces total plasma cholesterol and LDL levels by 15 to 25 per cent. Reductions of 10 to 15 per cent are often seen in the free-living situation.[26] Many heterozygous children achieve normal lipid levels on such treatment. Most adults do not. Biliary sequestrants, such as cholestyramine or colestipol, consistently reduce LDL levels further, frequently into the normal range. Adequate doses of cholestyramine (up to 24 g. per day) typically effect a 20 to 25 per cent reduction in plasma cholesterol over that achieved by diet alone.[31] Troublesome side effects are not infrequent but can be overcome in many subjects. Nicotinic acid may also be useful to further achieve a reduction of LDL levels and can be especially useful in Type IIb by also reducing VLDL levels. It decreases VLDL and LDL production. Its frequent side effects interfere with its general use, and we tend to restrict it to supplementing diet and biliary sequestrant therapy in subjects with marked LDL elevation, namely Type II homozygotes and severe heterozygotes. Levels of LDL may also be reduced by several other drugs, such as D-thyroxine, neomycin, and PAS, most likely by accelerating LDL removal. Either there is less experience with these drugs than with the biliary sequestrants, or they have proved more toxic so that they are not as widely used.

Control of the excess concentrations of the intermediate lipoprotein of Type III hyperlipoproteinemia is readily effected by reduction to ideal weight and its maintenance by a balanced diet containing proteins, fat, and carbohydrates in the proportions of 20:40:40. Cholesterol is also restricted to less than 300 mg. per day and the P:S ratio raised to 2:1. These dietary steps substantially reduce plasma cholesterol and triglyceride, but further impressive reductions can be achieved with clofibrate or nicotinic acid. The use of cholestyramine or related drugs is contraindicated here, as in other forms of hyperlipoproteinemia associated with excess VLDL, since the hypertriglyceridemia may be aggravated.

The isolated increases in VLDL of Type IV should be treated, when appropriate, by correction of the oft-present obesity followed by maintenance of ideal weight with a balanced 20:40:40 diet. Cholesterol is moderately restricted (300 to 500 mg. per day), and polyunsaturated fats are preferred. When diet alone is insufficient to treat the hypertriglyceridemia, clofibrate or nicotinic acid may be helpful.

The hypolipidemic therapy described so far has been confined to diet and drugs. Other more radical procedures have been developed, mainly with the objective of effectively reducing the lipids of the otherwise resistant Type II homozygote. Thus, repeated plasmapheresis and, more recently, plasma exchange using a continuous-flow blood cell separator have been employed, as have biliary diversion, intravenous hyperalimentation, and portacaval shunting.[21, 22, 27] The partial ileal bypass procedure, in the few homozygote Type II's in whom it has been evaluated, has not proved particularly successful. Of these various procedures, only the ileal bypass has been advocated for use in other than the Type II homozygote.[28]

## Toxic Effects of Long-Term Therapy (Table 5)

Hypolipidemic therapy for the prevention of CHD must be given indefinitely. Even if atherosclerotic disease and its sequelae per se are beneficially influenced by such treatment, some price inevitably has to be paid in the form of morbidity and even mortality from the long-term administration of hypolipidemic drugs to large groups of subjects. The risks of such treatment may outweigh the benefits. The results of the CDP are a good example.[14-17] Not only were several anticipated serious toxic side effects of drugs such as estrogens or DT4 encountered, but also several hitherto totally or largely unsuspected effects were uncovered. Thus, the use of clofibrate was associated with an increased incidence of various nonfatal cardiovascular events, such as definite or suspected pulmonary embolism or thrombophlebitis, certain serious arrhythmias, and intermittent claudication. Another important finding was that the clofibrate-treated group experienced more cholelithiasis. The use of nicotinic acid was associated with increased frequency of cardiac arrhythmias, as well as GI problems. Both clofibrate and nicotinic acid produced increases or decreases in many routine clinical chemical measurements, the significance of which is unclear but argues for further caution.

## Design and Implementation of Intervention Studies

What are the obstacles in the way of conducting a satisfactory trial of lipid lowering? We have already alluded to the need for a randomized, double-blind study design. It is especially important in the study of a disorder for which several major risk factors have been identified. Possible confounding influences through unintentional impact on other major risk factors are protected against by use of a double-blind design. Depending on the treatment being evaluated, it may be difficult to maintain the double-blind elements of a study. Symptoms associated with the treatment under evaluation may alert the physician and/or the patient. The former must be carefully shielded from data that may indicate whether a subject is on drug or placebo. An appropriate administrative structure must then be erected to protect the patient's safety.

Other formidable problems have to be faced. These relate to the infrequency with which new CHD events occur, even in so-called high-risk populations. Approximately one such event is experienced annually by 100 middle-aged males. About twice as many may be predicted for hypercholesterolemic males. Such frequencies mean that large study populations are required and long periods of follow-up are inevitable. Another important determinant of sample size and duration is the degree of cholesterol-lowering that is obtained. The impact of such considerations is dramatically illustrated by the report of the National Heart and Lung Institute Task Force on Arteriosclerosis, which, based on the Diet Heart Feasibility Study, concluded

Table 5.  Approved Hypolipidemic Agents*

| | Decrease Lipoprotein Synthesis | | Increase Lipoprotein Catabolism | | |
| --- | --- | --- | --- | --- | --- |
| | Nicotinic Acid | Clofibrate | Cholestyramine | D-Thyroxine | Sitosterol |
| Primary indication | ↑VLDL, ↑ILDL** (Types III, IV, & V) | ↑ILDL (Type III) | ↑LDL (Type II) | ↑LDL (Type II) | ↑LDL (Type II) |
| Other indications | ↑LDL (Type II) | ↑VLDL (Types IV & V) | | ↑ILDL (Type III) | |
| Initial dose | 100 mg. t.i.d. | 1 g. b.i.d. | 8 g. b.i.d. | 2 mg. q.i.d. | 30 ml. b.i.d. |
| Maintenance dose | 1–3 g. t.i.d. | 1 g. b.i.d. | 8–16 g. b.i.d. | 4–8 mg. q.d. | 30 ml. q.i.d. |
| Major side effects | Flushing Pruritus Nausea Diarrhea | | Constipation Nausea | Mild hypermetabolism Angina and cardiac irritability in patients with heart disease | Nausea Diarrhea |
| Other side effects | Glucose intolerance Hyperuricemia Hepatotoxicity Cardiac arrhythmias | Cholelithiasis Cardiac arrhythmias Pulmonary embolism Thrombophlebitis Claudication | Hyperchloremic acidosis Steatorrhea | Glucose intolerance Neutropenia | |
| Drug interactions | | Warfarin sodium | | Warfarin sodium | |

*Abbreviations: q.d. represents every day, b.i.d. twice a day, t.i.d. 3 times a day, q.i.d. 4 times a day, ↑ increase.
**ILDL = intermediate low density lipoprotein of Type III.

that a national dietary prevention study in a free-living population as a means of testing the lipid hypothesis was not logistically feasible.[29, 30] The various concerns included the large size of the study population (24,000 to 115,000), projected expenditures of 0.5 to 1.0 billion dollars, confounding of the study by likely modifications of other risk factors, and skepticism about how much lipid-lowering would actually be achieved in that context.

The Lipid Research Clinics, in formulating their primary prevention study, opted for recruiting so-called high-risk male subjects with primary Type II hyperlipoproteinemia (entry cholesterol > 95th percentile) and, using cholestyramine, aimed to reduce the cholesterol by 20 to 25 per cent over the reduction achieved by a cholesterol-restricted diet. About 400,000 to 500,000 age-eligible males are being screened to provide the 3500 to 4500 subjects to be recruited into this study. A follow-up of 7 years is projected. These numbers require 12 collaborating clinics and appropriate support facilities, and stringent attention to standardization of subject observation and laboratory measurements.

## Partial Ileal Bypass

It is not disputed that partial ileal bypass is capable, in selected subjects, of effecting a substantial reduction in plasma cholesterol. Buchwald et al. reported an average fall of ~40 per cent in their and others' experience.[28] As Thompson and Gotto pointed out, although it has been used and may be effective in Types II, III, and IV hyperlipoproteinemia, partial ileal bypass would not be considered by most physicians for use in Types III and IV, since several effective dietary and/or drug regimens are available for their control.[31]

As discussed, Type II hyperlipoproteinemia is often responsive to diet therapy, supplemented when necessary by biliary sequestrants such as cholestyramine. The modes of action of partial ileal bypass and cholestyramine appear to be closely related, both principally affecting bile acid excretion and cholesterol absorption. Despite statements that partial ileal bypass may effect a greater reduction in cholesterol than cholestyramine, a claim that requires further evaluation, few would consider an operative procedure with its inevitable risk as the treatment of choice, at least until a trial of medical treatment had failed. One immediate postoperative death due to myocardial infarction and ten deaths 2 to 90 months after the operative procedure have been reported by Buchwald et al. in their series of 101 patients.[28] It has to be established to what extent the procedure heightens the risk of death in hypercholesterolemic subjects at high prior risk for CHD. While it is tempting in the abstract to seek as great a degree of lipid-lowering as possible, the widespread use of an operative procedure associated with some morbidity and mortality to achieve a further decrement in the lipid levels can hardly be routinely justified when it is not yet known whether cholesterol-lowering, whatever its extent, is of real benefit to the hyperlipidemic patient.

Like any treatment, partial ileal bypass is not without its known side effects and hazards. The full appreciation of the impact of these and the possibility of additional ones await the careful long-term follow-up of larger numbers of subjects than the present experience of about 160 cases, most concentrated in one center. We would agree with Thompson and Gotto that consideration of the use of this operation should be limited to young adult patients with severe heterozygous Type II hyperlipoproteinemia which has not adequately responded to appropriate diet and drug therapy or who are genuinely unable to tolerate the medical regimen.[31] These considerations merely emphasize that children, heterozygous for Type II, should not be considered for treatment.

## References

1. Fredrickson, D. S., Levy, R. I., and Lees, R. S.: Fat transport in lipoproteins – An integrated approach to mechanisms and disorders. New Engl. J. Med. 276:32–42, 94–103, 148–156, 215–225, 273–281, 1967.
2. Fredrickson, D. S., and Levy, R. I.: Familial hyperlipoproteinemia. In Stanbury, J. B., Wyngaarden, J. B., and Fredrickson, D. S. (eds.): Metabolic Basis of Inherited Disease. 3rd ed. New York, McGraw-Hill, 1972.
3. Brown, M. S., and Goldstein, J. L.: Familial hypercholesterolemia: Genetic, biochemical, and pathophysiological considerations. Adv. Intern. Med. 20:273, 1975.
4. Morganroth, J., Levy, R. I., and Fredrickson, D. S.: The biochemical, clinical and genetic features of Type III hyperlipoproteinemia. Ann. Intern. Med. 82:158, 1975.
5. Fredrickson, D. S., Morganroth, J., and Levy, R. I.: Type III hyperlipoproteinemia: An analysis of two contemporary definitions. Ann. Intern. Med. 82:150, 1975.
6. Kannel, W. B., Castelli, W. P., Gordon, T., et al.: Serum cholesterol, lipoproteins, and the risk of coronary heart disease. The Framingham Study. Ann. Intern. Med. 74:1, 1971.
7. Keys, A.: Coronary heart disease in seven countries. Circulation 41(Suppl. 1):211, 1970.
8. Carlson, L. A., and Böttiger, L. E.: Ischaemic heart disease in relation to fasting values of plasma triglycerides and cholesterol. Lancet 1:865, 1972.
9. Wilhelmsen, L., Wedel, H., and Tibblin, G.: Multivariate analysis of risk factors for coronary heart disease. Circulation 48:950, 1973.
10. Stone, N. J., Levy, R. I., Fredrickson, D. S., and Verter, J.: Coronary artery disease in 116 kindreds with familial Type II hyperlipoproteinemia. Circulation 49:476, 1974.
11. Cornfield, J., and Mitchell, S.: Selected risk factors in coronary disease. Possible intervention effects. Arch. Environ. Health 19:382, 1969.
12. Oliver, M. F., et al.: Ischemic heart disease: A secondary prevention trial using clofibrate. Br. Med. J. 4:775, 1971.
13. Arthur, J. B., et al.: Trial of clofibrate in the treatment of ischemic heart disease. Br. Med. J. 4:767, 1971.
14. The Coronary Drug Project. Clofibrate and niacin in coronary heart disease. J.A.M.A. 231:360, 1975.
15. The Coronary Drug Project. Initial findings leading to modifications of its research protocol. J.A.M.A. 214:1303, 1970.
16. The Coronary Drug Project. Findings leading to further modifications of its protocol with respect to dextrothyroxine. J.A.M.A. 220:996, 1972.
17. The Coronary Drug Project. Findings leading to discontinuation of the 2.5 mg/day estrogen group. J.A.M.A. 226:642, 1973.
18. Miettinen, M., Turpeinen, O., Karvonen, M. J., et al.: Effect of cholesterol-lowering diet on mortality from coronary heart disease and other causes. A twelve-year clinical trial in men and women. Lancet 1:835, 1972.
19. Cornfield, J., Halperin, M., and Mitchell, S.: Effect of diet on coronary heart disease mortality. Lancet 2:438, 1973.
20. Heady, J. A.: A cooperative trial on the primary prevention of ischaemic heart disease using clofibrate: Design, methods, and progress. Bull. W.H.O. 48:243, 1973.

21. Starzl, T. E., Chase, H. P., Putnam, C. W., and Porter, K. A.: Portacaval shunt in hyperlipo-proteinemia. Lancet 2:940, 1973.
22. Thompson, G. R., Lowenthal, R., and Myant, N. B.: Plasma exchange in the management of homozygous familial hypercholesterolemia. Lancet 1:1208, 1975.
23. Levy, R. I., Bonnell, M., and Ernst, N. D.: Dietary management of hyperlipoproteinemia. J. Am. Diet. Assoc. 58:406, 1971.
24. Fredrickson, D. S., Levy, R. I., Jones, E., et al.: *The Dietary Management of Hyperlipopro-teinemia: A Handbook for Physicians*. U.S. Dept. of Health, Education and Welfare, Public Health Service. Washington, D.C., U.S. Government Printing Office, 1970.
25. Levy, R. I., and Rifkind, B. M.: Lipid lowering drugs and hyperlipidaemia. Drugs 6:12, 1973.
26. Levy, R. I., Fredrickson, D. S., Shulman, R., et al.: Dietary and drug treatment of primary hyperlipoproteinemia. Ann. Intern. Med. 77:267, 1972.
27. Torsvik, H., Fischer, J. E., Feldman, H. A., and Lees, R. S.: Effects of intravenous hyperalimentation on plasma-lipoproteins in severe familial hypercholesterolaemia. Lancet 1:601, 1975.
28. Buchwald, H., Moore, R. B., and Varco, R. L.: Surgical treatment of hyperlipidemia. Circulation 49(Suppl. 1), 1974.
29. National Heart and Lung Institute Task Force on Arteriosclerosis. U.S. Dept. of Health, Education and Welfare, Public Health Service. Washington, D.C., U.S. Government Printing Office, 1971.
30. Report of the Diet-Heart Review Panel of the National Heart Institute: Mass field trials of the diet-heart question: Their significance, timeliness, feasibility and applicability. AHA Monograph #28, New York, American Heart Association, Inc., 1969.
31. Thompson, G. R., and Gotto, A. M.: Ileal bypass in the treatment of hyperlipoproteinaemia. Lancet 2:35, 1973.

# Partial Ileal Bypass Operation in the Management of the Hyperlipidemias

HENRY BUCHWALD

*University of Minnesota Health Sciences Center*

Remember that to change thy mind and to follow him that sets thee right, is to be none the less the free agent that thou wast before.

Marcus Aurelius, *Meditations* VIII, 16

I have been asked to discuss what has been termed a controversial subject: the role, if any, of partial ileal bypass surgery in the management of the hyperlipidemias. I enlisted no co-authors. My long-term associate, Richard L. Varco, is an editor of this book. I do not wish any of my other co-workers to be held responsible for these remarks.

Facts are eloquence in science. I will, therefore, attempt to synthesize the known positive data, draw attention to the negative correlations, and discuss what appear to me to be the unanswered questions in this field. I will cite published material, readily available for inspection and analysis by the critical reader. Thus, with regard to the issues, I do not envision any controversy.

## Fifteen Facts

### Plasma Cholesterol Levels Are Exponentially Proportional to Atherosclerosis Risk

The complications of atherosclerosis account for the majority of deaths in the industrial countries of the Western World.[1] Approximately 600,000

625

coronary deaths occur in the United States yearly, and the combined cardiac, cerebral, and peripheral atherosclerotic vascular deaths in the United States account for 54 per cent of the national death rate, exceeding the combined death rates from cancer, accidents, and all other causes.[2] From a review of 787 articles, Katz, Stamler, and Pick[3] concluded that there is a direct correlation, throughout the world, of the national incidence of atherosclerosis and the circulating cholesterol concentration. These retrospective analyses were confirmed by the prospective data of the Framingham,[4] Albany,[5] and Los Angeles[6] studies. At Framingham, Cornfield derived an equation relating atherosclerotic risk to an exponential power of the plasma cholesterol level.[7] These exponents were in the range of 3.0 to 5.0. There is less definitive, but still good, evidence to relate atherosclerotic risk to the plasma triglyceride level.[8]

On the basis of these data, efforts have been initiated in those nations with relatively high average values to reduce lipid levels, particularly in those individuals whose circulating lipid concentrations are well above the respective national age and sex mean. In the management of the hyperlipidemias, primary concern has been given to persons with demonstrable atherosclerotic cardiovascular disease, e.g., patients who have had a myocardial infarction. A more logical approach may consist of providing lipid-lowering programs for younger and presently asymptomatic hyperlipidemics who have not yet developed symptoms of atherosclerosis. (Note: Levy and Rifkind use the term hyperlipoproteinemia rather than hyperlipidemia, in part because such a classification may prove to reflect etiologic mechanisms accurately. The atherosclerosis correlation statistics, however, have been developed for cholesterol levels and not lipoprotein levels. I prefer to refer to the lipid moiety per se, without deprecating the value of the lipoprotein classification system.[9])

### Dietary Therapy Reduces Circulating Cholesterol Levels by 6 Per Cent Net

We have previously reviewed the most quoted dietary lipid modification trials.[10] In 16 of the better studies, encompassing 2516 patients — 1370 free-living and 1146 confined individuals — followed a total of 1,305,804 patient-months, an average cholesterol-lowering of 12.68 per cent was realized. If Leren's[11] recommendation to subtract from this gross value the percentage cholesterol reduction found in the controls (~6 per cent) is used, the net cholesterol-lowering is 6 per cent. Confined subjects generally do better (−16.5 per cent gross for B diet in the National Diet Heart Study[12]) than the free-living population subjected to the temptations of our lipotrophic culture (−10.8 per cent gross for B diet in the National Diet Heart Study[12]). Currently, multiple studies with data for triglyceride reduction by dietary means are not available.

### Drug Therapy Can Reduce Circulating Cholesterol by 0 to 25 Per Cent and Triglyceride Levels by 0 to 47 Per Cent

The review previously cited[10] analyzed the best available papers on lipid modification by a single drug and by polypharmacy.

The average plasma cholesterol reduction in 13 studies of cholestyramine therapy was 22.3 per cent gross and 24.2 per cent patient-number weighted (1415 patient-months' experience). In a double-blind trial, Levy[13] found a 23 per cent cholesterol-lowering on cholestyramine therapy subsequent and in addition to the cholesterol reduction achieved by a diet program. The triglyceride response to cholestyramine has been variable. Fallon and Woods[14] found no reduction of either triglyceride or cholesterol in six patients with Type IV and V lipoprotein patterns. Bressler et al.[15] reported a significant triglyceride-lowering in six of seven individuals with hypertriglyceridemia.

Clofibrate, today the most commonly used drug in the pharmaceutical lipid-lowering armamentarium, is a fair triglyceride-lowering drug but has a poor cholesterol-lowering effect. Cholesterol-lowering in the two more prevalent hyperlipoproteinemias (II and IV) is, at best, about 15 per cent, with a high percentage of nonresponders (nine-study review[10]). The response with respect to the plasma triglyceride concentration in four reported study groups has been better: −18 per cent (Type II),[16] −45 per cent (Type III),[16] −18 per cent,[17] and −47 per cent.[18] Levy and associates[16] documented the type-specific triglyceride results listed above with 13 patients in each group. They showed a concomitant cholesterol-lowering of 9 per cent in the Type II's and 38 per cent in the Type III's. There are few Type III individuals in this world, and in his published data, Levy has demonstrated less than a 10 per cent cholesterol-lowering in Type II's on clofibrate. These results were obtained under optimal conditions: the patients were subject to hospital confinement and were studied for only 3 weeks. The termination report of the Coronary Drug Project concluded that clofibrate resulted in a mean decrease in the cholesterol concentration of only 6.5 per cent and a mean triglyceride-lowering of 22.3 per cent.[19] These figures, especially that for cholesterol reduction, are unimpressive.

In six studies, representing 14,910 patient-months of follow-up, the mean decrease in plasma cholesterol by nicotinic acid therapy was 23 per cent gross and 25 per cent patient-weighted.[10] In the Coronary Drug Project, cholesterol-lowering by nicotinic acid yielded a mean decrease of 9.9 per cent (26.1 per cent decrease for triglycerides).[19]

It makes little sense to review the data for D-thyroxine or estrogens, agents whose toxicity forced an early break in the code of the Coronary Drug Project and the removal of these drugs from the protocol.[20, 21] There are few studies on the combined use of two or more hypolipidemic agents.[22]

## Partial Ileal Bypass Therapy Can Reduce Circulating Cholesterol by Greater than 40 Per Cent and Triglyceride Levels by Greater than 50 Per Cent After Maximum Dietary Therapy

Citation of our actual data can be found in the recent cumulative review of 10 years of clinical experience.[23] Also in that publication are references for 11 confirmatory studies by other investigators.

No patient is considered for partial ileal bypass until he has completed 3

months of a dietary program tailored for his hyperlipidemia type. For 114
consecutive, heterozygous, hyperlipidemic individuals, followed for a minimum of 3 months after partial ileal bypass and with a preoperative postdietary mean plasma cholesterol concentration of 359 mg. per 100 ml., the
sequential postoperative cholesterol reductions from the respective postdietary baselines were: 40.3 per cent (3 months, n = 114), 39.3 per cent (1 year,
n = 87), 37.0 per cent (2 years, n = 60), 39.9 per cent (3 years, n = 43), 40.1
per cent (4 years, n = 28), 38.3 per cent (5 years, n = 16), 33.8 per cent (6
years, n = 12), 33.8 per cent (7 years, n = 8), 38.9 per cent (8 years, n = 5),
and 38.7 per cent (9 years, n = 4). Thus, the cholesterol-lowering action of
partial ileal bypass appears to be lasting; cholesterol levels have not re-
bounded, and the average sustained reduction is calculated to be 41.1 per
cent (Figure 1). This marked cholesterol response has been documented in
all of the lipoprotein types (Figure 2).

In our three homogyzous Type II patients, the results have not been
nearly as good, with mean 1-year postoperative cholesterol reductions of 13,
21, and 20 per cent. Balfour and Kim,[24] however, have shown a 42 per cent
and a 33 per cent cholesterol-lowering response sustained for better than 3
years in two homozygous Type II children.

Our triglyceride data are not as extensive as our cholesterol data; nevertheless, the changes in the triglyceride concentration are as well-
documented (Figure 3).[23] In the Type IV abnormality, we have recorded a
52.6 per cent triglyceride reduction 1 year after bypass in comparison to the
preoperative but postdietary baseline. The response of the "mixed" type
(i.e., subjects having lipid characteristics of both Type II and Type IV) has
been −16.5 per cent; of the Type IIb patients −16.7 per cent; and of the

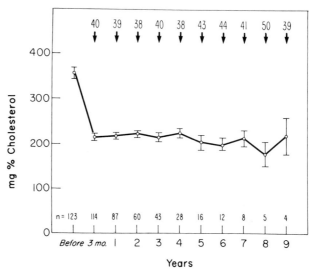

Figure 1.   Average plasma cholesterol concentrations before and after operation
(±1 SE), excluding the three homozygous Type II patients; number of patients at
each time interval given.

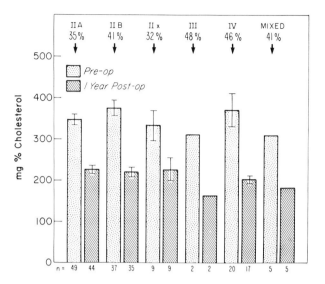

*Figure 2.* Average 1-year postoperative plasma cholesterol level response by lipoprotein type (± 1 SE); Type IIX = no triglyceride values before operation.

Type III−6 per cent. There has been a paradoxical triglyceride elevation of 21.2 per cent in the Type IIa individuals; however, the IIa postoperative triglyceride mean has remained within the accepted range of normal (<150 mg. per 100 ml.).

### *Partial Ileal Bypass Plus Diet Can Reduce Circulating Cholesterol By Greater Than 50 Per Cent (A Halving of the Pretreatment Value)*

In a cohort of 24 heterozygous Type II individuals, we demonstrated an 11 per cent mean cholesterol level reduction after 3 months on diet therapy

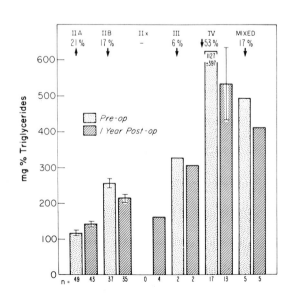

*Figure 3.* Average 1-year postoperative plasma triglyceride level response by lipoprotein type (± 1 SE); Type IIX = no triglyceride values before operation.

(423 mg. per 100 ml. to 379 mg. per 100 ml.). One year after partial ileal bypass, the mean cholesterol concentration for this group was 224 mg. per 100 ml., a 42 per cent greater lowering than after diet and 53 per cent down from the concentration existent prior to therapy.[23]

### Diet Therapy Morbidity, If Any, Is Minimal

Though Pearce and Dayton[25] have reported an increased incidence of gastrointestinal carcinoma in patients on a high intake of polyunsaturated fats, there are no data to support the presence of any danger in following the dietary prescriptions published for the hyperlipidemias by the National Heart and Lung Institute.[26]

### Drug Therapy Morbidity Is Considerable

The fewest drug side effects are associated with cholestyramine. There are no known complications following use of this bile acid–binding resin, though its potentiality for cholelithiasis induction has not been critically tested. The material is insoluble and must be taken in water or fruit juice three to four times daily; it is described as unpleasant to the taste by some individuals. Taken in adequate daily dosage, the drug can be associated with constipation, since bile acids are the body's natural cathartics.

The development of abnormal liver function[27] and myositis[28] have been described in association with the use of clofibrate. In addition, a significant increase in the incidence of thrombophlebitis and pulmonary embolization has been reported with the use of clofibrate, as well as an increase in the serum alkaline phosphatase, SGOT, CPK, and bilirubin, the development of cholelithiasis, breast tenderness, and a decreased libido.[19] The manufacturer warns physicians prescribing the drug that it potentiates Coumadin anticoagulants and causes nausea in 5 per cent of individuals on the medication.

The use of nicotinic acid has been limited by its predictable and rather potent side effects. Flushing of the skin occurs in nearly all patients initially started on therapy and persists in 10 to 15 per cent of individuals.[29] Other known side effects include an erythematous rash, pruritus, hyperpigmentation, gastrointestinal disturbances, hypertriglyceridemia, postural hypotension, and the more serious reactions of hyperuricemia and impairment of liver function, including jaundice.[29-31]

The complications of D-thyroxine have mediated against its greater use and, as previously stated, have led to its removal from the Coronary Drug Trial protocol.[20, 21] It can potentiate angina pectoris and arrhythmias, cause hypermetabolism, and even bring about functional hyperthyroidism.[29, 32-36] Estrogen therapy was demonstrated to cause feminization in men,[37] intravascular clotting,[38] and an increased frequency of sudden death.[39]

### The Mortality of Partial Ileal Bypass Has Been Less Than 1 Per Cent; The Morbidity Associated With This Procedure Has Been Minimal

To this time, our in-hospital mortality is 0.7 per cent.[10, 23] Our one immediate postoperative death occurred in a patient who had sustained three myocardial infarctions prior to his bypass and who died on the fourth postoperative day from his fourth infarction. No operative mortality associated with partial ileal bypass has been reported by other investigators.[40-47] Our late postoperative morbidity has been limited to four cases of bowel obstruction that necessitated operative intervention. Immediate in-hospital complications have consisted of minor wound problems (2 per cent), none of which prolonged hospitalization.

Diarrhea is the one unpleasant side effect of this operation; however, it has not been a significant or persistent problem in the majority of patients. On the basis of a patient survey taken 1 year after partial ileal bypass, 86 per cent of our patients had less than five bowel movements daily without the aid of bowel-controlling medications. Within 1 to 2 years, greater than 90 per cent of the patients experienced an increase in firmness and consistency of the stools. One patient, however, underwent operative restoration of bowel continuity elsewhere because of intractable diarrhea.[23] Helsingen and Rootwelt[41] report that postoperative diarrhea has been troublesome and has persisted for months or years. Sodal and associates[40] state that several of their patients were free of diarrhea after 2 to 10 months, whereas others displayed this symptom longer. Streuter[46] tends to regard postoperative bowel frequency as a minor and readily managed problem. The experience of Strisower[44] with respect to postoperative diarrhea is similar to our own. Brown[47] states that her patients have not had any difficulty controlling the number of stools. Miettinen[48] states that diarrhea has been a minor problem in his patients. Swan and McGowan[49] report that the postoperative diarrhea lessens with time and that they have been able to control it with medications to slow bowel transit time.

We have always instructed our patients to receive 1000 $\mu$g. of vitamin $B_{12}$ intramuscularly every 2 months for the rest of their lives, though $B_{12}$ absorptive capacity may be recovered in some individuals.[50, 51]

It is essential to differentiate the partial ileal bypass operation from the jejunoileal bypass performed in the management of morbid obesity. Partial ileal bypass does not cause nutrient malabsorption or significant weight loss. Neither is the partial bypass complicated by liver damage, establishment of a lithogenic bile, arthritic changes, or associated nephrolithiasis.

## Long-Term Acceptance of Dietary Therapy Has Been Documented To Be Poor

The difference in cholesterol response to dietary management in a free-living population versus a confined population has been cited; this difference is probably a result of subject compliance. Brown and Gren[52] calculated that, in order to achieve a reduction in plasma cholesterol concentration of 15 per cent or more, the saturated animal fat in the diet must be limited to no more than 25 g. per day. They concluded that this form of dietary management, although useful in the hospital setting, is usually not feasible for the nonhospitalized, healthy, active person who does not have the incentive of pain or physical disability. Difficulty with adherence to a dietary protocol in a prevention trial, in which repetitive reinforcement is offered by a physician, is likely to be amplified in lifelong, nontrial management, especially in asymptomatic individuals. Young individuals at work, in school, or at play will find it extremely difficult, if not at least occasionally impossible, to disregard the influence of their associates and the relative availability of less proper food products in order to follow a low-cholesterol, low–saturated fat dietary prescription.[52, 53]

### Long-Term Acceptance of Drug Therapy Is Difficult To Achieve

Clinicians know the problems inherent in maintaining certain individuals on a drug therapy program, even when discontinuation of the agent is associated with overt and distressing symptoms. Patient adherence to a drug regimen designed to affect a blood chemical abnormality over a lifetime may predictably become less than optimal. This failure to be faithful is even more likely if the side effects of the drug are annoying or distressing. The financial factor also is relevant (see below).

Furthermore, certain drugs are known to be associated with therapeutic escape, even under a supervised administration schedule. Levy and co-workers[16] have noted that, in the Type IV patients, discontinuation of clofibrate frequently resulted in "a marked rebound or overshoot of both triglycerides and cholesterol." The overshoot values were often considerably higher than control values, even though the patients were maintained on strict dietary management. In a later publication,[54] they again were cautious in their recommendation of clofibrate because of this rebound phenomenon.

### The Long-Term Effects of Partial Ileal Bypass Are Obligatory And Lasting

Over the last 12 years, the lipid-lowering effect of partial ileal bypass has been clinically documented as persistent.[23] It is reasonable to assume that it is lasting. The obligatory nature of this therapy can be critically important to the therapeutic result.

### The Cost of Dietary Therapy Is Reasonable

Except for the expense of low-fat meat products, a low-cholesterol, low-fat diet can be an economical one.

### The Current Cost Of Drug Therapy Is Formidable

Current prices of the average daily, weekly, monthly, and yearly consumption of therapeutically prescribed amounts of cholestyramine, clofibrate, and nicotinic acid are shown in Table 1. Thus, at current prices, 10 years of management by cholestyramine costs $6533, by clofibrate $1058, and by nicotinic acid $1168.

### An Operative Procedure Is A One-Time Expense

The average cost in the Midwest for a partial ileal bypass operation today, including hospitalization and professional fees, is about $2500.

TABLE 1. Current Cost of Drug Therapy

| Drug | Daily Dose | Cost | | | |
|------|-----------|------|------|------|------|
| | | *Daily* | *Weekly* | *Monthly* | *Yearly* |
| Cholestyramine | 24 g. | $1.79 | $12.53 | $54.45 | $653.35 |
| Clofibrate | 2 g. | .29 | 2.03 | 8.82 | 105.85 |
| Nicotinic acid | 4 g. | .32 | 2.24 | 9.73 | 116.80 |

### The Degree of Benefit Derived From Lipid Reduction May Be Positively Correlated with the Degree of Lipid Reduction Achieved

If the converse of the Cornfield equation[7] is valid, then a decrease in atherosclerotic risk is exponentially proportional to the degree of lowering of the plasma cholesterol. Using this equation (risk $\alpha$ [cholesterol]$^n$) with n = 2.7, a factual exponent in the Framingham study, we can calculate that a 15 per cent cholesterol reduction should yield a 35.5 per cent decrease in risk, a 20 per cent reduction 45.3 per cent lower risk, and a 50 per cent reduction an 84.6 per cent lower risk. Only combined partial ileal bypass and diet therapy can give a uniform and persistent cholesterol reduction greater than 50 per cent. By plotting Cornfield coordinates for the exponent 2.7 (that of middle-aged men in Framingham), the lethal risk from atherosclerosis in our partial ileal bypass series should have decreased from 2.75 times "normal" (i.e., of the Framingham men) before operation to 0.7 times normal risk after the procedure (Figure 4).

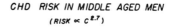

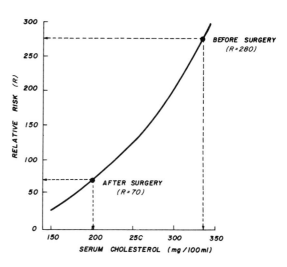

*Figure 4.* Risk of coronary heart disease in middle-aged men in the partial ileal bypass series plotted on the Cornfield coordinates.

## The Critical Unknowns

The positive correlation between atherosclerotic risk and the plasma cholesterol concentration has been fully substantiated by the handmaiden of modern science — statistics. It would seem to be a logical assumption that the converse of the lipid-atherosclerosis hypothesis, namely that cholesterol-lowering will reduce atherosclerotic risk, would be equally valid. Unfortunately, history has left us a legacy of apparently logical assumptions that subsequent investigations have proved to be riddled with fallacy.

There are substantial data showing that experimental atherosclerosis can be prevented, retarded, arrested, and reversed by cholesterol-lowering in animals, with some of the more convincing studies involving use of partial ileal bypass surgery.[55-65] Promising laboratory findings have stimulated the establishment of human studies. Though certain clinical reports[11, 66, 67] hint at amelioration of atherosclerosis after a reduction of the circulating cholesterol level, clearly we do not know the answers to the following questions: Does plasma cholesterol-lowering reduce atherosclerotic risk? Does plasma triglyceride-lowering reduce atherosclerotic risk? If the lowering of either, or both, of these lipid parameters influences risk, is a beneficial effect a function of the relative per cent lowering and/or the absolute postmanagement circulating cholesterol (triglyceride) concentration? Can favorable risk modification by lipid-lowering be brought about after the onset of manifest atherosclerotic disease (secondary prevention)? Can long-term risk be beneficially influenced before hemodynamically significant plaque deposition occurs (primary prevention)?

Investigators are attempting to find answers to some of these questions through scientific inquiry by clinical trials. The Coronary Drug Project showed that a 9.9 per cent cholesterol reduction and a 26.1 per cent triglyceride reduction by nicotinic acid in men aged 30 to 64 with one or more documented myocardial infarctions did not alter prognosis. The MRFIT study is an attempt to intervene primarily by modification of three risk factors: the plasma cholesterol, hypertension, and cigarette smoking. The Lipid Research Clinics represent a primary prevention trial of lipid modification by cholestyramine. And the Partial Ileal Bypass Program, which matches a control population against a diet plus operatively treated cohort, is currently funded for a secondary prevention trial. The climate of the times, which often demands therapy based on presumptive evidence prior to the availability of critical data, tragically may preclude completion of these trials before statistically sound end points are reached.

## References

1. Keys, A.: Coronary heart disease in seven countries. Circulation Suppl. *41*(I), 1970.
2. United States Department of Health, Education and Welfare, National Center for Health Statistics. Vital Statistics of the United States: 1968. Rockville, Maryland, Government Printing Office, 1971, p. 7.

3. Katz, L. N., Stamler, J., and Pick, R.: *Nutrition and Atherosclerosis*. Philadelphia, Lea and Febiger, 1958.
4. Dawber, T. R., Moore, F. E., and Mann, G. V.: Coronary heart disease in the Framingham study. Am. J. Publ. Health 47(II):4, 1957.
5. Doyle, J. T., Heslin, A. S., Hilleboe, H. E., Formel, P. F., and Korns, R. F.: A prospective study of degenerative cardiovascular disease in Albany: Report of three years' experience. I. Ischemic heart disease. Am. J. Publ. Health 47(II):25, 1957.
6. Chapman, J. M., Goerke, L. S., Dixon, W., Loveland, D. B., and Phillips, E.: The clinical status of a population group in Los Angeles under observation for two to three years. Am. J. Publ. Health 47(II):33, 1957.
7. Cornfield, J.: Joint dependence of risk of coronary heart disease on serum cholesterol and systolic blood pressure: Discriminant function analysis. Fed. Proc. 21:58, 1962.
8. Albrink, M. J., and Mann, E. B.: Serum triglycerides in coronary artery disease. Arch. Intern. Med. 103:4, 1959.
9. Fredrickson, D. S., Levy, R. I., and Lees, R. S.: Fat transport in lipoproteins: An integrated approach to mechanisms and disorders. New Engl. J. Med. 276:32,94,148,215,273, 1967.
10. Buchwald, H., Moore, R. B., and Varco, R. L.: Surgical treatment of hyperlipidemia. Circulation 49(Suppl. 1):122, 1974.
11. Leren, P.: The effect of plasma cholesterol-lowering diet in male survivors of myocardial infarction. Bull. N.Y. Acad. Med. 44:1012, 1968.
12. National Diet Heart Study. Circulation 37(Suppl. 1), 1968.
13. Levy, R. I.: Dietary and drug treatment of primary hyperlipoproteinemia. Ann. Intern. Med. 77:267, 1972.
14. Fallon, H. J., and Woods, J. W.: Response of hyperlipoproteinemia to cholestyramine resin. J.A.M.A. 204:1161, 1968.
15. Bressler, R., Nowlin, J., and Bogdonoff, M. D.: Treatment of hypercholesterolemia and hypertriglyceridemia by anion exchange resin. South. Med. J. 59:1097, 1966.
16. Levy, R. I., Quarfardt, S. H., and Brown, W. V.: The efficacy of clofibrate (CPIB) in familial hyperlipoproteinemias. Adv. Exp. Med. Biol. 4:377, 1969.
17. Jepson, E. M., Fahmy, M. F. I., Torrens, P. E., and Billimoria, J. D.: Treatment of essential hyperlipidaemia. Lancet 2:1315, 1969.
18. Krasno, L. R., and Kidera, G. J.: Clofibrate in coronary heart disease: Effect on morbidity and mortality. J.A.M.A. 219:845, 1972.
19. The Coronary Drug Project: Clofibrate and niacin in coronary heart disease. J.A.M.A. 231:360, 1975.
20. Special communication: Coronary Drug Project. Initial findings leading to modifications of its research protocol. J.A.M.A. 214:1303, 1970.
21. Special communication: Coronary Drug Project. Findings leading to further modifications of its protocol with respect to D-thyroxine. J.A.M.A. 220:996, 1972.
22. Levy, R. I., and Rifkind, B. M.: Diagnosis and management of hyperlipoproteinemia in infants and children. Am. J. Cardiol. 31:547, 1973.
23. Buchwald, H., Moore, R. B., and Varco, R. L.: Ten years' clinical experience with partial ileal bypass in management of the hyperlipidemias. Ann. Surg. 180:384, 1974.
24. Balfour, J. F., and Kim, R.: Homozygous type II hyperlipoproteinemia treatment, partial ileal bypass in two children. J.A.M.A. 227:1145, 1974.
25. Pearce, M. L., and Dayton, S.: Incidence of cancer in men on a diet high in polyunsaturated fat. Lancet 1:464, 1971.
26. National Heart and Lung Institute Diet Manuals, Bethesda, Maryland, 1973.
27. Symposium on Atromid: Proceeding of a conference held in Buxton (England), June 5–6, 1963. J. Atheroscler. Res. 3:341, 1963.
28. Langer, T., and Levy, R. I.: Acute muscular syndrome associated with administration of clofibrate. New Engl. J. Med. 279:856, 1968.
29. Eder, H. A.: Drugs used in the prevention and treatment of atherosclerosis. *In* Goodman, L. S., and Gilman, A. (eds.): *The Pharmacological Basis of Therapeutics*. 3rd ed. New York, Macmillan Company, 1965, p. 754.
30. Berge, K. G., Achor, R. W. P., Christensen, N. A., Mason, H. L., and Barker, N. W.: Hypercholesteremia and nicotonic acid: A long-term study. Am. J. Med. 31:24, 1961.
31. Parsons, W. B., Jr.: Studies of nicotinic acid use in hypercholesterolemia, changes in hepatic function, carbohydrate tolerance, and uric acid metabolism. Arch. Intern. Med. 107:653, 1961.
32. Drugs which lower the blood lipids. Med. Lett. Drugs Ther. 5:81, 1963.
33. Steinberg, D.: Chemotherapeutic control of serum lipid levels. Trans. N.Y. Acad. Sci. 24:704, 1962.

34. Eisalo, A., Ahrenberg, P., Nikkila, E. A.: Treatment of hyperlipidemia with D-thyroxine. Acta. Med. Scand. *173*:639, 1963.
35. Boyd, G. S., and Oliver, M. F.: Effect of certain thyroxine analogues on the serum lipids in human subjects. J. Endocrinol. *21*:33, 1960.
36. Mishkel, M. A.: Diagnosis and management of the patient with xanthomatosis: An experience with thirty-five cases. Quart. J. Med. *36*:107, 1967.
37. Russ, E. M., Eder, H. A., and Barr, D. P.: Influence of gonadal hormones on protein-lipid relationships in human plasma. Am. J. Med. *19*:4, 1955.
38. Jeffcoate, T. N. A., Miller, J., Roos, R. F., and Tindall, V. R.: Puerperal thromboembolism in relation to the inhibition of lactation by oestrogen therapy. Br. Med. J. 3:19, 1968.
39. Stamler, J., Pick, R., Katz, L. N., Pick, A., Kaplan, B. M., Berkson, D. M., and Century, D.: Effectiveness of estrogens for therapy of myocardial infarction in middle-age men. J.A.M.A. *183*:632, 1963.
40. Sodal, G., Gjertsen, K. T., and Schrumpf, A.: Surgical treatment of hypercholesterolemia. Acta. Chir. Scand. *136*:671, 1970.
41. Helsinger, N., Jr., and Rootwelt, K.: Partial ileal bypass for surgical treatment of hypercholesterolemia. Nord. Med. *82*:1409, 1969.
42. Miettinen, T.: Commentary. *In* Jones, R. J. (ed.): *Proceedings of the Second International Symposium on Atherosclerosis.* New York, Springer-Verlag, 1970, p. 304.
43. Rowe, G. G., Young, W. P., and Wasserburger, R. H.: The effect of reduced serum cholesterol on human coronary atherosclerosis. Circulation *40*(III):22, 1969.
44. Strisower, E. H., Kradjian, R., Nichols, A. V., Coggiola, E., and Tsai, J.: Effect of ileal bypass on serum lipoproteins in essential hypercholesterolemia. J. Atheroscler. Res. 8:525, 1968.
45. Fritz, S. H., and Walker, W. J.: Ileal bypass in the control of intractable hypercholesterolemia. Am. Surg. *32*:691, 1966.
46. Streuter, M.: Personal communication.
47. Brown, H. B.: Personal communication.
48. Miettinen, T.: Personal communication.
49. Swan, D. M., and McGowan, J. M.: Ileal bypass in hypercholesterolemia associated with coronary heart disease. Am. J. Surg. *116*:22, 1968.
50. Nygaard, K., Helsinger, N., and Rootwelt, K.: Adaptation of vitamin $B_{12}$ absorption after ileal bypass. Scand. J. Gastroenterol. 5:349, 1970.
51. Coyle, J. J., Varco, R. L., and Buchwald, H.: In preparation.
52. Brown, H. B., and Greene, J. G.: Diets suitable for reduction of serum cholesterol levels. The Cleveland Clinic Dietary Research Project. Cleveland Clin. Quart. 29:101, 1962.
53. Lewis, L. A., Brown, H. B., and Page, I.: Ten years' dietary treatment of primary hyperlipidemia. Geriatrics 25:64, 1970.
54. Levy, R. I., and Fredrickson, D. S.: The current status of hypolipidemic drugs. Postgrad. Med. *47*:130, 1970.
55. Buchwald, H.: The effect of ileal bypass on atherosclerosis and hypercholesterolemia in the rabbit. Surgery 58:22, 1965.
56. Buchwald, H., Bertish, J., and Moore, R. B.: Ileal bypass in the infant rabbit with pediatric clinical findings. Surg. Forum *20*:394 1969.
57. Buchwald, H., Moore, R. B., Bertish, J., and Varco, R. L.: Effect of ileal bypass on cholesterol levels, atherosclerosis and growth in the infant rabbit. Ann. Surg. *175*:311, 1972.
58. Okuboye, J. A., Ferguson, C. C., and Wyatt, J. P.: The effect of ileal bypass on dietary induced atherosclerosis in the rabbit. Can. J. Surg. *11*:69, 1968.
59. Scott, H. W., Jr., Stephenson, S. E., Jr., Younger, R., Carlisle, R. B., and Turney, S. W.: Prevention of experimental atherosclerosis by ileal bypass: Twenty-percent cholesterol diet and I-[131] induced hypothyroidism in dogs. Ann. Surg. *163*:795, 1966.
60. Scott, H. W., Jr., Stephenson, S. E., Jr., Younger, R., Hayes, C. W., Welborn, M. B., and Robbins, L. B.: Effects of distal intestinal bypass and other gastrointestinal operations on experimental hypercholesterolemia and atherosclerosis. Am. J. Surg. *115*:605, 1968.
61. Frost, J. W., Finch, W. T., Younger, R., Butts, W. H., and Scott, H. W., Jr.: Pilot study of the therapeutic effects of ileal bypass in dogs with experimentally established hypercholesterolemia and atherosclerosis. Surg. Forum *21*:398, 1970.
62. Shepard, G. H., Wimberly, J. E., Younger, R. K., Stephenson, S. E., Jr., and Scott, H. W., Jr.: Effects of bypass of the distal third of the small intestine on experimental hypercholesterolemia and atherosclerosis in rhesus monkeys. Surg. Forum *19*:302, 1968.
63. Scott, H. W., Jr., Stephenson, S. E., Jr., Hayes, C. W., and Younger, R. K.: Effects of bypass of the distal fourth of small intestine on experimental hypercholesterolemia and atherosclerosis in rhesus monkeys. Surg. Gynecol. Obstet. *125*:3, 1967.

64. Younger, R. K., Shepard, G. H., Butts, W. H., and Scott, H. W., Jr.: Comparison of the protective effects of cholestyramine and ileal bypass in rhesus monkeys on an atherogenic regimen. Surg. Forum 20:101, 1969.
65. Gomes, M. M., Kottke, B. A., Bernatz, P., and Titus, J. L.: Effect of ileal bypass on aortic atherosclerosis of white carneau pigeons. Surgery 70:353, 1971.
66. Rinzler, S. H.: Primary prevention of coronary heart disease by diet. Bull. N.Y. Acad. Med. 44:936, 1968.
67. Bierenbaum, M. L., Fleischman, A. I., Green, D. P., Raichelson, R. I., Hayton, T., Watson, P. B., and Caldwell, A. B.: The five year experience of modified fat diets on younger men with coronary heart disease. Circulation 42:943, 1970.

# 28

# Staging for Hodgkin's Disease and Malignant Lymphomas

HODGKIN'S DISEASE—THE
LAPAROTOMY-SPLENECTOMY
CONTROVERSY
  *by Mortimer J. Lacher*

THE RATIONALE FOR
"SELECTIVE" STAGING
LAPAROTOMY IN HODGKIN'S
DISEASE AND THE MALIGNANT
LYMPHOMAS
  *by Ralph E. Johnson*

## Statement of the Problem

*The issue concerns those circumstances in which a patient with a diagnosed lymphoma should undergo staging laparotomy. The yield, morbidity, and clinical rewards of the procedure are examined and data analyzed.*

*Evaluate the contribution made by the operative staging procedure as a function of the histologic-type Hodgkin's disease versus other malignant lymphomas. Does location of known involvement—groin versus neck—alter the value of staging?*

*Assess data regarding morbidity of operative staging.*

*Summarize and analyze data comparing clinical staging with operative staging.*

*Analyze the contribution made by operative staging to planning by the radiotherapist. If the radiotherapist uses total body nodal radiation for treatment, what case can be made for staging? Cite data regarding "sterilization" of an involved spleen by radiation. Discuss other visceral injury with splenic irradiation.*

*Discuss data indicating that splenectomy leads to enhanced tolerance to chemotherapeutic agents.*

# Hodgkin's Disease – The Laparotomy-Splenectomy Controversy

MORTIMER J. LACHER

*Memorial Sloan-Kettering Cancer Center*

## Introduction

Although staging laparotomy-splenectomy for patients with Hodgkin's disease has been under intense investigation since 1967, oncologists are still in a position of indecisiveness regarding its true usefulness. I have no doubts regarding the usefulness of staging laparotomy-splenectomy as a diagnostic tool.[16] In 1975 the weight of data is so heavy as to preclude any but minor differences among investigators with regard to staging laparotomy-splenectomy as a valuable procedure for precise delineation of intra-abdominal sites of involvement in patients with Hodgkin's disease.

Therefore, there is at least one conclusion that everyone can agree upon – namely, that the staging laparotomy-splenectomy procedure does more precisely outline the true extent of the Hodgkin's disease both prior to treatment and after treatment as part of a "second look" exercise. Reasonably accurate evaluation of the liver or spleen can only be accomplished by actual liver biopsy and splenectomy. Peritoneoscopy is no substitute for splenectomy.[10] Preoperative evaluations of liver and spleen are inaccurate. Of this there is no doubt, as can be attested in many of the references listed at the end of this article.

What, then, are the problems or the controversy, if you will, at this time? They are as follows: The major operative undertaking known as the staging laparotomy-splenectomy (which in females may include transposition of the ovaries) is technically tedious, complex, and potentially dangerous. If it has been decided to treat all patients with extensive radiation therapy and chemotherapy, no matter what the stage (anatomic extent of disease), then precise delineation of the extent of the Hodgkin's tumor below the dia-

641

phragm becomes immaterial. The operative effort then poses a needless immediate risk to the patient and possibly a potential future hazard. In children (aged 15 and under), especially, splenectomy, with its attendant risk of future serious and potentially fatal infections,[8, 30, 35] probably should be abandoned. In adults, the risk of infection after splenectomy appears to be unchanged.[6, 8, 11, 14, 38]

In adults, if there is no intent to "individualize" therapy for Stage I and Stage II patients as opposed to Stage III and Stage IV patients, or if one can decide on a therapeutic program without knowledge of the true state of the spleen and liver, then the staging laparotomy-splenectomy is truly useless. On the other hand, if the treatment program clearly delineates a course of lesser therapy for patients with disease limited to areas above the diaphragm, the laparotomy-splenectomy procedure is indispensible. In addition, splenectomy in adults may have therapeutic implications associated with prolonged survival. Until this issue is clarified, controversy and continued investigation must persist.

## A Historical Perspective

How did we get to this position? By 1969 the first published data of the Stanford group regarding initial staging laparotomy-splenectomy as well as post-therapy laparotomy clearly revealed previously unrecognized important facts.[12]

The staging laparotomy-splenectomy procedure, which also included liver biopsy and extensive node sampling, definitely improved our knowledge of the precise delineation of the intra-abdominal sites of Hodgkin's disease. The preoperative techniques for evaluation of the liver and spleen were shown to be frequently misleading and inaccurate. Interpretation of lymphangiography, on the other hand, had a high level of accuracy.[7, 12, 13, 24] This was true for patients who had been intensely treated as well as for those who had not yet received any therapy. Since the published work of Glatstein et al.[12] in 1969 of two "selected" groups of patients (37 previously untreated patients with Hodgkin's disease and 28 previously treated patients), no study has significantly changed their astute conclusions:

1. "Although the lymphangiogram has been an invaluable diagnostic tool for the detection of previously occult abdominal disease, it is not infallible." Furthermore, "... it should be stressed that the operative findings in general did confirm the [lymphangiographic] radiographic interpretations. . . ."

2. "It is disheartening to see how unreliable routine liver function studies have been for the detection of liver involvement. Laparotomy and wedge biopsy have provided much more reliable information about the status of the liver. Yet even liver biopsy, whether by the open wedge technique or the percutaneous needle technique, is not immune from sampling errors."

3. The inability to assess accurately the spleen prior to operation was also revealed. "Clinically palpable spleens in untreated patients were histologically involved by Hodgkin's disease in 13 of 17 cases (67%) but it is noteworthy that an almost equally high proportion were involved when the spleen was not palpated (10 of 20)."

A special bonus was achieved because "laparotomy and splenectomy also greatly simplify the administration of radiotherapy to the abdomen. With the spleen removed and the stump of the splenic pedicle identifiable radiographically by virtue of a surgically placed silver clip, it becomes possible to irradiate the nodes along the splenic pedicle with the left lower lobe of the lung and almost all of the upper half of the left kidney shielded." In addition, it was noted that none of the splenectomized patients to whom extended field radiotherapy had been administered required interruption of treatment because of thrombocytopenia, leukopenia, or anemia.

## Strengths and Weaknesses of the Staging Laparotomy

Simply stated, the lymphangiogram is usually interpreted accurately, but both false-negative and false-positive lymphangiograms have been demonstrated by laparotomy.[13] The lymphangiogram technique itself outlines only a limited group of lymph nodes. The mesenteric nodes and nodes in the porta hepatis and above the celiac axis cannot be evaluated preoperatively, as they are "not seen" on routine bipedal lymphangiography.

The operative sampling of lymph nodes, on the other hand, is not infallible, and much depends on the individuals who are doing the procedure, as well as on the individual problems of anatomic variation encountered from patient to patient. In the hands of the casual operator (working in some instances without a preoperative lymphangiogram) who fails to explore adequately the retroperitoneal space, to perform the necessary wedge biopsies of the liver, and who in some instances even avoids splenectomy, the procedure becomes meaningless.

Liver function studies, particularly at the time of the initial diagnosis of Hodgkin's disease, are especially misleading.[7, 10, 12, 36, 37, 39] Even after extensive histologic examination, interpretation of the liver biopsy material may still be confusing, but liver biopsy material is definitely more accurate than either biochemical liver function studies or isotope imaging.[20]

The spleen is involved in an inordinately high proportion of patients whose preoperative assessment would have led us to believe that it was free of disease.[7, 12, 19, 36, 37, 41, 42] In fact, the most convincing argument for the staging laparotomy has come from the results of the data collected by isotope imaging, by which almost 50 per cent of spleens (in one cooperative study) initially interpreted as clinically "negative" were actually shown to be involved with Hodgkin's disease after splenectomy and histologic evaluation.[19]

## *Precise Staging is Necessary Only if it Alters the Therapeutic Approach*

Accepting the conclusion that the laparotomy-splenectomy is indispensible for accurate staging, why do we have a persistent controversy regarding its value? The answer is quite simple. Although no new diagnostic technique has supplanted "operative" staging, new therapeutic concepts and techniques have intervened over the past 8 years to force us all to question seriously the value of precise staging.

If the choice is to "undertreat" with the use of precisely limited radiation therapy fields and to avoid the use of postradiation multidrug chemotherapy, then every effort must be made to delineate the true anatomic extent of the disease. On the basis of the currently available data, it can be stated that, among the clinical Stage II patients with disease presumably limited to the area above the diaphragm (but in at least two loci, such as the left neck and mediastinum), about one-fourth will actually have Hodgkin's tumor in the spleen.[1, 7, 12, 15, 21, 23, 24, 27, 32, 33, 34, 37, 40] In about 50 per cent of the patients presumed to be in Stage III or Stage IV (liver), the actual stage after laparotomy is reduced to a lesser Stage (i.e., Stage III to II, Stage IV to III or II).[21, 23, 24, 32]

The clinical Stage I patient, however, usually remains in the category after staging laparotomy, with only about 10 per cent (or less) of these patients recategorized to a higher stage.[23, 24, 32]

The therapeutic manipulation forced by the change in stage as a consequence of the laparotomy-splenectomy procedure has become the actual focal point for debate and controversy. In addition, Johnson's view[18] that radiation treatment, in the case of the "normal size" spleen, is *not* facilitated by splenic removal is another side issue in the current controversy.

Some groups have taken the view that the staging laparotomy does alter their therapeutic approach in at least one-third of the patients,[9, 15, 21, 27, 31, 33] and therefore accurate staging is crucial to the success of their program. Others have decided that radiation therapy to a "mantle" field covering the cervical and axillary nodes and the mediastinum, as well as to the upper abdomen (with or without chemotherapy), is sufficient for the nonoperated, clinical Stage I or Stage II patient.[18, 25] Still others have shown that radiation therapy followed by multiple drug chemotherapy in laparotomy-splenectomized patients results in more and prolonged relapse-free intervals.[28] This range of choices, in the absence of any long-term follow-up data, makes it difficult to choose a generally acceptable pathway without letting emotion lead the way.

One more intriguing issue has emerged from the unpublished data of a cooperative Hodgkin's disease study group.[16, 25] In that study, Stage I and Stage II patients after splenectomy (staging laparotomy) have a significantly better survival than an equivalent series of clinical Stage I and II patients treated in exactly the same fashion but with spleens intact. Interpretation of this phenomenon is not clear, and it has been the subject of much controversy. Nonetheless, it has been suggested that this effect is not related to better selection of cases through splenectomy but is in some way related to the splenectomy as a therapeutic procedure. Data of this nature force us to continue to consider splenectomy as part of the initial treatment of all patients with Hodgkin's disease.

## Summary

One can summarize some of the current policies and positions and their consequences as follows:

1. The laparotomy-splenectomy procedure does delineate disease more accurately than do current nonoperative techniques. In addition, splenectomy may be therapeutically advantageous.

2. Limiting laparotomy-splenectomy to patients with clinical Stage III and Stage IV disease ignores those patients in clinical Stage II whose actual anatomic Stage would be increased after laparotomy-splenectomy and who probably should receive chemotherapy with or without more extensive radiation therapy.[43] Those in clinical Stage I, without laparotomy-splenectomy, would tend to be overtreated. The consequences of this "overtreatment" should not be underestimated.[4, 5, 9]

3. If the correct therapeutic approach is unique to each stage, then the laparotomy-splenectomy is indispensible, because there is no other way to achieve acceptable staging accuracy. This is the position held by Hellman[15, 33] and others,[7, 21, 27, 31, 34, 40] and their view implies that staging changes the treatment protocol for at least one-third of the patients.

4. Others have reverted to the historical posture of the curative capacity of "radical radiotherapy" and have accepted Johnson's view that splenic radiation therapy is relatively easy and successful. For these therapists, splenectomy is immaterial. "Radical radiotherapy" is sufficient. It seems that we have come too far not to recognize that, if the original concepts of the "curative" nature of radical radiotherapy prevailed, there would be no relapses, no need for staging splenectomy, no need for post-treatment laparotomy, etc. Treating patients with "potential" tumor below the diaphragm only with extensive radiation therapy and failing to combine radiation therapy with chemotherapy merely retraces historical experience with its known record of relapse.

5. There is the probability that laparotomy-splenectomy will be dispensed with if one follows a therapeutic course of radiation therapy followed by multidrug chemotherapy, or if the treatment is chemotherapy alone. The only seriously disadvantaged patient would be the clinical Stage I patient. This patient might be considered overtreated if intense and extensive radiation and chemotherapy are used.

## A Proposal for Future Study

Since we now have a large historical base of intensely evaluated, meticulously treated, and carefully followed patients (The Cooperative Hodgkin's

Study Group)[16, 25] in which we can readily compare Stage "I" and Stage "II" patients with and without splenectomy, treated with involved field and extended field radiation therapy, it may be worthwhile to treat similar groups with the addition of at least 6 months of multidrug therapy.

For instance, let us compare patients carefully staged by laparotomy-splenectomy followed by involved field or extended field radiation therapy plus 6 months of chemotherapy with nonsplenectomized patients treated with involved field or extended field radiation therapy plus 6 months of multidrug chemotherapy. In that way we may be able to decide between lesser and more complex therapies to determine which is most advantageous for the patient.

Finally, it must be stated that, as the chemotherapeutic techniques continue to improve, the need for compulsive, accurate staging will disappear. The staging laparotomy controversy will then fade into the history of medicine and will be noted only as a milestone marker on the road to a more complete knowledge of the "unnatural" history of Hodgkin's disease, disrupted in so many ways by our calculated interventions.

## References

1. Aisenberg, A. C.: Editorial note: Hematogenous dissemination of Hodgkin's disease. Ann. Intern. Med. 77:810, 1972.
2. Aisenberg, A. C., Goldman, J. M., Raker, J. W., and Wang, C. C.: Spleen involvement at the onset of Hodgkin's disease. Ann. Intern. Med. 74:544, 1971.
3. Allen, L. W., and Ultmann, J. E.: Laparotomy and splenectomy in staging of Hodgkin's disease (abstract). Clin. Res. 18:398, 1970.
4. Al-Mondhiry, H., and Lacher, M. J.: Hodgkin's disease and leukemia. In Hodgkin's Disease. New York, J. Wiley & Sons, 1976.
5. Arseneau, J. C., Sponzo, R. W., and Levin, D. L.: Nonlymphomatous malignant tumors complicating Hodgkin's disease. New Engl. J. Med. 42:1119, 1972.
6. Cooper, I. A., Ironside, P. N. J., Madigan, J. P., Morris, P. J., and Ewing, M. R.: The role of splenectomy in the management of advanced Hodgkin's disease. Cancer 34:408, 1974.
7. Desser, R. K., Moran, E. M., and Ultmann, J. E.: Staging Hodgkin's disease and lymphoma: Diagnostic procedures including staging laparotomy and splenectomy. Med. Clin. North Am. 57:479, 1973.
8. Desser, R. K., and Ultmann, J. E.: Risk of severe infection in patients with Hodgkin's disease or lymphoma after diagnostic laparotomy and splenectomy. Ann. Intern. Med. 77:143, 1972.
9. DeVita, V. T., Jr., and Carbone, P. P.: Chemotherapeutic implications of staging in Hodgkin's disease. Cancer Res. 31:1838, 1971.
10. DeVita, V. T., Bagley, C. M., Jr., Goodell, B., O'Kieffe, D. A., and Trujillo, N. P.: Peritoneoscopy in the staging of Hodgkin's disease. Cancer Res. 31:1746, 1971.
11. Donaldson, S. S., Moore, M. R., Rosenberg, S. A., and Vosti, K. L.: Characterization of postsplenectomy bacteremia among patients with and without lymphoma. New Engl. J. Med. 287:69, 1972.
12. Glatstein, E., Guernsey, J. M., Rosenberg, S. A., and Kaplan, H. S.: The value of laparotomy and splenectomy in the staging of Hodgkin's disease. Cancer 24:709, 1969.
13. Glatstein, E., Trueblod, H. W., Enright, L. P., Rosenberg, S. A., and Kaplan, H. S.: Surgical staging of abdominal involvement in unselected patients with Hodgkin's disease. Radiology 97:425, 1970.
14. Goffinet, D. R., Glatstein, E. J., and Merigan, T. C.: Herpes zoster–varicella infections and lymphoma. Ann. Intern. Med. 76:235, 1972.
15. Hellman, S.: Current studies in Hodgkin's disease. What laparotomy has wrought. New Engl. J. Med. 290:894, 1974.
16. Hutchison, G. B.: Personal communication, Cooperative Hodgkin's Disease Study.

17. Ingelfinger, F. J.: Editorial: The fraudulent we. New Engl. J. Med. 285:1144, 1971.
18. Johnson, R. E.: Is staging laparotomy routinely indicated in Hodgkin's disease? Ann. Intern. Med. 75:459, 1971.
19. Johnston, G., Benua, R. S., Teates, C. D., Edwards, C. L., and Kniseley, R. M.: [67]Ga-citrate imaging in untreated Hodgkin's disease. Preliminary report of cooperative group. J. Nucl. Med. 15:399, 1974.
20. Kadin, M. E., Glatstein, E., and Dorfman, R. F.: Clinicopathologic studies of 117 untreated patients subjected to laparotomy for the staging of Hodgkin's disease. Cancer 27:1277, 1971.
21. Kirschner, R. H., O'Connell, M. J., Sutherland, J. C., et al.: Baltimore Cancer Research Center Public Health Service Hospital, Baltimore. Letter to the Editor. J.A.M.A. 225:635, 1973.
22. Lacher, M. J.: Laparotomy and splenectomy in Hodgkin's disease. Hosp. Pract. Aug., 1971, pp. 87–100.
23. Lacher, M. J., Paglia, M. A., Hertz, R. E., et al.: Staging laparotomy and splenectomy in Hodgkin's disease. MSKCC-Clin. Bull. 3:43, 1973.
24. Lacher, M. J.: Results of staging laparotomy (Memorial Hospital 1969–1972). Unpublished data.
25. Lee, B. J., and Nisce, L.: Personal communication.
26. Lowenbraun, S., Ramsey, J., Sutherland, J., and Serpick, A.: Diagnostic laparotomy and splenectomy for staging Hodgkin's disease. Ann. Intern. Med. 72:655, 1970.
27. Mitchell, R. I., Peters, M. V., Brown, T. C., and Rideout, D.: Laparotomy for Hodgkin's disease. Some surgical observations. Surgery 71:694, 1972.
28. Moore, M. R., Bull, J. M., Jones, J. E., et al.: Sequential radiotherapy and chemotherapy in the treatment of Hodgkin's disease. Ann. Intern. Med. 77:1, 1972.
29. Nahhas, W. A., Nisce, L. Z., D'Angio, G. J., and Lewis, J. L., Jr.: Lateral ovarian transposition. Obstet. Gynecol. 38:785, 1971.
30. Nixon, D. W., and Aisenberg, A. C.: Fatal Hemophilus influenzae sepsis in an asymptomatic splenectomized Hodgkin's disease patient. Ann. Intern. Med. 77:69, 1972.
31. O'Connell, M., Sklansky, D., Green, W., Abt, A., Kirschner, R., Ramsey, H., Murphy, L., and Wiernik, P.: Routine staging laparotomy in the management of Hodgkin's disease (abstract). Clin. Res. 21:562, 1973.
32. Paglia, M. A., Lacher, M. J., Hertz, R. E., et al.: Surgical aspects and results of laparotomy and splenectomy in Hodgkin's disease. Am. J. Roentgenol. Radium Ther. Nucl. Med. 117:12, 1973.
33. Piro, A. J., Hellman, S., and Moloney, W. C.: The influence of laparotomy on management decisions in Hodgkin's disease. Arch. Intern. Med. 130:844, 1972.
34. Prosnitz, L. R., Nuland, S. B., and Kligerman, M. M.: Role of laparotomy and splenectomy in the management of Hodgkin's disease. Cancer 29:44, 1972.
35. Ravry, M., Maldonado, N., Velez-Garcia, E., Montalvo, J., and Santiago, P. J.: Serious infection after splenectomy for the staging of Hodgkin's disease. Ann. Intern. Med. 77:11, 1972.
36. Rosenberg, S. A.: A critique of the value of laparotomy and splenectomy in the evaluation of patients with Hodgkin's disease. Cancer Res. 31:1737, 1971.
37. Rosenberg, S. A.: Updated Hodgkin's disease: Place of splenectomy in evaluation and management. J.A.M.A. 222:1296, 1972.
38. Schimpff, S., O'Connell, M., Greene, W., Young, V., and Wiernik, P.: American College of Physicians, Annual Meeting, Abstract No. 47, 1974.
39. Silverman, S., DeNardo, G. L., Glatstein, E., and Lipton, M. J.: Evaluation of the liver and spleen in Hodgkin's disease. II. The value of splenic scintigraphy. Am. J. Med. 52:362, 1972.
40. Smith, J., Pasmantier, M. W., Silver, R. T., Cornell, G., Coleman, M., and Cortese, A.: The staging of Hodgkin's disease. J.A.M.A. 224:1026, 1973.
41. Smithers, D. W.: Summary of papers delivered at the Conference on Staging in Hodgkin's disease (Ann Arbor). Cancer Res. 31:1869, 1971.
42. Turner, D. A., Pinsky, S. M., Gottschalk, A., Hoffer, P. B., Utmann, J. E., and Harper, P. V.: The use of [67]Ga-scanning in the staging of Hodgkin's disease. Radiology 104:97, 1972.
43. Ultmann, J. E.: Hodgkin's disease: Laparotomy or not? Letters to the Editor. Ann. Intern. Med. 76:320, 1972.

# The Rationale for "Selective" Staging Laparotomy in Hodgkin's Disease and the Malignant Lymphomas

RALPH E. JOHNSON

*National Cancer Institute, National Institutes of Health*

## *The Basis for Effective Cancer Therapy*

There are three fundamental prerequisites constituting the basis for effective therapeutic management of cancer. These have an orderly generic sequence—namely, defining the natural history of any neoplasm, locating ("staging") a given patient within the overall spectrum of his disease, and selecting an appropriately individualized treatment.

Many of the advances in oncology have evolved historically from trial and error, with failure of an empirically chosen therapy exerting a "feedback" effect on subsequently elected treatment. In other words, analysis of the mechanisms of treatment failure led to recognition of deficient understanding of the natural history of disease or of the assumed accuracy of the staging process.

This past decade has witnessed a remarkable interest in Hodgkin's disease and the malignant lymphomas. The efforts of many have illustrated an attempt to reverse the traditional "feedback" method of improving cancer therapeutics. Published articles have been increasingly directed toward more precise definition of the natural history and staging of patients. Unfortunately, perspective is lost on occasions as to the interrelationship between the three facets of cancer management outlined above. The intent of this paper is to focus attention on integration of the staging process in general,

649

and of staging laparotomy in particular, with our understanding of the natural history of and selection of treatment for Hodgkin's disease and the lymphomas.

## Hodgkin's Disease

Clinically, Hodgkin's disease has its initial manifestation within the lymphatic distribution depicted in Figure 1 in an overwhelming predominance of cases. Direct (contiguous) extension of tumor from lymph nodes into adjacent structures, such as lung or bone, occurs with some frequency, as does dissemination to nonadjacent organs. However, primary presentations in extranodal sites are relatively uncommon, constituting less than 5 per cent of newly diagnosed cases.

The advent of bipedal lymphography enhanced our ability to assess the extent of lymphatic involvement and thereby not only contributed to the understanding of the natural history of Hodgkin's disease but also influenced therapy when "silent" subdiaphragmatic involvement of lymph nodes was detected. However, any expectation that lymphography would prove a reli-

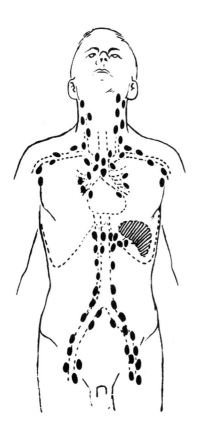

*Figure 1.* The distribution of lymph nodes which manifest the initial evidence of Hodgkin's disease in the vast majority of patients.

able guide to treatment selection was short-lived,[1] as false-negative studies proved commonplace. Only physicians neglecting to maintain observation of patients in whom irradiation below the diaphragm was withheld because of negative lymphography failed to appreciate the fallibility of this test for purposes of treatment decision making.

Disenchantment with lymphography was partially responsible for initiation of a prospective clinical trial of subdiaphragmatic irradiation in lymphogram-negative patients at the National Cancer Institute in 1965. The objective of this study was not to determine if the incidence of relapse could be reduced by such "prophylactic" irradiation, a prophecy which seemed self-fulfilling, but rather to determine if the prevention of relapse could improve long-term survival without incurring undue toxicity. The randomly assigned alternative consisted of secondary treatment in those cases involving relapse below the diaphragm when it was not prophylactically irradiated. The reduction in relapse rates after prophylactic irradiation below the diaphragm was quickly documented and eventually became extrapolated into superior survival.[2-4] Furthermore, data were obtained which in retrospect related directly to the role of pretreatment staging laparotomy in the therapeutic management of Hodgkin's disease.[5]

It is now apparent that two major situations must be considered when the potential contribution of staging laparotomy to treatment decision making is examined. These are concerned with the presence versus absence of clinical or radiographic evidence of involvement in the upper abdomen by disease. The pivotal question (and one too commonly ignored in many articles on staging laparotomy) is identical to that of lymphography—namely, are the results of laparotomy, when negative, sufficiently reliable to warrant elimination of empiric irradiation of the paralumbar lymph nodes and the remaining splenic pedicle? The answer to this question regarding the reliability of laparotomy is unequivocally "no," although to a lesser degree than for lymphography. Experience supporting this contention, although not yet reported in the literature, is accumulating in many centers throughout the world. Multiple personal communications to the author suggest that approximately one patient in five with supradiaphragmatic disease has clinically occult involvement below the diaphragm which is not detected by staging laparotomy. When irradiation is withheld, this results in an incidence of relapse far too high for automatic reliance upon random biopsy sampling of nodes for treatment decision making.

If one accepts the necessity of arbitrarily irradiating the paralumbar lymph nodes and splenic pedicle, despite a negative staging laparotomy, the critical issue becomes how frequently such treatment is altered by staging laparotomy. Approaching it in this light, we consider any of the following as acceptable indications for routine staging laparotomy (see exceptions and discussion below):

1. Marked enlargement of retroperitoneal lymph nodes demonstrated lymphographically or implied by gross displacement of the ureters/kidneys on intravenous pyelography.

2. Splenomegaly (despite recognition that some enlarged spleens are

histologically negative for Hodgkin's disease), or the occasional situation in which a normal-sized spleen is directly superimposed over the left kidney, so that effective renal shielding during splenic irradiation[6] is not possible.

3. Massive hepatomegaly or large defects on liver scan (as distinguished from inhomogeneous uptake[7]) when other causes are absent and needle biopsy of the liver does not provide an adequate explanation.

Our experience has clearly indicated that, under these conditions, staging laparotomy often modifies therapeutic management. In a group of 32 consecutive patients with splenomegaly or unequivocally positive lymphograms in the upper paralumbar area, radiotherapy was frequently followed by relapse. In 8 of these 32 cases, failure resulted from relapse in the upper abdomen (4 instances of extension to the liver and 4 instances of recurrence in upper abdominal lymph nodes or the spleen). Had staging laparotomy been performed, the information potentially obtained, together with splenectomy, would have been useful in retrospect in this group of patients. The high risk of liver involvement associated with massively involved spleens has now been confirmed by prospective staging laparotomy studies.[8, 9] This contrasts with the very low probability of unsuspected hepatic spread in patients without splenomegaly or positive lymphograms, as discussed below.

The three conditions outlined for staging laparotomy deserve reconsideration under two circumstances. The first is the presence of serious medical contraindications to operation or general anesthesia. The second is when systemic treatment with chemotherapy is to be used irrespective of the results of staging laparotomy. It has been possible to define prospectively such a cohort of patients[10] as those with a combination of unfavorable histology (mixed cellularity or lymphocyte depletion types) plus constitutional symptoms, irrespective of the clinical stage of disease. The great likelihood of extranodal dissemination in these cases warrants routine treatment with intensive combination chemotherapy.[11] This opinion is based not only on our own experience but also on the absence of any reports to date that such cases have an encouraging outlook when treated by radiotherapy alone.

Staging laparotomy does not contribute to therapeutic management with sufficient frequency to warrant routine use under the following conditions:

1. Already documented dissemination (Stage IV) of disease.

2. Decision to administer systemic chemotherapy empirically irrespective of operative staging results, as discussed above.

3. Presentations of Hodgkin's disease above the diaphragm when evidence (whether clinical or radiographic) of involvement below the diaphragm is lacking.

Amplification of the last point is required, for it is here that a major controversy exists with respect to staging laparotomy and its potential role in the management of Hodgkin's disease. In this area the literature is somewhat confusing. One needs to examine carefully the items listed in Table 1 to appreciate that absence of apparent involvement in the upper abdomen is a situation in which staging laparotomy is unlikely to make an important contribution to treatment decisions.

This conclusion is firmly supported by review of the consecutive series

### TABLE 1. Potential Contributions of Staging Laparotomy to Therapeutic Management of Hodgkin's Disease*

1. Detection of involved lymph nodes in sites not routinely irradiated when empiric radiotherapy is to be administered.

2. Removal of the spleen when markedly enlarged or superimposed over the left kidney, so that radiation nephritis is otherwise not avoidable.

3. Detection of hepatic involvement not discernible by percutaneous liver biopsy or peritoneoscopy.

*Preservation of fertility by transposition of the ovaries to the midline and purported improved tolerance to treatment as a consequence of splenectomy are viewed as quite conjectural benefits of staging laparotomy which do not justify its use.

of previously untreated patients with Hodgkin's disease admitted to the National Cancer Institute between 1965 and 1969. All patients have now been followed for more than 5 years since initial treatment, and the series includes 124 patients with supradiaphragmatic presentations (Stages Ia, IIa, and IIb) who were clinically staged without laparotomy but using bipedal lymphography and liver-spleen scans. When relapse due to abdominal extension occurred in patients not empirically irradiated below the diaphragm, laparotomy was nearly always performed to confirm relapse histologically and to "map" the areas of involvement. The study clearly demonstrated that prophylactic irradiation below the diaphragm reduced the relapse rate and improved survival. It also provided documentation that the treatment techniques used would have virtually never been altered with the use of routine staging laparotomy. The following points summarize the experience relevant to this latter statement:

1. Tumoricidal radiation doses to the paralumbar lymph nodes and spleen consistently prevented relapse of disease within the treated fields.

2. Relapse due to extension of disease to atypically located lymph nodes (e.g., porta hepatic or mesenteric) was not observed in any of the 124 patients.

3. Laparotomy at the time of relapse in patients not irradiated below the diaphragm uniformly documented disease confined to sites that would have been included within the fields of irradiation with prophylactic therapy.

4. Only 2 of the 124 consecutive patients have been found to have extension of disease to the liver upon relapse over a minimum observation time of 5 years.

This careful follow-up with restaging of patients by laparotomy upon relapse clearly indicates the absence of any indication for routine staging laparotomy in those patients with supradiaphragmatic presentations, *provided the paralumbar nodes and spleen are prophylactically irradiated.* The extremely low incidence of subsequent liver involvement also deserves emphatic stress, in that random probability dictates that microscopic (or minimal macroscopic) disease would have been detected in many of the 124 spleens had splenectomy been routinely performed before treatment. It is therefore apparent that minimal disease occultly present in normal-sized spleens shows a very poor correlation with hepatic spread, as contrasted with extensively involved spleens with splenomegaly.

Thus it seems to be well established that staging laparotomy in Hodgkin's disease is warranted when it is likely to serve as a guide to treatment decisions. Such is the case when there is clinical evidence of involvement in the upper abdomen, the absence of which implies that treatment decision making will rarely be altered by the results of staging laparotomy. Furthermore, there is no published information that therapeutic management of Hodgkin's disease has been improved except in "selected" cases, despite the well-recognized morbidity as well as occasional mortality from staging laparotomy.[12]

## Malignant Lymphomas with Extranodal Presentation

The non-Hodgkin's lymphomas, here referred to as malignant lymphomas, are usually classifiable at diagnosis as lymph node or extranodal in primary origin. This distinction is critical, since the biologic behavior and therapeutic management of the two types of presentation differ substantially.[13]

There are several features distinguishing primary extranodal lymphomas from the lymph node presentations. The extranodal lymphomas are quite ubiquitous, arising in nearly all organ systems. The most common sites are the gastrointestinal tract, skin, upper air passages, skeletal system, and connective or soft tissues. Two-thirds of extranodal lymphomas, both in our experience and in that recently described for a national survey,[14] present with involvement limited at the time of diagnosis to the primary site or with spread clinically restricted to the regional lymph nodes. This contrasts sharply with the clinically obvious dissemination in nearly all cases of lymph node presentations at the time of diagnosis.[15] The majority of pediatric cases of malignant lymphoma have extranodal presentations, whereas nodal presentations predominate in the adults.

Primary extranodal lymphomas confined to the site of origin have a reasonable prospect for cure with radiotherapy and/or operation.[14] However, the 5-year survival rate is reduced by a factor of two when regional lymphadenopathy is clinically apparent. Spread beyond the regional lymph nodes markedly differs from that in Hodgkin's disease in that a predictable pattern of dissemination is seldom observed. Rather, more remote spread is usually characterized by wide dissemination not unlike the metastatic pattern of carcinomas. This clinical impression has been reinforced by the pretreatment staging of the last 49 consecutive patients with primary extranodal lymphomas in our department (Table 2). When the Ann Arbor system of staging was used,[16] only one patient had dissemination beyond the regional lymph nodes which was confined to lymph nodes.

Systemic chemotherapy is not only mandatory as the primary form of treatment for patients with remote dissemination but in our opinion is also empirically warranted for the majority of patients with more localized

TABLE 2.  Ann Arbor Staging Distribution for 49 Consecutive Cases
of Extranodal Lymphoma

|  | Stage | | | |
| --- | --- | --- | --- | --- |
|  | I | II | III | IV |
| Number of cases | 11 | 22 | 1 | 15 |

presentations. Certainly the prognosis is sufficiently unfavorable when regional lymph node involvement is clinically apparent to employ adjuvant chemotherapy routinely. Some extranodal lymphomas, such as those primary in bone,[17] have a rather poor prognosis, even when clinically confined to the primary site. When this posture is accepted in terms of therapeutic management, staging laparotomy will not modify the treatment decision in most instances, and less invasive procedures, such as radioisotopic bone scanning, metastatic skeletal survey, bone marrow biopsy, and chest radiography, will suffice for pretreatment evaluation.

The one circumstance in which staging laparotomy has a definitive role for extranodal malignant lymphomas is for patients who present with intraabdominal tumors, such as a primary lesion of the gastrointestinal tract. Here, staging laparotomy not only serves to establish the diagnosis (occasionally permitting resection of the primary tumor) but also aids subsequent radiotherapy by defining the extent of the disease with metallic clips.

## Malignant Lymphomas with Lymph Node Presentation

It has been noted that most patients with lymph node presentations of malignant lymphoma have anatomically disseminated disease at the time of diagnosis. Our more recent experience with prospective operative staging of untreated patients has simply reinforced this clinical impression and is generally consistent with the data reported by others in emphasizing the systemic nature of these malignancies.[18]

Table 3 summarizes the results of operative staging for the last 105 consecutive patients with untreated lymph node presentations of malignant lymphoma. Only four patients were found to have involvement confined to a single lymph node region. In the category of diffuse histologic patterns, nearly all patients deserve to be viewed at the onset as having widely disseminated (Stage IV Ann Arbor) involvement. This was particularly emphasized for those with diffuse, poorly differentiated, lymphocytic histology; in this group 22 of 24 patients had proven bone marrow and/or liver involvement. It is patently misleading to believe that the 13 patients listed in the category of diffuse lymphocytic-histiocytic/histiocytic histology as having involvement confined to lymph nodes (Table 3) are truly staged with accuracy. Conventional radiotherapy has seldom controlled disease in patients of this type, the typical clinical course being one of rapid dissemination. Further-

TABLE 3.   Correlation Between Histology and Disease Extent for
105 Consecutive Untreated Lymph Node Presentations*

| Extent of Disease | Nodular Histology | | Diffuse Histology | |
|---|---|---|---|---|
| | PDL | L-H/H | PDL | L-H/H |
| Single lymph node area | 2 | 0 | 1 | 1 |
| Two or more nodal areas | 11 | 7 | 1 | 13 |
| Extranodal dissemination | 24 | 12 | 22 | 10 |

*Rappaport classification; PDL = poorly differentiated lymphocytic; L-H = lymphocytic-histiocytic; H = histiocytic type of lymphoma.

more, the staging evaluation was incomplete in 7 of the 13 cases because advanced local disease demanded immediate initiation of treatment. One is therefore left with the conclusion that lymph node presentations having a diffuse histologic pattern are so uniformly disseminated as to routinely require systemic treatment, excluding perhaps those anecdotal instances of disease localized to a single area. Consequently, staging laparotomy can in general be obviated as a prerequisite for treatment decisions.

Patients with nodular histologic patterns of lymph node presentations again are rarely seen when involvement is limited to a single area (Table 3). While a significant number of patients did not have detectable spread outside the lymphatic system, despite complete evaluation including staging laparotomy, the nodal involvement was usually one of anatomic generalization. Over two-thirds of patients in Table 3 with disease confined to lymph nodes in the nodular histology categories had extensive lymphatic involvement. Not only the nodes typically observed in Hodgkin's disease but also multiple nodes in other sites were involved, as shown in Figure 2. Despite absence of proven visceral spread, such disseminated disease throughout the lymphatic system mitigates against the type of "eradicative" radiotherapy used for Hodgkin's disease.

In the past, we attempted with little success a high-dose, total nodal irradiation approach in these patients with multiple areas of lymph node involvement. Not only was this extensive irradiation technically difficult and extremely depressive of bone marrow function, but also most patients eventually relapsed with extranodal dissemination, usually to the bone marrow. The clinician is again forced to recognize the systemic nature of the disease process when he is faced with patients having several areas of lymph node involvement with nodal presentations of malignant lymphoma. The logical implication of this understanding of the natural history of these lymphomas is that treatment itself must perforce be systemic, irrespective of what is found via invasive staging techniques such as laparotomy.

## Summary

An important role exists for staging laparotomy in treatment decision making for Hodgkin's disease when patients present with clinical evidence of involvement in the upper abdomen. In this situation, laparotomy has a

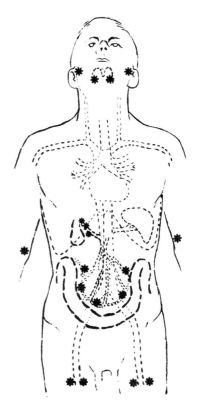

*Figure 2.* The lymph node chains which are frequently found to be involved by the malignant lymphomas of nodal origin, in addition to those areas of involvement observed in Hodgkin's disease.

considerable possibility of yielding information which will alter or facilitate treatment and should be routinely performed in the absence of medical contraindications or an a priori decision to employ systemic chemotherapy irrespective of laparotomy findings. In contrast, therapeutic management will rarely be modified by results of staging laparotomy in the absence of clinical disease in the upper abdomen.

The malignant lymphomas, whether nodal or extranodal in origin, again have selective indications for the use of staging laparotomy. The major value of laparotomy is for those patients with intra-abdominal presentations in whom operation not only serves to establish the diagnosis but also defines the extent of disease as an aid to potential subsequent radiotherapy. Staging laparotomy will not contribute to treatment decision making for the vast majority of patients with malignant lymphomas, however, since disseminated disease is the rule rather than the exception and systemic treatment is mandatory.

## References

1. Johnson, R. E., and Cook, P. L.: Hodgkin's disease: The negative lymphogram in guiding radiotherapy. Am. J. Roentgenol. *102*:883, 1968.
2. Johnson, R. E., Thomas, L. B., Schneiderman, M., Glenn, D. W., Faw, F., and Hafermann, M. D.: Preliminary experience with total nodal irradiation in Hodgkin's disease. Radiology 96:603, 1970.

3. Johnson, R. E., Glover, M. G., and Marshall, S. K.: Results of radiation therapy and implications for the clinical staging of Hodgkin's disease. Cancer Res. *31*:1834, 1971.
4. Johnson, R. E.: Updated Hodgkin's disease: Curability of localized disease. Total nodal irradiation. J.A.M.A. *223*:59, 1973.
5. Johnson, R. E.: Is staging laparotomy routinely indicated in Hodgkin's disease? Ann. Intern. Med. *75*:459, 1971.
6. Johnson, R. E.: Total nodal irradiation of Hodgkin's disease: Technical and clinical aspects. *In* Fletcher, G. (ed.): *Textbook of Radiotherapy*. Philadelphia, Lea & Febiger, 1974.
7. Johnson, R. E., Thomas, L. B., Johnson, S. K., and Johnston, G. S.: Correlation between abnormal baseline liver tests and long-term clinical course in Hodgkin's disease. Cancer *33*:1123, 1974.
8. Glatstein, E., Guernsey, J. M., Rosenberg, S. A., et al.: The value of laparotomy and splenectomy in the staging of Hodgkin's disease. Cancer *24*:709, 1969.
9. Prosnitz, L. R., Nuland, S. B., and Kligerman, M. M.: Role of laparotomy and splenectomy in the management of Hodgkin's disease. Cancer *29*:44, 1972.
10. Johnson, R. E., Thomas, L. B., and Chretien, P.: Correlation between clinico-histologic staging and extranodal relapse in Hodgkin's disease. Cancer *25*:1071, 1970.
11. DeVita, V. T., Serpick, A. A., and Carbone, P. P.: Combination chemotherapy in the treatment of advanced Hodgkin's disease. Ann. Intern. Med. *73*:881, 1970.
12. Meeker, W. R., Richardson, J. D., West, W. O., et al.: Critical evaluation of laparotomy and splenectomy in Hodgkin's disease. Arch. Surg. *105*:222, 1972.
13. Johnson, R. E., Ruhl, U., and Brereton, H.: Radiation therapy of malignant lymphomas: Rationale, techniques, and results. *In Proceedings of the XIth International Cancer Congress*. Amsterdam, Excerpta Medica. Inter. Cong. Series No. 354, Vol. 6:374, 1974.
14. Freeman, C., Berg, J. W., and Cutler, S. J.: Occurrence and prognosis of extranodal lymphomas. Cancer *29*:252, 1972.
15. Rosenberg, S. A., Diamond, H. D., Jaslowitz, B., and Craver, L. F.: Lymphosarcoma: Review of 1296 cases. Medicine *40*:31, 1961.
16. Carbone, P. P., Kaplan, H. S., Musshoff, K., Smithers, D. W., and Tubiana, M.: Report of the Committee on Hodgkin's Disease Staging Classification. Cancer Res. *31*:1860, 1971.
17. Boston, H. C., Dahlin, D. C., Ivins, J. C., and Cupps, R. E.: Malignant lymphoma (so-called reticulum cell sarcoma) of bone. Cancer *34*:1131, 1974.

# 29

# *Prevention of Wound Infections*

PROPHYLACTIC MEASURES FOR
WOUND INFECTIONS
  *by H. Harlan Stone*

## Statement of the Problem

*The multiple measures proposed for minimizing wound infection, while controversial, seem to be unsuited to analysis by the adversary approach. Therefore, the topic is adjudicated by a single author with special emphasis on firm data.*

*Do systemic antibiotics given prior to, during, or after operation help reduce the incidence of wound infections? If so, what antibiotic should be given? For all operations or for selected procedures? What are the criteria for patient selection and data which confirm the choices?*

*What are the reported frequencies of intra-abdominal infection with and without the use of prophylactic systemic antibiotics? Of subcutaneous wound infection? Cite prospective study data.*

*Discuss the frequency and significance of the complications of antibiotic administration, including fungal infections, overgrowth of resistant organisms, and long-term change in the hospital population of resistant organisms.*

*Do local irrigations help prevent intraperitoneal sepsis? Subcutaneous wound infection? Does addition of antibiotics to the irrigation fluid make a significant contribution to prevention of wound infection? Cite data.*

*Should the subcutaneous tissue be approximated routinely in an attempt to "eliminate dead space"? If so, what technique and suture material should be used? What are the data?*

*Discuss the value of delayed closure of the subcutaneous tissue and skin in general and in specific circumstances—for example, after ruptured appendix. What criteria are used for determining when it is "safe" to close the wound?*

*Is there demonstrated value of primary closure of the skin edges with tape rather than sutures?*

*Does the "wound protector" type of drape alter infection rates for abdominal procedures that are clean? Contaminated?*

*Is there value or harm in placing simple Penrose drains or suction-type drains in the subcutaneous tissue of either clean or contaminated wounds?*

# Prophylactic Measures for Wound Infections

## H. HARLAN STONE

*Emory University School of Medicine*

Wound infection has never been, is not now, and never will be caused by some stroke of fate.[1, 7, 26, 28, 69, 88, 106, 108, 115, 119] It is the direct result of finite and usually measurable factors acting on a given individual, who, in turn, himself varies in many and often easily identifiable characteristics from the accepted norm. Any study or survey of prophylaxis against wound infection should therefore address itself to a documentation and then to proper evaluation of these various aspects as well as those methods used to alter their adverse influence on wound healing.

There are three basic requisites to be satisfied in the evolution of a wound infection.[108] First, a bacterial *inoculum* must have reached the wound in sufficient quantity for that particular microbial species or mixture of species to contain at least the minimal virulence necessary for establishing an infection. Secondly, *nutrition* must be readily available for bacterial growth, regardless of whether it is present initially or is subsequently provided by blood and tissue breakdown products. Finally, patient *resistance* must in some way have been compromised by a failure to inherit a certain natural immunity, lack of prior contact with the pathogens for the development of specific acquired immunity, a poor local blood supply, or some combination of these or multiple other deficiencies.[1-3, 6-8, 10, 17, 21, 23, 26, 28, 40, 49, 59, 69, 76, 79, 83, 88, 95, 98, 106, 108, 113, 115, 119] Preventive measures, accordingly, should be aimed at correcting as many as possible of the several responsible deficits in each of these three areas.

## *Inoculum*

Bacterial inoculation can occur only during the time that the wound is open and for the several hours immediately thereafter, prior to the time that

661

a protective fibrin seal has formed between the approximated wound edges.[7, 17, 103] This coagulum, once dehydrated into a mature crust, is a highly effective barrier. Isolation of the wound below is then maintained until healing has been completed, that is, unless moisture softens the fibrin matrix and allows bacterial migration into the wound depths from the surface above.[106] In addition, most strains of pathogenic bacteria elaborate proteolytic enzymes that, when in aqueous solution, directly attack and break down the protein strands of the clot.[103]

Any measure that retards or delays the creation of a fibrin seal — e.g., drains, wet dressings, delayed primary wound closure, etc. — prolongs the period of susceptibility of the wound to bacterial inoculation.[12, 16, 18, 20, 25, 26, 30, 35, 48, 51, 53, 61, 67, 70, 71, 81, 82, 90, 97, 107, 108, 111, 118, 119, 122] During this interim, supplemental methods must be relied upon to reduce the likelihood of such contamination. Sterile dressings, properly applied and firmly secured, become an absolute necessity. Any break in strict aseptic technique uniformly leads to wound inoculation and thereby a greater risk of subsequent infection. The detrimental effect of an unnecessary drain on the incidence of later wound sepsis is primarily based on this mechanism of retrograde inoculation.[20, 26, 48, 53, 55, 56, 71, 81, 82, 106, 108, 118, 122]

## Protecting Against Inoculation

As the germ theory became more thoroughly understood and its basic concepts honored, surgery progressed from practices of antisepsis to those of asepsis.[62, 68, 119] Superior rates of primary healing and relatively uncommon instances of infection have followed the almost total avoidance of contamination by virulent hospital bacteria and contrast strikingly with the results obtained when attempts are made merely to reduce the magnitude of an already established inoculum.

Operations are now performed in areas where personnel traffic is limited, where garments worn by patient and operative team have not been in contact with other parts of the hospital, and where even the circulation of air is controlled with respect to direction, filtration, and horizontal stratification. The risk of inoculation from hospital workers is further reduced by the use of masks, head caps and/or hairnets, and, for those individuals involved directly with the operative wound or operative instruments, mechanically cleansed hands through scrubbing, sterile gloves, and germ-proof gowns.[14, 31, 38, 42, 52, 64, 69, 79, 104]

Prior to operation, the immediate vicinity of the wound is made at least *partially* sterile by scrubbing with an operative cleansing agent and/or topical application of a bactericidal prep solution.[14, 31, 79] During operation, this same area — i.e., where the disinfectant has been applied — is isolated from the remainder of the patient by means of sterile drapes; often the incised wound itself is separated from the body cavity to be explored by skin towels or a special plastic wound protector.[84] This latter maneuver is most important when there is risk of autoinoculation from active bacterial peritonitis, perforations of the colon or obstructed small bowel, or wounds of the stomach. In addition, attempts should always be made not to enter unnecessarily the lumen of colonized organs (e.g., decompressive enterotomy) or to dissect tissue planes known to harbor pathogenic microorganisms.[108]

The above are measures generally considered to be routine for preventing contamination of the clean operative wound during operation. Unfortunately, however, bacterial inoculation has often occurred prior to operation in cases of trauma or can be expected to occur during operation (i.e., autoinoculation) in cases involving perforation of a normally colonized organ or dissection into areas with an already established infection.[85, 108] It is for these wounds that additional techniques are indeed justified in an attempt to reduce the quantity of the bacterial inoculum and possibly even the virulence of the overall microbial flora that can be anticipated in the contaminant.

## REDUCING THE MAGNITUDE OF THE INOCULUM

The absolute quantity of bacterial inoculum can be lessened significantly through several different approaches. For convenience, these can be grouped into three major categories: mechanical, chemical, and electromagnetic.

### Mechanical

Debridement with removal of all gross contamination is relatively obvious.[33] However, all too frequently small particles of organic matter or bacteria-laden inert objects are overlooked, especially when there has been massive contamination, major contusion of local tissues, or an irregular wound with arborizing crevices. To offset this limitation in removal of so-called invisible contaminants, most surgeons resort to some form of wound washing.[33] However, unless the irrigant itself contains some antimicrobial agent, no reduction in incidence of wound infection has ever been achieved.[11, 15, 19, 33, 46, 47, 50, 58, 100, 101, 112] This has been demonstrated repeatedly by studies in the experimental animal as well as in the patient undergoing either formal operation or care of some traumatic wound. The same is true for peritoneal contamination.[22, 24, 27, 32, 60, 77, 78, 80, 99, 102, 114] To the contrary, some workers have shown that there is an even more widespread distribution of the bacterial inoculum when peritoneal lavage is used than would have taken place otherwise.[54, 60, 80, 114]

The cause for failure of irrigation methods appears to be a trapping of contaminating bacteria in the fibrin film that almost uniformly develops on the raw surface of any fresh wound or exposed serosal surface within a matter of only a few minutes.[33, 36, 92-94, 121] Scrubbing, proteolytic enzymes, detergents, and various other surface-active chemicals have been recommended as effective additives to eliminate this shortcoming.[64] Unfortunately, however, most agents or techniques used to free such microbes adhere to the wound surface and have been shown instead to produce an even greater infection rate because of their concomitant direct injury to the locally exposed tissues. Adverse reactions due to parenteral absorption of such agents must also be considered.[96]

Instead of attempting to decrease the magnitude of the bacterial inoculum after the wound or peritoneal cavity has already been contaminated, a better and certainly time-proven approach has been the preoperative reduction in absolute mass of any potential inoculum. That is the very reason for preparation of the skin and application of aseptic techniques.[14, 31, 38, 64, 104]

Another prime example is mechanical cleansing of the large bowel, whereby food with any residue is withheld from the diet for several days preoperatively, a cathartic is administered on the day prior to the scheduled operation, and cleansing enemas are given the night before and often even early in the morning on the day of operation.[95, 103] A proximal diverting colostomy certainly gives greater protection, yet this procedure generally is reserved for the first stage in operative correction of large bowel obstruction or colon perforation.[79, 95, 103] In essentially all operations involving the colon, the difference in rates of both wound infection and operative mortality, with and without such mechanical cleansing, is dramatic; indeed, it is the very reason that elective colon operations ever became accepted as practical and relatively safe procedures.[95]

## Chemical

Various chemicals, especially those with antibacterial properties, have further decreased the magnitude of the intraluminal inoculum and thus sepsis rates following large bowel operations. Initially, nonabsorbable agents (sulfonamides) with action only against the aerobic components of bowel flora were administered orally.[41, 89, 95] Improvement in incidence of infection was so striking that other and more effective oral antibiotics (neomycin and kanamycin) were either added to the initial regimen or substituted for the sulfonamide.[120] As a result, the aerobic bowel flora was almost eliminated. Nevertheless, it has been only in recent years that anaerobic species, representing more than 80 per cent of the fecal mass, were at last found to contribute significantly to infections of the wound and abdomen after colon operation.[10, 21, 49, 120] The addition of another oral antibiotic (erythromycin or clindamycin) with activity against anaerobes, particularly *Bacteroides fragilis*, to the preoperative regimen has further reduced the incidence of such infectious complications to the range of what is frequently taken to represent the acceptable norm in so-called clean operations.[120]

Direct application of antibacterial substances to the already contaminated wound has consistently been shown to reduce the magnitude of the bacterial inoculum and thus the incidence of subsequent infection.[45, 72-74, 107, 108, 111, 116] Medical texts are replete with lists of various agents that have been used throughout history to augment uncomplicated primary healing. However, most antimicrobial formulations have been shown to be more detrimental than truly beneficial if local irritation and systemic toxicity are also considered.[66, 119]

The first antimicrobial agents used to any great extent were the sulfonamides, which were applied topically to battlefield wounds incurred during the Second World War. Later work has mainly been concerned with the aminoglycosides (neomycin and kanamycin) and with different antibiotic mixtures.[42, 72-74, 107, 108, 111, 116] The delivery vehicle has never appeared to be of great importance, provided it is not noxious or irritating and the antibiotic is not bound to any component of the carrying media. Aqueous solutions and aerosol sprays of true antibiotics have been found to be remarkably effective in almost all laboratory and clinical trials in preventing the evolution of infection following primary closure of contaminated wounds. Previous wound infection rates of 60 to 70 per cent in such circumstances have been cut to a fifth or sixth, that is, to between 10 and 15 per cent.[108]

Critical, however, to any significant improvement in the infection rate has been the choice of topical antimicrobial agent. It must be soluble in an aqueous solution, penetrate the fibrin coagulum on the wound surface, and be active against the anticipated pathogens. Failure to protect against infection is usually caused by some deficiency in one of these three areas.

Similar benefits have been reported with respect to the intraperitoneal instillation of antibiotics (cephalothin, neomycin, and kanamycin) and the resultant lessened likelihood of developing bacterial peritonitis.[22, 24, 32, 77, 78, 80, 99, 102] Irrigation of the peritoneal cavity with such antibiotic solutions, either once during operation or several additional times during the postoperative phase, has been said to curtail significantly both the incidence and the consequences of intra-abdominal sepsis in cases in which major peritoneal contamination has occurred. Almost identical results, however, have been noted to follow the preoperative or intraoperative administration of parenteral antibiotics (cephalosporins and aminoglycosides) in similarly contaminated cases.[99, 102] In fact, blood and peritoneal fluid concentrations of antibiotic have appeared to equilibrate within a very few minutes in such individuals.[99] Since no randomized studies or valid comparative data have ever been presented to support or refute these claims of added benefit, the advantage of intraperitoneal antibiotics over parenteral administration can only be considered to represent a clinical impression.[99]

Another aspect to be considered is the systemic toxicity of antibiotic that has been suddenly absorbed from the peritoneal cavity. Blood levels peak at many times the therapeutic and toxic concentrations.[96] Adverse reactions, such as aminoglycoside-induced myoneural blockade and its resultant respiratory arrest, may be much more life-threatening than the original infection being treated.[39, 96] Accordingly, the dangers of intraperitoneal administration of the more potent antibiotics (aminoglycosides) seem to greatly outweigh any additional advantage gained through direct application of antibiotic onto infected or contaminated peritoneum.

One chemical, often forgotten, is universally provided in the air we breathe—oxygen. Its killing effect on anaerobic species is probably the main reason why the technique of delayed primary wound closure works so well.[110] Previously, the tiny fresh granulations observed on a 3- to 5-day old wound were thought to make any exposed surface much more resistant to infection.[62, 108, 109] However, on reanalysis of reported data, reductions in the incidence of wound infection as obtained by delayed primary closure were found to correlate almost exactly with the presence of anaerobic species in the contaminant.[108] In fact, no measurable change in infection rate could be demonstrated with respect to clean operative wounds or wounds inoculated only with aerobic species.

A similar benefit of atmospheric oxygen has been reported in patients with peritoneal contamination by bowel contents as well as in cases of established peritonitis.[110] The duration of exposure of the abdominal parietes to air was found to be inversely proportional to the incidence and number of surviving anaerobes.[110] These benefits, only subjectively appreciated, may well have been a major factor in the initial popularity of hydrogen peroxide as an irrigant for infected wounds.

### Electromagnetic

Many of the criteria used to establish the diagnosis and to identify the causes of postoperative wound infection were the products of a multicenter study supported by the National Academy of Sciences.[88] The basic conclusion reached was that electromagnetic energy—in the form of ultraviolet light—would indeed eliminate sufficient numbers of pathogenic bacteria to the point at which wound and intra-abdominal infection rates could be reduced significantly. However, the small magnitude of this improvement has never seemed to justify the additional trouble and expense that would be required to implement such an anti-infectious program.

Other forms of electromagnetic energy are frequently used for sterilization of medications, body implants, and operative instruments. However, risks of radiation injury appear to preclude direct exposure of human tissues to their action.

## REDUCING THE VIRULENCE OF THE INOCULUM

Certain bacterial species are known to be considerably more virulent than others. Unfortunately, the hospital environment is the single area in which factors in natural selection have been so altered as almost to insure the evolution of more pathogenic strains.[8, 26, 69] The concentration of resistance-deprived patients, the widespread administration of antimicrobial agents, prolonged exposure of massive wounds and body cavities, a common reliance upon invasive monitoring devices, and the close physical contacts of infected patients and carriers with the general patient population make the hospital a place where the most dangerous of all of the usual pathogens have been amassed amid a system which permits their distribution to potential hosts.[8, 26, 52, 69, 106]

In order to protect the operative candidate from such bacteria, a shortened preoperative stay will significantly lessen his chances of acquiring these new species as part of his own endemic flora, whether in the bowel or on the body surface.[106] Should contemplated operation be delayed, then it is safest to have the patient spend the extra preoperative days at home rather than in the hospital.

If the patient already harbors pathogenic bacteria, either in his nasopharynx or on a granulating surface, an otherwise clean operation should be postponed until antibiotics have eradicated the carrier state and all superficial wounds have completely healed. Proceeding immediately with an elective operation almost guarantees a 50 per cent wound infection rate.[106] Skin preparatory measures are indeed effective in these cases, but never to the extreme degree required to eliminate all surface bacteria.

## Nutrition

Bacteria, like other forms of life, must have a source of food. Death is certain otherwise.[106] Blood clots, various accumulations of extracellular fluid, necrotic tissue, and buried organic matter provide sufficient nutrition for bacterial growth. It is therefore the responsibility of the surgeon himself to prevent such nourishment from becoming available to those pathogens that may have already reached the wound. Dedication to this principle is best exhibited by the technical expertise of the proficient surgeon. His low infection rate is not the result of luck but is achieved by strict adherence to these basic tenets.[16, 106]

All grossly necrotic tissue is removed, while creation of additional areas of ischemia is avoided by pinpoint ligature or electric coagulation. Never should sizable masses of tissue be caught up in a single big suture or large areas be cauterized to insure control of bleeding.[26] Blood products routinely collect in potential cavities, yet these so-called dead spaces must not be sutured excessively; otherwise, tissue necrosis and foreign body reaction may well increase the amount of local pabulum for bacterial culture and thus lead to an increased risk of infection.[29] Nevertheless, hemostasis should always have been achieved prior to final wound closure.

Suture material not only is a foreign body but also may itself cause local irritation and tissue necrosis.[34, 87, 117] Chromic sutures and plain catgut are notoriously of this type, even though a part of the cellular injury is due to the preservative solution in which the sutures are packaged. The ideal strand is an inert monofilament or, better yet, no suture at all.[57, 105] Considerable success has in fact been reported with sutureless wound closure. By the application of strips of adhesive directly to the skin, wound edges can be pulled together.[37, 43] Unfortunately, no similar method has been developed that could be adapted to deeper structures.

## Host Resistance

Host resistance is a difficult thing to define.[1, 2] It includes pathogen- and toxin-specific antibodies, an effective phagocytic system composed of circulating leukocytes as well as migrating and fixed tissue histiocytes, local resistance residing in the individual cells of a given organ, and many other less well understood factors.[1, 2, 76, 98] Nevertheless, one common denominator to all host defense mechanisms is an adequate circulatory system. In fact, the resistance to infection of any fresh wound parallels relatively closely the density of its capillary network. Any reduction in local blood supply, as might occur with vasoconstriction, etc., causes an equivalent reduction in local resistance to infection.[17] Perhaps it is this association with tissue vascularity that explains the predisposition to infection of patients in shock, of tissues such as cortical bone and subcutaneous fat,[59] and of ischemic organs anywhere in the body.[83]

The overall resistance to infection of any given individual varies considerably, not only in comparison to other members of the same species but also with respect to fluctuations in his own defense mechanisms that are constantly changing in an almost cyclically regulated rhythm.[3] Few things can be done to augment this resistance; yet shock, stress, various poisonous medications, and bacterial toxins can significantly impair host defenses.[98, 109] Nevertheless, one treatment modality can remarkably increase local wound and organ resistance to infection — parenteral prophylactic antibiotics.[17, 85, 86] If such an agent is given sufficiently ahead of the microbial insult, protective blood and/or tissue levels of antibiotic will already be present and can thereby preclude both bacterial colonization and subsequent infection.[17, 65, 86]

## PROPHYLACTIC ANTIBIOTICS

A relatively large number of studies have confirmed conclusively the value of prophylactic antibiotics for selected operative patients — provided the drug is given prior to the time that the incision has been made, is distributed relatively rapidly to the tissues anticipated to be contaminated, is not protein-bound, and has antibacterial activity which will cover those species making up the inoculum.[4, 5, 13, 17, 44, 46, 63, 65, 85, 86, 91, 99, 108, 118] Failure of various agents in the past has been the result of delayed initiation of therapy, poor delivery to those tissues at risk due to simultaneous shock or dehydration, and absence of the appropriate antibacterial spectrum.[9, 44, 65, 71, 75, 91, 92, 108, 121]

Table 1 demonstrates the need for timely administration of the prophy-

**TABLE 1.   Prophylactic Antibiotics —
Parenteral Cefazolin in Abdominal Surgery**

| Area of Operation | Time of Antibiotic Administration | | | |
|---|---|---|---|---|
| | Preoperatively | | Postoperatively | |
| | 12 hours | 1 hour | 1 to 4 hours | Never |
| Gastroduodenal | 5 | 10 | 9* | 5 |
| Biliary | 10 | 13 | 11 | 15 |
| Colon | 26* | 17 | 21 | 20 |
| Total patients | 40 | 40 | 40 | 40 |
| Infection | 2 | 2 | 9 | 7 |
| Incidence (per cent) | 5 | 5 | 23 | 18 |

*One patient had operations in both areas at the same time.

lactic antibiotic. Treatment begun after the wound was closed gives the same infection rate as if antibiotic had not been given at all. On the other hand, any significant reduction in the incidence of wound infection can be expected only in those cases with an already high infection rate. The latter, as reflected in Table 2, is frequently noted in elective colon and biliary tract operations, but not when operations are performed on the stomach and duodenum.

The choice of specific antibiotic to be used for prophylaxis is primarily a function of its activity against pathogens likely to make up the operative inoculum, as well as its ability to diffuse or penetrate into those areas of the body at greatest risk. Once these requirements have been satisfied, then the safest of all available agents is selected according to the incidence of allergic reactions and minimal potential for organ toxicity. Cost is generally the last consideration, for effectiveness and safety must always be assured.

There are only two presently acceptable indications for the parenteral administration of prophylactic antibiotics:[17, 85] first, when the likelihood of an infection is so great that such measures are definitely warranted in an effort to reduce wound morbidity, shorten the hospital stay, and decrease overall patient as well as third-party expense. Elective colon and gallbladder operations are excellent examples. The other major indication is based upon a uniformly catastrophic end result if postoperative sepsis follows a particular operation. This is reflected in exorbitantly high mortality rates whenever the wound or area of operative dissection becomes infected, e.g., insertion of an aortic graft or open heart operation. There are almost no other valid reasons.

As with any other treatment modality, antibiotics do cause serious complications.[63, 75] Such should always be expected. Once the problem has been recognized, the responsible drug must be discontinued immediately

**TABLE 2.  Prophylactic Antibiotics in Elective Surgery — Incidence of Wound Infection**

| | Time of Antibiotic Administration | |
| --- | --- | --- |
| | *Preoperative* *1 to 12 hours* | *Postoperative or Never* |
| Gastroduodenal | 15 | 14° |
| Infection | 1 | 1 |
| Incidence (per cent) | 6 | 7 |
| Biliary | 23 | 26 |
| Infection | 0 | 6 |
| Incidence (per cent) | — | 23 |
| Colon | 43° | 41 |
| Infection | 2 | 8 |
| Incidence (per cent) | 5 | 20 |
| Total patients | 81 | 81 |
| Infection | 3 | 15 |
| Incidence (per cent) | 4 | 19 |

°One patient had operations in both areas at the same time.

and appropriate corrective measures begun. Any allergy, as manifested by urticaria or the even more accelerated anaphylaxis, is most common with penicillin and its related compounds. Oto- and nephrotoxicity are the major complications of aminoglycoside therapy, while certain other agents can cause a depression in one or more individual components of the bone marrow.

Superinfection with nonbacterial pathogens is always a potential risk, even though it is seldom if ever noted after a brief course of antibiotics. Candida sepsis is the typical example.[109] Equally feared, and possibly more threatening to the community at large, is the evolution of resistant bacterial strains that can subsequently spread to other susceptible patients and create a life-threatening hospital epidemic.[69] This happened in the 1940's following the widespread use of penicillin as a prophylactic panacea.

In general, the product of the absolute number of bacteria in the inoculum multiplied by the total virulence of the individual bacterial species participating in that inoculum must reach a certain ill-defined minimum before infection is possible. The presence of an excellent source for microbe nourishment and significant impairment in host resistance merely set this bacterial threshold at a much lower level than would otherwise be the case.

It is the surgeon's responsibility to limit the mass of the bacterial inoculum, as well as the availability of nutrient media upon which such bacteria thrive. Usually the quality of the host defense mechanism has been established long before operation. Nevertheless, the selective use of prophylactic antibiotics can significantly improve the patient's resistance to infection when certain specified conditions are met.

# *References*

1. Alexander, J. W.: Surgical infections – pathogen versus host. J. Surg. Res. 8:225, 1968.
2. Alexander, J. W.: Host defense mechanisms against infection. Surg. Clin. North Am. 52:1367, 1972.
3. Alexander, J. W., Dionigi, R., and Meakins, J. L.: Periodic variation in the antibacterial function of human neutrophils and its relationship to sepsis. Ann. Surg. 173:206, 1971.
4. Alexander, J. W., McGloin, J. J., and Altemeier, W. A.: Penicillin prophylaxis in experimental wound infection. Surg. Forum 11:299, 1960.
5. Alexander, J. W., Sykes, N. S., Mitchell, M. M., and Fisher, M. W.: Concentration of selected intravenously administered antibiotics in experimental surgical wounds. J. Trauma 13:423, 1973.
6. Altemeier, W. A.: The bacterial flora of acute perforated appendicitis with peritonitis. Ann. Surg. 107:517, 1938.
7. Altemeier, W. A.: The significance of infection in trauma. Bull. Am. Coll. Surg. 57:7, Feb., 1972.
8. Altemeier, W. A., Hummel, R. P., Hill, E. O., and Lewis, S.: Changing patterns in surgical infections. Ann. Surg. 178:436, 1973.
9. Barnes, J., Pace, W. G., Trump, D. S., and Ellison, E. H.: Prophylactic postoperative antibiotics. Arch. Surg. 79:190, 1959.
10. Beazley, R. M., Polakavetz, S. H., and Miller, R. M.: Bacteroides infections on a university surgical service. Surg. Gynecol. Obstet. 135:742, 1972.
11. Belzer, F. O., Salvatierra, O., Jr., Schweizer, R. T., and Kountz, S. L.: Prevention of wound infections by topical antibiotics in high risk patients. Am. J. Surg. 126:180, 1973.
12. Berliner, S. D., Burson, L. C., and Lear, P. E.: Use and abuse of intraperitoneal drains in colon surgery. Arch. Surg. 89:686, 1964.
13. Bernard, H. R., and Cole, W. R.: The prophylaxis of surgical infection: The effect of

prophylactic antimicrobial drugs on the incidence of infection following potentially contaminated operations. Surgery 56:151, 1964.

14. Bornside, G. H., Crowder, V. H., Jr., and Cohn, I., Jr.: A bacteriological evaluation of surgical scrubbing with disposable iodophor-soap impregnated polyurethane scrub sponges. Surgery 64:743, 1968.

15. Brockenbrough, E. C., and Moylan, J. A.: Treatment of contaminated surgical wounds, with a topical antibiotic. Am. Surg. 35:789, 1969.

16. Brown, P. W.: The prevention of infection in open wounds. Clin. Orthop. 96:42, 1973.

17. Burke, J. F.: The effective period of preventive antibiotic action in experimental incisions and dermal lesions. Surgery 50:161, 1961.

18. Burke, J. F., and Bondoc, C. C.: A method of secondary closure of heavily contaminated wounds providing "physiologic primary closure." J. Trauma 8:228, 1968.

19. Casten, D. F., Nach, R. J., and Spinzia, J.: An experimental and clinical study of the effectiveness of antibiotic wound irrigation in preventing infection. Surg. Gynecol. Obstet. 118:783, 1964.

20. Cerise, E. J., Pierce, W. A., and Diamond, D. L.: Abdominal drains: Their role as a source of infection following splenectomy. Ann. Surg. 171:764, 1970.

21. Clark, L. P., Marshall, H. A., and Ackerman, N. B.: The role of bacteroides as an infectious organism. Surg. Gynecol. Obstet. 138:562, 1974.

22. Cohn, I., Jr., and Cotlar, A. M.: Intraperitoneal kanamycin. Ann. Surg. 155:532, 1962.

23. Conolly, W. B., Hunt, T. K., and Dunphy, J. E.: Management of contaminated surgical wounds. Surg. Gynecol. Obstet. 129:593, 1969.

24. Crook, J. N., Cotlar, A. M., Bornside, G. H., and Cohn, I.: Intraperitoneal cephalothin in the treatment of experimental appendiceal peritonitis. Am. Surg. 34:736, 1968.

25. Crowson, W. N., and Wilson, C. S.: An experimental study of the effects of drains on colon anastomoses. Am. Surg. 39:597, 1973.

26. Cruse, P. J. E., and Foord, R.: A five-year prospective study of 23,649 surgical wounds. Arch. Surg. 107:206, 1973.

27. Currie, D. J.: Continuous peritoneal lavage. Surg. Gynecol. Obstet. 135:951, 1972.

28. De Haan, B., Ellis, H., and Wilks, M.: The role of infection on wound healing. Surg. Gynecol. Obstet. 138:693, 1974.

29. de Holl, D., Rodeheaver, G., Edgerton, M. T., and Edlich, R. F.: Potentiation of infection by suture closure of dead space. Am. J. Surg. 127:716, 1974.

30. Dillon, M., and Postlethwait, R. W.: Pre- and postoperative prophylactic use of cephaloridine: A study of 201 cases. Am. J. Surg. 122:61, 1971.

31. Dineen, P.: An evaluation of the duration of the surgical scrub. Surg. Gynecol. Obstet. 129:1181, 1969.

32. DiVincenti, F. C., and Cohn, I., Jr.: Prolonged administration of intraperitoneal kanamycin in the treatment of peritonitis. Am. Surg. 37:177, 1971.

33. Dunphy, J. E.: Editorial: Wound irrigation versus wound debridement. Ann. Surg. 181:12A, June, 1975.

34. Edlich, R. F., Panek, P. H., Rodeheaver, G. T., Turnbull, V. G., Kurtz, L. D., and Edgerton, M. T.: Physical and chemical configuration of sutures in the development of surgical infection. Ann. Surg. 177:679, 1973.

35. Edlich, R. F., Rogers, W., Kasper, G., Kaufman, D., Tsung, M. S., and Wangensteen, O. W.: Studies in the management of the contaminated wound. I. Optimal time for closure of contaminated open wounds. II. Comparison of resistance to infection of open and closed wounds during healing. Am. J. Surg. 117:323, 1969.

36. Edlich, R. F., Smith, Q. T., and Edgerton, M. T.: Resistance of the surgical wound to antimicrobial prophylaxis and its mechanisms of development. Am. J. Surg. 126:583, 1973.

37. Edlich, R. F., Tsung, M. S., Rogers, W., Rogers, P., and Wangensteen, O. H.: Studies in management of the contaminated wound. I. Technique of closure of such wounds together with a note on a reproducible experimental model. J. Surg. Res. 8:585, 1968.

38. Ericson, C., Juhlin, I., and Willard, L. O.: Removal of the superficial bacterial flora of the hands—A comparison between different antibacterial preparations and soap. Acta Chir. Scand. 134:7, 1968.

39. Eugel, H. L., and Denson, J. S.: Respiratory depression due to neomycin. Surgery 42:862, 1957.

40. Feller, I., Richards, K. E., and Pierson, C. L.: Prevention of postoperative infections. Surg. Clin. North Am. 52:1361, 1972.

41. Fior, W. M., and Jonas, A.: The use of sulfanilylguanidine in surgical patients. Ann. Surg. 114:19, 1941.

42. Ford, C. R., Peterson, D. E., and Mitchell, C. R.: An appraisal of the role of surgical face masks. Am. J. Surg. 113:787, 1967.

43. Forrester, J. C., Zederfeldt, B. H., Hayes, T. L., and Hunt, T. K.: A comparison by ten-siometry and scanning electron microscopy. Br. J. Surg. 57:729, 1970.
44. Fullen, W. D., Hunt, H., and Altemeier, W. A.: Prophylactic antibiotics in penetrating wounds of the abdomen. J. Trauma 12:282, 1972.
45. Gibson, R. M.: Application of antibiotics in surgical practice using the aerosol technique. Br. Med. J. 1:1326, 1958.
46. Gingrass, R. P., Close, A. S., and Ellison, E. H.: Effect of various topical and parenteral agents on the prevention of infection in experimentally contaminated wounds. J. Trauma 4:763, 1964.
47. Glotzer, D. J., Goodman, W. S., and Geronimus, L. H.: Topical antibiotic prophylaxis in contaminated wounds. Arch. Surg. 100:589, 1970.
48. Goldstein, H. S., Kredi, R., Cecil, F., and Wolcott, M. W.: Drains at the suture line. Surgery 60:908, 1966.
49. Gorbach, S. L., and Bartlett, J. G.: Anaerobic infections. New Engl. J. Med. 290:1177, 1237, 1289, 1974.
50. Gray, F. J., and Kidd, E.: Topical chemotherapy in prevention of wound infection. Surgery 54:891, 1963.
51. Grosfeld, J. L., and Solit, R. W.: Prevention of wound infection in perforated appendicitis: Experience with delayed wound closure. Ann. Surg. 168:891, 1968.
52. Gryska, P. F., and O'Dea, A. E.: Postoperative streptococcal wound infection. J.A.M.A. 213:1189, 1970.
53. Haller, J. A., Shaker, I. J., Donahoo, J. S., Schnaufer, L., and White, J. J.: Peritoneal drainage versus non-drainage for generalized peritonitis from ruptured appendicitis in children; a prospective study. Ann. Surg. 177:595, 1973.
54. Hamer, M. L., Robson, M. C., Krizek, T. J., and Southwick, W. O.: Quantitative bacterial analysis of comparative wound irrigations. Ann. Surg. 181:819, 1975.
55. Hanna, E. A.: Efficiency of peritoneal drainage. Surg. Gynecol. Obstet. 131:983, 1970.
56. Hermann, G.: Intraperitoneal drainage. Surg. Clin. North Am. 49:1279, 1969.
57. Hermann, R. E.: Abdominal wound closure using a new polypropylene monofilament suture. Surg. Gynecol. Obstet. 138:84, 1974.
58. Hopson, W. B., Britt, L. G., Sherman, R. T., and Ledes, C. P.: The use of topical antibiotics in the prevention of experimental wound infection. J. Surg. Res. 8:261, 1968.
59. Hofman, E., and Reback, T. F.: Subcutaneous space contamination. Am. Surg. 24:364, 1958.
60. Hovnanian, A. P., and Saddawi, N.: An experimental study of the consequences of intraperitoneal irrigation. Surg. Gynecol. Obstet. 134:575, 1972.
61. Hudspeth, A. S.: Elimination of surgical wound infections by delayed primary closure. South. Med. J. 66:934, 1973.
62. Hunter, J.: A Treatise on the Blood, Inflammation, and Gunshot Wounds. Philadelphia, J. Webster, 1817, p. 180.
63. Karl, R. C., Mertz, J. J., Veith, F. J., and Dineen, P.: Prophylactic antimicrobial drugs in surgery. New Engl. J. Med. 275:305, 1966.
64. Kundsin, R. B., and Walter, C. W.: The surgical scrub—Practical consideration. Arch. Surg. 107:75, 1973.
65. Ledger, W. J., Sweet, R. L., and Headington, J. T.: Prophylactic cephaloridine in the prevention of postoperative pelvic infections in premenopausal women undergoing vaginal hysterectomy. Am. J. Obstet. Gynecol. 115:766, 1973.
66. Leveen, H. H., Falk, G., Borek, B., Diaz, C., Lynfield, Y., Wynkoop, B. J., Mabunda, G. A., Rubricius, J. L., and Christoudias, G. C.: Chemical acidification of wounds. An adjuvant to healing and the unfavorable action of alkalinity and ammonia. Ann. Surg. 178:745, 1973.
67. Lipton, S., Estrin, J., Kamath, M. L., Haq, I., and Berkowitz, S.: Surface hydrogen ion concentration as a determinant in timing delayed closure of wounds. Surg. Gynecol. Obstet. 139:189, 1974.
68. Lister, J.: On a new method of treating compound fractures. Lancet 1:357, 1867.
69. Lorian, V., and Topf, B.: Microbiology of nosocomial infections. Arch. Intern. Med. 130:104, 1972.
70. Manz, C. W., LaTendresse, C., and Sako, Y.: The detrimental effect of drains on colonic anastomoses; an experimental study. Dis. Colon Rectum 13:17, 1970.
71. Magarey, C. J., Chant, A. D. B., Rickford, C. R. K., and Margarey, J. R.: Peritoneal drainage and systemic antibiotics after appendectomy. Lancet 2:179, 1971.
72. Matsumoto, T., Dobeck, A. S., and Kovoric, J. J.: Topical spray of antibiotic in simulated combat wounds. IV. Dose factor. Arch. Surg. 97:61, 1968.

73. Matsumoto, T., Hardaway, R. M., Dobeck, A. S., and Nayes, E. H.: Antibiotic topical spray applied in simulated combat wounds. Arch. Surg. 95:288, 1967.

74. Matsumoto, T., Hardaway, R. M., Dobeck, A. S., Nayes, E. H., and Heisterkamp, C. A.: Antibiotic topical spray in simulated combat wounds. II. Neomycin-bacitracin-polymixin B, and penicillin. Arch. Surg. 96:786, 1967.

75. McCabe, W. R.: Antibiotics and their complications in surgery. Am. J. Surg. 116:327, 1968.

76. MacKaness, G. B.: Cell-mediated immunity to infection. Hosp. Pract. 5:73, Sept., 1970.

77. McKenna, J. P., Currie, D. J., MacDonald, J. A., Mahoney, L. J., Finlayson, D. C., and Lanskail, J. C.: The use of continuous postoperative peritoneal lavage in the management of diffuse peritonitis. Surg. Gynecol. Obstet. 130:254, 1970.

78. McMullan, M. H., and Barnett, W. O.: The clinical use of intraperitoneal cephalothin. Surgery 67:432, 1970.

79. NATO Handbook. *Emergency War Surgery.* Washington, D.C., U.S. Government Printing Office, 1959, p. 207.

80. Noon, G. P., Beall, A. C., Jr., Jordan, G. L., Jr., Riggs, S., and DeBakey, M. E.: Clinical evaluation of peritoneal irrigation with antibiotic solution. Surgery 62:73, 1967.

81. Nora, P. F., Vanecko, R. M., and Bransfield, J. J.: Prophylactic abdominal drains. Arch. Surg. 105:173, 1972.

82. Olsen, W. R., and Beaudoin, D. E.: Wound drainage after splenectomy. Am. J. Surg. 117:615, 1969.

83. Park, S. K., Brody, J. I., Wallace, H. A., and Blakemore, W. S.: Immunosuppressive effect of surgery. Lancet 1:53, 1971.

84. Paskin, D. L., and Lerner, H. J.: A prospective study of wound infections. Am. Surg. 35:627, 1969.

85. Polk, H. C., Jr.: Diminished surgical infection by systemic antibiotic administration in potentially contaminated operations. Surgery 75:312, 1974.

86. Polk, H. C., Jr., and Lopez-Mayor, J. F.: Postoperative wound infection: A prospective study of determinant factors and prevention. Surgery 66:97, 1969.

87. Postlethwait, R. W., Willigan, D. A., and Ulin, A. W.: Human tissue reaction to sutures. Ann. Surg. 181:144, 1975.

88. Postoperative wound infections: The influence of ultraviolet irradiation of the operating room and of various other factors, National Academy of Sciences–National Research Council, Division of Medical Sciences, Ad Hoc Committee of the Committee on Trauma. Ann. Surg. 160 (Suppl. 2):1, 1964.

89. Poth, E. J., and Knotts, F. L.: Succinyl sulfathiazole: A new bacteriostatic agent locally active in the gastrointestinal tract. Proc. Soc. Exp. Biol. Med. 48:129, 1941.

90. Prusak, M., Edlich, R. F., Payne, T. J., Madde, J., Edgerton, M. T., and Wangensteen, O. H.: Studies in the management of the contaminated wound. IX. Quantitation of the Evans blue dye content of open and primarily closed surgical wounds. Am. J. Surg. 125:585, 1973.

91. Pulaski, E. J., Minckes, J. R., and Beatty, G. L.: Acute appendicitis: Tetracycline prophylaxis and wound infection. Antibiot. Med. Clin. Ther. 3:392, 1956.

92. Robson, M. C., Edstrom, L. E., Krizek, T. J., and Groskin, M. G.: The efficacy of systemic antibiotics in the treatment of granulating wounds. J. Surg. Res. 16:299, 1974.

93. Rodeheaver, G., Edgerton, M. T., Elliott, M. B., Kurtz, L. D., and Edlich, R. F.: Proteolytic enzymes as adjuncts to antibiotic prophylaxis of surgical wounds. Am. J. Surg. 127:564, 1974.

94. Rodeheaver, G. T., Smith, S. L., Thacker, J. G., Edgerton, M. T., and Edlich, R. F.: Mechanical cleansing of contaminated wounds with a surfactant. Am. J. Surg. 129:241, 1975.

95. Roettig, L. C., Glasser, B. F., and Barney, C. O.: Definitive surgery of the large intestine following war wounds. Ann. Surg. 124:755, 1946.

96. Sakurai, K., Kolb, L. B., Naiman, J. G., and Martin, J. D., Jr.: Effects of calcium ion on kanamycin activity. Am. Surg. 31:165, 1965.

97. Schrock, T. R., Deveney, C. W., and Dunphy, J. E.: Factors contributing to leakage of colonic anastomoses. Ann. Surg. 177:513, 1973.

98. Serafin, D., Stone, H. H., Kolb, L. D., and Martin, J. D., Jr.: Alterations in reticuloendothelial functions as produced by the administration of bacterial toxins. Am. Surg. 34:714, 1968.

99. Sharbaugh, R. J., and Rambo, W. M.: Cephalothin and peritoneal lavage in the treatment of experimental peritonitis. Surg. Gynecol. Obstet. 139:211, 1974.

100. Singleton, A. O., Davis, D., and Julian, J.: The prevention of wound infection following contamination with colon organisms. Surg. Gynecol. Obstet. 108:389, 1959.

101. Singleton, A. O., and Julian, J.: An experimental evaluation of methods used to prevent infection in wounds which have been contaminated with feces. Ann. Surg. *151*:912, 1960.
102. Smith, E. B.: Adjuvant therapy of generalized peritonitis with intraperitoneally administered cephalothin. Surg. Gynecol. Obstet. *136*:441, 1973.
103. Spelman, A. E.: Healing of intestinal anastomosis. Am. J. Surg. *66*:309, 1944.
104. Sprunt, K., Redman, W., and Leidy, G.: Antibacterial effectiveness of routine hand washing. Pediatrics *52*:264, 1973.
105. Stone, H. H.: Nonsuture closure of cutaneous lacerations, skin grafting and bowel anastomosis. Am. Surg. *30*:177, 1964.
106. Stone, H. H.: The second edge of the sword. South. Med. J. *64*:472, 1971.
107. Stone, H. H., and Hester, T. R., Jr.: Topical antibiotic and delayed primary closure in the management of contaminated surgical incisions. J. Surg. Res. *12*:70, 1972.
108. Stone, H. H., and Hester, T. R., Jr.: Incisional and peritoneal infection after emergency celiotomy. Ann. Surg. *177*:669, 1973.
109. Stone, H. H., Kolb, L. D., Currie, C. A., Geheber, C. E., and Cuzzell, J. Z.: Candida sepsis: Pathogenesis and principles of treatment. Ann. Surg. *179*:697, 1974.
110. Stone, H. H., Kolb, L. D., and Geheber, C. E.: Incidence and significance of intraperitoneal anaerobic bacteria. Ann. Surg. *181*:705, 1975.
111. Stone, H. H., Sanders, S. L., and Martin, J. D., Jr.: Perforated appendicitis in children. Surgery *69*:673, 1971.
112. Taylor, F. W.: An experimental evaluation of operative wound irrigation. Surg. Gynecol. Obstet. *113*:465, 1961.
113. Thadepalli, H., Gorbach, S. L., Broido, P. W., Norsen, J., and Nyhus, L.: Abdominal trauma, anaerobes, and antibiotics. Surg. Gynecol. Obstet. *137*:270, 1973.
114. Thoroughman, J. C., Walker, L. G., Jr., and Collins, J.: Spreading organisms by peritoneal lavage. Am. J. Surg. *115*:339, 1968.
115. Todd, J. C.: Wound infection: Etiology, prevention, and management including selection of antibiotics. Surg. Clin. North Am. *48*:787, 1968.
116. Turk, D. C.: Laboratory studies of a multiple antibiotic spray. Can. Med. Assoc. J. *80*:194, 1959.
117. Van Winkle, W., Jr., Hastings, J. C., Barker, E., Hines, D., and Nichols, W.: Effect of suture materials on healing skin wounds. Surg. Gynecol. Obstet. *140*:7, 1975.
118. Vinnicombe, J.: Appendicectomy, wound infection, drainage, and antibiotics. Br. J. Surg. *51*:328, 1964.
119. Wangensteen, O. H., Wangensteen, S. D., and Klinger, C. F.: Some pre-Listerian and post-Listerian antiseptic wound practices and the emergency of asepsis. Surg. Gynecol. Obstet. *137*:677, 1973.
120. Washington, J. A., II, Dearing, W. H., Judd, E. S., and Elveback, L. R.: Effect of preoperative antibiotic regimen on development of infection after intestinal surgery: Prospective, randomized, double-blind study. Ann. Surg. *180*:567, 1974.
121. Waterman, N. G.: Editorial: Antibiotics and serum protein binding. Surg. Gynecol. Obstet. *138*:244, 1974.
122. Yates, J. L.: An experimental study of the local effects of peritoneal drainage. Surg. Gynecol. Obstet. *1*:473, 1905.

# 30

# *Renal Vascular Hypertension — Operative versus Nonoperative Treatment*

RENOVASCULAR
HYPERTENSION — THE CASE FOR
MEDICAL MANAGEMENT
*by W. Gordon Walker*

OPERATIVE TREATMENT
OF RENOVASCULAR HYPERTENSION
*by Ronald J. Stoney,*
*Robert J. Swanson, Roy E. Carlson,*
*and Dorothee L. Perloff*

## Statement of the Problem

*This discussion deals with selection of patients for operative intervention, long-term results, and possible nonoperative management of hypertension secondary to renal vascular disease.*

*If hypertension is clearly of renovascular etiology and operatively correctable but readily controlled by antihypertensive agents, should an operation be done? Analyze the data supporting that decision.*

*Evaluate all factors influencing selection for operation, including age, type of lesion, arteriographic findings, degree of renal insufficiency, bilateral versus unilateral disease, associated cardiovascular disease, and previous drug failure.*

*Discuss the differences in success rates for potentially remediable arteriosclerotic lesions versus fibromuscular dysplasias. What are the criteria of success? What percentage of patients were restored to normal diastolic and systolic blood pressures? What percentage still required drugs? In what percentage was blood pressure unaltered by operation?*

# Renovascular Hypertension—The Case for Medical Management

W. GORDON WALKER

*The Johns Hopkins University School of Medicine*

If renovascular hypertension is defined according to the most rigid criteria used in the cooperative study[1] as "diastolic hypertension secondary to renovascular disease...responding favorably to operative treatment, i.e., cured or improved," it is not possible to debate the relative merits of operative vs. medical management. Operative treatment becomes a means of defining the disease.[1] The early work of Howard,[2] however, and subsequently the studies of Stamey and many others[3-9] have established a set of diagnostic criteria permitting preoperative diagnosis with a reasonable degree of certainty. The presence of these criteria in a hypertensive patient establishes a high probability that the hypertension is attributable to an ischemic lesion in the kidney and that operative correction of the ischemia will lead to cure or amelioration of the hypertension. Given this diagnostic capability and the present availability of drugs that are extremely effective in the treatment of hypertension, it is reasonable to ask whether operative therapy represents a uniquely superior mode of treatment or whether the alternative of medical management of this condition is more desirable.

## *Requisite Criteria for Evaluating Efficacy of Alternate Modes of Therapy*

The unequivocal establishment of the superior efficacy of any form of therapy requires a prior knowledge of the natural history of the disease

677

under study.[10] Hence, for renovascular hypertension, informed judgment regarding the benefits of either medical or operative therapy requires prior quantitative information defining morbidity and mortality of untreated renovascular hypertension. This is not available; hence, unambiguous determination of the absolute benefits of either operative or medical therapy for this form of hypertension cannot be made with certainty. Relative superiority can be established. The assumption that is implicit in writings on renovascular hypertension is that the long-term prognosis in untreated cases is at least no better than that for essential hypertension of comparable levels of severity. A possible consequence of this assumption is that it may be permissible to compare the results of any therapeutic approach to renovascular hypertension with those from a comparable or matched group of untreated patients with essential hypertension. This suggests that a prospective study could easily be designed to resolve the issue of operative vs. medical therapy. Ethically, such a study cannot be justified or defended[10]; it presents the same problems as any controlled study that includes a group of untreated patients denied therapy that may be reasonably expected to prolong life. This issue is a difficult one that is not unique to the study of hypertension. The problem and its possible solutions have been considered in some detail by Meier.[10]

All available evidence dealing with the impact of elevated blood pressure on health indicates that morbidity and mortality increase as blood pressure increases; hence, the inclusion of an untreated group in any hypertensive study designed to evaluate therapy is precluded on ethical grounds. Any study directed toward evaluation of different therapeutic approaches to hypertension is subject to this constraint, and such studies must be confined to comparison of alternate regimens that are known or generally thought to be effective. To date, no prospective study has been reported that undertook a comparison of the results of medical vs. operative therapy of renovascular hypertension. Published reports that include data on patients treated medically and those treated operatively usually present a medical group that, for one reason or another, was judged unsuited for operation. When such data are used to compare medical and operative results, they will be heavily biased in favor of operative treatment because the medical group usually contains a relatively high proportion of high-risk patients in whom operation is thought to be ill advised. Data are not available to permit any clear assessment of the relative efficacy of operative vs. medical management of renovascular hypertension for the reasons outlined above. Nevertheless, a review of published experience with operative and medical treatment of renovascular hypertension permits important inferences to be made about the role of medical management of this condition. Despite the inadequacies of these published data, they offer impressive support for the superiority of medical therapy in a large segment of patients with renovascular hypertension. The published experience with the two modes of therapy is reviewed briefly below and the relevant findings supporting medical management summarized.

## Operative Treatment of Renovascular Hypertension

This therapeutic approach has been considered in detail in another chapter, and only that information which is pertinent to a comparison with medical therapy is reviewed briefly here. Relevant information includes operative mortality rate, results of operation, i.e., number of patients "cured" and number improved, annual mortality rate during postoperative follow-up, and, when available, the degree of permanence of the "cure." Data on the operative treatment of more than 1200 patients with renovascular hypertension are available from the literature. Although there are significant differences among the groups comprising the individual reports, the results are sufficiently consistent to provide a reasonably accurate picture of what can be expected from operation if the results reported from most studies involving relatively large numbers of patients are used.

The report of Morris et al.[12] describing the results of operative treatment in 432 patients cited an acute operative mortality rate of 7 per cent with an annual death rate of 6 per cent* for the 5-year period following surgery. Follow-up arteriographic studies in the operative group revealed that 10 per cent, or 24 of 245 patients studied postoperatively, had complete occlusion of the reconstructed vessel, and an additional 13 patients, or 5 per cent, had some degree of stenosis. Sixty-eight per cent of the group undergoing operation were surviving at 5 years. At 1 year following operation, 41 per cent were normotensive, and an additional 40 per cent were significantly improved. However, after a lapse of 5 years following operation, only 18 per cent were normotensive, and the proportion adjudged either improved or cured had fallen to 44 per cent. Atherosclerosis was the basis for the renal arterial obstruction in 73 per cent, and fibromuscular hyperplasia comprised 12 per cent of the total clinical material. Thus, this study identifies an acute operative mortality of 7 per cent, a technical failure rate of reconstructive operation that appears to lie somewhere between 10 and 15 per cent, and an annual mortality rate of 6 per cent after acute postoperative deaths are excluded. In addition, with continued follow-up the number of "cures"—those individuals who maintain normal blood pressure during the postoperative follow-up period—appears to decrease at a rate of approximately 20 per cent per year. The authors do not present data on the number of patients at risk during each of the follow-up years, so these figures can only be regarded as approximate. They do, however, establish that individuals exhibiting a satisfactory response to operation at 1 year are exposed to continuing risk of recurrence of hypertension.

Dustan et al.[15] reported an acute operative mortality rate of 10 per cent

---

*The authors reported an annual mortality rate of 3 to 5 per cent in the text, but calculation of the annual rate from their data in Figure 9 after deaths in the first 30 postoperative days are excluded yields an annual mortality rate of 6.3 per cent.

in 99 patients subjected to operation for renovascular hypertension. At the time of her report, all patients had been followed for between 1 and 6 years, and an additional 12 patients had died during follow-up. All but one of these deaths appeared to be related to the vascular disease, yielding an overall mortality rate for this group of 20 per cent, although the data are not presented in a manner that permits estimation of the annual mortality rate. In the operative group, 44 of the patients had maintained blood pressures in the normal range during follow-up, and 15 patients had arterial pressures that were substantially below preoperative levels. Operative treatment was without benefit in 17 patients. The results of Shapiro and associates[17] were less good, although the series was small. The follow-up period ranged between 1 and 6 years for this group, and at the time of the report, 35 per cent were dead and 30 per cent were reported as either normotensive or exhibiting marked improvement.

The largest experience is reported in the cooperative study.[11, 13, 14] Operative treatment of 502 patients yielded a mortality rate of 6.8 per cent. This group was sufficiently large, however, that stratification yielded subsets of sufficient size to permit accurate estimates of operative mortality rates within these subgroups. Thus, when the underlying etiology was arteriosclerosis, the mortality rate exceeded 9 per cent; when it was fibromuscular hyperplasia, the mortality rate was only 3.4 per cent. Even more striking is that the mortality rate approached 25 per cent in those individuals with arteriosclerotic renovascular disease who had angina pectoris or a myocardial infarction, or significant renal impairment. Similarly, combined operative procedures in the arteriosclerotic group led to mortality rates that in some instances equaled or exceeded 25 per cent. Although the atherosclerotic category of renovascular disease accounted for only 50 per cent of the total population in this large study, this category accounted for 82 per cent of the operative deaths. Evaluation of operative results 1 year after operation revealed that 196 of the 384 patients listed as classifiable were cured. If one considers the complete group of 502 patients and assumes that all of the unclassifiable patients had normal blood pressures,[1] this yields a cure rate at 1 year of 55 per cent; a correspondingly lower percentage results if the unclassifiable patients are excluded from the cured category. An additional 12 per cent were improved in this series. The results following nephrectomy were better than those after reconstructive surgery, because of the large percentage of anatomic failure in the reconstructive surgery group. Anatomic failures in this study, judged by thrombosis at the repair site demonstrated by arteriography, were significantly more frequent than in Morris' study.[12] The authors make an important point when they note that 21 per cent of the 226 "best defined surgical candidates," with all of the diagnostic criteria indicating unilateral curable renal vascular hypertension, still failed to benefit from operation and were classed as failures. Analysis of the results of this large study is continuing and should provide valuable information about the long-term operative results.

All these studies are consistent in their main findings. When careful diagnostic techniques are employed preoperatively to insure the best possible selection of patients for operation, the cure rate, as judged by the presence of a normal blood pressure 1 year after operation, may be expected to be between 40 and 50 per cent, with an additional 15 to 20 per cent showing improvement but continuing to exhibit some hypertension. The mortality rate for the operative procedure averages about 7 per cent for the entire group of patients at risk, but within this group several subsets may be identified which exhibit much higher operative mortality rates. Patients with evidence of coronary artery disease or with peripheral vascular disease who may require additional procedures or patients who have bilateral abnormalities of the vascular supply to the kidneys represent particularly high operative risk groups. In some instances that risk exceeds 25 per cent. The risk of operation appears to be lowest in the group with fibromuscular dysplasia, and long-term results are also best in this group. Long-term mortality data are not abundant, but an annual mortality rate as high as 6 per cent is reported; the data also indicate a progressive tendency for the hypertension to return. Finally, even the most careful preoperative diagnostic work-up has thus far been unable to reduce the failure rate (lack of significant blood pressure response to operation) below 25 to 30 per cent.

## Medical Treatment of Renovascular Hypertension

Fewer data on long-term follow-up of patients with renovascular hypertension who have been managed medically with antihypertensive drugs are available. Reports dealing with medical management of renovascular hypertension represent patients who were judged to be unsuitable operative candidates for a variety of reasons and hence were placed on a drug regimen for control of hypertension. As a result, these patients tend to be older, with more pronounced evidence of other cardiovascular abnormalities, and must be regarded as the high-risk group. Nevertheless, review of these data is instructive and permits some fairly definite conclusions.

Sheps et al.,[16] reviewing the experience with medical management in 54 patients, provide the most detailed account of the results of medical therapy. Of their patients, 32 had atheromatous disease and 22 had fibromuscular hyperplasia. The average age was 48.6 years, and the average blood pressure prior to beginning therapy was 195/117 mm. Hg. The average follow-up was 20 months. Sixty-five per cent were maintained normotensive on standard antihypertensive regimens. Five deaths during a mean period of follow-up of slightly less than 2 years yielded an overall mortality rate for the period of 9 per cent, a figure not really different from the annual mortality rate reported by Morris et al.[12] for a large operatively treated group. The mean blood pressure in the group reported by Sheps et al.[16] at the most recent follow-up was 154/93 mm. Hg, indicating quite acceptable control of hypertension and significant improvement over the pretreatment levels.

Shapiro et al.[17] reported on 72 patients treated medically. This group appears somewhat more heterogeneous with regard to the results of diagnostic studies; the principal criterion for the diagnosis of renovascular hypertension seemed to be identifiable renal arterial stenosis on arteriography. The group not operated upon was, on the average, 8 years older than patients from the same series who were admitted to operation, and there was a greater preponderance of males. Details of medical therapy are not given; follow-up ranged between 1 and 6 years, but the average period of follow-up was not given. Forty per cent of the group treated medically (29 patients) were dead at the time of the last follow-up.

Dustan[15] reported 32 patients with renovascular hypertension treated medically who had a history of long-standing hypertension. Coronary and cerebral vascular disease were more common in this group. She reports in detail on 10 of these patients in whom medical therapy was carefully supervised. Results were excellent; blood pressure dropped from a mean pretreatment level of 200/112 mm. Hg to 167/87 mm. Hg in response to medical therapy. Only one death was recorded. The mean period of follow-up was 20 months. Owen[18] includes a brief account of 83 patients treated medically. Although details of the medical management were not included, 5-year results indicated that normal blood pressure was achieved with treatment in 37 per cent of the patients. The overall 5-year mortality in this group was 34 per cent.

The above studies present an aggregate total of 219 patients who were treated medically. While it is not possible to give the precise period of follow-up of all patients, the mean follow-up appears to have been between 2 and 3 years. Sixty-three of these patients died during the total period of follow-up, representing an overall mortality rate of 28 per cent. This figure does not differ markedly from the operative survival data presented by Morris et al.[12] and is, indeed, no greater than the acute operative mortality data for the arteriosclerotic high-risk group reported in the cooperative study.

It is evident that the blood pressure can be effectively controlled by medical management. Sheps[16] was able to achieve a normal pressure in 65 per cent of his patients, and in the group reported by Dustan,[15] in which management was carefully supervised, normal diastolic blood pressures were achieved in 8 of 10 patients. Thus, the number of patients rendered normotensive in these two studies clearly exceeded the incidence of cures reported for operatively treated patients. This fact takes on added significance when it is considered that these are results reported in the high-risk group of patients. Since the majority of these patients had either bilateral renal lesions or evidence of extensive cardiovascular disease in other organs, this 2-year mortality rate compares very favorably with the direct operative mortality rate ranging between 22 and 25 per cent for comparably high-risk patients in the cooperative study. It also appears that the results of medical management of renovascular hypertension can be compared favorably with those of medical treatment of the more severe forms of essential hypertension and that medical management clearly confers a life expectancy that is superior to that in patients with untreated essential hypertension.[19, 22]

# The Conservative Approach to the Management of Renovascular Hypertension

Review of the foregoing evidence offers little support for the unequivocal superiority of operative treatment for renovascular hypertension. Indeed, the available mortality data would suggest that medical management is preferable in patients in whom renovascular hypertension is due to atherosclerosis. The operative mortality is sufficiently high in this latter group that prolonged follow-up with demonstration of a marked reduction in annual mortality rate is required to justify the risk in this patient group, particularly when the renovascular hypertension is complicated by evidence of vascular disease in other organs. It is unfortunate that such long-term follow-up data are so scarce despite numerous reports of operative treatment in large groups of patients. Indeed, those data available[12, 18] suggest a continuing and relatively high annual mortality rate in this group of operatively treated patients. In view of this, it would seem that medical therapy is the treatment of choice in patients diagnosed as having renovascular hypertension secondary to atheromatous disease. Operation should only be considered when such patients are refractory to medical management or when progression of the renal vascular lesion threatens to destroy renal function.

The case for medical management of renovascular hypertension due to fibromuscular hyperplasia cannot be so strongly supported. The argument for operation as an alternative to long-term medical management, with its attendant difficulties, has some force. Nevertheless, the risks of operation and the documented evidence of responsiveness to medical management lend some support to an alternate approach that would involve an initial trial of medical management, particularly in those cases in which the hypertension is mild or the presence of bilateral disease foreshadows an increased risk for operation.

The report of Pinedo et al.[21] introduces a new element for consideration in the treatment of renovascular hypertension. In addition to reporting superior results with medical management (81 per cent surviving 5 years on medical therapy and 67 per cent surviving for a comparable period following operation), they report remarkable results with anticoagulant therapy. Of 30 patients who were operated on and so treated postoperatively, no deaths were observed during the follow-up period. The report is brief, details of patient selection are not available, and the results must be accepted with caution. Nevertheless, they are sufficiently impressive to require independent verification.

Finally, on the basis of available evidence, it would appear that the word "cure" may be inappropriate in describing operative results. The tendency to increased recurrence of hypertension with time suggests that the cures may be relatively short-lived. Thus, the argument that operation offers the prospect of avoiding the inconvenience of long-term medication loses much of its force. When this is considered in concert with the acute operative mortality which the patient must face, the case for operation is seriously weakened.

One fact that emerges quite clearly from this review is the need for much greater and more careful reporting of long-term therapeutic results for *both* medical and operative therapy. It is to be hoped that the long-term results of the cooperative study will provide a more adequate data base upon which to design therapy for the patient with renovascular hypertension.

## References

1. Maxwell, M. H., Bleifer, K. H., Franklin, S. S., and Varady, P. D.: Cooperative study of renovascular hypertension. Demographic analysis of the study. J.A.M.A. *220*:1195, 1972.
2. Howard, J. E., Berthrong, M., Sloane, R. D., and Yendt, E. R.: Relief of malignant hypertension by nephrectomy in four patients with unilateral vascular disease. Trans. Assoc. Am. Phys. *66*:164, 1953.
3. Stamey, T. A., Nudelman, I. J., Schwentker, F. M., and Hendricks, F.: Functional characteristics of renovascular hypertension. Medicine *40*:347, 1961.
4. Connor, T. B., Berthrong, M., Thomas, W. C., and Howard, J. E.: Hypertension due to unilateral renal disease, with a report on a functional test helpful in diagnosis. Bull. Johns Hopkins Hosp. *100*:241, 1957.
5. Winer, B. M., Lubbe, W. F., Simon, M., and Williams, J. A.: Renin in the diagnosis of renovascular hypertension. J.A.M.A. *202*:139, 1967.
6. Del Greco, F., Simon, N., Goodman, S., and Roguska, J.: Plasma renin activity in primary and secondary hypertension. Medicine *46*:475, 1967.
7. Meyer, P., Ecoiffier, J., Alexander, J. M., Devaux, C., Guize, L., Menard, J., Biron, P., and Milliez, P.: Prognostic value of plasma renin activity in renovascular hypertension. Circulation *36*:570, 1967.
8. Michelakis, A. M., Foster, J. H., Liddle, G. W., Rhamy, R. K., Kuchel, O., and Gordon, R. D.: Measurement of renin in both renal veins, its use in diagnosis of renovascular hypertension. Arch. Intern. Med. *120*:444, 1967.
9. Munck, O., Faarup, P., Gammelgaard, P. A., Ladefoged, J., Mathiesen, F. R., and Pedersen, F.: Characteristics of renovascular hypertension. Data on renal blood flow and analysis of factors predicting the effect of surgery. Scand. J. Clin. Lab. Invest. *22*:288, 1968.
10. Meier, P.: Statistics and medical experimentation. Biometrics *31*:511, 1975.
11. Simon, N., Franklin, S. S., Bleifer, K. H., and Maxwell, M. H.: Cooperative study of renovascular hypertension. Clinical characteristics of renovascular hypertension. J.A.M.A. *220*:1209, 1972.
12. Morris, G. C., Jr., De Bakey, M. E., Crawford, E. S., Cooley, D. A., and Zanger, L. C. C.: Late results of surgical treatment for renovascular hypertension. Surg. Gynecol. Obstet. *122*:1255, 1966.
13. Franklin, S. S., Young, J. D., Maxwell, M. H., Foster, J. H., Palmer, J. M., Cerny, J., and Varady, P. D.: Operative morbidity and mortality in renovascular disease. J.A.M.A. *231*:1148, 1975.
14. Foster, J. H., Maxwell, M. H., Franklin, S. S., Bleifer, K. H., Trippel, O. H., Julian, O. C., De Camp, P. T., and Varady, P. T.: Renovascular occlusive disease. Results of operative treatment. J.A.M.A. *231*:1043, 1975.
15. Dustan, H. P., Page, I. H., Poutasse, E. F., and Wilson, L.: An evaluation of treatment of hypertension associated with occlusive renal arterial disease. Circulation *27*:1018, 1963.
16. Sheps, S. G., Osmundson, P. J., Hunt, J. C., Schirger, A., and Fairbairn, J. F., II: Hypertension and renal artery stenosis: Serial observations on 54 patients treated medically. Clin. Pharmacol. Ther. *6*:700, 1965.
17. Shapiro, A. P., Perez-Stable, E., Scheib, E. T., Bron, K., Moutsos, S. E., Berg, G., Misage, J. R., Bahnson, H., Fisher, B., and Drapanas, T.: Renal artery stenosis and hypertension. Observations on current status of therapy from a study of 115 patients. Am. J. Med. *47*:175, 1969.
18. Owen, K.: Results of surgical treatment in comparison with medical treatment of renovascular hypertension. Clin. Sci. Molec. Med. *45*:95s, 1973.

19. Farmer, R. G., Gifford, R. W., Jr., and Hines, E. A.: Effect of medical management of severe hypertension. A follow-up study of 161 patients with group 3 and group 4 hypertension. Arch. Intern. Med. *112*:118, 1963.
20. Peart, W. S.: Results of medical versus surgical treatment of renovascular hypertension. Clin. Sci. Molec. Med. *45*:89s, 1973.
21. Pinedo, H. M., De Graeff, J., and Struyvenberg, A.: Prognosis in arteriosclerotic renovascular hypertension. Clin. Sci. Molec. Med. *45*:309s, 1973.
22. Keith, N. M., Wagener, H. P., and Barker, N. M.: Some different types of hypertension: Their course and prognosis. Am. J. Med. Sci. *197*:332, 1939.

# Operative Treatment of Renovascular Hypertension

RONALD J. STONEY,
ROBERT J. SWANSON,
ROY E. CARLSON,
and DOROTHEE L. PERLOFF

*University of California, San Francisco, School of Medicine*

The initial interest in hypertension caused by impaired circulation to the kidney stemmed from the classic experiments of Goldblatt in 1934.[1] Within 4 years, isolated case reports of human hypertension resulting from renal vascular impairment appeared.[2,3] However, only in the past two decades has the syndrome of renovascular hypertension become recognized as a remediable clinical entity. During this era, the initial enthusiasm for operative treatment (revascularization of the ischemic kidney or nephrectomy) has been tempered by awareness of morbidity and mortality involved in studying and operating upon these patients. The availability of potent antihypertensive medications (including beta blockers which interfere with renin release, and experimentally, the angiotensin II and converting enzyme antagonists) has further diminished the urgency of operating on many patients, since often the blood pressure can be effectively controlled. Uncertainty concerning the proper diagnostic and therapeutic approach to the problem of renovascular hypertension has resulted.

In the face of these uncertainties, our continued enthusiasm for reconstructive vascular procedures in preference to drug therapy of renovascular hypertension in *selected* patients is based on:

1. Careful selection of hypertensive patients for evaluation
2. Accurate definition of pathologic lesions producing renal artery obstruction
3. Clear understanding of the natural history of these renovascular lesions
4. Identification of the physiologic derangements caused by renal ischemia

687

5. Employment of reliable and safe autogenous reconstructive techniques which we have perfected over a 20-year period

The recognition of renal artery lesions which could produce hypertension depends on precise arteriographic demonstration of the renal vasculature. Translumbar aortography, advanced by dos Santos in 1929[4] and used for delineating occlusive disease of the terminal aorta and its branches, was first applied to the renal arteries. Precise arteriographic assessment was not always achieved by this method. The Seldinger technique for arteriography introduced in 1953[5] using percutaneous, retrograde arterial catheterization has proved safe, simple, and effective when used for renal artery visualization.[6]

The initial operations in the 1950's demonstrated that in some hypertensive patients, removal of the renal arterial lesions or nephrectomy did not cure or improve their hypertension, suggesting a need for more precise identification of the characteristics of renovascular hypertension preoperatively. The renin-angiotensin-aldosterone system has been shown in experimental animals and humans to be activated by renal ischemia, but its role in the maintenance of hypertension is still not proved. Currently, selective renal vein blood samples are obtained using the Seldinger technique and are assayed for renin concentration. Ratios between the renin concentrations in the right and left renal veins greater than 1.5 to 1.0 suggest renal ischemia on the higher side and provide functional evidence that the renal arterial lesion is in fact responsible for the hypertension.

## Patient Selection

Careful renal arteriography and selective renal vein renin determination are the definitive diagnostic procedures currently available to demonstrate and evaluate an obstructing lesion of the renal artery which may be causing hypertension. These diagnostic measures should be applied only to patients in whom eventual surgical management of the hypertension is contemplated or feasible. Thus, patients with mild or borderline hypertension, elderly patients without significant renal functional impairment whose blood pressure is easily controlled, and patients with disabling complications of generalized vascular disease will benefit little, if at all, from a revascularization operation and so are not considered candidates for diagnostic studies. Those patients who are likely to have renovascular hypertension as suggested by certain features of the *history, physical examination,* and routine laboratory *screening studies* should be studied. These features are:

1. History or suspicion of renal trauma or embolism
2. Abrupt onset or acceleration of existing hypertension
3. Hypertension difficult to control medically
4. Severe accelerating hypertensive retinopathy
5. Abdominal or flank bruit
6. Other manifestation of occlusive peripheral vascular disease

7. Evidence of hyperaldosteronism

8. Sudden unexplained renal failure with hypertension

Our routine laboratory screening includes urinalysis, serum electrolytes, rapid-sequence intravenous urogram, and in some patients, the isotope renogram. The latter two are particularly valuable in patients with unilateral renal ischemia, as the ischemic kidney is often *smaller* than the contralateral normal kidney and *slower* in concentrating and excreting radiopaque contrast material or the isotope labeled tracer. However, Foster[7] reported that 30 per cent of patients with proved renovascular hypertension had a "normal" intravenous urogram.

## Pathology

The vascular lesions causing renovascular hypertension impair blood flow and affect arteriolar perfusion, resulting in renal ischemia that initiates the renin-angiotensin-aldosterone system. Fibromuscular dysplasia and atherosclerosis are the two most common pathologic findings affecting the renal arteries and causing hypertension.

### FIBROMUSCULAR DYSPLASIA (FMD)

This arterial disorder of unknown etiology has been found in all age groups but is most common in young adults (less than age 40) and children, predominantly females. Although the renal artery is the usual site of involvement, FMD has been described in several extrarenal arteries, including the internal carotid, mesenteric, and iliac. The natural history of this arterial lesion is not completely defined, but both progression of existing lesions and development of new lesions have been observed by serial arteriography.[8] The accepted terminology now in use is based on a classification of the location of the involvement within the layers of the arterial wall and the predominant cell type observed.[9]

1. *Intimal fibroplasia*, a rare form of the disease, consists of intimal deposits of fibrous tissue and reduplication of the internal elastic lamella.

2. *Medial fibromuscular dysplasia* consists of areas of medial thinning, fibrosis, and loss of the internal elastic lamella, with aneurysm formation alternating with septate fibrous ridges which protrude into the lumen. A variation of this lesion, *medial hyperplasia,* contains areas of smooth muscle hypertrophy and perimedial fibroplasia of the outer media and disruption of the external elastic lamella, together with multiple irregular stenoses of the lumen and, occasionally, dissection. Medial hyperplasia is the most common manifestation of the disease affecting the renal arteries.

3. *Periarterial or subadventitial fibroplasia* is quite rare and consists of focal collagen deposits between medial and adventitial layers, resulting in localized, smooth luminal narrowing.

The presence and extent of fibromuscular dysplasia are easily demonstrated by arteriography, aided by techniques which *elongate* and *uncoil* the renal arteries. Deep inspiration and oblique positioning may provide profile views of the lesions. Selective renal arteriograms are helpful in defining the extent of the disease in the branch arteries.

More than one half of patients have bilateral lesions, although not necessarily of equal severity.[10] At the time of diagnosis, the patients are usually young and their hypertension is usually of *short* duration. Consequently, cardiac, cerebral, or renal complications are rare, making these patients excellent operative candidates, as they respond to revascularization of the kidney with prompt and sustained relief of hypertension.

## ATHEROSCLEROSIS

The atheromatous intimal lesion of plaque produces eccentric or concentric narrowing of the lumen at the renal artery orifice and may involve the proximal one third of the main renal artery. Since the lesion is usually confined to the intima and innermost portion of the media, a cleavage plane between the involved and normal artery is present and permits the selective removal of atheroma from the remaining arterial wall. The plaque usually ends abruptly and can be clearly separated from the distal, uninvolved intima.

Atherosclerosis is a progressive, systemic, degenerative vascular disease that affects arteries supplying many organs other than the kidney. Vascular involvement of other critical organ systems, such as the brain, heart, and abdominal viscera, as well as the lower extremities, occurs in patients with atherosclerotic renovascular hypertension. The presence of extrarenal atherosclerosis adversely affects the results and safety of surgery in this patient group because:

1. The duration of hypertension is frequently long (more than 3 years) in these older patients, which accelerates the development of intrarenal arteriolar nephrosclerosis. The impairment of renal function and renal atrophy that result cannot be alleviated surgically, since the intrarenal lesion is not accessible for repair.

2. The disease is bilateral in more than one half of patients studied, and variable narrowing of the renal arteries makes identification of the specific, causative lesion difficult. Failure to cure or improve hypertension sometimes results because all the responsible lesions producing renal ischemia are not identified and removed.

3. Extrarenal atherosclerosis affecting other critical organs may impair their perfusion during renal revascularization operations, and their subsequent failure may increase postoperative morbidity and mortality.

4. Associated atherosclerotic involvement of the abdominal aorta adjacent and distal to the renal branches may require additional surgical resection and grafting procedures. Lengthy aortic occlusion necessary to complete these additional procedures may result in prolonged ischemia to the kidneys, viscera, or lower limbs, further increasing the operative risk.

5. Advanced age (50 to 70 years) and additional risk factors, including obesity, chronic pulmonary disease, tobacco usage, hypercholesterolemia, and diabetes, are frequently found in this group and adversely affect the patient's response to operative treatment of hypertension.

A variety of other less common renal artery lesions that may produce renovascular hypertension in certain instances must be considered.

## Renal Artery Aneurysm

These saccular or fusiform lesions result from medial degeneration of the arterial wall, commonly associated with atherosclerosis but which may be congenital or an isolated manifestation of fibromuscular dysplasia. Aneurysms may be intrarenal but are usually found in the middle or distal portion of the main renal artery or the principal renal branches. Atherosclerotic aneurysms are frequently calcified, a feature which may protect the patient from spontaneous aneurysm rupture. Rupture of a renal artery aneurysm usually results in loss of the kidney and may be associated with a mortality rate of 10 to 25 per cent. Thrombosis of the renal artery, embolization of aneurysmal contents to the renal parenchyma, and dissection are also potential complications of renal artery aneurysm.

Various mechanisms have been advanced to explain the hypertension associated with renal artery aneurysms:

1. Compromise of adjacent renal artery branches producing segmental ischemia
2. Embolization of aneurysm contents to the intrarenal vasculature, causing ischemia, infarction, or both
3. Alteration in blood flow and pressure in the renal vasculature

Some renal artery aneurysms are *not* associated with hypertension, however.

## Aortic Dissection

Atherosclerosis, luetic aortitis, Marfan's syndrome, and cystic medial necrosis of the aorta are all associated with thoracic aortic dissection. Type III dissection may involve the upper abdominal aorta and its branches, resulting in narrowing or occlusion of the renal artery orifice. Hypertension may result or be worsened by the resulting renal ischemia.

## Arteriovenous Malformations

Intrarenal arteriovenous malformations are rare but produce focal renal ischemia by shunting blood through the lesion itself rather than to portions of the parenchyma. Hypertension is produced in these patients by initiation of the renin-angiotensin mechanism.

### Homotransplant Renal Artery Stenosis

Two lesions have been described in this category following renal homotransplantation:

1. Stenosis at the arterial anastomosis (renal graft-to-host artery), resulting from trauma, such as clamping, from foreign body reaction, or from mechanical distortion or angulation.
2. Inflammation of unknown etiology, encasing the renal artery and the kidney itself but which may be a manifestation of the altered immune response in the host.

Both reactions result in severe hypertension in the renal transplant recipient without impairing function of the renal graft itself. Arteriography is necessary to define this curable lesion and should be employed in a renal transplant recipient with recurrent hypertension.

## Selection of Patients for Operation

A patient whose hypertension is "cured" when renal ischemia is alleviated by reconstruction of a diseased renal artery clearly *had* renovascular hypertension. How, then, do we select the patient with renovascular hypertension for operation? Before a patient is considered for a revascularization procedure for renovascular hypertension, he should have met the criteria outlined previously for selection for arteriography. Ideally, the operative risk should be low and the potential gain (cure or improvement in hypertension) high: (1) The candidate should be less than 60 years old and physiologically sound. (2) Moderate-to-severe diastolic hypertension not readily controlled should be present. (3) The duration of hypertension should be short, preferably less than 5 years. (4) Few, if any, vascular complications secondary to hypertension or associated atherosclerosis should be present.

However, young patients (35 years or less) with mild hypertension stand to gain much if their disease is cured, as they avoid a lifetime of medication which at best can maintain only a few patients at consistently normotensive levels. On the other hand, occasional older patients with abrupt onset or acceleration of longstanding hypertension have derived great benefit from operation, particularly from preservation of renal parenchyma. Further, patients with accelerating hypertension and progressive impairment of renal function are also candidates for operation to remove responsible renovascular lesions, though their risk is higher. Hypertension may only be improved, not cured, and renal impairment may be stabilized or improved slightly in this type of patient.

Increasing experience with beta adrenergic blocking agents such as propranolol suggests that absolute drug failures in the treatment of renovascular hypertension are rare, but difficulty in drug control of hypertension constitutes an important reason to consider a patient for arteriography and operation. On the other hand, those patients whose blood pressure is easily controlled are less frequently evaluated for a curable cause of hypertension. Additional experience with operative results in these patients will define more clearly the appropriate diagnostic and therapeutic approaches.

In Table 1, the operative results in all atherosclerotic patients alive one year after corrective operation are classified by duration of hypertension, severity of hypertension, and age at the time of operation. Among those patients with a duration of hypertension less than 5 years, 72 per cent benefited from operation; while among those with known duration of hypertension greater than 5 years, only 56 per cent benefited from operation. In this latter group, more patients fell into the "improved" rather than the "cured" category. The benefits from operation, however, did not appear related to the age or severity of hypertension in this atherosclerotic group. Among the patients with FMD (Table 1), the results from surgery did not correlate with duration of hypertension or age at the time of operation.

The lesion to be removed must be surgically accessible, and the adjacent aorta and major branches should preferably be uninvolved in the disease process. An arterial stenosis must be demonstrated radiographically; when an appropriate collateral network is also present, renal ischemia is certain and the likelihood of a surgical cure is excellent.[11] Other radiographic findings suggesting a lesion producing renovascular hypertension are:

1. Greater than 75 per cent narrowing of the renal arterial lumen
2. Poststenotic dilatation
3. Renal atrophy or focal infarction
4. Delayed filling or hypoperfusion of the kidney

Additional evidence that the renal artery lesion present radiographically is causing hypertension by producing renal ischemia and initiating the renin-angiotensin mechanism must be demonstrated. The renal vein renin determination is the best physiologic test currently available.[12, 13] Selective renal vein renin determinations from each kidney are compared. A ratio of 1.5 to 1.0 strongly suggests that the kidney with the higher renin is ischemic and is causing hypertension. As peripheral venous renin is not consistently elevated even in patients with severe renal ischemia and elevated renal vein renins, this test is not reliable for screening hypertensive patients.[14]

Furthermore, many factors influence renin output, including sodium intake, state of hydration, previous antihypertensive therapy, oral contraceptives, posture, and activity immediately prior to renal vein sampling.[15] When these variables are not standardized, the absolute level of plasma renin may be misleading. Patients with branch renal artery disease and segmental renal ischemia should have renal venous samples obtained from the segmental vein draining the affected area to avoid dilution of renin levels due to mixing in the main renal vein.

Recently, the isotope renogram and perfusion flow studies have been improved and computerized, providing data on relative renal plasma flow as well as absolute renal perfusion. Early experience using these observations suggests a correlation with renin determinations, but this needs further evaluation.

## TABLE 1. Renovascular Hypertension Surgical Results (1 Year Follow-Up) U.C.S.F.*

| | Atherosclerosis Obliterans 96 Patients | | | | Fibromuscular Dysplasia 102 Patients | | |
|---|---|---|---|---|---|---|---|
| | Total | BP decreased | No change | | Total | BP decreased | No change |
| **Duration of Hypertension** | | | | | | | |
| <5 years | 64 | 46 | 18 | <5 years | 80 | 69 | 11 |
| >5 years | 32 | 18 | 14 | >5 years | 22 | 19 | 3 |
| | 96 | 64 | 32 | | 102 | 88 | 14 |
| **Severity of Hypertension** | | | | | | | |
| Grade I–II | 61 | 39 | 22 | Grade I | 43 | 37 | 6 |
| Grade III–IV | 35 | 25 | 10 | Grade II | 42 | 37 | 5 |
| | | | | Grades III and IV | 17 | 13 | 4 |
| | 96 | 64 | 32 | | 102 | 87 | 15 |
| **Age** | | | | | | | |
| <45 | 20 | 10 | 10 | <25 | 18 | 17 | 1 |
| >45 | 76 | 54 | 22 | 25–45 | 61 | 51 | 10 |
| | | | | >45 | 23 | 19 | 4 |
| | 96 | 64 | 32 | | 102 | 87 | 15 |

*University of California Medical Center, San Francisco, California.

The editors have posed the question, "If hypertension is clearly of renovascular etiology and surgically correctable but readily controlled by antihypertensive agents, should an operation be done?" The answer depends on the patient. We advocate medical treatment for an elderly, debilitated patient with extensive atherosclerosis involving many organ systems in addition to the kidneys, since his operative risk is high and morbidity is considerable. If he has had longstanding hypertension, the atherosclerotic lesion is more likely to be the result rather than the cause of the hypertension. On the other hand, a young patient with recent onset of severe hypertension and a focal lesion of the renal artery due to either fibromuscular dysplasia or atherosclerosis should undergo a revascularization operation. Success is highest in this type of patient, and prolonged drug use with its attendant problems is avoided.

The operation for this patient has two objectives: (1) to preserve or improve renal function and (2) to improve the quality of life. DeBakey has pointed out the beneficial effect of renovascular reconstruction on renal function.[16] The natural history of untreated disease causing renovascular hypertension is understood; progressive stenosis and occlusion occur, resulting in renal infarction and atrophy, especially in patients with atherosclerosis obliterans.

## *Technique*

The technique used for renal revascularization varies, but the principles are governed by the disease process itself.

### ATHEROSCLEROSIS

Endarterectomy is fundamental in relieving atherosclerotic stenosing lesions at many sites, including the renal arteries. Our experience began in 1952, and initially we employed the transrenal method, but subsequently adopted the transaortic route. Bilateral lesions or multiple renal artery lesions are frequently encountered and are expeditiously handled through the latter route.[17]

Use of bypass grafts or synthetic material is favored by others,[18] but the reported failure rate is high[19] and risks of infection and false aneurysm formation attendant to prosthetic vascular repairs are always present.

Nephrectomy, polar or unilateral, is now used only for patients with advanced renal atrophy or infarction. However, an occasional patient who exhibits many risk factors for revascularization will tolerate flank nephrectomy satisfactorily if operation is selected because of failure to control the renovascular hypertension medically.

TABLE 2.    U.C.S.F.* Experience with Ex Vivo Renal Artery Reconstruction—
1973–1975

| No. of Patients | Cured | Improved | Failed |
|---|---|---|---|
| 14† | 8 | 3 | 1 |

*University of California Medical Center, San Francisco.
†Two patients with less than 2 months follow-up.

## FIBROMUSCULAR DYSPLASIA

Resection and either bypass or replacement grafts are usually employed for these lesions, as they are not amenable to endarterectomy. Our initial technique, segmental resection and reanastomosis, was discarded when suture line stenosis appeared late (1 to 5 years) owing to excessive tension. Autogenous grafts (aortorenal) employing segments of the internal iliac artery have been used for more than 10 years at the University of California Medical Center, San Francisco.[17, 20] The autogenous saphenous vein aortorenal graft has produced excellent early results, as reported by Foster[21] and Ernst,[22] but long-term follow-up of their cases showed graft degeneration appearing in as many as 35 per cent of their vein grafts.[7, 23, 24]

The disease involves the renal artery branches in approximately 15 per cent of patients with renovascular hypertension due to fibromuscular dysplasia, and microvascular repair following excision of the diseased renal artery is required. The size of the branched internal iliac autograft closely approximates the renal artery and its branches and is an ideal replacement graft. The kidney is temporarily removed, cooled, and perfused while the repair is performed and then is reimplanted. A high success rate (Table 2) is reported with this technique, which permits cure of hypertension and preservation of the kidney, for lesions once thought inoperable and, therefore, previously treated with drug therapy or nephrectomy.[25]

## Results of Operative Therapy

Table 3 reviews the mortality rate in our hospital and in the Cooperative Study.[26] The greatest risk of death occurs in patients with atherosclerotic

TABLE 3.    Renovascular Hypertension—Operative Mortality

| Study | Atherosclerosis Obliterans | Fibromuscular Dysplasia |
|---|---|---|
| U.C.S.F. | | |
| 1953–1962 | 11/52   (21%) | |
| 1963–1975 | 1/80   (1.2%) | 1/84   (1.2%) |
| Cooperative Study[26] | 28/300 (9.3%) | 6/179 (3.4%) |

TABLE 4.   Fibromuscular Dysplasia — Operative Results

| Study | Follow-up | No. of Patients | Cured | Improved | Failed |
|-------|-----------|-----------------|-------|----------|--------|
| Foster[22] | 6 mo.–11 yr. | 44 | 72% | 24% | 4% |
| Fry[25] | 6 mo.–13 yr. | 113 | 51% | 43% | 6% |
| U.C.S.F. | 5–12 yr. | 45 | 49% | 42% | 9% |

renovascular hypertension, since they are older, have more risk factors, and suffer from generalized vascular disease. Improved patient selection and operative techniques can reduce the risk in the atherosclerotic group, as was achieved at U.C.S.F. in the period 1963 to 1975. In our hospital, the only death following renal artery reconstruction for FMD was from a cerebral hemorrhage from a ruptured intracranial aneurysm.

The operative results in patients with FMD are summarized in Table 4. Three large series are reported with follow-up data from 6 months to 12 years. Nearly all operations involved the use of autogenous aortorenal grafts and resulted in cure or improvement in more than 90 per cent of the patients.

The operative results for patients with atherosclerotic lesions causing renovascular hypertension in comparable series are listed in Table 5. A failure rate approaching one third is evident and reflects problems in patient selection, evaluation of location and extent of lesions, and the presence of intrarenal (inaccessible) lesions which were not removed. Perhaps of more interest is Table 6, which shows distinct differences in blood pressure response between patients with focal or diffuse atherosclerosis.

Two additional objectives of operation are not emphasized in the foregoing tables. First, the restoration of renal parenchymal mass in patients who exhibited mild-to-moderate, but reversible, atrophy owing to their occlusive renal artery disease. Eleven of 132 patients in the U.C.S.F. series who underwent surgical treatment of hypertension secondary to atherosclerosis of their renal arteries were found to have renal atrophy (kidney less than 10.5 cm. in long axis). In 5 of these patients, revascularization resulted in a substantial increase in renal size (average 1.6 cm.). Unilateral nephrectomy was required in the remaining 6 patients with occlusion of renal artery branches and infarction already present.

Second, impaired renal function, as measured by creatinine clearance and creatinine elevations, was not common in the U.C.S.F. series. However,

TABLE 5.   Atherosclerotic Renovascular Hypertension — Operative Results
(1 to 15 Year Follow-Up)

| Study | No. of Patients | Cured | Improved | Failed |
|-------|-----------------|-------|----------|--------|
| Foster[21] | 78 | 53% | 36% | 11% |
| Fry[22] | 68 | 28% | 41% | 31% |
| U.C.S.F. | 105 | 35% | 31% | 36% |

TABLE 6.   Atherosclerotic Distribution and Location of Lesion–
University of Michigan[24]

|  | No. of Patients | Cured | Improved | Failed |
|---|---|---|---|---|
| Focal | 32 | 31% | 56% | 13% |
| Generalized | 36 | 25% | 28% | 47% |

°Data from Ernst, C. B., Stanley, J. C., Marshall, F. F., and Dry, W. J.: Renal revascularization for arteriosclerotic renovascular hypertension: prognostic implications of focal renal arterial vs. overt generalized arteriosclerosis. Surgery 73:859, 1973.

as has been reported by others,[16] we found improvement in renal function in more than one half of those patients following operation. Furthermore, progressive renal failure or uremia has not appeared in the follow-up period.

Recurrence of disease appears in operated patients regardless of the type of renal artery occlusive disease. Since progression of disease is slow,[8] many years may pass during which the patient may experience significant benefit from operative treatment. In some patients, new lesions can subsequently be repaired using techniques of ex vivo perfusion and microvascular repair.

Certain risks do exist for the patient who undergoes a renovascular reconstructive procedure for hypertension. In addition, there is a small chance of failure and the problem of recurrent disease may eventually negate a successful initial operative result. Why then should one encourage operation rather than drug therapy for a patient who can be treated medically?

Ease of blood pressure control is not necessarily a deterrent to repair. However, if it is difficult to control or even refractory, the alternative of operative therapy should be considered. Hunt and Strong[27] followed 214 patients with renovascular hypertension. Only 18 were initially referred for operative treatment because of accelerated hypertension, the young age of the patient, or failure to accomplish satisfactory blood pressure control with vigorous medical regimens. Eighty-two additional patients treated medically for 1 to 3 months were subsequently operated upon because of failure to maintain a diastolic blood pressure below 100 mm. Hg.

The patient who may be easily controlled by drug therapy may also possess many of the characteristics associated with a potential cure of hypertension following operation: (1) young age; (2) short duration of hypertension; (3) absence of renal parenchymal disease; (4) evidence that the lesion is functionally significant and is producing renal ischemia and initiating the renin-angiotensin mechanism; and (5) demonstration of a focal, accessible renal artery stenosis. If operation is not advocated for such an individual, he is deprived of the high probability of cure, is committed to a lifetime of drug therapy, and is susceptible to progression of the disease, which may alter response to treatment and cause subsequent parenchymal damage that results in functional impairment and renal atrophy.

Thus, operative correction of functionally significant occlusive renal artery lesions should be performed in selected patients to preserve renal function rather than pursuing medical therapy. Of the 100 patients reported by Hunt[27] who had operation for renovascular hypertension, late renal failure with death occurred in only 3, one of whom had demonstrated recurrent atherosclerotic stenosis 5 years following successful operation. However, of the 114 patients treated medically, renal failure caused death in 8 patients, and 4 of 7 additional patients whose blood pressure response became unsatisfactory on medication developed renal failure necessitating dialysis or renal transplantation. Thus renal failure and its complications occurred in 13 per cent of medically treated patients, compared to 3 per cent of surgically treated patients.

We also advocate operation rather than drug therapy to improve the *quality of life* for the patient. The ongoing expense of medical therapy and problems with compliance are encumbrances that affect the life of the medically treated patient. We know that these factors are minor in a patient whose blood pressure is controlled by one tablet of a diuretic daily. However, these problems become significant when multiple drugs and complicated dose schedules are necessary. The side effects of antihypertensive medical regimens are experienced by many patients so treated and include postural hypotension, impotence, tachycardia or bradycardia, nasal congestion, diarrhea, nightmares, and weakness associated with hypokalemia.

Finally, the problem of satisfactory blood pressure control must be considered. In any group of hypertensive patients, 20 to 25 per cent of the group do not have a normal blood pressure (140/90 or less) at any one time in spite of a vigorous medical regimen and efforts to insure compliance.

Many factors must therefore be weighed when considering medical therapy for a patient with renovascular hypertension. When the adverse effects on the life style of the medically treated patient are contrasted with the improved quality of life reported in patients cured of hypertension by operation, the operative treatment of renovascular hypertension appears clearly justified.

# References

1. Goldblatt, H., Lynch, J., Hanzal, R. F., and Summerville, W. W.: Studies on experimental hypertension. I. The production of persistent elevation of systolic blood pressure by means of renal ischemia. J. Exper. Med. 59:347, 1934.
2. Leadbetter, W. F., and Burkland, C. E.: Hypertension in unilateral renal disease. J. Urol. 39:611, 1938.
3. Freeman, G., and Hartley, G., Jr.: Hypertension in a patient with a solitary ischemic kidney. J.A.M.A. 111:1159, 1938.
4. Dos Santos, M. R., Jamas, M. M., and Caldos, R. J.: L'arteriographie des membres, de l'aorte et de ses branches abdominale. Bull. Mem. Soc. Nat. Chir. 55:587, 1929.
5. Seldinger, S. I.: Catheter replacement of the needle in percutaneous arteriography. Acta Radiol. 39:368, 1953.
6. Dean, R. H., Burks, H., Wilson J. P. et al.: Deceptive patterns of renal artery stenosis. Surgery 76:872, 1974.
7. Foster, J. H., Dean, R. H., Pinkerton, J. A., and Rhaney, R. K.: Ten years' experience with the surgical management of renovascular hypertension. Ann. Surg. 177:755, 1973.

8. Sheps, S. G., Kincaid, O. W. and Hunt, J. C.: Serial renal function and angiographic observations in idiopathic fibrosis and fibromuscular stenosis of the renal arteries. Am. J. Cardiol. *30*:55, 1972.

9. Harrison, E. G., Jr., McCormack, L. J.: Pathologic classification of renal arterial disease in renovascular hypertension. Mayo Clinic Proc. *46*:161, 1971.

10. Stanley, J. C., and Fry, W. J.: Renovascular hypertension secondary to arterial fibrodysplasia in adults. Arch. Surg. *110*:922, 1975.

11. Ernst, C. B., Bookstein, J. J., Montie, J., et al.: Renal vein renin ratios and collateral vessels in renovascular hypertension. Arch. Surg. *104*:495, 1972.

12. Bourgoignie, J., Kurz, S., Catanzaro, F. J., et al.: Renal venous renin in hypertension. Amer. J. Med. *48*:332, 1970.

13. Fitz, A.: Renal vein renin determinations in the diagnosis of surgically correctable hypertension. Circulation *36*:942, 1967.

14. Del Greco, F., Simon, N. M., Goodman, S., and Roguska, J.: Plasma renin activity in primary and secondary hypertension. Medicine *46*:475, 1967.

15. Marks, L. S., and Maxwell, M.: Renal vein renin: value and limitations in the production of operative results. Urol. Clin. North Am. 2:311, 1975.

16. DeBakey, M. E., Morris, G. C., Jr., Morgen, R. O., et al.: Lesions of the renal artery. Surgical technique and results. Am. J. Surg. *107*:84, 1964.

17. Wylie, E., Perloff, D. L., and Stoney, R. J.: Autogenous tissue revascularization technics in surgery for renovascular hypertension. Ann. Surg. *170*:416, 1969.

18. Morris, G. C., Jr., DeBakey, M. E., Crawford, E. S., et al.: Late results of surgical treatment for renovascular hypertension. Surg. Gynecol. Obstet. *122*:1255, 1966.

19. Kaufman, J. J., Maxwell, M. H., and Moloney, P. J.: Synthetic bypass grafts in the treatment of renal artery stenosis. Surg. Gynecol. Obstet. *126*:53, 1968.

20. Lye, C. R., String, S. T., Wylie, E. J., and Stoney, R. J.: Aortorenal arterial autografts. Arch. Surg. *110*:1321, 1975.

21. Foster, J. H., Oates, J. A., Rhamy, R. K., et al.: Hypertension and fibromuscular dysplasia of the renal arteries. Surgery *65*:157, 1969.

22. Ernst, C. B., Stanley, J. C., Marshall, F. F., and Fry, W. J.: Autogenous saphenous vein aortorenal grafts: a ten year experience. Arch. Surg. *105*:855, 1972.

23. Stanley, J. C., Ernst, C. B., and Fry, W. J.: Fate of 100 aortorenal vein grafts: characteristics of late graft expansion, aneurysmal dilatation, and stenosis. Surgery *74*:931, 1973.

24. Ernst, C. B., Stanley, J. C., Marshall, F. F., and Fry, W. J.: Renal revascularization for arteriosclerotic renovascular hypertension: prognostic implications of focal renal arterial vs. overt generalized arteriosclerosis. Surgery *73*:859, 1973.

25. Belzer, F. O., Salvatierra, O., Palubinskas, A., and Stoney, R. J.: Ex vivo renal artery reconstruction. Ann. Surg. *182*:456, 1975.

26. Franklin, S. S., Young J. D., Jr., Maxwell, M. H., et al.: Operative morbidity and mortality in renovascular disease. J.A.MA. *231*:1148, 1975.

27. Hunt, J. C., and Strong, C. G.: Renovascular hypertension: mechanisms, natural history and treatment. *In* Lavagh, J. H. (ed.): Hypertension Manual: Mechanisms, Methods, and Management. New York, Yorke Medical Books, 1974, p. 509.

# INDEX

Page numbers in *italics* indicate illustrations; page numbers followed by (t) indicate tables.

**701**